Immediate Help for:

D0580608

Nursing Care Plans

PAIN
Clinical Manual For Nursing Practice

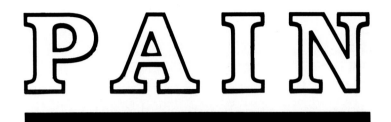

PAIN

Clinical Manual For Nursing Practice

Margo McCaffery, R.N., M.S., F.A.A.N.
Consultant in the Nursing Care of Patients with Pain
Santa Monica, California

Alexandra Beebe, R.N., M.S., O.C.N.
Founder and Director
InControl: Cancer Pain Care Associates
Washington, D.C.

illustrated

The C.V. Mosby Company

St. Louis • Baltimore • Philadelphia • Toronto   1989

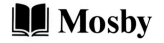 **Mosby**

Editor: Linda L. Duncan
Assistant Editor: Susie Baxter
Project Manager: Mark Spann
Cover Design: Elise A. Stimac

Printed in the United States of America

The C.V. Mosby Company
11830 Westline Industrial Drive, St. Louis, Missouri 63146

Library of Congress Cataloging-in-Publication Data

McCaffery, Margo.
   Pain : clinical manual for nursing practice / Margo McCaffery,
Alexandra Beebe.
      p.   cm.
   Includes index.
   ISBN 0-8016-3248-X
   1. Pain—Nursing—Handbooks, manuals, etc.   I. Beebe, Alexandra.
II. Title.
   [DNLM: 1. Pain—nursing.   WY 150 M478p]
RT87.P35M325   1989
616′.0472—dc19
DNLM/DLC
for Library of Congress   89-2849
                                                              CIP

VT/VH/VH   9   8   7   6

Preface

Purposes of This Clinical Manual

From the vast and expanding literature on pain, this clinical book provides a selection of basic information, tools, and specific techniques that the nurse and other caregivers may use to assess and help the patient with pain. Emphasis is placed on specific strategies that may be used with patients of all ages in all clinical settings.

The intention is to contribute to the re-education of those whose basic education addressed pain in a limited fashion, as well as to assist students to apply theory and develop skill in helping the patient with pain. Primarily, however, the focus is on developing the foundations of nursing's unique contribution to the care of patients with pain. We are convinced that it is through the efforts of the nurse that most patients with pain will receive assistance. Nurses probably spend more time with patients with pain than any other health team members. Consequently, nurses are in a unique position to observe the patient with pain, identify and attempt to obtain what the patient may need, and work with the patient to use effectively what the nurse and other health team members have to offer. This manual will help nurses identify their particular areas of accountability in the care of patients with pain.

This is truly meant to be a *clinical manual*. It covers a significant portion of what the nurse on a one-to-one basis can *do* with or for the patient with pain. We hope that in busy clinical situations, nurses and other caregivers will be able to refer to this manual, quickly locate helpful information, and find it presented in a manner that enables them to use it immediately. The size (standard 8½ by 11 inch pages) and spiral binding facilitate use in the clinical setting, including ease of duplicating pages. Through this manual, we hope to promote the use of current knowledge about assessment and relief of pain. Information is presented in a manner that will help the reader to:

- Locate the specific information needed for a given patient by referring to suggestions regarding patients and situations for which a specific approach may be appropriate.
- Understand exactly how to use the information through clear, brief, simple suggestions along with patient examples and immediate help sections in each chapter.
- Provide the patient/family with necessary information by duplicating patient/family teaching points directly from this manual.
- Formulate a nursing diagnosis, document the problem, and write a nursing care plan.
- Communicate effectively with other health team members to obtain their understanding and cooperation in helping the patient with pain by applying current knowledge and substantiating this with specifically identified references and the annotated references.

Ultimately this manual is meant to help the patient with pain by assisting his caregivers, particularly his nurses, to use the knowledge currently available about the assessment and relief of pain. We believe that relief from pain is not only humane but also a legitimate therapeutic goal, having a significant impact on the patient's physical and emotional well-being. Unrelieved pain may have many detrimental effects on the individual, including retarded recovery from illness or surgery.

Audience for This Manual

This clinical manual is intended primarily for nursing students and practicing nurses in all areas of clinical practice, but the information may be useful for anyone giving direct care to a patient with pain, e.g., social workers, physicians, pharmacists, physical therapists, and hospice volunteers.

Unfortunately, pain relief tends to remain a low priority in many clinical situations. Traditionally pain has been viewed as a symptom of something that could be diagnosed and then cured or controlled. In the last 15 years in North America, health professionals have gone one step further and addressed the issue of what can be done about pain per se while diagnosis and treatment are taking place and what can be done for the patient when the cause of pain cannot be controlled. Thus, the science of pain is new. Consequently, many health team members have been taught little about how to bring comfort and relief to the patient with pain. (In fact, many health team members have actually been taught ineffective, unsubstantiated, and inaccurate methods of assessing and relieving pain.) The busy practicing nurse often lacks the time, skill, or knowledge to assess and help the patient with pain, and caring for the patient with pain may become frustrating.

This manual will help nursing students bridge the gap between theory and actual clinical practice. To provide additional assistance to nursing students who are beginning to develop skills or practicing nurses who want to expand their skills, study guides for each chapter are provided at the end of the book.

This manual focuses on strategies that nurses can use in a relatively independent manner—strategies that require clinical nursing judgment. Some pain relief methods do require a physician's prescription, such as analgesics, but the pain relief methods are ones that the nurse often identifies the need for, obtains a prescription for if necessary, carries out with or for the patient with pain, evaluates the effectiveness of, and attempts to implement any changes indicated. In particular, this book identifies the nurse's *active* role in the pharmacological management of pain, an area traditionally physician oriented. Observations of the patient's responses to analgesic prescriptions are viewed as an independent nursing function, along with the nurse's responsibility to select appropriate analgesics from those prescribed, combine analgesics, identify and avoid those that are unhelpful, and implement PRN prescriptions in a preventive, around the clock manner based on individual assessment.

Limitations of This Manual

This manual applies theory; it does not provide an extensive review of research or the theoretical bases of pain assessment and relief. It does provide basic theoretical explanations along with the most relevant research findings.

The authors are acutely aware of the many useful approaches to assessment and relief of pain that are omitted in this manual; for nurses whose interest in pain goes beyond this manual (and hopefully there will be many) and for nurses caring for patients who present pain problems too difficult to resolve with strategies suggested in this manual, there are countless articles and books, many of which are listed in the selected readings and annotated references sections at the end of the chapters.

Content and Framework of This Manual

The chapters in this manual and the content within each chapter follow the problem-solving process, or nursing process. Chapter 1 is an exception since it provides an introduction to the subject of pain control. It addresses the brief history of professional interest in pain, the differences between the nurse's and the physician's approach to the patient with pain, and the authors' philosophy about pain control.

Chapter 2 begins the nursing process, focusing on assessment. It contains information on common problems in assessing individual patients, classifications and definitions of the major types of pain, and practical assessment tools. Chapter 3 includes nursing diagnoses and broadly focuses on the problem-solving process. Pain theories that underlie information in the following chapters are discussed briefly.

Nursing interventions are contained in Chapters 4 through 11. Pharmacological interventions are covered in Chapter 4. Noninvasive pain relief measures are covered in Chapter 5 on cutaneous stimulation, Chapter 6 on distraction, Chapter 7 on relaxation, and Chapter 8 on imagery. Nursing interventions for more specialized situations are discussed in Chapter 9 on chronic nonmalignant pain, Chapter 10 on pain in children, and Chapter 11 on pain in the elderly. Due to the lack of definitive research, information about pain in the elderly is limited.

Chapter 12 focuses on evaluation. This is followed by the study guide. The latter is intended to assist the reader in gaining skills in using the nursing approaches discussed in each chapter. It may be particularly helpful for the nursing student. "Immediate Help" sections are included in most chapters to facilitate implementation of material in situations where time is limited.

Each chapter on specific nursing interventions (Chapters 4 through 8) incorporates the problem-solving process by including a definition of the intervention, benefits and limits, appropriate and inappropriate situations, specific directions for using the interventions, patient/family teaching points, identification and handling of complications or problems, methods of obtaining the understanding and cooperation of other health team members, and nursing care plans.

The content for each chapter is focused on what is *practical* for both the practicing nurse and the patient with pain. Especially important aspects are designated as "Key Points." An effort is made to include approaches that are not too time consuming, are not too difficult to learn, require minimal equipment or else require items that tend to be readily available in most homes or hospitals, are as low risk as possible, and have a reasonable chance of being effective, based on research and/or the authors' experiences teaching patients and practicing nurses.

Annotated references and selected readings are listed at the end of the chapter. To conserve space and enhance readability, extensive footnoting within the text is avoided except in Chapter 4 on analgesics and other pharmacological approaches. Nurses work constantly with physicians who legally prescribe the analgesics. Justification and documentation of the nurse's suggestions are often essential to effective communication with the physician. Therefore, within the text of this chapter there are many references or footnotes, especially to medical and pharmacology journals. Those sources that are particularly helpful in documenting newer or less commonly used pharmacological approaches are specifically noted.

The term *patient* or *person*, rather than client, is used since the intended use of this manual is in the clinical setting where the majority of health team members use the term *patient*. However, the authors wholly subscribe to the philosophy underlying reference to the patient as client, i.e., consumer of care with basic rights to know, accept, or reject care.

In keeping with tradition and simplicity, the masculine pronoun is used in reference to the patient, unless the patient is identified in an example as female. For similar reasons, the feminine form is used in reference to the nurse.

In attempting to provide practical assistance in busy clinical situations, we do not in any way intend to discount the seriousness of a patient's pain or the complex nature of pain. Hopefully this impression is averted by our repeated focus on suggestions for individualizing approaches and evaluating their effectiveness.

The authors look forward to developing the content of this book further in future editions, especially pain in the elderly. Both of us frequently speak on the topic of pain, and have extended to our audiences an open invitation to write or telephone regarding patients with pain. Many patient examples in this book are a result of these interactions. We are grateful to those who contacted us, and we invite you, the reader, to contact us for assistance and make comments and suggestions to us personally.

Margo McCaffery, R.N., M.S., F.A.A.N.
Consultant in the Nursing Care of Patients with Pain
1458 Berkeley St, Apt 1
Santa Monica, CA 90404
Telephone: (213) 828-7251

Alexandra Beebe, R.N., M.S., O.C.N.
On sabbatical

Acknowledgments

Although writing a book is a lonely task, it is truly never done alone. Many people helped us in many ways, some as professional colleagues and some as friends and family.

A very special thank you goes to our library researcher, Lucie Ferrell. This is the second book she has researched for Margo and the first for both of us. We cannot imagine writing a book without her. No computer-generated research could ever achieve what Lucie can do in a library.

Somehow the manuscript must be on paper, and there are various ways of accomplishing this. We chose computers. In January of 1987, neither one of us knew how to make our computers engage in word processing. Craig Colbert, Margo's computer consultant, and Dolores Stammer, Alexandra's consultant, were available by telephone 24 hours a day and provided compassionate consulting. We literally could not have written the book without them.

Together we express our appreciation to our many colleagues for their insights and ideas. Both of us encounter hundreds of nurses each year, since we participate in many educational programs. We are impressed with the willingness of nurses to share their experiences. Sometimes it is only a comment, a question, or a story told hurriedly in a hallway. These pages reflect many such encounters.

Other times we selected specific nurses and asked them for a critical review of what we had written. They not only responded readily and conscientiously, giving enormous time, energy, and knowledge, but also responded with enthusiasm that encouraged us. Colleagues who contributed invaluable ideas include Judith Beyer, Jo Eland, Shoosh Lettick, Noreen Meinhart, Madelyn Miscally, Judith A. Paice, Susan C. Schafer, Sandy Sentivany, Carol Wenzl, Fran Wiley, and Donna Wong.

Many people at Mosby contributed to the publication of this book. Paul Koren is particularly important to us because he initiated the idea of our publishing with Mosby. And, we are indebted to our editors Linda Duncan and Susie Baxter for their efforts and encouragement.

For each of us, writing this book resulted in considerable social isolation. Yet there were those who continued to maintain contact and to tolerate our behavior although they probably questioned our sanity at times. Each of us would personally like to thank certain people.

Margo makes the following acknowledgments. I thank my family for enduring me: my daughter, Melissa McCaffery; my mother, Mary Katharine Smith; my brother, Don Smith; and especially my husband, Rick Brewer, for his love and presence. To those friends who kept calling when there was little response and who were still there and ready to be friends when the writing was over, I am deeply grateful: Elaine, Lee and Ren, Bill, Carol, Jo, and especially Noreen with whom I have shared so much for so many years and Mark for the special meaning he gives to friendship.

Alexandra would like to acknowledge the following. Special thanks to my sister, Schuyler Savage, for her courage in speaking the truth and for her unwavering belief in my ability to complete this project. My appreciation to the following friends who were so generous with their encouragement and support: Camilla, Debbie, Dolores S., Connie, Eleanor, Joyce, and Dolores R.

We don't know how other people really feel about writing a book, but we found that for two years it demanded the greatest effort we have ever exerted. We were always supportive of each other, and frequently we both depended on humor to save us. Typically when we were the most stressed, feeling the most hopeless, and really unable to believe that it would ever end, we laughed. Each of us has a rather large collection of cartoons sent by the other.

Contents

Perspectives on Pain: History, Current Status, and Developing the Nurse's Role

Unquestionably, pain is extremely prevalent. Pain is a universal human experience, and it is the most frequent reason that people seek health care. However, no data exist that accurately reveal the incidence of either brief or prolonged pain of any sort. The frequency and perhaps the severity of pain may even be increasing as progress in medical science increases survival from birth through old age.

HISTORICAL PERSPECTIVE ON PAIN CONTROL

Traditionally, pain has been viewed as a symptom for which a cause is diagnosed, and pain is then eliminated by cure or control of the cause. However, during the last 15 to 20 years in North America, health professionals have looked beyond this approach to what can be done in the meantime to help the patient with pain. That is, how do we help the patient with pain during the process of diagnosis and cure or control of the cause of pain? What can we do for the patient whose pain cannot be cured or controlled? Such a patient might have an end-stage illness, but the person might live for months with pain. The patient might have a normal life expectancy with a non–life-threatening cause for pain, such as arthritis or peripheral neuropathy. How do we help people with these various sorts of pain? The palliative, as well as the curative, approach is now seen as important.

Relief from pain has probably been a concern of mankind since the beginning of time, but health professionals have not until recently devoted much clinical effort or research to pain relief. The study of pain, algology, is in its infancy. Before the introduction of the gate control theory in 1965 by Melzack and Wall, very little appeared in the professional literature about pain. Today there are countless books on the subject, and professional journals in all the health care disciplines regularly feature articles on pain.

Not only must information about pain control be disseminated but also *pain control must be recognized as a priority.* Historically, this has not been the case.

The question of responsibility or accountability for pain relief was studied in the late 1960s and early 1970s, and the conclusion was drawn that health care systems did not hold health team members accountable for pain relief (Fagerhaugh, 1974; Fagerhaugh and Strauss, 1977; Strauss et al, 1974; Weiner, 1975). This problem continues today. The nurse may work in a system, such as a hospital or home care agency, and the nurse personally may want to relieve the patient's pain; however, the nurse may discover that the system does not actually regard pain relief as a high priority. The importance of assessing and relieving pain may be verbalized, but other indications may be lacking.

Interestingly, most high priorities have fairly predictable indicators, such as standardized "paper work." For example, delivery of medications to the patient is a legitimate high priority and one for which the nurse is held accountable by the hospital. Very predictable paper work goes into this: the physician writes and signs prescriptions that are transferred to various places such as Kardexes, and all medications are usually recorded on a standardized medication record, easily located in the patient's chart, so that all health team members can quickly access this information.

By contrast, such is not the case with pain. Many clinical areas where patients with pain are cared for do not have standardized pain assessment records nor do they have a systematic method of recording all pain relief measures for the individual patient and whether they have been safe and effective. Thus information about the problem of pain and possible solutions are not easily identified and transmitted quickly to other members of the health team. Furthermore, if pain relief measures are not implemented (e.g., a PRN analgesic is not given), the nurse is not as likely to be questioned about this as she is if she fails to administer scheduled medications, such as penicillin q6h.

Unfortunately, the studies of responsibility for pain management reveal that health team members are held accountable for controlling the patient's *expression* of pain, which may include the patient asking for an analgesic, moaning, saying he hurts, or splinting the painful area. These expressions of pain could be controlled by relieving the pain; however, since the health team usually is not held responsible for pain relief, an attempt may be made to control the expression of pain without relieving the pain. This may take the form of statements such as "Try to take control of yourself," "It's not as bad as you think," and "You're going to have to learn to handle this yourself." In essence, we are saying to the patient "We are not responsible for relieving your pain, you are responsible for your being quiet about it." We are asking the patient to suffer in silence, to learn to live with his pain and leave us alone. Obviously, this is not good quality patient care: while it is a problem for all health professionals, it is a special problem for nurses. Nurses spend more time with patients with pain than do any other health team members. The nursing profession must come to grips with its unique contribution to the care of patients with pain.

CURRENT STATUS OF PAIN CONTROL

Overall, some progress has been made in the last 15 to 20 years. Health professionals have begun to focus on pain control. This progress is reflected in the following six ways:

1. Widespread development of programs that explicitly state pain control as a high priority. Certainly some clinical areas or hospitals may make an effort to make pain relief a high priority; however, only a few state that pain control is a high priority. That is, if a patient is referred to such a program, pain control definitely will be addressed. These are:

Hospice programs. The first operating hospice in the United States began in 1974. In the late 1980s there are hundreds of hospice programs of various types throughout the United States. Every hospice program states that pain control is one of its primary goals.

Multidisciplinary pain clinics. Nerve block clinics for pain relief have existed for many years, but today we have hundreds of pain clinics, many of them partially multidisciplinary. In the early 1960s there were probably only two multidisciplinary pain centers in the United States, one at The University of Washington in Seattle (directed by John Bonica) and the other at The City of Hope Medical Center in Duarte, California (directed by Benjamin Crue, Jr.).

Childbirth education programs. Regardless of the type of preparation for childbirth, almost always one explicit goal is to make labor and delivery a more positive and comfortable experience. Many of these programs, e.g., Lamaze, Kitzinger, and Bradley, grew rapidly during the 1970s and early 1980s.

2. Founding of professional organizations concerned with pain management. The International Association for the Study of Pain (IASP) was founded in 1974. National chapters were founded shortly thereafter, including the Canadian Pain Society (CPS) in 1976 and the American Pain Society (APS) in 1978. Regional groups have been formed, e.g., the Western Pain Society in the United States. The IASP and its chapters have as their goal the promotion of education and research on pain.

The International Pain Foundation, formed in 1986, has as its goal the support of public and professional education about pain disorders and their treatment.

The National Hospice Organization (NHO), formed in 1978, promotes quality care for terminally ill persons and their families. It is dedicated to integrating hospice into the U.S. health care system.

Many of the prepared childbirth programs also have national organizations, e.g., the American Society for Psychoprophylaxis in Obstetrics.

3. Publication of professional journals that focus primarily or exclusively on pain management. Such publications include the *Journal of Pain and Symptom Management, The Clinical Journal of Pain, Pain Management,* and *Pain.*

4. National and international meetings with pain as the primary topic. These are fairly common now and include meetings every 3 years for the IASP and yearly for the APS and NHO.

In May 1986, health professionals and lay persons participated in a consensus development conference on pain sponsored by the National Institutes of Health (NIH) (Engber, 1986a). The following were noted in the consensus statement:

Progress has been made since the last conference in 1979, including new commitment to utilizing a multidisciplinary team approach for chronic pain, advances in pharmacological techniques, and increased research in nonpharmacological methods.

Deficiencies continue in the clinical management of pain, including undermedication of patients, especially children, with acute pain and those with prolonged pain due to malignancy, overmedication of people with chronic nonmalignant pain, inadequate education of health professionals, and inadequate communication between professionals and patients.

The nurse's role is stated as the key link in facilitating communication between the patient, family, and health team. The role of the nurse includes teaching the patient about pain, scheduling medications in relation to the individual's needs, and using nonpharmacological pain relief methods.

In July 1988, the First International Symposium on Pediatric Pain, sponsored by the IASP, APS and others, was held in Seattle, Washington.

5. Worldwide concern for cancer pain control. The World Health Organization (WHO) recognizes cancer pain relief as a worldwide priority. Their booklet, *Cancer Pain Relief,* discusses the prevalence of cancer pain, education and training, legislative factors, and specific pharmacological guidelines.

6. National initiatives for improving cancer pain management. The Wisconsin Initiative for Improving Cancer Pain Management is a voluntary statewide network of health care professionals that began in 1985 with the goal of improving the assessment and management of cancer pain (Engber, 1986b). The following projects are now part of this statewide effort: a cancer pain hotline; a network of physicians, nurses, pharmacists, and hospice personnel serving as patient advocates and resources for health professionals; a question and answer patient education booklet; medical education activities; and a statewide newsletter, *Cancer Pain Update,* distributed to health professionals. Reports and updates on the initiative are discussed in the *Journal of Pain and Symptom Management.* Interest has been expressed in starting similar initiatives in other states.

Information about some of the above, e.g., addresses and telephone numbers, is included at the end of the chapter in the "Resources" section.

In addition, there has been a dramatic increase in books on pain and articles in journals representing the various health care disciplines. Considerably more research is being done on assessment and relief of pain by a variety of approaches, both pharmacological and nonpharmacological.

URGENT NEED FOR REEDUCATION OF HEALTH PROFESSIONALS

The newness of the science of pain has practical implications regarding professional education. It takes years for a new science to gain acceptance and for the body of knowledge to be disseminated and incorporated in basic education. Hence many health professionals practicing

today were taught very little about pain relief, and much of what little they were taught may very well have been wrong. It is often disconcerting for these health care providers to be reeducated about pain control. Many of the current approaches are different from what they were taught originally and sometimes are even the opposite of what they have conscientiously been doing.

Health professionals who received inadequate or inaccurate education about pain control very often *are unaware of their lack of knowledge about pain control.* They have been doing what they were taught. Because the sensation of pain is subjective and cannot be measured by anyone except the person who feels it, the health professional may not always realize when their efforts have not been effective. If the health care provider does not believe what the patient says or if the patient is not carefully assessed, it may appear that efforts to relieve pain are successful when in fact they are not. It is difficult at times to convince health professionals of the need for reeducation. Because of misconceptions about how to assess pain and a lack of knowledge about the pharmacology of analgesics, situations that at first seem simple can easily be misunderstood and can lead to faulty conclusions about a patient.

Patient Example

John, 20 years old, was hospitalized 2 days ago for fractures and lacerations following an automobile accident. Within the last 24 hours he has become a "problem" for the staff. The analgesics prescribed for him are meperidine (Demerol) 50 mg IM or PO q4h. He has become a "clock watcher" and "prefers the needle to the pill." He jokes with the staff and is often smiling or watching TV. He has many visitors throughout the day and evening. He says he never really gets good pain relief, but about 30 minutes after he receives the injectable narcotics he is usually on the telephone laughing and talking with his friends. The staff is convinced that he does not hurt as much as he says because he does not act like he is in pain. The staff also believes his preference for the injection over the pill and his regular requests by the clock are indications that he was or is becoming a drug abuser.

These *inaccurate conclusions* are a result of the staff's failure to understand this patient's effective coping mechanisms for handling pain and stress, in addition to their lack of pharmacological information about the analgesics prescribed. These inaccurate conclusions interfere with effective treatment and evaluation of John's pain. Reeducation of all health team members is *essential* if adequate pain control is to be achieved.

THE NURSE'S UNIQUE ROLE

No distinct line can be drawn between what different health team members do for the patient with pain. There seems to be much overlap in the functioning of team members, as well there should be if a multidisciplinary approach is being used.

From a practical point of view, the nurse's unique role in the care of people with pain can be distinguished from other members of the health team because of the nurse's sheer presence with the patient: the nurse spends more time with people with pain than does any other health team member. Although the care of patients with pain ideally is multidisciplinary, in most cases *nursing care is the cornerstone*. In well-developed programs of pain control, such as hospice, this role of the nurse is well-recognized.

The nurse's role in the care of people with pain most often includes carrying out pain relief methods with and for the patient, identifying the need for change or additional methods, obtaining them, and assessing the impact on the patient. It is usually through the nurse that the most patients can receive the best pain control.

When the nurse is knowledgeable of pharmacological approaches to pain control along with noninvasive methods, such as relaxation and cutaneous stimulation, there is a unique opportunity to individualize these interventions for the patient.

OUR BELIEFS ABOUT PAIN RELIEF AND THE PATIENT'S RIGHTS

Our beliefs about pain relief and the patient's rights form the foundation of our suggested approaches to the care of people with pain. Some of these beliefs have been presented before (McCaffery, 1979), and we continue to be committed to them. These beliefs are not, however, truths. They are simply an honest statement of what we have become convinced of as we have cared for people with pain. We hope that the statements will enable the reader to understand our underlying philosophy and will provoke thought and discussion among nurses. Above all, we urge others to address the issue of the patient's rights.

We believe that pain control:
1. Is a legitimate therapeutic goal.
2. Contributes significantly to the patient's physical and emotional well-being.
3. Must rank high in the list of priorities in patient care.
4. Is patient controlled, i.e., the patient is the final authority about assessment of pain and all methods of pain control to the extent that it is safe and that communication, including nonverbal, is possible.

We believe that the patient has a right:
1. To decide the duration and intensity of pain he is willing to endure or tolerate.
2. To be informed of all possible methods of pain relief along with the favorable and unfavorable consequences, as well as the controversial aspects.
3. To choose which pain control method(s) he wishes to try.

4. To choose to live with or without pain.*

We also recognize that the health care provider has a right to refuse to treat a patient with pain by a method that the health care provider deems harmful.

RESOURCES
Publications

The Journal of Pain and Symptom Management (expansion of PRN forum)
Quarterly
Elsevier Publishing Co, Inc
Journal Fulfillment Department
PO Box 882, Madison Square Station
New York, NY 10160-0200

The Clinical Journal of Pain
Quarterly
Raven Press Books, Ltd
1140 Avenue of the Americas
New York, NY 10036

Pain Management
Bimonthly
CORE Medical Journals
3131 Princeton Pike, Bldg 2A
Lawrenceville, NJ 08648

Cancer Pain Relief, 1986
74 page booklet
WHO Publications Center USA
49 Sheridan Ave
Albany, NY 12210

Principles of Analgesic Use in the Treatment of Acute Pain and Chronic Cancer Pain: A Concise Guide to Medical Practice, 1987
9 page booklet
American Pain Society
1615 L Street NW, Suite 925
Washington DC 20036
(202) 296-9200

Questions and Answers about Pain Control
43 page booklet written for the general public.
Contact local division of American Cancer Society.

Organizations

IASP (International Association for the Study of Pain)
Membership includes subscription to the journal *Pain,* monthly.
Information may be obtained on pain societies in other countries, e.g., Canada, Italy.
IASP Secretary
909 NE 43rd St, Suite 306
Seattle, WA 98105-6020
(206) 547-6409

---

*There may be exception to this right if it endangers another person. For example, the mother's right to take certain medications for the sole purpose of her own comfort during pregnancy or labor and delivery may be questioned if these medications endanger the health or life of the baby. Likewise, there may be questions about an individual's right to take an analgesic that also sedates him while he is driving a vehicle or operating machinery that could injure other people if operated improperly.

International Pain Foundation
 909 NE 43rd St, Suite 306
 Seattle, WA 98105-6020
American Pain Society
 Information may be obtained on regional chapters.
 5700 Old Orchard Road, 1st Floor
 Skokie, IL 60077-1024
 (708) 966-5595
National Hospice Organization
 1901 N Fort Myer Dr, Suite 307
 Arlington, VA 22209
 (703) 234-5900
HospiceLink, sponsored by the Hospice Education Institute.
 Provides a listing of local hospice programs and answers
 general questions.
 (800) 331-1620
National Headache Foundation
 5252 N Western Ave
 Chicago, IL 60625
 Excellent newsletter, membership for professionals and general public.
Pharmaceutical Companies that manufacture analgesics have a
 variety of free resources on pain control. Many companies
 have toll-free numbers, or a pharmacist would have the
 phone number of the local sales representative. Some drug
 companies have programs for indigent patients.

REFERENCES AND SELECTED READINGS

Engber, D: Report on the NIH consensus development conference on pain, *J Pain Sympt Manag* 1:165-167, Summer
1986a

Engber, D: Wisconsin initiative for improving cancer pain management: progress report, *J Pain Sympt Manag* 1:58-59, Winter 1986b

Fagerhaugh, SY: Pain expression and control on a burn unit,
Nursing Outlook 22:645-650, Oct 1974

Fagerhaugh, SY, and Strauss, A: Politics of pain management:
staff-patient interaction, Menlo Park, Cal, 1977, Addison-Wesley
Publishing Co

Liebeskind, JC, and Melzack, R: The international pain foundation: meeting a need for education in pain management, *Pain*
30:1-2, 1987

McCaffery, M: Nursing management of the patient with pain,
New York, 1979, JB Lippincott Co

Strauss, A, Fagerhaugh, SY, and Glaser, B: An organizational-
work-interactional perspective, *Nursing Outlook* 22:560-566,
Sept 1974

Weiner, CL: Pain assessment on an orthopedic ward, *Nursing
Outlook* 23:508-516, Aug 1975

CHAPTER

2

Assessment

If patients could always tell us that they hurt and we could accept this as fact, the assessment and treatment of pain would be a great deal simpler than they are. However, we do not always readily believe and help people who say they hurt. Furthermore, not all people can or will tell us about their pain. Some people who hurt may deny pain or refuse pain relief. These complexities of assessing pain initially and performing ongoing assessments that enable us to refine the relief of pain are addressed here along with an overview of simple classifications and treatment approaches to major types of pain problems and specific assessment tools that may be easily used in the clinical setting.

MISCONCEPTIONS THAT HAMPER ASSESSMENT OF PATIENTS WHO INDICATE THEY HAVE PAIN

Virtually all of us grow up thinking in certain ways that cause us to erroneously doubt others who indicate they have pain. Unfortunately, these misconceptions are sometimes reinforced in our professional education. Since almost everyone is prone at times to discount another's report of pain, it is essential to become aware of the misconceptions that cause us to doubt the patient with pain so that we can accomplish the following goals:

- Prevent ourselves from acting on our misconceptions. Many of our misconceptions are well-entrenched in our thinking from early childhood. They may be emotional reactions that are not possible or easy to eliminate and may creep into our thinking no matter how well we understand them logically. Therefore we simply hope to prevent them from having a detrimental effect on what we actually do for the patient. When we think in these ways, ideally we will recognize it and stop ourselves before we act.

- Help others, e.g., health team and family, think through reasons that they may unjustifiably doubt the patient.
- Identify our *professional* responsibility to the patient who says he has pain.

The misconceptions covered in this chapter apply to all types of pain. Extensions of and additions to them are discussed later in relation to chronic nonmalignant pain, children, and the elderly. The misconceptions overlap to some degree. An understanding of the first one below is, however, basic to comprehending the others.

Authority about Pain: Health Team vs. Patient

Misconception: The health team is the authority about the existence and nature of the patient's pain sensation.

Correction: The person with the pain is the only authority about the existence and nature of that pain, since the sensation of pain can be felt only by the person who has it.

The basic question is "Whose pain is it?" The answer, of course, is that it is the patient's pain. The content of this entire book revolves around a thorough understanding of the fact that the patient is the only authority about his pain.

Sometimes the issue of who is the authority about pain unfortunately boils down to a battle between the health team or family and the patient. Members of the health team or the family may erroneously believe that they can determine whether the patient hurts and just how much he hurts—regardless of what the patient says about it. This is the most detrimental attitude that one can have if the intention is to help the patient.

The most important and most difficult aspect of helping the patient with pain is to accept and appreciate that only the patient can feel the pain. The sensation of pain is completely subjective. The health team would rather deal with a symptom that can be detected and measured objec-

IMMEDIATE HELP FOR ASSESSMENT

Quick Assessment in Situations where Patients are Unable to Tolerate Lengthy Questions

Time involved: Reading time, 5 minutes; implementation time, about 10 minutes.

Sample situation: Mr. M., 65 years old, with lung cancer and widespread metastasis is admitted to your floor. He is not able to concentrate long enough to answer many questions. He grimaces frequently and cries out saying "It hurts, please give me something." His wife states that he is not swallowing anything by mouth.

Possible solution: Assess pain with minimal number of questions in order to give initial analgesic safely.

Expected outcome: Patient states he is comfortable. Further pain assessment is completed at a later time so that a detailed plan of care may be implemented.

Tell the patient that you are going to work to get him comfortable as quickly as possible but that you must get some information first:

1. Point (on his body) to where the pain is.
   Mr. M. points to his lower back.
2. Is this the same location for the pain over the last several days?
   Mr. M. says that this is the same area that has bothered him over the last week, but it has gotten much worse since yesterday evening.

3. On a 0 to 10 scale (0 = no pain, 10 = worst pain), what number would you give your pain right now?
   Mr. M. becomes very agitated and yells "It is unbearable." This is a good enough answer under the circumstances.
4. What medication were you taking at home, and did it help the pain?
   Mrs. M. tells you that her husband was taking morphine 90 mg q4h with Motrin 800 mg q6h. He has not been able to swallow anything since late last night, so he has had nothing for pain since then. Prior to this, the medication was keeping the pain well controlled.

Due to Mr. M.'s condition, it was appropriate to ask only the most essential questions to initiate an analgesic regimen. The above four questions give you important baseline data and establish an initial narcotic dose.

Using a flow sheet, the immediate goal is to establish pain control quickly. Using Mr. M.'s words ask "Is the pain more bearable now?" Once Mr. M. is comfortable, additional questions from the initial pain assessment tool may be filled in, and a long-term plan of care may be reviewed with the patient and his wife.

---

tively. It is reassuring to read a pathology report or get back some numbers from the lab; however, when the symptom is pain, we must ask the patient about it. We have no direct measure of the pain sensation—no pain thermometer. When we treat the patient with pain, we must again ask him about his pain to determine if we have succeeded. We do not know about pain or the effect of our treatment of it unless we get this information from the patient. Caring for patients with pain can be a humbling experience.

Remember too that patients do not like the fact that the pain sensation is subjective. Sooner or later, most patients with pain realize that they cannot prove their pain. Their only hope is to find someone who will believe them.

Because the pain sensation is subjective, considerable research has been devoted to developing assessment tools that help the patient communicate information about the sensation of pain. Many tools have been developed for adults and recently for children as young as 3 years of age.

Still, some patients, such as a baby, a confused or sedated patient, or a patient who speaks a different language, are not able to communicate about pain. With these patients it is necessary to make an educated guess about what pain may be felt. This may be based on our knowledge of the physical pathology and the type of pain

other patients have told us they experienced from comparable physical causes. We may also be able to obtain some notion of pain by observing nonverbal behaviors such as crying, restlessness, or rigid posture. However, we must remember that here we are merely guessing about pain and we must be ever ready to revise our guess based on additional information from the patient and from others who know the patient and new information about the patient's pathology.

Thus some patients may be unable to communicate about pain, and others with pain may deny it or refuse pain relief (discussed later in this chapter). Whenever the patient is able to indicate he has pain, we believe the patient's statements are the most valid measurement of pain.

Because pain is subjective, the definition of pain we propose for use in clinical practice, originally proposed in 1968 (McCaffery, p. 95) is "Pain is whatever the experiencing person says it is, existing whenever the experiencing person says it does." Specifically this definition means that when the patient *indicates* he has pain, the health team responds positively. The patient's report of pain is either believed or given the benefit of the doubt. This is the professional response. Each health team member is entitled to his or her personal opinion about whether the patient is telling the truth about his pain. However, the issue is professional responsibility, which is to accept the patient's report of pain and to help the patient in a responsive and positive manner.

This approach to pain is difficult to accept. People look at the definition proposed and its implications and voice the fear that if they believe every person who says he has pain or if they give every person the benefit of the doubt, they will be fooled. Indeed they will be fooled sooner or later. Pain is subjective, and being fooled is simply a reality in dealing with something that can never be proved or disproved. This point must be acknowledged by all members of the health team. The risk of being fooled does not justify doubting the patient or withholding pain relief. Furthermore, the risk of malingering, discussed below, is not as high as we usually think. Nevertheless, caring for the patient with pain is truly a humbling experience. Here and in other areas of caring for the patient with pain, the subjectivity of pain affects all who care for patients with pain.

No matter which approach we use in responding to the patient's report of pain, we will eventually make a mistake. If we doubt some patients and withhold treatment, we may avoid being fooled by the minority who are addicts, abusers, or malingerers, but we will eventually fail to help someone who does have pain. On the other hand, if we give everyone the benefit of the doubt and try to relieve pain in all who say they have it, we will be fooled by some who are addicts, abusers, or malingerers, but we will never fail to help someone who does have pain. Either way, we will make a mistake. Therefore we must address our professional responsibility and consider which mistake we can afford. (Of course, some addicts and abusers do have pain that requires narcotics for relief, see pp. 74-76.)

What may happen if we do not believe or respond positively to the patient's report of pain? Pain specialists are very specific about the issue of believing or accepting the patient's report of pain. For example, the booklet *Cancer Pain Relief* published by the World Health Organization, 1986, which represents the combined efforts of pain specialists from throughout the world, lists simply and clearly as the first of eight steps for assessing cancer pain "Believe the patient's complaint of pain" (p. 14). This statement is not discussed—there are no exceptions. The point is made that to ignore the main steps in clinical assessment of cancer pain is the major cause of misdiagnosis and inappropriate management.

One study of children showed that pain caused by cancer was experienced for as long as 821 days before initiation of cancer therapy (Miser et al, 1987). Obviously, failure to believe or respond to the patient's report of pain may cause us to miss a diagnosis until the disease is too far advanced for treatment or to delay treatment until the outcome is poor.

An equally disastrous outcome may be seen almost daily in the clinical situation when a patient's report of pain is ignored because it is doubted, an altogether too familiar scene. The patient says he hurts, and the health team doesn't really believe this. They do little to help, and the patient senses that they do not believe him and concludes that they will not do much to help him; however, he still hurts and wants pain relief. He reacts to this situation with anger and perhaps some sadness or depression and may become irritable and demanding. Perhaps he changes his story because the truth did not work. He may exaggerate or lie to get others to believe him and help him. The health team sees this change in behavior and becomes frustrated, perhaps believing that the patient is manipulative. Thus evolves the adversarial relationship, with the health team and patient disagreeing about whether the patient has pain. Enormous emotion and energy are wasted on the part of both patient and health team over something that can never be proved or disproved.

Whenever this occurs, ask why it is difficult to believe that this patient hurts. Many of the more common answers are covered below. Ideally, these can be discussed with the health team, and the result will be a positive approach, based either on believing the patient or being willing to give him the benefit of the doubt. However, this doesn't always happen. If the health team continues in the adversarial relationship, it is essential to remember the following:

- An adversarial relationship is not a therapeutic one. It is doubtful that anything helpful can be done for the patient in the context of an adversarial relationship.
- Every time the patient indicates that he hurts and the health team indicates that they do not believe this, the health team is calling the patient a liar. This is insulting and degrading and is not a professional approach to the patient. It is an unethical and unprofessional response to a client's stated need.
- If we are unable to respond professionally and positively to the patient, it is our responsibility to consult with or refer the patient to those who can respond positively to his expressed needs. Referral or consultation is the same approach we use for any health/illness problem presented by a patient when we do not know how to treat it or are not able to do so.

Patient Credibility: Personal Values vs. Professional Responsibility

Misconception: Our personal values and intuition about the trustworthiness of others is a valuable tool in identifying whether a person is lying about pain.

Correction: Personal values and intuition may serve us well in our social lives, but they do not constitute a professional approach to the patient with pain. Further, the patient's credibility is not on trial, and the health team is not called upon to judge this.

In our daily personal lives, it is not uncommon for us to make tentative judgments about those we meet even briefly. It is almost unavoidable to encounter someone without having some impression of him or her, including whether the person is honest and dependable. When we are unsure, we may or may not decide to take the risk of depending on the person.

What information we use to make these judgments and decisions may be largely unconscious or at least difficult to specify. On the other hand, sometimes visual impact alone causes us to be cautious of a person. For example, if you are walking alone at dusk in a strange neighborhood with no one else on the street except some strange looking person walking toward you, you may decide to avoid any risk associated with this person by crossing to the other side of the street to put distance between the two of you. You may be wrong about the person's character, but in daily life decisions such as this may help us avoid being taken advantage of by others, e.g., being hurt or robbed. Such decisions may cause little or no harm to others. In our professional activities, however, such judgments are a disservice to the patient.

Because the sensation of pain is totally subjective, it is understandable how health team members might inadvertently rely on personal biases and judgments about human nature to determine the truthfulness of a patient's report of pain. When the patient reporting pain lives an entirely different life-style from ours, it may be tempting to invoke personal judgments. The patient may even engage in activities that are illegal or that we consider immoral. Although we have the right to choose not to socialize with such a person in our personal lives, we have no right as health professionals to be punitive or withhold appropriate treatment. As professionals we have the responsibility to provide, at the very least, humane care.

Putting aside personal values so that the highest quality of care can be provided for the patient is not always easy. Sometimes it helps a health team member if he is allowed to acknowledge that the patient is not exactly someone he would invite home to dinner.

Pain and Emotion: Reaction vs. Cause

Misconception: Pain is largely an emotional or psychological problem, especially in the patient who is highly anxious or depressed or who has an unclear physical cause for pain.

Correction: An emotional reaction to pain does not mean that pain is caused by an emotional problem. Pain will not simply disappear or necessarily be any less intense if the patient stops being anxious or depressed. Similarly, if a diagnosis of cancer causes the patient to become upset, this does not mean that cancer is mostly a psychological problem that can be treated with appropriate psychotherapy. Furthermore, inability to diagnose a physical cause for the pain does not mean that there is no physical cause for pain, a misconception further discussed below in relation to known physical causes of pain.

Pain almost always results in some degree of anxiety or depression. To experience pain without any emotional response would be abnormal. However, the relationship between pain and anxiety or depression is complicated and unclear. Although anxiety or depression is rarely the sole cause of pain, it certainly affects how the patient handles pain. For example, anxiety or depression probably makes pain more difficult to bear and adversely affects the patient's outlook and motivation or ability to be involved in his own pain control.

Intensity of pain, however, is *not* nearly as likely to be affected by anxiety or depression as is the patient's ability to handle pain. A study of cancer patients showed that depressed patients were not more likely to have more intense pain than those who were not depressed. The depression associated with cancer pain did not alter the patient's reports of the intensity of pain. However, depression did affect the patient's perception of life's quality (Cleeland, 1984; see also pp. 237-238 on the relationship between depression and chronic nonmalignant pain). Thus the intensity of pain is not likely to subside simply because anxiety and depression are alleviated.

Anxiety is usually associated with brief pain, whereas depression tends to accompany prolonged pain; an element of both is usually present with all pain. When anxiety or depression is caused by pain, the preferred treatment is to relieve the pain. In other words, if a patient is anxious because of severe pain, he should not be given a tranquilizer or sedative. Rather, every effort should be made to relieve his pain.

An appreciation of the fact that pain is not simply a psychological problem, but rather a physical problem accompanied by emotional responses, is especially important in understanding the difference between narcotic addiction and use of narcotics for pain relief (see discussion of addiction on pp. 67-71). Although it is usually clearly understood that a patient in the emergency room with bloody lacerations and multiple fractures needs narcotics to relieve pain and not to meet a psychological need, this distinction may be less obvious to the observer after the patient begins to heal. Weeks later when the patient still has musculoskeletal pain from nonunion fractures, the anxiety and depression accompanying this pain and the continued requests for narcotics to relieve the pain may be misunderstood as an example of using narcotics to meet psychological needs. The use of narcotics for psychological (or psychic) reasons rather than for an approved medical reason such as pain relief would fit the definition of narcotic addiction. Such a patient might erroneously be labeled a narcotic addict unless it is understood that pain is primarily a physical problem with psychological effects.

Malingering: Lies vs. Truth

Misconception: Lying about the existence of pain, malingering, is common.

Correction: Very few people who say they have pain are lying about it. Outright fabrication of pain is rare (Hendler, 1984; Leavitt and Sweet, 1986; Reesor and Craig,

1988). Malingering does exist, but it simply is not as likely as many of us believe.

Regarding pain, the malingerer may be defined as a person who says that pain is present when it is not, i.e., he fakes pain or pretends to have pain, usually to avoid or gain something. The malingerer does not feel pain but tries to make others believe that he does. It is a conscious lie because the malingerer by definition does not imagine pain and does not believe he has it. An example of malingering on a small scale is the person who does not want to accept a dinner invitation and uses the excuse of having a headache when in fact he does not have a headache.

The fear of being duped by the malingerer has bothered practitioners for years. Many attempts have been made to devise a test that would detect the malingerer, but none has been proved effective. Therefore we must accept the reality that believing the patient with pain could result in our believing someone who is deliberately lying to us about having pain. This vulnerability seems unavoidable. Although by believing a malingerer we may aid him to accomplish his goals, our professional responsibility is to treat patients with respect and believe them or give them the benefit of the doubt.

Great care must be taken to avoid inaccurate labeling of patients as malingerers. Patients with chronic nonmalignant pain are especially likely to be inaccurately diagnosed as malingerers (see p. 238). Patients may be labeled as malingerers simply because the cause of the pain is unknown or the patient fails to respond to treatment (i.e., patients with vague or unresponsive symptoms seem likely to be labeled malingerers).

Interestingly, documented cases of malingering usually involve patients with textbook symptoms. The patient may identify expected symptoms on the basis of the way he is physically assessed by the physician or he may actually go to the library and read about the condition. If the patient's intent is to fool the health team, it makes sense that he would try to do as good a job as possible.

Sometimes malingering is confused with psychogenic pain or secondary gain. However, malingering, secondary gain, and psychogenic pain are three separate conditions. Further, all of them except malingering involve feeling pain. Psychogenic pain may hurt as much as any type of pain of primarily physical origin. The patient with pain who receives secondary gain may also have a very painful condition.

Secondary Gain: Apparent Benefits of Pain vs. Intensity or Existence of Pain

Misconception: The patient who obtains benefits or preferential treatment because of pain is receiving secondary gain and does not hurt as much as he says he does or may not hurt at all.

Correction: The patient who uses his pain to his advantage is not the same as a malingerer and may still hurt as much as he says he does. Secondary gain may be an inaccurate conclusion, since what is secondary gain for one person is not for another.

Secondary gain is defined as any practical or emotional advantages that result from having the symptom of pain, especially financial compensation and preferential treatment at home or work, including special favors or attention from friends or family. By definition, the patient has pain and is not malingering, i.e., is not lying about the presence of pain. It may not always be easy to distinguish between malingering and secondary gain because the sensation of pain is totally subjective, and both malingering and secondary gain result in benefits to the patient. However, it is important to remember that malingering involves lying about the existence of pain and is relatively uncommon. By contrast, with secondary gain pain is assumed to be present, and secondary gain may be a fairly common component of the prolonged pain experience.

Secondary gain need not be negative. The term *secondary gain* usually has negative connotations of involving gains that could be more appropriately achieved by behaviors other than reporting pain. When this is true, secondary gain may be a disability (discussed below). Certain secondary gains, however, are appropriate, such as attention and assistance from others when pain limits activity or financial compensation for a work-related injury resulting from unsafe conditions.

In daily life, secondary gain from pain is not unusual. Just as a person may lie about having a headache to avoid accepting a dinner invitation, so may a person use an already existing headache to decline the dinner invitation. In both cases the person wants to avoid attending the dinner, but in one case the excuse is malingering (lying) and in the other case the excuse is based on fact.

Obviously, if pain is prolonged and if the patient begins to use pain as a means of handling many problems or inconveniences of daily life, secondary gain may become a disability. For example, if the patient has chronic low back pain, he may begin to use this to avoid a job or spouse he does not like. Rather than find a new job or go to work and find ways to make the job better, he may use the pain as an excuse to stay at home. When he has disagreements with his wife, he may use the pain as an excuse to avoid her by taking a nap or resting, rather than finding ways to resolve the conflict. Using pain to handle these significant problems disables the patient to the extent that he becomes increasingly isolated and less able to function in life.

Whenever the patient uses pain to deal with many problems, this may result in a disability that requires treatment. The question becomes how can problems of daily living be handled more constructively. Vocational counseling, family therapy, and assertiveness training may be helpful. Many structured pain management programs include these therapies, recognizing that it is not unusual for people with prolonged pain to be accused of or to actually use pain to their advantage.

However, it is extremely important to be sure that secondary gain has been accurately diagnosed. The question is not whether the patient has pain. The patient is given the benefit of the doubt. Even if the patient exaggerates his pain to obtain secondary gain, this still does not mean he has no pain at all. In fact, exaggeration of pain may not be for secondary gain but may reflect ineffective coping mechanisms or may be for the purpose of obtaining appropriate treatment for the pain. Exaggeration may be due to the failure of others to believe the patient when he tells the truth about his pain or due to the patient lacking effective coping styles and being overwhelmed by the pain (see further discussion, p. 237). Possible exaggeration may be prevented or minimized by ensuring that the existence of pain is acknowledged to the patient.

Accurate diagnosis of secondary gain involves not only recognizing that the presence of pain is not in question but also recognizing that certain behaviors are not always secondary gain. What is secondary gain for one person is not necessarily secondary gain for another. The patient's responses to pain may appear to be for secondary gain, but this may or may not be the case. For example, the patient may use pain as a reason to rest. Resting at work may enable him to avoid a task he does not like, such as doing inventory on supplies. Thus he may be using his pain for secondary gain. However, it is also possible that in spite of disliking doing the inventory, the patient does have pain and may benefit from pacing himself and resting at that time. If the latter is true, pain is not being used for secondary gain. In both instances the behavior of resting is the same and the disliked task is avoided, but in only one instance is the diagnosis of secondary gain appropriate.

It is often erroneously assumed that patients who are awaiting litigation after an injury or who are receiving worker's compensation are likely to prolong or exaggerate their pain to benefit from financial secondary gain. Numerous studies have failed to support this view (Dworkin et al, 1985; Melzack, Katz, and Jeans, 1985; see also p. 238). Financial gain from pain may in fact be appropriate financial compensation for an injury.

Accurate assessment of secondary gain is not necessarily simple. Useful assessment guidelines may include observing whether the patient *regularly* uses his pain to avoid activity that he would not want to engage in even if he did not have pain or to obtain benefits that he could not without the pain. If the patient does this regularly and often, secondary gain may be a disability in need of treatment. In discussing with the health team the possibility that the patient receives secondary gain from pain that might be more appropriately obtained in other ways, important points are:

- Secondary gain from pain is not the same as malin-

gering, nor does it mean that pain is psychogenic, i.e., caused solely by mental events.
- Pain with demonstrable physical cause, including severe pathology, may be used for secondary gains.
- What is secondary gain for one person is not for another. Accurate assessment of whether a behavior is for the purpose of secondary gain may be difficult.
- Secondary gain is not always inappropriate, e.g., financial gain or attention resulting from pain may be necessary or justifiable.
- The occasional use of pain to obtain certain advantages is not unusual and does not necessarily warrant any special treatment.
- Secondary gain from pain becomes a problem for which the patient requires assistance when it disables him, i.e., when the patient uses pain instead of a more constructive method of solving daily problems. The patient should then be approached with suggestions for alternatives to solving his specific problems of daily living, e.g., marital conflict or job placement. The patient should not be berated for using pain as a solution nor should he be accused of faking or exaggerating pain.

Cause of Pain: Known vs. Unknown Physical Cause

Misconception: All "real" pain has an identifiable physical cause.

Correction: All pain is real, regardless of its cause. Almost all pain has both physical and mental components. The absence of an identifiable physical cause of pain does not mean the pain is purely psychogenic.

It is easier to believe a patient's report of pain when he has a physical diagnosis that corresponds to what he says. We are mistakenly tempted to rely more on identifiable cellular pathology than the patient's statement of what he feels.

Because the sensation of pain is subjective, our thinking about a physical cause may inadvertently disintegrate into a fallacy. If this happens with the health team, it is helpful to state the problem, saying that it seems that we are thinking the following misconception: "If there is pain, there is a cause. If there is a cause, we can find it. If we can't find the cause, there is no pain and no pain relief is needed." Such thinking is based on the absurd assumption that our own assessment and the diagnostic tests we use are infallible.

In addition to stating the problem clearly, using an analogy (something similar to the situation but not as threatening) may also help promote more logical thinking. For example, you might say "If a patient came into the emergency room vomiting blood but our assessment revealed no cause for the vomiting and bleeding, would we then doubt that the patient was vomiting and bleeding and do nothing about it?" The point is that vomiting and bleeding, unlike the pain sensation, are objective and potentially life threatening, so we do not dare indulge in the omnipotent thinking expressed in relation to pain. We must remind ourselves and others that just as patients may bleed or vomit without our knowing why, so may they have pain without our being able to identify a cause. Our failure to identify the cause in no way justifies saying that the problem does not exist or does not deserve treatment. Once again, we find that the subjectivity of pain haunts us and that caring for patients with pain is indeed a humbling experience.

In the absence of a readily identifiable physical cause for pain, another interesting and unjustifiable type of thinking tends to occur. We may begin to speculate about whether the pain is imaginary, "all in his head," or psychogenic.

The matter becomes even more complicated if the patient is very anxious or depressed about his pain. In the absence of a diagnosed physical cause for pain, it may be reasoned that these emotions indicate a largely psychological cause of the pain. The patient then faces an almost insoluble problem. Anxiety and depression normally associated with pain become even more intense when the patient realizes that the physical cause cannot be found and that the staff is beginning to doubt his pain. The more upset the patient becomes, the more basis the staff seems to have for suspecting that his pain is psychological in origin. The vicious cycle continues with the patient becoming more anxious or depressed and the staff becoming more sure that the pain is psychogenic.

To have pain acknowledged and validated, particularly by the diagnosis of a physical cause, is extremely important to both staff and patient. Until this happens the staff may become confused and the patient may fear abandonment by the staff or fear that he is losing his sanity. To help both the patient and the health team understand the reality of this situation, it may help to examine the possible extremes.

The general causes of pain may be conceptualized on a continuum from pain that is totally psychogenic to pain that is totally physical. "Pure" psychogenic pain may be defined as a localized sensation of pain caused solely by mental events, with no physical findings to initiate or sustain the pain. Pure psychogenic pain is extremely rare. However, the term *psychogenic* is used loosely, and this leads to misunderstandings about its frequency.

For example, in the literature, tension headache is often referred to as psychogenic headache. Yet when a stressful situation is followed by a headache, it does not mean that the person's brain perceived the stressful environment and immediately converted it into a pain in the head. It is not pure psychogenic pain. Very soon after the stress is perceived, physical changes occur, usually in the form of contraction of the muscles in the neck and scalp, ischemia, accumulation of toxins, and further muscle contraction. Thus what may be called psychogenic headache is actually caused by both mental and physical events, not

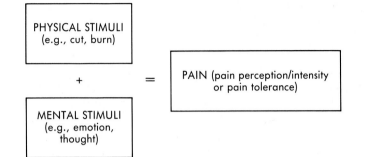

FIGURE 2-1 Most pain results from a combination of both physical and mental events. Rarely is pain purely psychogenic (mental) or purely physical in origin. Pain results from a total body response.

one or the other. In this instance, the intensity of pain, pain perception, is influenced by both physical and mental events.

By contrast, pure physical pain is a localized sensation of pain caused solely by physical events not accompanied by mental events. Again, this is extremely rare. It is unusual to have a cut or burn that hurts and to have no thoughts or feelings about it. The person is going to think something about the pain. The accompanying mental events may render the pain more bearable if the patient thinks that the pain will be relieved and he will recover. However, if the mental events involve the fear that no help will be available and that death is imminent, pain may be very difficult to tolerate. In this instance, pain tolerance, as opposed to pain intensity, is influenced by both physical and mental events.

The most successful approach to pain control is to assess and treat both the physical and mental causes. Most localized sensations of pain are a combination of *both* physical and mental events (Figure 2-1). No pain is imaginary, and calling pain imaginary certainly does not make it go away. The final word on imaginary versus real pain may well be a quote from a collection of letters to the *New England Journal of Medicine* (Moskow, 1987, p. 68): "Pain occurring in unicorns, griffins, and jabberwockies is always imaginary pain, since these are imaginary animals; patients on the other hand, are real, and so they always have real pain."

Pain Behavior: Acute Pain Model vs. Adaptation

Misconception: Visible signs, either physiological or behavioral, accompany pain and can be used to verify its existence and severity.

Correction: Even with severe pain, periods of physiological and behavioral adaptation occur, leading to periods of minimal pain or no signs of pain. Lack of pain expression does not necessarily mean lack of pain. How must the patient behave for us to believe he has pain?

In the acute pain model, certain signs of pain exist at

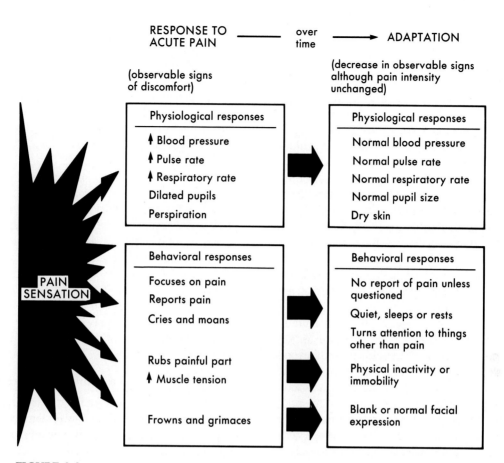

RESPONSE TO ACUTE PAIN ⎯⎯⎯ over time ⎯⎯→ ADAPTATION

(observable signs of discomfort)

(decrease in observable signs although pain intensity unchanged)

Physiological responses	Physiological responses
↑ Blood pressure	Normal blood pressure
↑ Pulse rate	Normal pulse rate
↑ Respiratory rate	Normal respiratory rate
Dilated pupils	Normal pupil size
Perspiration	Dry skin

PAIN SENSATION

Behavioral responses	Behavioral responses
Focuses on pain	No report of pain unless questioned
Reports pain	Quiet, sleeps or rests
Cries and moans	Turns attention to things other than pain
Rubs painful part	Physical inactivity or immobility
↑ Muscle tension	
Frowns and grimaces	Blank or normal facial expression

FIGURE 2-2 Acute pain model vs. adaptation.

Modified from Brunner, LS, and Suddarth, DS: Textbook of medical-surgical nursing, ed 6, Philadelphia, 1988, JB Lippincott.

the onset of sudden, severe pain. Physiologically the patient may have increased heart rate, perspiration, pallor, or increased blood pressure. Behaviorally, the patient may talk about the pain, cry, moan, tense his skeletal muscles, or rub the painful part. However, the acute pain model usually exists only briefly. Both physiological and behavioral adaptation occur, sometimes within seconds or minutes. In other words, the patient may continue to hurt just as badly, but behavioral and physiological signs of pain will cease to exist, at least for certain periods (Figure 2-2).

Physiologically, the body seeks equilibrium. Certain physiological responses could not be sustained without there finally being physical harm to the person. Thus these parameters usually return to near normal for periods. Occasionally, a patient may go into shock from severe pain, but most patients show physiological adaptation.

Behaviorally there is also adaptation. The pain may continue to be just as severe as it was at its onset, but if the pain remains that severe for days, the patient is not likely to continue to scream for the entire time. Patients minimize their controllable behavioral expressions of pain for a number of reasons, including the following:

- To be a "good patient." The patient may realize that the health team is more or less responsible for keep-

ing him quiet and that they do not like to hear him cry or make persistent requests for pain relief.
- To avoid being a "sissy," i.e., to maintain a favorable self-concept. If the patient values a stoic response to pain or notes that those around him do, he may be embarrassed to even talk about pain except to selected individuals and only at certain times. A sudden increase in pain may lead to a gasp or grimace, but the patient may strive to bring this under control quickly.
- Exhaustion. Pain is fatiguing. After the patient has been in pain for hours, or certainly for days, he becomes too tired to talk and cry about the pain and so tired that he falls asleep. Many health team members are taught to equate sleep with pain relief. While the sleeping patient may not have a conscious awareness of pain, he may have a dream-state awareness, and more importantly, he will be in pain when he awakens—unless there has been a miracle cure. Double-blind analgesic studies have been done since the 1950s, and in these studies when the patient in the hospital is evaluated for pain relief at hourly intervals, he is awakened because it is well known that even patients with severe pain may sleep. Or a patient with pain may close his eyes and remain very

still, appearing to be asleep, but actually may be only trying to make pain bearable by conserving energy or concentrating on something else. Many behaviors diminish as a result of sheer exhaustion.

- Distraction. The patient may laugh and joke with visitors, walk them to the elevator, and then walk to the nurse's station to request an analgesic. If distraction is not understood, this patient will be misunderstood. As discussed in Chapter 6, distraction is a potent method of making pain more bearable, but it does not make pain go away. While the patient made the effort to distract himself with his visitors, he probably became exhausted from this plus the ongoing pain. Now that the distraction has ceased, his pain is back in the center of his awareness, difficult to tolerate, and he is tired. The patient now needs another form of pain relief that allows him to rest, and hence he requests an analgesic.

For a variety of reasons, adaptation will occur, and the patient's behavioral and physiological response to pain will become minimal or cease to exist for periods, even if the pain is severe. Lack of response to pain does not necessarily mean a lack of pain. If we adhere to the acute pain model in assessing a patient with pain, at some point we are likely to think or say "He doesn't act like he's in pain." Whenever you think or say this or hear others say it, ask "How would this person have to act for us to believe he has pain?" This is not an easy question to answer honestly. One of the first things that most people acknowledge is that laughter is not appropriate. The patient who smiles when he asks for a narcotic is not very likely to be believed. It usually seems more appropriate if the patient frowns or becomes tearful. Decreased activity is also preferred. In home care the patient who goes to work usually finds this is held against him in the form of people saying "If he can go to work, it couldn't be that bad." In the hospital, the patient who walks the halls and visits other patients is not likely to be freely given a strong analgesic. The likelihood of receiving a narcotic injection is increased, however, if he goes to bed, curls up in the fetal position, and frowns.

It is apparent that we do not really wish to reinforce, encourage, or require the behaviors that are apt to convince us that the patient hurts. In fact, we actually want to encourage the behaviors that ordinarily make us doubt the patient. Requiring the patient to act as if he is in pain is embarrassing to patients, but many learn that they must alter their behavior to be believed and helped by the health team and their own families. If we require the patient to look or act like he is in pain, we may even help reinforce a disability. By doubting the patient's pain when he goes to work but believing him when he stays in bed, we inadvertently reinforce inactivity and lower the quality of life.

For many years it has been known in pain research that behavioral and physiological signs are unreliable indices of pain severity, and the patient's self-report of pain has been accepted as the most successful way to quantify pain (Houde, 1982). Unfortunately, in daily clinical practice we seem reluctant to follow this simple guideline.

Occasionally, behavioral management techniques, such as operant conditioning, are used to minimize the patient's expression of pain. However, this is not to be confused with pain relief and is done only in carefully selected patients who understand and consent to such an approach. For example, it may be clear that a patient focuses on his pain and discusses it to such an extent that others avoid him or that he is unable to focus attention on other ways of handling problems. In some pain management programs this is discussed with the patient, and the importance of focusing on other approaches to life's problems is explained. With the patient's understanding and cooperation, discussion of pain by the patient may be limited to a certain time of day or to one particular person, focusing the rest of the time on other solutions to problems.

Pain Perception: Predictability vs. Variability

Pain perception may be defined as the least experience of pain that a person can recognize. Simply, it is the point at which a given stimulus is felt as painful and the amount of pain felt beyond that point.

Misconception: Comparable physical stimuli produce comparable pain in different people. The severity and duration of pain can be predicted accurately for everyone on the basis of the stimuli for pain.

Correction: Comparable stimuli in different people do *not* produce the same intensities of pain. Comparable stimuli in different people produce different intensities and durations of pain. There is no direct and invariant relationship between any stimulus and the perception of pain.

It is tempting to believe that we can predict severity and duration of pain, probably because we like to know what to expect. However, such a belief will produce erroneous conclusions. Patients who experience more pain for longer periods may be erroneously judged as exaggerating. Any health team member with experience in caring for patients with certain painful procedures or diseases will be able to develop some fairly accurate conclusions about the range of intensity and duration of pain for most people exposed to a certain painful condition; however, this is merely a range of possibilities and there will always be exceptions.

Health team members tend to expect that postoperative pain following cholecystectomy, laminectomy, or thyroid lobectomy will be moderate to severe for 1 to 2 days and subside substantially or be resolved within 3 to 4 days. A study of 88 patients on a typical postsurgical unit revealed that in 31% of patients, pain persisted beyond the fourth day because of complications and that the patients received inadequate analgesia for this (Melzack et al, 1987).

The fact that pain intensity and duration vary, sometimes considerably, between individuals exposed to comparable painful conditions may be best appreciated by a review of current theories of the underlying mechanisms of pain. For example, the gate control theory (pp. 36-37) clearly indicates that a comparable stimulus in different people will be subject to a variety of different factors that influence whether that stimulus will reach awareness and be felt as painful. Pain may be decreased, or the gate partially closed to pain, so to speak, if there is stimulation over the large-diameter afferent fibers such as rubbing, inhibition from the brain stem due to sensory input from distraction, or inhibition from the cortex due to knowledge that the pain will end soon. In a person exposed to the same stimuli but without inhibition from these areas, the pain is much greater.

Similarly, the endorphins (see pp. 37-38) help explain why pain intensity and duration vary from one person to another. The endorphins are familiar to both lay persons and health team members and provide a fairly easily understood explanation of why people feel pain differently. For example, simply knowing that different people have different levels of natural narcotics in their bodies and that this level may be influenced by a variety of factors, such as duration of pain and stress, helps us realize that individuals having the same disease or surgical procedure are likely to feel different intensities of pain and require different amounts of narcotic for relief. Those with a high level of endorphin probably will feel less pain and need less narcotic than those with a low level.

Pain Tolerance: High vs. Low

Pain tolerance may be defined as the duration or intensity of pain that a person is *willing* to endure. A high pain tolerance means that pain must be very intense or last a long time before the person finds it intolerable or wants pain relief. A low pain tolerance means that mild or brief pain is intolerable to the person and results in a desire for relief.

Misconception: People with pain should be taught to have a high tolerance for pain. The more prolonged the pain or the more experience a person has with pain, the better his tolerance for pain.

Correction: Pain tolerance is the individual's unique response, varying between patients and varying in the individual patient from one situation to another. People with prolonged or recurrent pain tend to have an increasingly low pain tolerance. The patient's tolerance for pain is not a matter to be judged as right or wrong by the health team. Respect for the patient's pain tolerance is crucial for adequate pain control.

Pain tolerance may be stable for the individual, but there seem to be great variations between individuals. However, pain tolerance may vary considerably within the individual. Under certain circumstances a person's pain tolerance may increase or decrease. For example, if an analgesic makes the patient drowsy, then he may tolerate pain during visiting hours so he can be alert to converse with his family, but he may not be willing to tolerate the same degree of pain at bedtime or during meals.

Pain tolerance may also be affected by the patient's own goals or by what he thinks others value. For example, during childbirth the mother may tolerate what she rates as severe pain without any anesthesia or analgesia either because she wants to be alert for the delivery and spare her unborn baby any possible ill effects of medications or because she believes that her husband would be ashamed of her if she requested analgesia.

Pain tolerance is probably also influenced by the specific combination of pain intensity and duration for the particular situation. The patient may tolerate mild pain for a long time but tolerate severe pain for only a brief time.

Prolonged or recurrent experience with pain tends to lower pain tolerance because pain tends to be inadequately controlled. If the patient with prolonged pain had repeated experiences with having the pain quickly and adequately controlled, the patient might be confident about pain management and be able to learn to use noninvasive or self-management pain relief methods. However, the patient who goes to the emergency room with recurrent migraine headaches or is hospitalized for recurrent sickle cell crises or exacerbations of low back pain is likely to learn two things that decrease pain tolerance: (1) how severe the pain may be, and (2) how difficult it is to get pain relief. With many memories such as these, the patient with prolonged or recurrent pain faces each period of pain with increasing fear and depression and fewer resources with which to bear the pain.

Pain tolerance is an important aspect of adequate pain control. Patients are often asked to rate their pain on a scale such as 0 to 10, discussed in this chapter in the section on assessment tools (pp. 22-23). The patient is also asked to identify the rating that represents an acceptable level of pain. This is a significant index to the patient's pain tolerance, i.e., the severity of pain he is willing to endure. In titrating analgesics or identifying the effectiveness of other pain relief measures, the patient's tolerance for pain is extremely important. Although we would like to reduce pain to zero at all times, this is not always possible. By identifying the level of pain relief that is satisfactory to the patient, it may be possible to identify a more realistic immediate goal.

The following are distinct entities in the individual patient but are often very difficult to assess separately:
- Pain intensity (perception).
- Pain tolerance.
- Pain expression.

Whenever possible, the nurse distinguishes between these, remembering that pain tolerance is probably more relevant to establishing pain control than either the intensity of pain or the manner in which the patient expresses pain. For example, two patients may rate their pain at 4 on a scale of 0 to 10. Both may be lying in bed watching television. These data cover pain intensity and pain expression but do not tell us if that level of pain is tolerable to either patient. Therefore we do not know if further pain relief is needed. Obviously one patient may find pain of 4 easily tolerated, but the other patient may find it unbearable. Further, although we do not know if the rating of 4 in both patients means equal pain, this does not matter, since our intention is not to compare one patient with another, nor is it our purpose to judge whether the patient should tolerate the pain.

In many cultures a value judgment is placed on pain tolerance. Often a high pain tolerance is admired. Men are usually expected to tolerate more pain than women and adults to tolerate more pain than children. Although each of us is entitled to our personal value regarding pain tolerance in ourselves and others, as a health professional we have no right to impose that value judgment on the patient. Inadvertently imposing our personal values or cultural beliefs may lead to erroneous conclusions, such as believing that men who report pain need relief more desperately than do women who report pain.

Placebos: Faked or Imagined Pain vs. Real Pain

A placebo may be defined as any medical treatment (medication or procedure, including surgery) or nursing care that produces an effect in a patient because of its implicit or explicit intent and not because of its specific nature or therapeutic properties (physical or chemical properties). When a patient responds to a placebo in accordance with its intent he is said to be a placebo reactor for that occasion. His response is called a positive placebo response.

Misconception: When the patient reports relief following a placebo, this means that the patient is a malingerer or the pain is "all in his head."

Correction: There is no evidence in the literature to justify using a placebo to determine the presence or absence of pain or to determine whether pain is physical or psychogenic in origin; in fact, to do so raises serious ethical and legal questions. The only accurate conclusion about a person who reacts positively to a placebo is that he very much wants pain relief and that he trusts something or someone to help him obtain it (Goodwin et al, 1979; McCaffery, 1979).

Using a placebo in this inappropriate way usually requires the nurse to lie to the patient about what medication he is getting. This deception may destroy the patient's trust in the health care team and ultimately the hospital. The question of damage to the nurse-patient relationship is important to consider, because although the physician

TABLE 2-1 Myths about Placebos

Are the Following Statements True or False?	Answer
1. When a person reports pain relief from a placebo, it may be concluded that:	
a. He is a malingerer.	False
b. There is no physical reason for his pain.	False
c. He is easily duped or is neurotic.	False
2. Placebos are capable of relieving severe pain caused by obvious physical stimuli.	True
3. Patients who benefit from placebos may be intelligent, educated, and mentally healthy.	True

may prescribe a placebo, it is the nurse who gives it and often must answer the patient's questions about it. Each nurse must decide for herself how she will react if she is asked to administer a placebo under these circumstances.

However, placebos are appropriate and important in research situations. In these instances, the patient is told about and gives his informed consent to the use of a placebo.

Suggestions for dealing with a prescription for a placebo may include the following strategies:

- Discuss with the physician his reason for using a placebo.
- Use research to reinforce the point that using a placebo to diagnose pain is inappropriate.

     Fact: A minimum of a third of all people with obvious physical stimuli for pain (e.g., abdominal surgery, cancer pain) report adequate relief from a placebo (Lasagna et al, 1954; Goodwin et al, 1979).

     Fact: Although the mechanism underlying placebo analgesia is not well understood, it does have a physiological basis, possibly involving an increase in endorphins (Grevert et al, 1983; Levine et al, 1978).

- Point out that the patient receives a printout of drugs received during hospitalization. He may discover that he has been deceived. He may discuss his distrust of the health care team with his friends and recommend that they avoid the physician involved and the hospital. Presently, as hospitals are competitively marketing their services and trying to build community support, potential loss of business may be your strongest argument.
- Suggest other strategies to better control the patient's pain. For example, implement a flow sheet or daily diary (see pp. 27 and 30) to plan for changes or alternatives.
- If the physician continues to insist that a placebo be given, you have the right to refuse to give it. Let your supervisor know about your action so that you will have administrative support.

Table 2-1 summarizes some of the myths about placebos. How many of these statements can you answer

TABLE 2-2 Misconceptions about Assessment of Patients Who Indicate They Have Pain

Misconception	Correction
1. The health team is the authority about the existence and nature of the patient's pain sensation.	The person with pain is the only authority about the existence and nature of that pain, since the sensation of pain can be felt only by the person who has it.
2. Our personal values and intuition about the trustworthiness of others is a valuable tool in identifying whether a person is lying about pain.	Personal values and intuition do not constitute a professional approach to the patient with pain. The patient's credibility is not on trial.
3. Pain is largely an emotional or psychological problem, especially in the patient who is highly anxious or depressed.	Having an emotional reaction to pain does not mean that pain is caused by an emotional problem. If anxiety or depression is alleviated, the intensity of pain will not necessarily be any less.
4. Lying about the existence of pain, malingering, is common.	Very few people who say they have pain are lying about it. Outright fabrication of pain is considered rare.
5. The patient who obtains benefits or preferential treatment because of pain is receiving secondary gain and does not hurt as much as he says or may not hurt at all.	The patient who uses his pain to his advantage is not the same as a malingerer and may still hurt as much as he says he does. Also, secondary gain may be an inaccurate diagnosis.
6. All real pain has an identifiable physical cause.	All pain is real, regardless of its cause. Almost all pain has both physical and mental components. Pure psychogenic pain is rare.
7. Visible signs, either physiological or behavioral, accompany pain and can be used to verify its existence and severity.	Even with severe pain, periods of physiological and behavioral adaptation occur, leading to periods of minimal or no signs of pain. Lack of pain expression does not necessarily mean lack of pain. How must the patient act for us to believe he has pain?
8. Comparable physical stimuli produce comparable pain in different people. The severity and duration of pain can be predicted accurately for everyone on the basis of the stimuli for pain.	Comparable stimuli in different people do *not* produce the same intensities of pain. Comparable stimuli in different people will produce different intensities of pain that last different periods. There is no direct and invariant relationship between any stimulus and the perception of pain.
9. People with pain should be taught to have a high tolerance for pain. The more prolonged the pain or the more experience a person has with pain, the better is his tolerance for pain.	Pain tolerance is the individual's unique response, varying between patients and varying in the same patient from one situation to another. People with prolonged pain tend to have an increasingly low pain tolerance. Respect for the patient's pain tolerance is crucial for adequate pain control.
10. When the patient reports pain relief following a placebo, this means that the patient is a malingerer or that the pain is psychogenic.	There is not a shred of evidence anywhere in the literature to justify using a placebo to diagnose malingering or psychogenic pain.

correctly? Take responsibility for correcting these myths among the health team members in your clinical setting. Table 2-2 summarizes the misconceptions about assessment of patients who indicate that they have pain.

PATIENTS WITH PAIN WHO DENY PAIN OR REFUSE PAIN RELIEF

People who hurt may have a variety of reasons for denying pain or refusing analgesics. Strong indications that such a patient might indeed have pain include patient behaviors such as frowning or rigid posture, pathology such as tumor encroachment on a nerve, or knowledge about the stimuli involved such as the discomfort usually reported from a procedure. This possibility should be explored with the patient. Usually the nurse or another health team member must initiate conversation with the patient about this, since the patient, for whatever reason is avoiding discussion.

The definition of pain that we propose, "Pain is what-

ever the experiencing person says it is, existing whenever the experiencing person says it does," (McCaffery, 1968, p. 95) is appropriate for patients who *indicate* that they have pain. When a patient denies pain despite other indications, it is important not to take the patient's word for it without exploring the reasons for his denial.

Following are examples of frequent reasons that patients may deny or refuse analgesics. In each case, the nurse must introduce the subject and explore reasons along with possible solutions to the problems that are causing the patient to deny pain or refuse analgesics.

Communication/Language Problems

Some patients may not ordinarily use the word *pain;* therefore they may deny pain when asked about it. To avoid misinterpretation of terms, use other words such as *hurt, discomfort, aches, soreness,* or *pressure.*

Language barriers in patients who do not speak English, who are retarded, or who are too young to verbalize may also result in denial of pain or analgesics. For example, one mentally retarded adult used the word "headache" for all pain. The nurse took this description literally and failed to realize that the patient had abdominal pain.

Fears Related to Analgesics

Some patients may be so afraid of analgesics, especially narcotics, that they refuse pain medications. Patients have the right to choose to feel pain or refuse analgesia; however, it is important that this decision is based on accurate information and not on unfounded fears and misconceptions.

Following are possible reasons and some suggested solutions for patients who refuse pain medication (each of these is discussed in more detail in Chapter 4). The patient may not readily articulate these concerns, in which case the nurse may need to initiate a discussion about the issues presented below. A helpful question to begin the discussion is "How do you feel about taking medications for relief of your pain/discomfort?"

- Fear of addiction. Stress to the patient that addiction does not happen when people take narcotics to relieve pain. Ask the patient "Would you want to take medication if you were not in pain?" If the patient answers no, then you may assure him that addiction is very unlikely.

  For the patient with prolonged pain, it is important to define addiction, distinguishing the psychological dependence from the physiological problems that might occur (see Chapter 4, pp. 67-72).
- Fear that taking pain medication now will result in it not working later on. This is a very common fear in patients who have prolonged pain, such as those with cancer. Explain that tolerance to analgesia can be handled. It is appropriate to take whatever the patient needs now to control pain. Later, if needed, the dose can be increased safely and effectively.
- Fear of sedation. If sedation does occur, it often stops after several days of the same dose of medication. If, however, it continues, dose adjustments or stimulants such as caffeine may be tried.
- Fear of loss of control and/or "strange feelings." Try to identify and address specific fears. Explain that narcotics are not a "truth serum," which result in the patient doing or saying things against his will. If the patient experiences any feelings that he does not like, he may be switched to a different narcotic. Stress that the patient's response to medication is continuously monitored and that he is never started on medication and then expected to just "put up with" whatever happens.
- Fear of shots. Injections scare many people, and some would rather put up with the pain than receive a shot. Explore the possibility of using other routes of administration, e.g., PO, SL, IV infusion, or rectal suppositories. Many times the IM route is prescribed because it is what the physician is most comfortable with, when in fact the patient could easily tolerate an alternate route.

  If there is no choice but to administer an injection, ice to the site immediately before injecting the medication may reduce discomfort. Avoid meperidine (Demerol) and hydroxyzine (Vistaril) given together in an injection. Meperidine can be irritating to the tissue, and hydroxyzine may cause extreme pain at the injection site.

Inadvertent Denial

Some patients may state that they feel fine in the presence of the health care team, especially the physician. They do not want to take up the physician's time or divert him from other more important symptoms. The patient often feels better when the physician is present. In fact visitors of any sort may improve the patient's mood. He does not mean to deny pain, but because a visit may be distracting and reassuring for the patient, when asked at that time he may state that he feels fine.

It may be helpful to describe the patient's behavior before and after the appointment with the physician. The physician may then talk with the patient about inconsistencies between his statements and his behavior and encourage him not to hesitate to share reports of pain.

Some patients are simply *not able to isolate pain as part of their total discomfort.* This is especially true in the person who is chronically debilitated with prolonged pain that has gradually increased. For example, an older person may experience joint pain and stiffness which have slowly increased over many years. The patient may have many additional physical and emotional miseries such as constipation, nausea, grief, and fear. It may be difficult to sort out that part of these miseries is physical pain. The nurse may be instrumental in assessing this by asking the patient about inconsistencies between his behavior and his denial of discomfort. Ask the patient if he would agree to a trial dose of analgesics for 24 hours to see if he notices any improvement in his general comfort. Stress that these medications can always be stopped, but that they may make a tremendous difference if part of the patient's general discomfort is pain.

In some patients, the desire to recover or live longer is so strong that they may deny any negative symptom, such as pain. Some may deny to themselves that they have pain. They may try to convince themselves that they are really doing much better. The nurse may encourage a fighting spirit, but she may also address the fact that comfort is an appropriate goal to work toward so that the patient will have the energy to continue to fight. Careful discussion and probing is important; other members of the health care team, such as a chaplain or psychologist, may be consulted.

Deliberate Cover-up

A patient may desire to please the physician or nurse. Because they have tried to help him, he wants to express his gratitude by fulfilling a "good patient" role. Express your desire to know the truth. Discuss with the patient that you, he, and other health team members are working together as a team to control his pain, but you depend on him to give you accurate information about the effects of a treatment. Assure him that you will not abandon him.

Some patients deliberately deny pain because they do not want to look like "a sissy." These may be people who are uncomfortable with saying "I hurt, please help me." Discuss what part of this acknowledgment bothers the patient. Reassure him that pain is appropriate for whatever condition he has or procedure he has undergone. Emphasize that the use of analgesics and other measures will help to increase function and/or speed recovery. Administer analgesics on a regular schedule or routinely offer them to the patient.

Some patients fear that the consequences of admitting pain may lead to diagnostic procedures, prolonged hospitalizations, and additional expenses. It is important to discuss the risks involved and options available.

A patient may say different things about his pain to different people: *do not assume manipulation.* In some instances, the patient may be trying to protect his family. He may only admit pain to certain members of the health care team because he trusts them or knows them better. In an attempt to avoid being a sissy, he may try not to talk with everyone about his pain.

In other cases, the family may report pain, while the patient denies it. The patient may be in awe of the health care team. The family may feel helpless. Discussion with the family and patient may be helpful.

In summary, after exploration of the possible reasons for denial of pain, we may find that, in fact, the patient does not hurt. However, if the patient does have pain, he still has a right to choose to hurt. Hopefully, this decision will be based on accurate information and not on myths and misconceptions.

MAJOR TYPES OF PAIN: CLASSIFICATION AND TREATMENT APPROACHES

Pain specialists usually classify pain in two major categories—acute and chronic. Some type of classification system for various types of pain is helpful in the assessment of the patient with pain, since it provides a framework for understanding the major differences in patients' pain experiences and for identifying differences in approaches to pain relief recommended by pain specialists.

Classification of Types of Pain

Several classification systems for types of pain exist, and each tends to reflect a philosophy or concept of treatment approaches (e.g., Classification of Chronic Pain,

1986; Crue, 1985). The classification system that we use is a simplified adaptation of several others. There are two major categories of pain.

1. Acute Pain

The critical, distinguishing characteristics of acute pain are that:
- It subsides as healing takes place, i.e., it has a predictable end.
- It is of brief duration, at least less than 6 months.

In most clinical areas the terminology *acute pain* means sudden, severe pain. In any discussion of pain as a speciality, it is important to remember that this customary definition does not apply. In fact, in the language of the pain specialist and throughout this text, acute pain not only has the above characteristics but also may be either sudden or slow in onset and may be of any intensity, ranging from mild to severe. Acute pain may include anything from a simple pin prick to a traumatic amputation of a limb. Other examples include a fractured bone, streptococcal throat infection, and postoperative pain.

2. Chronic Pain

Chronic pain is prolonged, usually 6 months or longer, but there is disagreement about how long pain should exist before being called chronic. It is clear that several distinctly different types of chronic pain exist, but there is controversy over exactly how they should be defined and classified. Following is one way to distinguish between different types of prolonged pain:

a. Recurrent acute pain with potential for recurrence over a lifetime or a prolonged period, e.g., migraine headaches and sickle cell crises. These are self-contained episodes of pain that can be predicted to end. However, they tend to recur. In some people the recurrence may be frequent, e.g., a migraine once a week. In between episodes, the patient is virtually pain free.

b. Ongoing time-limited pain, or chronic acute. This pain has the potential for lasting months, perhaps years, but has a high probability of ending. This type of pain occurs almost daily over a long period. Examples of this may include cancer or burn pain. This pain may last for many months before the condition is cured or controlled and pain subsides, or the pain may end only with the death of the patient.

c. Chronic nonmalignant pain, sometimes referred to as chronic "benign" pain (discussed in Chapter 9). When the patient is severely disabled by the pain, it may be called chronic intractable benign pain syndrome. This type of pain usually occurs almost daily and has existed for 6 months or longer. Intensity may range from mild to very severe. Critical, distinguishing characteristics of this type of pain are that it:
- Is due to non–life-threatening causes.
- Is not responsive to currently available methods of pain relief.

• May continue for the remainder of the patient's life.

Examples include a wide variety of very different pain problems such as rheumatoid arthritis, peripheral neuropathy, phantom limb pain, diffuse myofascial pain, vascular diseases of the limbs such as Raynaud's disease, ankylosing spondylitis, and low back pain from various causes.

Treatment Approaches Recommended by Pain Specialists

Following is a brief review of treatment approaches recommended by those who specialize in pain control. Considerable controversy exists among pain specialists regarding certain forms of treatment and the type of treatment appropriate for specific painful conditions. Therefore this overview is a general guideline to the differences in pain control for the different categories of pain problems.

Perhaps the most important characteristic of pain that tends to determine recommended approaches to pain relief is whether an end to the pain can be predicted. If pain has a fairly predictable end, either by control of the cause or by death, a more aggressive approach to pain control is used than if the pain has no predictable end. Thus in the relief of postoperative pain, recurrent acute pain of sickle cell crises, chronic cancer pain, and the pain of any terminal illness, many pain specialists recommend an aggressive approach that includes liberal use of narcotics. When narcotics are used, an appropriate dose and interval is strongly encouraged. Thus the patient should receive as much narcotic as often as needed to relieve the pain.

When the pain has no predictable end and is not life threatening, a more conservative approach is advised. Traditionally narcotics have been avoided, although recently there have been reports of the successful use of oral narcotics daily in selected patients. Certainly surgical procedures for pain relief are avoided unless the procedure is clearly indicated. Until recently, far too many patients had the unfortunate experience of having multiple laminectomies for the purpose of relieving low back pain, only to find that pain was much worse after these procedures.

One current concept of the treatment of pain distinguishes between a centralist and peripheralist view of chronic pain (Crue, 1985). The centralist view suggests that the mechanism for certain chronic pain conditions is in the central nervous system, not in the periphery as the peripheralist would believe. The centralist view maintains that there is no longer any stimulus for pain originating at the site of pain, and therefore treatment should not be aimed at the periphery. Nerve blocks, for example, would be inappropriate. This view does, however, recognize the peripheral input of chronic pain in certain conditions such as cancer, in which a nerve block might well be helpful. The merit of the centralist view is that some types of pain, such as phantom limb pain and other neuralgias, respond well to drugs that act centrally, such as the anticonvulsants.

ASSESSMENT TOOLS

In the assessment process, the nurse gathers information from the patient that allows her to understand his experience and its effect on his life. The information obtained guides the nurse in planning and evaluating strategies for care. Pain is rarely static; therefore its assessment is not a one-time process but is ongoing.

The assessment of pain is a beginning step in understanding and working toward the patient's goals. Unfortunately, this crucial step may be neglected. In a study of 353 hospitalized medical-surgical patients who experienced pain, fewer than half of the patients recalled a health team member asking them about their pain (Donovan et al, 1987).

There are numerous methods of assessing pain. The McGill Pain Questionnaire is one well-known method; however, it is complex, time-consuming, and appropriate for research situations, not general clinical use (Melzack, 1975). More recently, a short form of the McGill questionnaire was developed for use in research when time with patients is limited (Melzack, 1987). Several articles review other tools commonly used (Chapman et al, 1985; Karoly, 1985; McGuire, 1984; Syrjala and Chapman, 1984).

The purpose of this section is to present two tools that are *practical* in any clinical setting and *easily adapted* to an individual patient's needs: (1) initial pain assessment tool and (2) pain flow sheet.

Initial Pain Assessment Tool

Ten sections comprise this tool (Figure 2-3, copyright McCaffery, 1982b; also appeared in Meinhart and McCaffery, 1983), which provides initial information from which a plan of care may be developed. The authors encourage the reader to copy the tool directly from p. 21 and to adapt it according to the forms already used in your clinical setting. All information is obtained directly from the patient whenever possible; no one else really knows the location, intensity, and other characteristics of the pain. If anyone other than the patient provides information, it should be noted, e.g., wife states patient is restless when he sleeps. Each of the ten sections is discussed in detail below.

I. Location

Using the front, back, and side view figures, the patient is asked to place a mark where the pain is. If there is more than one site of pain, use letters, e.g., A, B, C, to distinguish the different sites. If the patient is unwilling or unable to mark the figures on the tool, ask him to trace or point to the areas on his body that hurt, and then you or a family member can mark the figure for him.

INITIAL PAIN ASSESSMENT TOOL

Date_____

Patient's Name_____ Age_____ Room_____

Diagnosis_____ Physician_____

Nurse_____

I. LOCATION: Patient or nurse mark drawing.

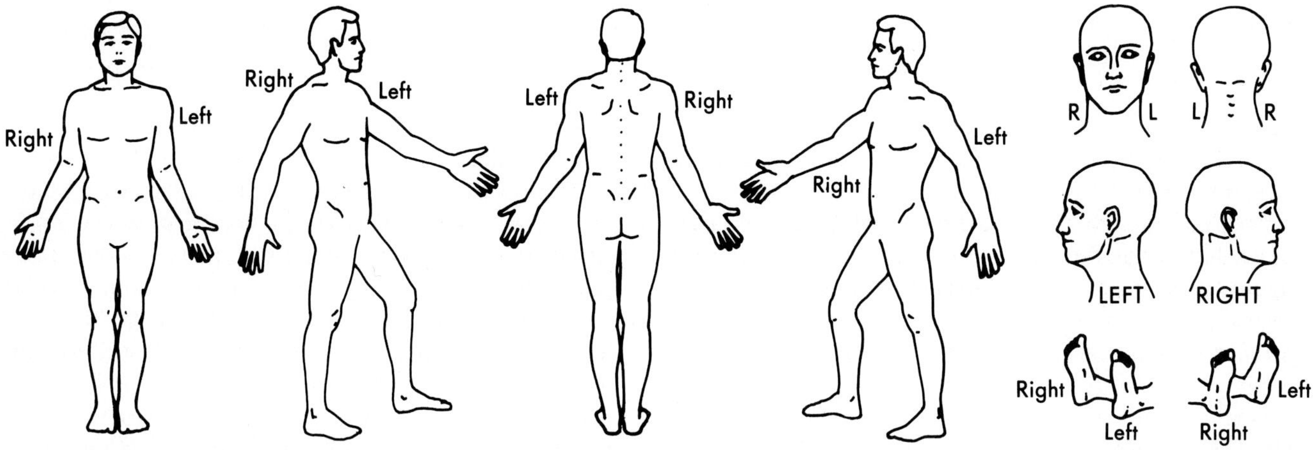

II. INTENSITY: Patient rates the pain. Scale used _____

  Present:_____
  Worst pain gets:_____
  Best pain gets:_____
  Acceptable level of pain:_____

III. QUALITY: (Use patient's own words, e.g. prick, ache, burn, throb, pull, sharp)_____
_____

IV. ONSET, DURATION VARIATIONS, RHYTHMS:_____

V. MANNER OF EXPRESSING PAIN:_____
_____

VI. WHAT RELIEVES THE PAIN?_____
_____

VII. WHAT CAUSES OR INCREASES THE PAIN?_____
_____

VIII. EFFECTS OF PAIN: (Note decreased function, decreased quality of life.)
  Accompanying symptoms (e.g. nausea)_____
  Sleep_____
  Appetite_____
  Physical activity_____
  Relationship with others (e.g. irritability)_____
  Emotions (e.g. anger, suicidal, crying)_____
  Concentration_____
  Other_____

IX. OTHER COMMENTS:_____
_____

X. PLAN:_____
_____

■ May be duplicated for use in clinical practice. From McCaffery, M, and Beebe, A: PAIN: CLINICAL MANUAL FOR NURSING PRACTICE, St. Louis, 1989, The C.V. Mosby Company.

FIGURE 2-3 Initial pain assessment tool.

KEY POINT: When asking a patient about the location of pain, do not rely solely on a verbal description of the location. Ask the patient to point to or trace with two fingers the area of pain. Verbal descriptions of pain location can be confusing and nonspecific.

II. Intensity

Naturally the person experiencing the pain is the only one who knows its intensity. In this step of the assessment process, the goal is to translate the patient's description of intensity into numbers or words that provide as objective a description as possible for a subjective experience.

Various numerical scales may be used and include 0 to 5, 0 to 10, or 0 to 100, where 0 equals no pain, and the largest number equals the worst pain. The patient is asked "What number would you give your pain right now?" Additional questions include "What number on a 0 to 10 scale would you give your pain when it is the worst that it gets and when it is the best that it gets?" "At what number is the pain at an acceptable level for you?" This last question is particularly important because it acknowledges each person's individuality in tolerating pain. On a 0 to 10 scale, 3 may be an acceptable level of pain control for some people but unacceptable for others. The number that is acceptable to the patient then becomes the goal that you both work toward initially, perhaps hoping to do better eventually. The goal is to relieve as much pain as possible. A pain rating of 0 twenty-four hours a day is the ideal but not always realistic.

Advantages to using a numerical scale to describe pain intensity include:
- Consistency in interpretation and communication of pain rating. Verbal or written statements of a patient's exact numerical pain rating, e.g., 8 on a 0 to 10 scale, are likely to be more consistently reported among health team members than a word description, e.g., "a lot of pain."
- Clearer understanding of the patient's experience. A patient who states his pain is 100 when asked what number he would give it on a 0 to 10 scale clearly communicates it's severity and helps us understand far better than with a descriptive phrase such as "the pain is very bad."
- Method of evaluating the effectiveness of an intervention. Using a numerical rating scale clearly documents the effectiveness of interventions, e.g., pain reduced from 7 to 3 when a relaxation technique is used in addition to pain medication. On the other hand, if a patient's pain is the most severe at 9, and the least severe it gets is 7 two hours after PO pain medication, it is quickly evident that more effective interventions need to be explored with the patient.

When asked to use a numerical scale to rate their pain, some patients may ask "What is the right answer?" It is important to stress that there is no "right or wrong" answer, that the patient is the one experiencing pain,

therefore he is the only one who knows what that number should be.

Some patients are unable to use a numerical scale to rate their pain; the numbers do not make sense to them, or it is too hard for them to apply numbers to their experience. In this case, the following choice of descriptive words may be helpful for the patient to use:
- No pain.
- A little pain.
- A lot of pain.
- Too much pain.

These four phrases may then be converted to a 0 to 3 scale for documentation and communication among health team members: 0 equals no pain, 1 equals a little pain, 2 equals a lot of pain, and 3 equals too much pain.

A visual analog scale is considered to be the more sensitive and reliable method of measuring pain intensity (Chapman et al, 1985; Syrjala and Chapman, 1984; Wallenstein et al, 1980). However, it has been our experience that progression is not as easily understood horizontally as it is vertically. A vertical progression, i.e., from bottom to top, may be a more familiar concept to patients and therefore easier to apply to pain intensity. For example, a temperature on a thermometer increases from bottom to top, and a container fills with fluid from bottom to top. If a patient has trouble verbalizing a numerical scale, Figure 2-4 may be shown to help the patient understand the concept. If necessary the patient can mark his rating directly on the scale.

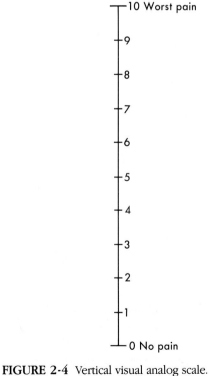

FIGURE 2-4 Vertical visual analog scale.
■ May be duplicated for use in clinical practice. From McCaffery, M, and Beebe, A: PAIN: CLINICAL MANUAL FOR NURSING PRACTICE, St. Louis, 1989, The CV Mosby Company.

KEY POINT: *Which* scale or phrase used to rate pain intensity is not as important as applying the following guidelines:

- Use what makes sense to the patient.
- Use the same scale every time with the same patient.
- Specify the parameters of whatever scale is used each time it is used so that the meaning of the pain rating is clear. For example, a rating of 5 is meaningless unless it is followed by a statement of the scale used, e.g., 5 on a scale of 0 to 10 (0 = no pain, 10 = worst pain) or 5 on a scale of 0 to 5 (0 = no pain, 5 = worst pain).

How do you get health team members to use a pain rating scale? If you are just beginning to implement a pain rating scale in your clinical setting, one of the best ways is to be a role model. Use the scale whenever you communicate verbally or on paper with physicians, other nurses, or other health team members. The specific, concise, and consistent data gained from a scale will be one of its selling points.

III. Quality

Ask the patient to describe his pain. This may be very difficult to do. Questions such as "What words would you use to describe your pain?" or "What would you do to me to have me feel the pain that you have?" may help the patient if he states that the pain is indescribable.

If the patient still has trouble describing his pain, the 15 descriptors used in the short-form McGill Pain Questionnaire may be helpful (Melzack, 1987):

- Throbbing.
- Shooting.
- Stabbing.
- Sharp.
- Cramping.
- Gnawing.
- Hot-burning.
- Aching.
- Heavy.
- Tender.
- Splitting.
- Tiring-exhausting.
- Sickening.
- Fearful.
- Punishing-cruel.

Descriptions of the pain may be helpful in determining its origin and implementing effective measures for its control. For instance, burning, shocklike pain may indicate injury to the nerve tissue. This type of pain often does not respond to narcotic analgesics (see Chapter 4, p. 119).

IV. Onset, Duration, Variations, and Rhythms

Assessment of this section might include such questions as "How long have you had this pain?" "Has its intensity or quality changed since you first noticed it?" "Is there any event or activity that changes the nature of the pain, for example, movement, being involved in a hobby, or visiting with family?" "Is the pain better or worse at certain times or certain hours during the day or night?"

V. Manner of Expressing Pain

Learning the patient's expression of pain is particularly important if the patient cannot communicate, is very young, or is unable to hear. Family members who know the patient's expression of pain will be able to tell you what clues they look for, e.g., a facial expression or body posture. In patients who cannot verbally communicate, these indications may be all we have to assess pain and evaluate interventions. However, for the patient who can communicate, facial expressions or body posture should be used only as clues to the presence of pain, not as sole indicators. Ask the patient and trust what he tells you. However, remember some patients hesitate to admit pain.

VI. What Relieves the Pain?

If a patient is hospitalized, there may be specific pain-relieving methods that he used successfully at home. He may assume that these are not possible to continue upon admission. Discussing these methods may result in their being easily incorporated into his plan of care. For instance, listening to music to enhance the effects of a bedtime analgesic can easily be included, even when sharing a hospital room, by using a headset on a portable tape player.

VII. What Causes or Increases the Pain?

Knowledge of the things that make pain worse allows planning care so that these increases in pain are avoided. For instance, if lying on the hard table for radiation treatments increases the pain, a patient may plan to take an extra dose of analgesic before leaving home so that it has taken effect by the time he arrives for his treatment.

VIII. Effects of Pain

Asking the patient what effect his pain has on each of the areas listed indicates the extent that it is interfering with his daily life. Answers to these questions also indicate any need to control other symptoms. It is helpful to be specific when asking questions about the effects of pain. For example, "Is physical activity limited because of pain?, If so, how?" "Does pain interfere with sleep?" "How does it interfere?" "Is getting to sleep at night a problem?" "How many consecutive hours do you sleep?" "Do you awaken throughout the night because of pain?"

IX. Other Comments

It may be helpful to ask the patient "Is there anything else that you can tell me that may help us work with you to get the best possible control of your pain?"

X. Plan

This communicates the initial plan for pain control. Examples of using an initial pain assessment tool are shown in Figures 2-5 and 2-6.

INITIAL PAIN ASSESSMENT TOOL FOR MR. T. Date _4/10/87_

Patient's Name _Mr. T._   Age _45_ Room _Surgical unit_

Diagnosis _Spleenectomy_   _12 hrs. post-op_ Physician _____
Pin insert for fractured (L) femur
Nurse _____

I. LOCATION: Patient or nurse mark drawing. A= Spleenectomy pain   B= Fractured femur

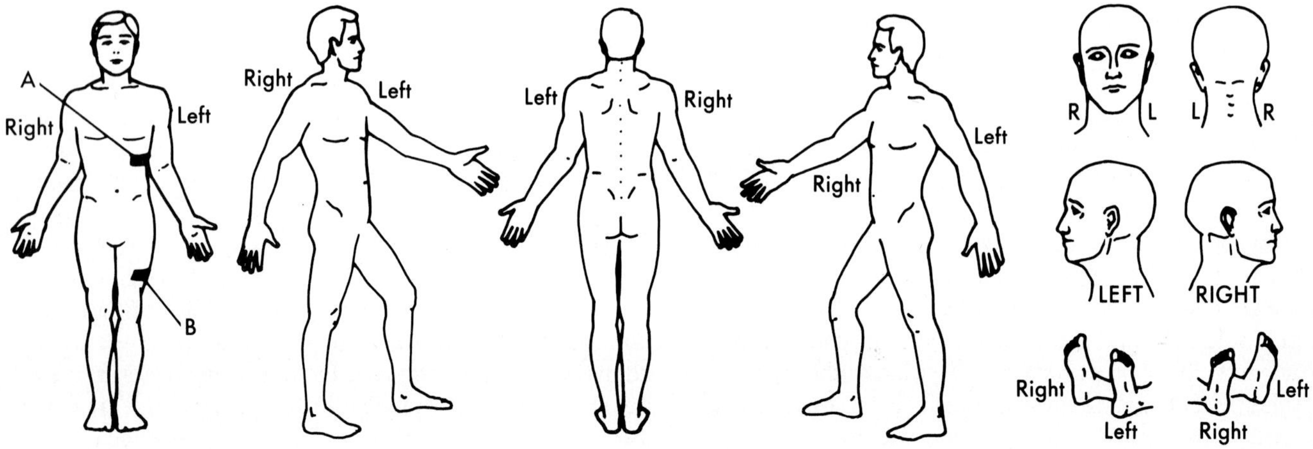

II. INTENSITY: Patient rates the pain. Scale used _0-10 (0= no pain, 10= worst pain)_

Present: _Site A=8; Site B=6. 2 hours after Demerol 75 mg IM._
Worst pain gets: _Site A=10 when cough; Site B=10 when try to shift position._
Best pain gets: _Site A and B=6 when lies totally still._
Acceptable level of pain: _2-3 could move more and sleep._

III. QUALITY: (Use patient's own words, e.g. prick, ache, burn, throb, pull, sharp) _____
A — deep aching.   B — sharp throbbing.

IV. ONSET, DURATION VARIATIONS, RHYTHMS: _Pain in site B felt right after accident._
Movement increases pain at both sites.

V. MANNER OF EXPRESSING PAIN: _Clenching side rails, grimacing. Pt. readily_
describes pain and states he is not comfortable.

VI. WHAT RELIEVES THE PAIN? _Has not felt relief since coming out of surgery._
Lying totally still decreases pain from 8 to 6.

VII. WHAT CAUSES OR INCREASES THE PAIN? _Movement, coughing increases pain_
_to 9-10._

VIII. EFFECTS OF PAIN: (Note decreased function, decreased quality of life.)
Accompanying symptoms (e.g. nausea) _Nausea when got OOB, pain ↑ to 9._
Sleep _Difficulty falling asleep, wakes up approximately every hour due to pain._
Appetite _Just started clear liquids._
Physical activity _Been in chair once. Pain ↑ to 9._
Relationship with others (e.g. irritability) _Can't talk with wife because of pain._
Emotions (e.g. anger, suicidal, crying) _____
Concentration _____
Other _____

IX. OTHER COMMENTS: _Knows importance of getting OOB, but states can't_
stand pain.

X. PLAN: _Evaluate response to Demerol IM. Suggest change to higher_
dose or different route. Goal: pain rating of 2-3.

FIGURE 2-5 Initial pain assessment tool completed for Mr. T.

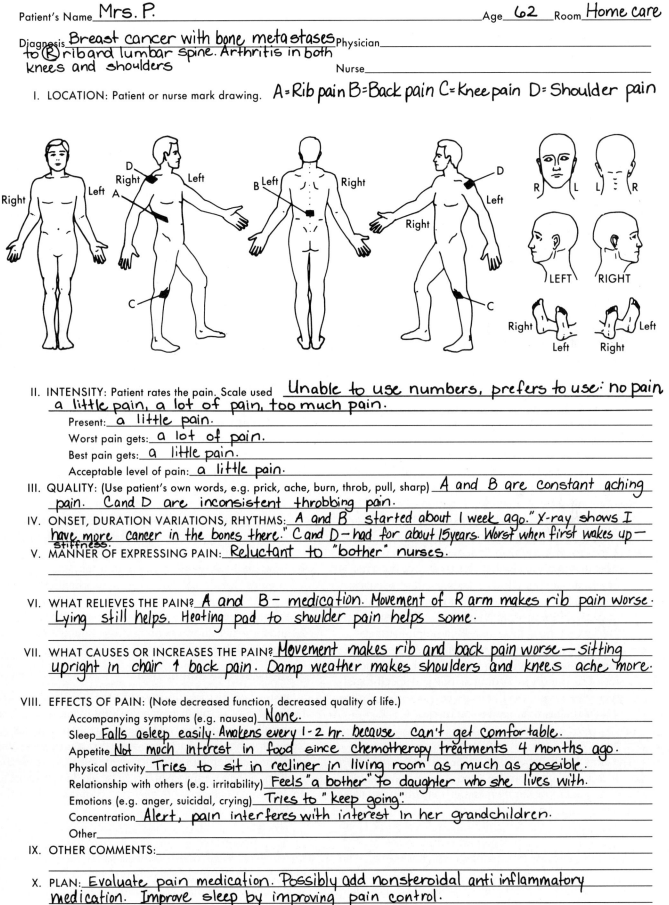

INITIAL PAIN ASSESSMENT TOOL FOR MRS. P.   Date 5/2/87

Patient's Name Mrs. P.   Age 62 Room Home care

Diagnosis Breast cancer with bone metastases Physician_____
to Ⓡ ribard lumbar spine. Arthritis in both
knees and shoulders   Nurse_____

I. LOCATION: Patient or nurse mark drawing. A=Rib pain B=Back pain C=Knee pain D=Shoulder pain

II. INTENSITY: Patient rates the pain. Scale used Unable to use numbers, prefers to use: no pain
a little pain, a lot of pain, too much pain.
    Present: a little pain.
    Worst pain gets: a lot of pain.
    Best pain gets: a little pain.
    Acceptable level of pain: a little pain.

III. QUALITY: (Use patient's own words, e.g. prick, ache, burn, throb, pull, sharp) A and B are constant aching
pain. C and D are inconsistent throbbing pain.

IV. ONSET, DURATION VARIATIONS, RHYTHMS: A and B started about 1 week ago." X-ray shows I
have more cancer in the bones there." C and D — had for about 15 years. Worst when first wakes up —
stiffness.

V. MANNER OF EXPRESSING PAIN: Reluctant to "bother" nurses.

VI. WHAT RELIEVES THE PAIN? A and B — medication. Movement of R arm makes rib pain worse.
Lying still helps. Heating pad to shoulder pain helps some.

VII. WHAT CAUSES OR INCREASES THE PAIN? Movement makes rib and back pain worse — sitting
upright in chair ↑ back pain. Damp weather makes shoulders and knees ache more.

VIII. EFFECTS OF PAIN: (Note decreased function, decreased quality of life.)
    Accompanying symptoms (e.g. nausea) None.
    Sleep Falls asleep easily. Awakens every 1-2 hr. because can't get comfortable.
    Appetite Not much interest in food since chemotherapy treatments 4 months ago.
    Physical activity Tries to sit in recliner in living room as much as possible.
    Relationship with others (e.g. irritability) Feels "a bother" to daughter who she lives with.
    Emotions (e.g. anger, suicidal, crying) Tries to "keep going".
    Concentration Alert, pain interferes with interest in her grandchildren.
    Other_____

IX. OTHER COMMENTS:_____

X. PLAN: Evaluate pain medication. Possibly add nonsteroidal anti inflammatory
medication. Improve sleep by improving pain control.

FIGURE 2-6 Initial pain assessment tool completed for Mrs. P.

Pain Flow Sheet

The flow sheet (copyright McCaffery, 1982b; also appeared in Meinhart and McCaffery, 1983) allows ongoing evaluation of assessment. Although it is most frequently used to evaluate the safety and effectiveness of analgesics, it is also appropriate for nonpharmacological methods of pain control. Columns may be added for this, or these methods may be included in the "other" column.

The only safe and effective way to administer an analgesic is to monitor the patient's response to the medication and make changes based on these responses. The flow sheet is a tool that allows quick documentation of such responses along with easy retrieval of information for continuous evaluation.

Appropriate Uses of the Flow Sheet

Situations in which the use of a flow sheet may be appropriate include the following:

- Initial doses of any new prescription of analgesic. Although initial doses are based on as much pharmacological knowledge and individual history as possible, initial doses are still "educated guesses" because each person reacts differently to medication. However, follow-up with a flow sheet so that changes can be made immediately results in a guess being tailored or titrated into a safe and effective analgesic regimen. A new prescription of analgesic not only includes any change in choice of drug but also any change in dose, interval, or route of administration.

- Some part of the analgesic regimen is causing the health team to be unsure or fearful of its administration. For example, a high dose of narcotic may cause nurses to hesitate giving what is prescribed. A flow sheet that provides easy access to the patient's respiratory rate can be quickly reassuring. If you suggest a new route of narcotic administration to a physician, reassuring him that the patient will be closely monitored with a flow sheet may be a helpful strategy.

- A patient's pain changes, or a complicated pain situation results in ineffective pain control. Documentation of responses according to time and specific analgesic given may help the team gain a clearer picture of adjustments that need to be made.

Characteristics of the Pain Flow Sheet

The flow sheet provides a quick and easy evaluation tool. It is a tool that can be used in the home setting where the patient or family member may fill in information in the columns.

A suggested format for a flow sheet is on p. 27. However, the form may be changed according to the individual patient's needs or the setting in which it is used. The columns that would probably remain regardless of the situation would be Time, Pain Rating, and Plan and Comments.

An explanation of the flow sheet columns follows.

Time. Initially most routes are assessed hourly, if possible, except for IV, which is monitored every 10 minutes until safety and effectiveness are established.

Pain rating. A footnote about this column appears at the bottom of the form. It is important to explain which scale is used at the top of the form so that everyone is consistent and clear about its meaning.

Analgesic. This column should include the name of the drug, dose, and route. If this form is used to evaluate nonpharmacological pain control methods, simply use "Pain Control Method" instead.

Respirations, pulse, blood pressure, level of arousal. Respiratory status is the most important physiological parameter to monitor to determine safety of a narcotic analgesic. A dramatic decrease in respiratory rate, e.g., from 12 to 6, 30 minutes after a narcotic is given IM requires immediate dose reduction with close patient evaluation. A less dramatic decrease in respirations, e.g., from 12 to 10 may occur when the patient sleeps and requires no dose adjustment. The flow sheet clearly documents these different responses.

Pulse and blood pressure are rarely monitored unless a patient's respiratory status becomes unstable. A certain amount of sedation may be noted initially; however, it usually subsides. Unless respirations change, the presence of sedation does not automatically warrant a change in analgesic regimen.

Other. Additional parameters may need to be assessed and evaluated. Examples of these are noted at the bottom of the form and depend on the individual patient situation.

Plan and comments. This column may include strategies for improving or maintaining pain control.

Examples of using a pain flow sheet are shown on pp. 28 and 29, which show continuing assessment and evaluation of Mr. T. and Mrs. P.

Additional Assessment Tool

Instead of the tools discussed above, a daily diary kept by the patient or family may be helpful in gathering data, especially if the patient is at home. On p. 30 is a suggested format for the daily diary (copyright McCaffery, 1980; also appeared in Meinhart and McCaffery, 1983). As with the tools mentioned previously, it may be altered to adjust to an individual situation. It may be accompanied by the patient/family teaching point, p. 31.

The diary may be particularly helpful for the patient to bring to the next office visit or to show to the home health nurse. Every hour does not need to be recorded; however, it is important to note when medication is taken or when an activity alters a previous pain rating. A completed diary on Mrs. A. is shown on p. 32.

Text continued on p. 33.

FLOW SHEET—PAIN

Patient _____ Date _____

*Pain rating scale used _____

Purpose: To evaluate the safety and effectiveness of the analgesic(s).

Analgesic(s) prescribed: _____

Time	Pain rating	Analgesic	R	P	BP	Level of arousal	Other†	Plan & comments

*Pain rating: A number of different scales may be used. Indicate which scale is used and use the same one each time. For example, 0-10 (0 = no pain, 10 = worst pain).

†Possibilities for other columns: bowel function, activities, nausea and vomiting, other pain relief measures. Identify the side effects of greatest concern to patient, family, physician, nurses.

FLOW SHEET—PAIN FOR MR. T.

Patient _Mr. T_ Date _4/10/87_

*Pain rating scale used _0 to 10 (0 = no pain, 10 = worst pain)_

Purpose: To evaluate the safety and effectiveness of the analgesic(s).

Analgesic(s) prescribed: _Demerol 75 mg IM q4th prn. Later changed to morphine IV._

Time	Pain rating	Analgesic	R	P	BP	Level of arousal	Other†	Plan & comments
4/10 9 AM	A = 8 B = 6	Demerol 75mg IM	22			Awake "Really hurts" clenching side rails.		Site A = splenectomy Site B = ① femur change to different analgesic to ↓ pain
9 30 A	A = 7 B = 6		18			Ask if he can have more pain med.		
9 45 A	A = 8 B = 7	Morphine 10mg IV bolus Tylenol gr X supp.	22			Alert. Asking about new med.		Evaluate morphine + tylenol
10 AM	A = 5 B = 5		18			States pain is easing some.		
10 30 A	A = 5 B = 3	Morphine 10mg IV bolus	16			Eyes closed. Open immed. when name called.		IV bolus repeated only last 45-50 min. + pain rating remains high
11 AM	A = 3 B = 2		14			Eyes closed. Opens immed. when name called. Feels "much better."		
11 15 A	A = 3 B = 1	Morphine infusion begun at 20mg/hr	18			Alert. Talking with wife.		
1 PM	A = 2 B = 1		16			Answers questions easily.		
2 PM		Morphine 10 mg IV bolus	22			Alert. Anxiety ↑ with effort to get into chair		Bolus given to get pt. into chair.
2 15 P	A = 4 B = 3	20mg/hr continues Tylenol gr X po	18			Sitting in chair. States pain much better with bolus.		Continue current plan

*Pain rating: A number of different scales may be used. Indicate which scale is used and use the same one each time. For example, 0-10 (0 = no pain, 10 = worst pain).

†Possibilities for other columns: bowel function, activities, nausea and vomiting, other pain relief measures. Identify the side effects of greatest concern to patient, family, physician, nurses.

FLOW SHEET—PAIN FOR MRS. P.

Patient __Mrs. P._____ Date __5/2/87_____

*Pain rating scale used __No pain, a little pain, a lot of pain, too much pain. Unable to use a__
__numerical scale.__

Purpose: To evaluate the safety and effectiveness of the analgesic(s).

Analgesic(s) prescribed: __Morphine 5-10 mg PO q 4h. ATC; Trilisate 1500 mg PO bid._____

Time	Pain rating	Analgesic	R	P	BP	Level of arousal	Other†	Plan & comments
10 AM	A lot of pain.	Morphine 10mg PO	18			Sleepy. Answers questions appropriately		Improve pain relelf, without ↑ sedation.
						States she does not like to sleep so much.		Begin anti inflammatory med.
11 AM	A lot of pain.	Trilisate 1500mg. PO	16			Very drowsy. Lies with eyes closed. Awakens easily but goes back to sleep.		
12 N			14			Eyes closed.		
1 PM	A little pain.		16			Talking with family Falls back to sleep easily.		
2 PM	A little pain.	Morphine 10mg. PO	16					
3 PM	A little pain.					Opens eyes when name called.		
6 PM	No pain.	Morphine 5mg PO	14			Eyes closed. Easily awakend.		↓ Morphine to try to
11 PM	No pain	Trilisate 1500 mg PO	14					↓ sedation
12 MN	No pain.							

*Pain rating: A number of different scales may be used. Indicate which scale is used and use the same one each time. For example, 0-10 (0 = no pain, 10 = worst pain).

† Possibilities for other columns: bowel function, activities, nausea and vomiting, other pain relief measures. Identify the side effects of greatest concern to patient, family, physician, nurses.

DAILY DIARY

Name _____ Date _____

Time	Pain rating scale	Medication type & amount taken	Other pain relief measures tried or anything that influences your pain	Major activity being done: lying sitting standing/walking
12 MIDNIGHT				
1 AM				
2				
3				
4				
5				
6				
7				
8				
9				
10				
11				
noon 12				
1				
2				
3				
4				
5				
6				
7				
8				
9				
10				
11				

Comments: _____

_____

_____

■ May be duplicated for use in clinical practice. From McCaffery, M, and Beebe, A: PAIN: CLINICAL MANUAL FOR NURSING PRACTICE, St. Louis, 1989, The CV Mosby Company.

Patient/Family Teaching Point: Use of Daily Diary

TO: _____ (patient's name)   DATE: _____

Filling out a daily diary will help us understand how pain affects your daily activities. With this information, we can work together toward the best possible control of your pain.

An explanation of the columns in the diary follows.

Pain rating. Use whatever pain rating you and the health team have decided is easiest for you to use. The scale you are to

use is _____.

Medication. Fill in the name of the medication and the amount you take at the time noted in the far left column.

Other pain relief measures. Fill in any measures that you might use to get good control of the pain. This might include your favorite hobby, listening to music, or use of heat or cold over the painful area.

Major activity being done. It is important for us to know how well you sleep and if walking or other activities have an effect on your pain.

Have the diary available when you see the nurse or doctor next. **Remember**: You are the only one who can tell us what your pain is like. The more you tell us about your pain, the more information we have to plan with you ways to make the pain better.

Additional comments: _____

_____

If you have any questions or problems with the diary, contact:

_____ (RN or MD name)   Phone _____

_____ (Nurse's name)

■ May be duplicated for use in clinical practice. From McCaffery, M, and Beebe, A: PAIN: CLINICAL MANUAL FOR NURSING PRACTICE, St. Louis, 1989, The CV Mosby Company.

DAILY DIARY

Name __Mrs. A__ Date __3/10/88__

Time	Pain rating scale 0-10 (0 = no pain, 10 = worst pain)	Medication type & amount taken	Other pain relief measures tried or anything that influences your pain	Major activity being done: lying sitting standing/walking
12 MIDNIGHT				sleep (10 PM)
1 AM				
2				
3				
4				
5				
6	6 Very stiff	Motrin 600mg Tylenol 650mg	Heating pad to low back.	Remains in bed.
7:30	3		Aim shower head at low back × 5 min.	OOB - Shower + dress.
8				Breakfast.
9				Standing + walking for light housework.
10	4	Tylenol 650 mg		
11				Listen to radio - reclining on sofa.
noon 12		Motrin 600mg		Sitting - lunch.
1	3			
2				Shopping - standing/walking.
3				
4	5		Does stretching exercises	Swimming in heated pool.
5	3		Ice pack to lower back.	Reclining on sofa.
6	2	Motrin 600mg Tylenol 650mg		Watch TV - reclining.
7:30	2			Supper - sitting.
8				Read + watch TV.
9				
10		Tylenol 650 mg		Bedtime.
11				

Comments: __Since I'm taking so much additional Tylenol, is it possible to increase Motrin?__

*Daily diary for Mrs. A.: Mrs. A. has rheumatoid arthritis. Stiffness in her lower back is especially bad upon awakening early in the morning. Heat to the area helps first thing in the A.M. while cold packs help later in the day after exercise Recording activities and medication helped the home health nurse and Mrs. A. determine that an increase in Motrin might help. No side effects from lower dose were noted, so Motrin was increased to 800 q6h.

SUMMARY

This chapter has addressed the important components of pain assessment. Misconceptions that hamper accurate assessment have been discussed, and three practical assessment tools, appropriate in any clinical setting, have been presented.

REFERENCES AND SELECTED READINGS

Cancer pain relief, World Health Organization, 1986

Chapman, DD, Casey, KL, Dubner, R, et al: Pain measurement: an overview, *Pain* **22**:1-31, 1985

Classification of chronic pain, *Pain* (suppl) **3**:S1-S226, 1986

Cleeland, CS: Assessing pain in cancer: the patient's role. In Management of cancer pain, pp 17-21, New York, 1984, HP Publishing Co, Inc

Crue, BL, Jr: Multidisciplinary pain treatment programs: current status, *Clin J Pain* **1**:31-38, 1985

Daut, RL, and Cleeland, CS: The prevalence and severity of pain in cancer, *Cancer* **50**:1913-1918, 1982

Donovan, MI: Clinical assessment of cancer pain. In McGuire, DB, and Yarbro, CH, eds: Cancer pain management, pp 105-131, Orlando, 1987, Grune & Stratton

Donovan, M, Dillon, P, and McGuire, L: Incidence and characteristics of pain in a sample of medical-surgical inpatients, *Pain* **30**:69-78, 1987

Dworkin, RH, et al: Unraveling the effects of compensation, litigation, and employment in treatment response in chronic pain, *Pain* **23**:49-59, 1985

Goodwin, JS, Goodwin, JM, and Vogel, AA: Knowledge and use of placebos by house officers and nurses, *Ann Intern Med* **91**:106-110, 1979

Grevert, P, Albert, LH, and Goldstein, A: Partial antagonism of placebo analgesia by naloxone, *Pain* **16**:129-143, 1983

Hendler, N: Depression caused by chronic pain, *J Clin Psychiatr* **45**:30-38, Mar 1984

Houde, RW: Methods for measuring clinical pain in humans, *Acta Anaesth Scand* (suppl) **74**:25-29, 1982

Infante, MC, and Mooney, NE: Interactive aspects of pain assessment, *Orthoped Nurs* **6**:31-34, 1987

Karoly, P: The assessment of pain: concepts and procedures. In Karoly, P, ed: Measurement strategies in health psychology, pp 461-519, New York, 1985, Wiley Interscience

Lasagna, L, Mosteller, F, von Felsinger, JM, and Beecher, HK: A study of the placebo response, *Am J Med* **16**:770-779, 1954

Leavitt, F, and Sweet, JJ: Characteristics and frequency of malingering among patients with low back pain, *Pain* **25**:357-364, 1986

Levine, JD, Gordon, NC, and Fields, H: The mechanism of placebo analgesia, *Lancet* **2**:654-657, 1978

McCaffery, M: Nursing practice theories related to cognition, bodily pain, and man-environment interactions, Los Angeles, 1968, University of California at Los Angeles Students' Store

McCaffery, M: Nursing management of the patient with pain, ed 2, Philadelphia, 1979, JB Lippincott Co

McCaffery, M: Unpublished material, 1980

McCaffery, M: Would you administer placebos for pain? *Nursing* **12**:80-85, Feb 1982

McCaffery, M: Unpublished material, 1982b

McGuire, DB: The measurement of clinical pain, *Nurs Res* **33**:152-156, 1984

Meinhart, NT, and McCaffery, M: Pain: a nursing approach to assessment and analysis, 1983, Norwalk, Conn, Appleton-Century-Crofts

Melzack, R: The McGill pain questionnaire: major properties and scoring methods, *Pain* **1**:275-299, 1975

Melzack, R: The short-form McGill pain questionnaire, *Pain* **30**:191-197, 1987

Melzack, R, Abbott, FV, Zackon, W, Mulder, DS, and Davis, MWL: Pain on a surgical ward: a survey of the duration and intensity of pain and the effectiveness of medication, *Pain* **29**:67-72, 1987

Melzack, R, Katz, J, and Jeans, ME: The role of compensation in chronic pain: analysis using a new method of scoring the McGill pain questionnaire, *Pain* **23**:101-112, 1985

Miser, AW, McCalla, J, Dothage, JA, Wesley, M, and Miser, JS: Pain as a presenting symptom in children and young adults with newly diagnosed malignancy, *Pain* **29**:85-90, 1987

Moskow, SB: Hunan hand and other ailments, Boston, 1987, Little, Brown & Co

Perry, SW, Cella, DF, Falkenberg, J, et al: Pain perception vs pain response in burn patients, *Am J Nurs* **87**:698, 1987

Reesor, KA, and Craig, KD: Medically incongruent chronic back pain: physical limitations, suffering, and ineffective coping, *Pain* **32**:35-45, 1988

Sanford, KD, and Schlicher, CM: Pain management, are your biases showing? *Nurs Life* **6**:47-51, 1986

Shacham, S, Reinhardt, LC, Raubertas, RF, and Cleeland, CS: Emotional states and pain: intraindividual and interindividual measures of association, *J Behav Med* **6**:405-419, 1983

Syrjala, KL, and Chapman, CR: Measurement of clinical pain: a review and integration of research findings. In Benedetti, C, Chapman, CR, and Moricca, G, eds: Advances in pain research and therapy, pp 71-101, vol 7, New York, 1984, Raven Press

Wallenstein, SL: Measurement of pain and analgesia in cancer patients, *Cancer* **53**:2260-2264, 1984

Wallenstein, SL, Heidrich, G, Kaiko, R, and Houde, RW: Clinical evaluation of mild analgesics: the measurement of clinical pain, *Br J Clin Pharmacol* **10**:319S-327S, 1980

CHAPTER

3

The Process of Nursing
People with Pain

Included in this chapter are discussions of:
• Nursing process.
• Nursing diagnosis.
• Pain theories (gate control, endorphins and non-opioid pathways, and multiple opioid receptor site theory).
• Guidelines for pain control.

NURSING PROCESS: A PROBLEM-SOLVING APPROACH

The process of nursing involves a systematic, scientific approach to care for patients and families. In order to deliver effective and safe care to patients with pain, the nurse collects data; identifies the problem; plans, implements, and evaluates nursing interventions; and makes appropriate modifications based on evaluation. Problem-solving in this manner is referred to as the nursing process.

The nursing process allows the nurse to be responsive to individual human needs. The components of this process are not mutually exclusive; they overlap, and each provides information for the other, sometimes resulting in a readjustment or revision of a previous step in the nursing process (Figure 3-1). Following are the five components of this process (Campbell, 1984; Carpenito, 1983).

1. Assessment

Subjective data, i.e., symptoms, and objective data, i.e., signs, are gathered that include not only physical information but also psychological and social aspects of the individual patient which may influence his perception of and

response to pain. Assessment is an ongoing process that is carried out by history taking, observation, interviewing, and physical examination.

2. Problem Identification

Gathering data helps the nurse decide on the nature of the problem. Once the existence and extent of a problem are identified, a nursing diagnosis is made.

3. Planning

The approach, or planning step identifies the goals and sets the priorities that both the patient and the nurse determine to work toward.

4. Intervention

Implementing an intervention involves executing a nursing measure that will diminish, resolve, or prevent the defined problem. A nursing measure for a patient with pain may include:
a. Nursing treatments, e.g., facilitating hygiene, initiating a relaxation technique, and coordinating home health care.
b. Nursing observations, e.g., baseline respirations before administering a narcotic.
c. Health education, e.g., correcting a patient's or family's misconceptions about pain and its treatment and teaching the concept of patient controlled analgesia.
d. Medical treatments performed by the nurse, e.g., administering a prescribed narcotic.

5. Evaluation

This step determines the effectiveness of nursing care in diminishing, resolving, or preventing the defined

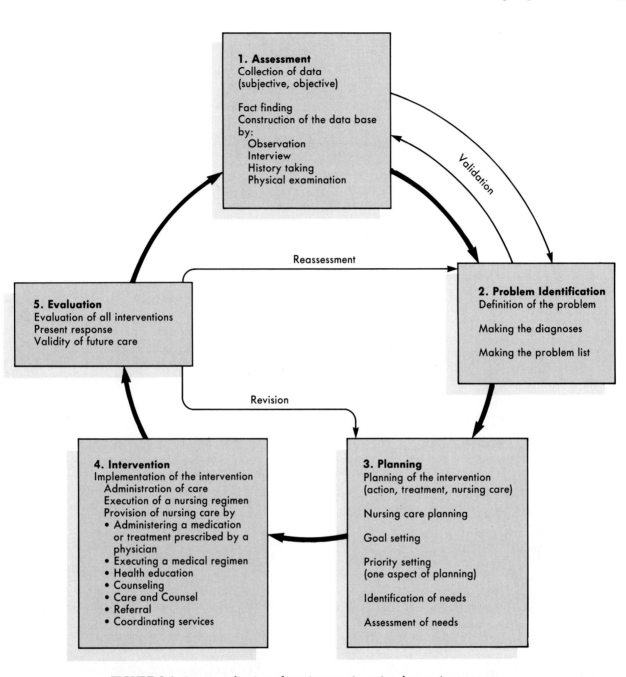

FIGURE 3-1 Conceptualization of nursing practice using the nursing process.
Modified from Reeder, SJ, and Martin, LL: Maternity nursing, ed 16, Philadelphia, 1987, JB Lippincott.

problem and predicts the need for future nursing actions. For example, evaluation of the safety and effectiveness of a narcotic analgesic includes monitoring a patient's response using a flow sheet. Evaluation includes ongoing assessment and may involve revisions of the plan of care.

In this book the major components of the nursing process are discussed primarily as follows: assessment in Chapter 2, nursing diagnosis in Chapter 3, nursing interventions in Chapters 4 to 9, and evaluation in Chapter 12.

Chapters 10 and 11 identify special considerations in these areas for children and the elderly.

The nursing care plans in this book are set up to incorporate the five components of the nursing process. Column I is assessment, column II is potential nursing diagnoses, column III is planning/intervention, and column IV is evaluation/expected outcomes. Refer to the inside cover of the book for a list of all the nursing care plans which utilize a number of the nursing diagnoses already discussed.

NURSING DIAGNOSES RELATED TO PAIN

When a problem is identified and possible etiology established, a nursing diagnosis is stated. Nursing diagnoses allow nurses to identify the health alterations of individuals in a systematic manner. Nursing diagnosis is defined as

...a statement that describes a health state or an actual or potential alteration in a person's life processes (physiological, psychological, sociocultural, developmental, and spiritual). The nurse uses the nursing process to identify and synthesize clinical data and to order nursing interventions to reduce, eliminate, or prevent health alterations which are in the legal and educational domain of nursing (Carpenito, 1983, p. 4).

As of 1988 (Proceedings of the Eighth National Conference of the North American Nursing Diagnosis Association), 98 diagnoses have been approved by the North American Nursing Diagnosis Association for use in nursing practice. The following two are directly associated with the care of patients with pain:

- Chronic pain.
- Pain.

Because pain, especially if it is prolonged, may affect all aspects of a person's life, the following 18 diagnoses may be especially appropriate for patients with pain:

- Anxiety.
- Constipation.
- Ineffective individual coping.
- Diversional activity deficit.
- Fatigue.
- Fear.
- Knowledge deficit (specify).
- Impaired physical mobility.
- Powerlessness.
- Feeding self-care deficit.
- Bathing/hygiene self-care deficit.
- Dressing/grooming self-care deficit.
- Toileting self-care deficit.
- Sexual dysfunction.
- Sleep pattern disturbance.
- Social isolation.
- Spiritual distress (distress of the human spirit).
- Altered thought processes.

This is by no means an exhaustive list, but as the nurse collects data and evaluates her plan, this list should alert her to the potential for pain to disrupt many aspects of a person's life.

PAIN THEORIES

Although the exact mechanism for the transmission and perception of pain is not known, neurophysiological, psychological, and sociological research has contributed to the formation of pain theories. By definition, a theory does not represent actual fact; instead it stimulates

thought and provides a basis for research. For the nurse who cares for patients with pain, pain theories offer a conceptual framework for research and for specific pain-relieving methods.

Although several theories exist, three will be briefly reviewed below. Those wishing further discussion and study are referred to the selected readings at the end of the chapter.

1. Gate Control Theory as a Conceptual Framework

The gate control theory, originally proposed in 1965 (Melzack and Wall, 1965), is not presented from a neurophysiological standpoint; instead parts of the theory that are especially useful in clinical practice are discussed below as a *conceptual framework*.

The gate control theory is particularly relevant to nursing practice in that it presents:

- An integrated conceptual model for appreciating the many factors that contribute to individual differences in the experience of pain.
- A conceptualization of categories of activity that may form a theoretical base for developing various pain relief measures.

Table 3-1 summarizes aspects of the theory that are useful in clinical practice. The middle column of the table shows three general categories of activity that may contribute to pain relief, i.e., three ways to close or partially close the gate so that impulses felt as painful are less likely to reach a level of awareness. These three aspects of the theory are discussed below in relation to pain control measures.

1. Cutaneous stimulation may relieve pain. The gate control theory proposes that activation of large diameter nerve fibers may alleviate pain. Since the skin is heavily endowed with such fibers, many types of tactile stimulation have the potential for pain relief. Specific types of cutaneous stimulation, such as massage or vibration, are obvious examples of the direct application of this theory. However, an element of touch and cutaneous stimulation also may be involved in other pain relief measures. Distraction may include rhythmic rubbing of a body part experiencing pain, or relaxation may be enhanced by a backrub.

2. "Normal" or excessive sensory input may relieve pain. It appears that the reticular system in the brainstem can inhibit incoming stimuli, including pain, if the person is receiving sufficient or excessive sensory input. The brainstem may then project inhibitory impulses that help close the gate to the transmission of impulses felt as painful. To accomplish this, elaborate distraction strategies may be devised. Sensory restriction, especially monotony, is avoided. This may enable the patient to "tune out" pain. Most pain relief methods involve some degree of sensory input. Some are excellent sources of sensory stimuli. Guided imagery, for example, involves intense

TABLE 3-1 Nursing Practice Aspects of the Gate Control Theory of Pain

Major Contributions

1. An integrated conceptual model for appreciating the many factors that contribute to individual differences in the experience of pain.
2. Conceptualization of categories of activity that may form a theoretical base for developing various pain relief measures.

Nature of the Gate

The transmission of potentially painful impulses to the level of conscious awareness may be affected by a gating mechanism, possibly located at the spinal cord level of the CNS.

Structures Involved	No Pain or Decreased Intensity of Pain	Pain
Spinal cord (?)	Results from CLOSING THE GATE by:	Results from OPENING THE GATE by:
Nerve fibers	1. Activity in the *large diameter nerve fibers,* e.g., caused by skin stimulation.	1. Activity in the *small diameter nerve fibers,* e.g., caused by tissue damage.
Brainstem	2. Inhibitory impulses from the *brainstem,* e.g., caused by sufficient or maximal sensory input arriving through distraction or guided imagery, or	2. Facilitory impulses from the *brainstem,* e.g., caused by insufficient input from a monotonous environment, or
Cerebral cortex and thalamus	3. Inhibitory impulses from the *cerebral cortex* and *thalamus,* e.g., caused by anxiety reduction based on learning when the pain will end and how to relieve it.	3. Facilitory impulses from the *cerebral cortex* and *thalamus,* e.g., caused by fear that the intensity of pain will escalate and will be associated with death.

concentration on imaginary sensory experiences. It is even possible that the enigma of causing brief pain to relieve chronic pain can be explained on the basis of brainstem activities. Intense stimulation of trigger points, by needling, for example, could increase input to the brainstem, which would close the gates to pain from other body areas (Melzack, Stillwell, and Fox, 1977).

3. Accurate information about the cause and relief of pain, a sense of control, or a decrease in anxiety or depression, may relieve pain. The gate control theory suggests that pain can be alleviated by inhibitory signals from the cerebral cortex and thalamus. Thoughts, emotions, and past experiences stored in these structures may result in impulses that affect the transmission of pain impulses. Therefore pain may be relieved by reducing unnecessary sources of anxiety about pain and by increasing the patient's feeling of confidence and control with respect to pain relief. Often this is accomplished through the nature of the nurse's relationship with the patient with pain or through certain patient teaching. Of course, most other methods of pain relief also contribute, directly or indirectly, to anxiety reduction and increased understanding of the pain experience.

2. Endorphins and Nonopioid Pathways

In the mid 1970s, the body's own internally secreted narcotic-like substances called endorphins were identified (Snyder, 1977). The term *endorphin* is a combination of the words "endogenous" and "morphine," meaning morphine within. It is believed that an impulse from the brain triggers the release of endorphins. They lock into the narcotic receptors at nerve endings in the brain and spinal cord to block the transmission of a pain signal, preventing the impulse from reaching consciousness.

Endorphin research has helped us understand that pain perception and the need for analgesia vary from one individual to another. Differences in the amount of endorphin present in different individuals and the probability that other factors increase or decrease endorphin levels help explain the differences in pain perception (Janal et al, 1984; Tamsen et al, 1982).

Preliminary research suggests that the following factors tend to increase or decrease endorphin levels (Clark et al, 1986; Emrich, 1981; Janal et al, 1984; Tamsen et al, 1982; Terenius, 1984; Whipple and Komisaruk, 1985):

↓ Endorphins	↑ Endorphins
Prolonged pain	Brief pain
Recurrent stress	Brief stress
Prolonged use of morphine or alcohol	Physical exercise
	Massive trauma
	Acupuncture, some types
	Transcutaneous electric nerve stimulation, some types
	Placebos, possibly
	Sexual activity

It may be tempting to assume that because endorphins are "natural" substances, they therefore have more benefits and fewer side effects than the narcotics that we administer. In fact we have not isolated anything that might be of more benefit than the narcotics presently administered. This certainly raises the question of the benefit of spending considerable time, energy, and expense to increase the patient's own endorphins.

Although there was considerable excitement initially over the endorphins, there are few clinically useful conclusions from this research (McGrath and Unruh, 1987).

There remains hope for the discovery of new analgesic drugs based on these narcotic-like substances (Terenius, 1984).

Endorphin-mediated analgesia appears not to be the only system that may produce pain relieving effects. There is evidence that nonopioid pathways may produce relief in patients with clinical pain (Janal et al, 1984; Walker and Katz, 1981; Young and Chambi, 1987).

3. Multiple Opioid Receptor Theory: Practical Aspects

How can a drug relieve pain in the same manner as a narcotic but also wipe out or antagonize another narcotic? The theory of multiple opioid receptor sites helps explain such events. Effective use of narcotics, especially the narcotic agonist-antagonists, depends on a basic understanding of this theory.

KEY POINT: Effective use of butorphanol (Stadol), nalbuphine (Nubain), and pentazocine (Talwin) requires a basic understanding of the three opioid receptor sites—mu, kappa, and sigma.

The theory of multiple opioid receptor sites is one of the most recent theories related to pain relief, and surprisingly little has been written about it in the health science literature. Therefore it is unfamiliar to most clinical practitioners and somewhat difficult to understand initially. Like all theories, it is not fact; it is an idea generated by the need to explain something and is meant to stimulate thought and research. However, the reality is that narcotics relieve pain in a variety of ways—ways that may complement, compete, or be specific in ways we do not yet fully understand.

Overview of Multiple Opioid Receptor Theory

In the central nervous system (CNS) at the spinal and supraspinal levels, theory suggests that narcotics may bind to, or occupy, multiple opioid receptor sites at the ends of nerves (Buprenorphine, 1976; Houde, 1979; Jaffee and Martin, 1985; Martin et al, 1976; Millan, 1986; Offermeier and Van Rooyen, 1984; Physicians' Desk Reference, 1987; Rogmagnoli and Keats, 1980; Wood, 1982; Yaksh et al, 1987). Three receptor sites have practical implications for effective use of narcotics. Table 3-2 lists three opioid receptor sites and their activities as follows (see also the box below for definition of terms used in the table):

1. *Mu* (μ) receptor site. Activity consists of supraspinal and probably spinal analgesia, respiratory depression, physical dependence, tolerance, constipation, and euphoria.
2. *Kappa* (κ) receptor site. Activity consists of spinal level analgesia and sedation, but no respiratory depression and no physical dependence.
3. *Sigma* (σ) receptor site. Activity consists of vasomotor stimulation and probable psychotomimetic effects (mimics psychosis, e.g., hallucinations).

Drugs bind to opioid receptor sites with varying degrees of affinity, or strength, i.e., some bind very tightly, referred to as "pure," and others bind less tightly, referred to as "partial." When a drug binds to a receptor site, the action may be pure or partial agonist or antagonist (Table 3-2):

1. When an *agonist drug* binds to the receptor site, activity occurs, i.e., an agonist *turns on the activity,* or
2. When an *antagonist drug* binds to the receptor site, activity is antagonized or blocked, i.e., an antagonist *turns off or blocks the activity.*

Table 3-2 lists analgesia as an activity at the mu and kappa receptor sites. Therefore when an agonist drug binds to either of these sites, pain relief will occur. Table 3-2 shows morphine, meperidine, and several other narcotics binding as agonists at the mu receptor site and not binding as agonist or antagonist to the other two receptor sites. Thus these drugs relieve pain mainly by action at the mu receptor.

Definitions: Opioid Receptor Site Theory

Opioid: Narcotic- or opiate-like drug; includes natural, synthetic, and endogenous drugs.

Receptor site: That portion of a nerve cell to which a drug can bind. There are several different opioid receptor sites, e.g., mu, kappa, and sigma.

Agonist: In large enough doses this type of drug binds to a specific receptor site and initiates activity at that receptor site. Types of agonists:

a. *Pure agonist:* Binds tightly with the receptor site and produces the near maximal activity possible at that receptor site.

b. *Partial agonist:* Binds with the receptor site less tightly than a pure agonist, producing less effect than a pure agonist.

Antagonist: In large enough doses this type of drug binds to a specific receptor and blocks activity at that receptor; or it displaces the agonist at the receptor site, thereby stopping the receptor's activity. Types of antagonists:

a. *Pure antagonist:* Binds tightly with the receptor site and stops or blocks activity at that receptor site.

b. *Partial antagonist:* Binds with the receptor site less tightly than a pure antagonist, stopping or blocking less of the activity at that receptor site.

Spinal analgesia: Pain relief with awareness; results from binding of opioids to receptor sites at the spinal level. The kappa opioid receptor provides spinal analgesia.

Supraspinal analgesia: Pain relief that affects awareness and other cortical and brainstem functions such as respirations; results from binding of opioids to receptor sites at the supraspinal level. The mu opioid receptor provides supraspinal analgesia.

TABLE 3-2 Practical Summary of Actions at Opioid Receptor Sites

Opioid Receptor Site	Activity	Drug Action Agonist (On)	Drug Action Antagonist (Off)
Mu (μ)	Analgesia, respiratory depression, physical dependence, tolerance, constipation, euphoria	Pure: e.g., morphine, methadone, codeine, fentanyl, hydromorphone (Dilaudid), meperidine (Demerol) Partial: buprenorphine (Buprenex)	Pure: naloxone (Narcan), naltrexone (Trexan) Partial: butorphanol (Stadol), nalbuphine (Nubain), pentazocine (Talwin)
Kappa (κ)	Analgesia, sedation, no physical dependence, no respiratory depression	Butorphanol (Stadol), buprenorphine (Buprenex), nalbuphine (Nubain), pentazocine (Talwin)	Pure: naloxone (Narcan), naltrexone (Trexan)
Sigma (σ)	Vasomotor stimulation, psychotomimetic effects (e.g., hallucinations, paranoia)	Butorphanol (Stadol), pentazocine (Talwin)	Antagonists not very effective at this site

When an antagonist drug attaches to the mu or kappa sites, analgesia at these sites will be blocked; or an antagonist drug can displace an agonist drug that is attached to the mu or kappa site, reversing analgesia along with other effects such as respiratory depression.

The purest narcotic antagonists are naloxone (Narcan) and naltrexone (Trexan). These antagonize, or block, activity at all three opioid receptor sites, but their strongest antagonist effect is at the mu and kappa sites. Naloxone is commonly used as an antidote for narcotic overdose, particularly to reverse respiratory depression and sedation, but it also reverses analgesia and other activities at the mu and kappa sites. Naltrexone, which is also an antagonist at the mu and kappa sites, is like a long-acting naloxone. It is used mainly during narcotic rehabilitation to block the effect of any narcotics taken impulsively by the recovering narcotic addict.

Table 3-2 shows that three drugs, butorphanol, nalbuphine, and pentazocine, result in analgesia by binding as agonists at the kappa site. Thus they relieve pain mainly by action at the kappa, not the mu, site. Butorphanol, nalbuphine, and pentazocine are also shown as partial antagonists at the mu site, meaning they can antagonize some of the analgesia and other effects of morphine and other pure agonists at the mu site. Buprenorphine is shown as an agonist at both the mu and kappa sites, so it relieves pain at two receptor sites.

Clinical Application of Opioid Receptor Theory

Two Groups of Narcotics. Pain relief from narcotics can result from drug occupation of receptors of more than one type. Currently, two types of narcotics are marketed in the United States:
1. Pure narcotic agonists, such as morphine and codeine, occupy the mu site and do not antagonize activity at other receptor sites.
2. Narcotic agonist-antagonists occupy the kappa site for pain relief and antagonize the effects of pure agonists at the mu site. Only three are available:

- butorphanol (Stadol)
- nalbuphine (Nubain)
- pentazocine (Talwin)

(Buprenorphine [Buprenex] is also a narcotic agonist-antagonist but is unlike the others in this group. It does not antagonize at the mu site except at very high doses in very physically dependent persons. Also, although respiratory depression is rare with this drug, it is the only one in which narcotic-induced respiratory depression cannot be completely reversed by naloxone.)

Potential Problems with Narcotic Agonist-antagonists. If the narcotic antagonist property of butorphanol, nalbuphine, and pentazocine is not understood, these drugs may cause the following difficulties:

- *They may precipitate withdrawal in a person who has been on pure narcotic agonists for a week or more.* After a course of narcotic agonists, the person may become physically dependent, i.e., if the narcotic is abruptly discontinued, the person experiences withdrawal. Narcotics with an antagonist property may precipitate withdrawal by abruptly blocking the action of the pure agonist. Therefore the three narcotic agonist-antagonists mentioned must be used with caution after a person has been on pure narcotics for a week or longer. A physically dependent person may be carefully switched from a narcotic agonist to an agonist-antagonist, but it may take up to 10 days or longer of small, daily decreases in the agonist accompanied by small, daily additions of the agonist-antagonist.

- *Given along with pure narcotics, they may eventually antagonize analgesia from the pure narcotics.* Initially, giving the two narcotic groups together may be additive, and it is difficult to predict when the agonist-antagonist will begin to reverse analgesia of the agonist. Early in narcotic therapy, a decision should be made about which group of narcotics will be used. A person can be switched from a narcotic agonist-antagonist to a narcotic agonist without much difficulty, except for some possible initial decrease in analgesia until the agonist-antagonist is excreted.

Benefits of the Narcotic Agonist-antagonists. Because all four of the narcotic agonist-antagonists (buprenorphine, butorphanol, nalbuphine, and pentazocine) act mainly at the kappa site where there is no respiratory depression, they usually cause only limited respiratory depression, and there is a ceiling on the amount of respiratory depression they cause. Beyond a certain dose, additional respiratory depression does not occur; therefore an increase in dose usually results in more pain relief without more respiratory depression. For further explanation and clinical examples, see Chapter 4 (pp. 85-86).

Future Applications of Multiple Opioid Receptor Theory

Greater understanding of the actions, location, and other characteristics of the various opioid receptor sites may play an important role in developing a more perfect analgesic and in refining methods of using analgesics. Perhaps it will be possible to identify an opioid receptor site with excellent analgesia and no side effects and then develop a drug that would attach to that site only.

Understanding of the opioid receptor sites may enable us to determine the most appropriate drug for a certain route of administration. For example, an analgesic with affinity for only spinal opioid receptor sites might be the most logical choice for epidural or intrathecal administration.

Tolerance to analgesia may be more easily controlled by identifying which drugs act at the various opioid receptor sites. Alternating drugs that act at different opioid receptor sites may delay tolerance. Of course, further research may yield unexpected findings. Already a search for understanding endorphins and opioid receptor sites has revealed that there are nonopioid analgesic systems. Humans apparently also have natural nonnarcotic substances that provide pain relief. The current status of research into human analgesic systems has been called the tip of the iceberg.

GUIDELINES FOR PAIN CONTROL

Following is a general introduction to the pain control methods discussed in Chapters 4 through 11. Certain attitudes and approaches that are important to communicate to a patient with pain and his family are summarized in the box at the top of the page. Occasionally the nurse must accept the fact that the desired relationship between herself and the patient is unlikely to develop. She does not desert the patient but makes every effort to promote a relationship between the patient and someone else.

Deciding which pain control measures to use with which patient can be difficult. Because pain experience is highly individual, its treatment must be likewise. In-depth

---

Important Attitudes Communicated by the Nurse to the Patient and Family

1. I care.
2. I believe you about your pain.
3. I respect the way you are reacting to the pain.
4. I want to explore with you what you think will help relieve your pain.
5. I want to discuss with you what your pain means to you.
6. I am willing to stay with you even if I fail to help control your pain.
7. If you cannot relate to me, I will try to find someone else for you.

Summary of Guidelines for Using and Individualizing Pain Control Measures

1. Use a variety of pain control measures.
2. Use pain control measures before pain becomes severe.
3. Include what the patient believes will be effective.
4. Consider the patient's ability or willingness to be active or passive in the application of pain control measures.
5. Institute and modify pain control measures on the basis of the patient's response.
6. If the pain control measure is ineffective the first time it is used, consider encouraging the patient to try it at least one or two more times before abandoning it.
7. Be open-minded about what may control pain.
8. Keep trying.
9. Do no harm.

---

discussions of the goals and guidelines for individualizing pain control measures are discussed in each of the chapters that follow. The box above summarizes these guidelines.

REFERENCES AND SELECTED READINGS

Buprenorphine: *Med Lett Drugs Ther* 28-56, May 23, 1986

Campbell, C: Nursing diagnosis and intervention in nursing practice, ed 2, New York, 1984, John Wiley & Sons

Carpenito, LJ: Nursing diagnosis: application to clinical practice, Philadelphia, 1983, JB Lippincott

Clark, WC, Yang, JC, and Janal, MN: Altered pain and visual sensitivity in humans: the effect of acute and chronic stress. In Kelly, DD, ed: Stress-induced analgesia, *Ann NY Acad Sci* 467:116-129, 1986

Emrich, HM, ed: The role of endorphins in neuropsychiatry. In Ban, TA, et al, eds: Modern problems of pharmacopsychiatry, pp 1-292, vol 17, New York, 1981, Basal

Hoffert, M: The gate control theory re-revisited, *J Pain Sympt Manag* 1:39-41, Winter 1986

Houde, RW: Analgesic effectiveness of the narcotic agonist-antagonists, *Br J Clin Pharmacol* 7:297S-308S, 1979

Jaffee, JH, and Martin, WR: Opioid analgesics and antagonists. In Gilman, AG, et al, eds: Goodman and Gilman's the pharmacological basis of therapeutics, ed 7, pp 491-553, New York, 1985, Macmillan Publishing Co

Janal, MN, Colt, EWD, Clark, WC, and Glusman, M: Pain sensitivity, mood and plasma endocrine levels in man following long-distance running: effects of naloxone, *Pain* 19:13-25, 1984

Kim, MJ, McFarland, GK, and McLane, AM: Pocket guide to nursing diagnoses, ed 3, St. Louis, 1989, The CV Mosby Company

Kosten, TR, and Kleber, HD: Control of nociception by endogenous opioids. In Aronoff, GM, ed: Mediguide to pain 8:1-5, New York, 1987, DellaCorte Publications

Martin, WR, Eades, CG, Thompson, JA, et al: The effects of morphine and nalorphine-like drugs in the nondependent and morphine-dependent chronic spinal dog, *J Pharmacol Exp Ther* 197:517-532, 1976

Melzack, R, Stillwell, DB, and Fox, EJ: Trigger points and acupuncture points for pain: correlations and implications, *Pain* 3:3-23, 1977

Melzack, R, and Wall, PD: Pain mechanisms: a new theory, *Science* 150:971-979, 1965

McGrath, PJ, and Unruh, AM: Pain in children and adolescents, Amsterdam, 1987, Elsevier

Millan, MJ: Multiple opioid systems and pain, *Pain* 27:303-347, 1986

Offermeier, J, and Van Rooyen, JM: Opioid drugs and their receptors: a summary of the present state of knowledge, *S Afr Med J* 66:299-305, Aug 1984

Pasternak, GW: Multiple morphine and enkephalin receptors and the relief of pain, *JAMA* 259:1362-1367, Mar 1988

Physicians' Desk Reference, ed 41, Oradell, NJ, 1987, Medical Economics Co Inc

Proceedings of the Eighth National Conference of the North American Nursing Diagnosis Association, St. Louis, Mar 13-16, 1988

Rance, MJ: Multiple opiate receptors—their occurrence and significance, *Clin Anaesthesiol* 1:183-199, Apr 1983

Riordan, MP: Validation of the defining characteristics of the nursing diagnosis, alteration in comfort: pain. In McLane, AM, ed: Classification of nursing diagnoses: proceedings of the seventh conference, pp 221-228, St. Louis, 1987, The CV Mosby Company

Rogmagnoli, A, and Keats, AJS: Ceiling effect for respiratory depression by nalbuphine, *Clin Pharmacol Ther* 27:478-485, Apr 1980

Snyder, SH: Opiate receptors and internal opiates, *Sci Am* 236:44-56, 1977

Tamsen, A, Sakurada, T, Wahlstrom, A, et al: Postoperative demand for analgesics in relation to individual levels of endorphins and substance P in cerebrospinal fluid, *Pain* 13:171-183, 1982

Terenius, L: The endogenous opioids and other central peptides. In Wall, PD, and Melzack, R, eds: Textbook of pain, pp 133-141, Edinburgh, 1984, Churchill Livingstone

Walker, JB, and Katz, RL: Non-opioid pathways suppress pain in humans, *Pain* 11:347-354, 1981

Whipple, B: Methods of pain control: review of research and literature, *Image: J Nurs Scholar* 19:142-146, Fall 1987

Whipple, B, and Komisaruk, BR: Elevation of pain threshold by vaginal stimulation in women, *Pain* 21:357-367, 1985

Wood, PL: Multiple opiate receptors: support for unique mu, delta and kappa sites, *Neuropharmacology* 21:487-497, 1982

Yaksh, TL, Durant, PAC, Gaumann, DM, Stevens, CW, and Mjanger, E: The use of receptor-selective agents as analgesics in the spinal cord: trends and possibilities, *J Pain Sympt Manag* 2:129-138, Summer 1987

Young, RF, and Chambi, VI: Pain relief by electrical stimulation of the periaqueductal and periventricular gray matter. Evidence for a non-opioid mechanism, *J Neurosurg* 66:364-371, 1987

Pharmacological Control of Pain

A Multidisciplinary Approach

What is your role and responsibility in this situation?

Mrs. M. has end-stage breast cancer. She is admitted to your unit for pain control. The admitting orders read:
Demerol 50 mg IM q4h PRN for pain.
You have already assessed Mrs. M.'s pain. You know the dose of Demerol is inadequate and the route and drug choice are inappropriate.

It is unacceptable for health care professionals to allow this kind of undertreatment of pain and inappropriate prescribing to continue. As professionals with a knowledge base in assessment, treatment, and evaluation, nurses must articulate their suggestions for optimal pain control to all members of the health care team. It is our responsibility to obtain the best pain control possible for patients, and it is part of our role to work toward this in whatever clinical setting we practice.

The responsibility for pharmacological control of pain rests with the *entire* health care team. Each member possesses a unique body of information, but some knowledge is shared by all. The key people involved are most often the physician, the nurse, and the patient. Usually all three possess some information about the pharmacology of analgesics, yet each makes a unique contribution to pharmacological control. For example, the physician's prescription of analgesic is influenced by the patient's physical pathology; the nurse's recommendations about

changes in analgesics are based on her assessment of the patient's responses; and the patient, who is the only one who can feel the pain, contributes by communicating information about his pain.

For these reasons, this chapter addresses pharmacological control of pain as a multidisciplinary process. Since the information and recommendations in this chapter are pertinent to all members of the health team, they are not labeled as nursing care guidelines (as they are in other chapters).

The nurse's immediate role and responsibility in the above situation is to communicate her assessment and suggestions effectively to the physician so that Mrs. M. can begin on a medication schedule that satisfies her and that effectively controls the pain.

To assist the nurse in making her significant contribution to the multidisciplinary approach, this chapter presents specific information that enables her to:
• Be knowledgeable in the pharmacological control of pain.
• Be able to effectively communicate this knowledge with the physician and other health team members.
• Cite research and articles that are particularly helpful in documenting a point or backing up a suggestion.

THE ROLE AND RESPONSIBILITY OF THE NURSE

The nurse plays a key role in assuring good pain control for people with unrelieved pain. She is with the patient more than any other health team member and is

■ Generic drug names are used throughout the text. The reader is referred to the inside back cover for a list of frequently used generic and trade names.

Text continued on p. 47.

IMMEDIATE HELP FOR PHARMACOLOGICAL CONTROL OF PAIN

Making the Best of Inadequate Analgesics

Time involved: Reading time, 10 minutes; decision time, 10 to 15 minutes; implementation time, variable.

Sample situation: For Mr. R., 25 years old, this is the fifth day following surgical repair of a gunshot wound to the abdomen. The surgical site is infected, drains were inserted at 8:00 AM, and the patient's pain has not been well controlled during the 8 hours since then.

Analgesics ordered: meperidine 50 mg IM q3h PRN pain; promethazine 50 mg IM q3h PRN pain or nausea; acetaminophen 650 mg PO q4h PRN pain or fever; Percodan (approximately 5 mg oxycodone plus aspirin 325 mg) one tablet q4h PRN mild to moderate pain.

It is 4:00 PM and you have just seen the patient for the first time. He is alert, breathing well (respirations 16 per minute), and tells you his pain is awful now and that today the "pain shots" help even less than before. The medication record shows that he received both meperidine and promethazine at 7:30 AM and 12 noon. The chart includes a notation, made about 1 hour following each injection, that the pain was not relieved. The physician was notified both times, but the orders have not been changed. No side effects were noted. Acetaminophen and Percodan have also been given separately on previous days with poor pain relief but no side effects noted.

Possible solution: While you continue to try to contact the physician, make better use of the available orders.

Expected outcome: Better pain relief, although it probably will not be satisfactory.

DON'Ts

1. Do not tell the patient that the analgesics given should have relieved his pain.
2. Do not tell the patient he simply must endure the pain.
3. Do not tell the patient that postoperative pain should not be severe after 3 days.
4. Do not tell the patient nothing else can be done to help him.
5. Do not tell the patient that narcotics must be tapered to avoid addiction.

DOs

1. Assure the patient you know he hurts as much as he says he does.
2. Tell the patient you will continue to try to contact the physician to get the prescriptions changed.
3. Tell the patient that in the meantime you will try to use the present analgesics in a way that provides somewhat better pain relief.
4. Answers to the following questions are basic to getting better results from inadequate prescriptions. Here they are answered in relation to Mr. R. Use your patient's responses and charted information to document your assessment and the rationale for your actions.
   - Is the patient experiencing any undesirable side effects from the present analgesics? No side effects were noted from meperidine, promethazine, acetaminophen, or Percodan.
   - After the administration of each analgesic, is the patient still in pain? Yes. Document in the chart that following administration of each analgesic no side

effects are noted but pain is not relieved, e.g., following meperidine IM, pain is still mild to moderate. State that Percodan and/or acetaminophen need to be added to relieve the remaining mild to moderate pain. Therefore it appears both safe and necessary to give two or more analgesics at the same time.
   - Is there a medication that may be causing increased pain and therefore should be eliminated? Yes. Research shows that promethazine makes some people more sensitive to pain.
   - How often can the analgesics be given, and can pain be predicted to continue? The prescription allows meperidine every 3 hours and Percodan and acetaminophen every 4 hours. Yes, pain can be expected to be ongoing, i.e., it will return. Document that the PRN prescriptions are needed to relieve and prevent the return of severe pain, and they need to be implemented around the clock, given as often as the order allows.
   - Are any of the analgesics incompatible? That is, are there any analgesics ordered that would be dangerous to combine?

     Giving two or more pure narcotic agonists, such as meperidine and oxycodone, at the same time results in additive analgesia and depressant effects. Document that additive analgesia is needed and that additive depressant effects, e.g., decreased respirations, are not expected since no depressant effects have been noted from the single administration of a narcotic, but both analgesic and depressant effects will be monitored hourly.

     The two nonnarcotics involved, acetaminophen and aspirin, are compatible. Further, combining nonnarcotics with narcotics is a safe and pharmacologically sound method of pain relief. Document that the patient is already receiving a narcotic-nonnarcotic combination (Percodan) with no adverse effects, and that the prescriptions allow the administration of both narcotics and nonnarcotics.

     Document that promethazine is neither a narcotic or nonnarcotic, but is known to be sedating and as a phenothiazine it tends to increase undesirable narcotic side effects such as respiratory depression, sedation, and hypotension. Therefore it will be omitted initially.
   - What can the patient have right now? All of them.
   - Which analgesics are the most effective? Probably, in descending order, meperidine, Percodan, and acetaminophen. Promethazine has no proven value in pain relief.
5. Plan to give as many available analgesics as often as is allowed, as long as it appears to be safe to do so. Keep a flow sheet (p. 27) to document safety and degree of pain relief. Following is the plan for Mr. R.

   4:00 PM—Meperidine 50 mg IM; Percodan one tablet; acetaminophen 650 mg PO.

   6:00 PM—Enough time has elapsed to evaluate the effect of the analgesics administered at 4:00 PM. Now ask the patient if he thinks promethaine would increase or decrease his pain. If

Continued.

Making the Best of Inadequate Analgesics—cont'd.

he thinks it might help, give it, but evaluate it on the flow sheet. If pain relief increases within the next 30 to 60 minutes, plan to give promethazine with meperidine injections, beginning with the 10:00 PM dose.

7:00 PM—Meperidine 50 mg IM (continued q3h at 10 PM, 1:00 AM, etc.).

8:00 PM—Percodan one tablet; acetaminophen 650 mg PO (continued q4h at 12 midnight, 4:00 AM, etc.).

6. Adjust the number and frequency of analgesics given on the basis of the patient's response regarding pain relief and side effects. If he has no side effects and if pain relief is better but still inadequate, continue the above plan of administering as many analgesics as often as possible and continue to try to contact the physician.

7. Show the results of the flow sheet to the physician and to other nurses.
   • Encourage the nurses to continue to use your plan.
   • Encourage the physician to use the information to provide better analgesic prescriptions. Suggest a longer acting narcotic at a more effective dose, e.g., morphine 10 mg IM q3h or a gradual switch to methadone 10 to 20 mg PO or levorphanol 2 to 4 mg PO. Suggest regular administration of all analgesics at frequent enough intervals to keep pain from increasing.

Summary of Guidelines: When Available Analgesics Result in Inadequate Pain Relief, How Can the Nurse Temporarily Make Them Work as Well as Possible?

Caution: Never use these guidelines as a substitute for contacting the patient's physician, persistently presenting to the physician an organized assessment of the patient's response to present analgesic prescriptions, and providing appropriate references that support changes that seem appropriate for the patient.

Purpose of these simple guidelines: To provide *temporary* assistance when available analgesics are not providing adequate pain relief. In reality there are times when a patient is in pain and access to appropriate analgesics is not possible. Multiple reasons for this exist, in both hospital and home care. The physician may not agree to change the prescriptions, he may be temporarily unavailable for consultation, or he may prescribe analgesics that are not available in that community or at that time (nights and weekends are especially difficult). The patient may have lost his medication or run out because he failed to have it refilled.

Simple guides to improving pain relief when existing analgesics are inadequate revolve around two questions:

1. *What are the logical choices?*
   • *Look at all medications the patient is currently taking.*

   • *Identify all narcotic and nonnarcotic analgesics.* If they have been prescribed they can usually be given simultaneously or alternately, but review exceptions below.
   • *Identify any narcotics that are incompatible.* This is rarely a problem. All pure narcotic agonists may be given simultaneously. Such practice is safe and fairly common, but it is not necessarily rational. However, clinicians seem to feel safer giving relatively small doses of several different narcotics than giving a large dose of one narcotic. Simply be aware that over time narcotic agonist-antagonists (Stadol, Talwin, and Nubain) given along with pure narcotics may reduce the analgesia of pure narcotics, so discontinue one or the other. Most of the time, after a few days of administration, it is best to choose the pure narcotic, but not always.
   • *Identify any nonnarcotics that are incompatible.* Although most of the current concern is that one nonnarcotic, especially aspirin, will decrease the effectiveness of another, the most serious danger is that chronic simultaneous use of more than one nonnarcotic will increase side effects. Certainly, for a few days there seems to be little danger in simultaneous administration of nonnarcotics, especially acetaminophen with any other nonnarcotic.
   • *Identify any drug given as a "potentiator" of narcotic analgesia, and consider eliminating it.* Most popular "potentiators" are most accurately viewed as sedatives, tranquilizers, or antiemetics. Some popular potentiators merely sedate, and some, such as the phenothiazines, actually increase pain and potentiate narcotic-related side effects. When additional analgesia is needed, most of the time the most effective and safest approach is simply to increase the narcotic dose, rather than add a so-called potentiator. Never confuse sedation with pain relief.
   • *Give narcotics with nonnarcotics.* This is logical and safe, particularly if the patient has taken both without incident.

   If a given nonnarcotic is safe for the individual and if a given narcotic is safe for the individual, there is absolutely no known reason to suspect that simultaneous administration of both narcotic and nonnarcotic will pose any danger. There is every reason to suspect that the combination will be beneficial and safe.

2. *Once you identify the rational choices, what do you do?*
   • Give narcotics and nonnarcotics on a regular basis around the clock, maintaining the best analgesic blood level you can.
   • Evaluate safety and effectiveness with the flow sheet, and adjust dose, interval, and drug choice accordingly.

IMMEDIATE HELP FOR PHARMACOLOGICAL CONTROL OF PAIN

Patient in Home Care Setting Unexpectedly Unable to Take Oral Analgesics

Time involved: Reading time, 4 minutes; implementation time, about 10 minutes.

Situation: Patient of any age being cared for at home with moderate to severe pain controlled with oral analgesics is now unexpectedly unable to swallow or has uncontrolled nausea and vomiting. His next dose of analgesics is due in 1 hour, and he cannot take it orally, even in liquid form. Moderate to severe pain will occur unless analgesics can be administered by another route, but no provision has been made for this, e.g., there are no drugs or equipment for IM, SC, IV, or rectal administration. It would take 2 hours or longer to obtain such drugs or equipment. How can the oral analgesics he has been taking be used to provide pain relief now?

Possible solution: Take all oral forms of analgesics due in the next oral dose, dissolve them in warm water, and administer rectally.

Expected outcome: Pain relief will be satisfactory, but perhaps not ideal. Pain may increase somewhat, but moderate to severe pain will not occur.

How to Use Oral Analgesics Rectally in an Emergency

- Obtain the physician's approval for changing the route of administration.
- Instruct the patient or family via telephone or do this yourself if you are in the home at the time:
  1. Assemble all the oral analgesics to be given at the next dose, including narcotics and nonnarcotics.
  2. Review the ingredients and formulations.
  Caution: The only known exception to the following instructions concerns sustained-release formulations. Be especially alert to sustained-release morphine (MS Contin, Roxanol SR). If sustained-release morphine is included, administer only a portion of the dose due since dissolving the tablets will convert morphine to immediate-release morphine with a duration of approximately 4 hours. Thus if sustained-release morphine doses are given every 8 hours, each dose would be divided in half and given every 4 hours.

  Although there is no research to support this practice, many home care nurses report that satisfactory analgesia can be obtained from any of the oral analgesics by converting them to the rectal route as explained here. Some medications are more irritating than others, but hopefully this is only a temporary measure. Oral analgesics given rectally with successful pain relief include tablets of oxycodone plus acetaminophen, hydromorphone, liquid or tablets of morphine, methadone, and several of the NSAIDs.
  3. Place the tablets in a small, but strong container, e.g., cup, and crush them with the bowl of a small spoon.
  4. Measure a teaspoon (5 ml), or more if necessary, of very hot tap water. Pour over the crushed tablets. Mix or crush further until fairly well dissolved. Let it sit while you find the equipment needed to insert it into the rectum. It should be about body temperature when it is inserted. Warm again if it gets cold or hardens.
  5. Several types of equipment may be improvised for rectal insertion of the liquid. An ideal arrangement is a syringe with a short length of small-lumen rubber catheter attached. If this is not available, any of the following will suffice if the patient is placed in a position where gravity can assist, e.g., bending over or lying on his side:
     a. Any equipment used to administer enemas. The main problem is likely to be that the tubing is so long that some of the medication is lost by adhering to the sides of the tubing. Using more water to dissolve the tablets may help.
     b. Douche equipment, with some modification of the usual tip for insertion. Again, long tubing may be a problem.
     c. Baster (pointed tube with bulb attached, often used for basting turkey) or rubber ear syringe (not used much anymore, but it has a small rubber tip and a bulb). With either of these, immediately prior to insertion into the rectum, suction up the liquid, point the open end upward, and squeeze out as much air as possible without losing the liquid. Maintain that amount of bulb compression until the tube is inserted in the rectum. Then compress completely and withdraw.
     d. Any clean, small lumen rubber tubing attached to a funnel.
     e. If all else fails, a plastic straw may be attached to a funnel shaped of aluminum foil or wax paper.
  6. Lubricate the end of the tubing prior to insertion. A water-soluble lubricant (e.g., K-Y Jelly) is best, but if it is not available, use a small amount of any lubricant such as Vaseline, butter, or cooking oil.
  7. Slowly insert the tube about 1½ inches into the rectum.
  8. After the liquid has been inserted, position the patient on his left side for better absorption.
  9. Get a pain rating from the patient at the time the medication is given rectally, and then at half-hour intervals. If pain is not relieved or has increased after 1 hour, give another dose rectally. If there is no relief after 1 hour, consider giving 50% to 100% of the previous rectal dose. If there is some relief but not enough, consider giving an additional 25% of the previous dose.

Quick Alternatives to Liquid Form of Rectal Administration

1. Except for sustained-release tablets, the tablets or capsules themselves may simply be inserted about 1½ inches into the rectum. If lubricant is necessary, moisten with water or use a water-soluble lubricant such as K-Y Jelly. Absorption takes longer, since the tablets must first dissolve, and seems less reliable than the liquid formulation. However, small tablets or those without a coating may work well.
2. If the volume is small, put the crushed tablet in an empty capsule. Simply empty any capsule for use unless the patient is allergic to whatever it contained. Again, absorption may take longer than with the liquid formulation.

IMMEDIATE HELP FOR PHARMACOLOGICAL CONTROL OF PAIN

Maximal Use of Nonprescription Analgesics when Prescription Analgesics Are Unavailable*

Time involved: Reading time, 3 minutes; implementation time, after ingredients are obtained, 5 minutes.

Situation: Unexpected moderate to severe pain of known cause, e.g., dislocated shoulder or broken bone from accidental fall, occurring in a healthy adult patient. A physician is contacted, but it will be 2 hours or longer before the patient can be seen by the physician. Also, due to time, location, and other factors, it is not possible to obtain any prescription analgesic. Using nonprescription analgesics available from a general store, what can be done to obtain maximal analgesia on a one-time only basis?

Possible solution: Consider a combination of the following, if available, and obtain the physician's consent.

Expected outcome: Significant pain relief, but it may not be sufficient.

Maximal Pain Relief with Nonprescription Drugs

1. Acetaminophen 1000 mg in liquid form, if possible, or tablets (three regular tablets or two "extra strength" tablets).
2. Ibuprofen 800 mg (four tablets of 200 mg each).
3. Antacid (1 teaspoon of a concentrated liquid, if possible).
4. Caffeine 100 to 200 mg (a strong cup of brewed coffee, or one to two "keep awake" nonprescription tablets).
5. Carbonated beverage, e.g., 7-Up, or one with caffeine, e.g., Pepsi.
6. Alcohol, e.g., wine, gin. (Many social drinks combine a carbonated beverage with alcohol, e.g., gin and tonic. A social drink may be relaxing or distracting.)

Caution: Use of the above should be restricted to emergencies or "one time only." Consult a physician and determine the patient's previous response to each ingredient. Drugs that have produced unwanted side effects should be eliminated.

Rationale: No research supports the safety or effectiveness of the above combination. Separate research studies suggest that these ingredients would be an effective combination, and they are pharmacologically compatible, i.e., they may be given together. Regarding each item, the rationale is as follows:

1. Acetaminophen relieves pain in a manner different from other nonnarcotics. It is well tolerated, i.e., side effects are unlikely. Combinations of acetaminophen and aspirin have been approved for sale as nonprescription analgesics. Patients on NSAIDs are allowed to take acetaminophen.

2. Ibuprofen is an NSAID somewhat similar to aspirin but better tolerated, e.g., fewer GI upsets. The maximal recommended single dose of ibuprofen when it is prescribed by a physician is 800 mg. (The nonprescription recommended dose is limited to 400 mg.) If ibuprofen is unavailable or undesirable for any reason, aspirin can be substituted in a dose of 1000 mg. Aspirin could be given along with ibuprofen and the other ingredients. Omitting it from the above list may be unnecessary, but it could increase the risk of GI upset and it could decrease the effectiveness of the ibuprofen (probably to a limited extent). There are no data on the combination of ibuprofen and aspirin as a single dose. They are sometimes combined in the treatment of rheumatoid arthritis. The recommendation in this instance to give either aspirin or ibuprofen, but not both, is merely a qualified guess. On a single dose basis for analgesia only, ibuprofen may do what aspirin does but with fewer side effects. Adding aspirin to the ibuprofen may increase the risks more than the analgesia (possibly is a duplication of effort).

3. Antacids are recommended in combination with NSAIDs to prevent stomach upset. Antacids may also hasten the absorption of NSAIDs.

4. Caffeine, in doses of 100 to 200 mg, has been shown to increase the effectiveness of both acetaminophen and aspirin. If the patient does not ordinarily consume caffeine beverages, he probably is not tolerant to them so the dose should be kept to the minimum of 100 mg to prevent side effects, such as nervousness. If the patient is a regular user of caffeine, e.g., 4 cups or more of coffee a day, the larger dose of 200 mg may be advisable.

5. Carbonation seems to result in a much faster onset of action, probably by helping to dissolve tablets and promoting absorption.

6. Alcohol has some analgesic as well as tranquilizing and sedating properties. If the patient drinks alcohol enough to be familiar with his response to it, it can be given in the amount usually tolerated. However, it does increase the likelihood of GI irritation, especially along with aspirin.

Nausea or anxiety: If the patient has a history of vomiting in response to varied stimuli (a "weak stomach"), give a nonprescription antiemetic or sedative. Most over-the-counter (OTC) antiemetics are sedating. Sedation alone may decrease nausea or anxiety. An OTC product for "motion sickness" or anything for an allergy or cold may help, e.g., one that contains diphenhydramine (Benadryl). There is some indication that diphenhydramine is analgesic or potentiates analgesia. If needed, give it prior to or along with the analgesic combination.

---

*Or, when the physician won't return your call, when the physician has refused to prescribe anything, when the pharmacy loses the prescription, or other frustrating situations.

in a position to constantly assess and evaluate the effectiveness of the pain treatments.

Nursing behaviors that result in an *active role* in the use of medications for pain control include:
- Choosing the appropriate analgesic.
- Determining whether to give it.
- Evaluating its effectiveness.
- Obtaining a change in analgesic prescriptions if needed.

These behaviors involve the application of assessment skills and knowledge about analgesics to each individual patient situation. Table 4-1 elaborates on the nurse's role in relation to medications for pain relief.

Nurses also often suggest changes in analgesics. To accomplish this effectively, the following areas must be addressed:

1. *Articulate a concise pain assessment.* Continuing with the example on p. 42, the nurse might report "Mrs. M. rates her pain at 9 on a 0 to 10 scale (0 = no pain, 10 = worst pain). Upon movement her pain increases to 10. The best the pain gets is 6 when she lies totally still. Pain does not get below 6 even after she takes meperidine 50 mg IM q4h. She has been without sleep for the last 2 days because of the pain.

2. *Use an equianalgesic chart when suggesting dose changes.* This is discussed in detail starting on pp. 76-80. Tables 4-4 and 4-11 (pp. 61 and 78-79) list equianalgesic doses for mild to moderate and moderate to severe pain.

Share a copy of these tables with physicians and other health team members. Have them available, especially Table 4-11, so that they are easily accessible, e.g., post one in a central place such as the medication room or chart room in your clinical setting. Carry one with you. A laminated pocket-size one is provided inside the front cover for your convenience.

3. *Supply reference and research articles to back up suggestions.* In Mrs. M.'s case, and for any patient receiving meperidine, the following articles might be made available to the physician and other health team members:

> Kaiko, R, et al: Central nervous system excitatory effects of meperidine in cancer patients, *Ann Neurol* 13: 180-185, Feb 1983. This article discusses the potential toxic effects and mood changes associated with meperidine.
> McCaffery, M: Problems with meperidine, *Am J Nurs* 84:525, Apr 1984. Reviews Kaiko's article and discusses clinical implications of inappropriate use of meperidine.
> McCaffery, M: Giving meperidine for pain—should it be so mechanical? *Nursing* 17:61-64, Apr 1987.

4. *Address misconceptions held by the health care provider, patient, and family.* In Mrs. M.'s case, or any patient on IMs and/or narcotics, these might include the following (both of these misconceptions are discussed in greater detail later in this chapter):

TABLE 4-1 Nurse's Power and Responsibility in Relation to Medication for Pain Relief

Nurse is Expected to:	Comments
1. Determine whether the analgesic is to be given and, if so, when.	1. Many analgesics are on PRN basis (PRN means use clinical judgment). Assess and apply knowledge. Based on this assessment, a PRN analgesic order may be given around the clock (ATC), on a regular basis, e.g., q3h.
2. Choose the appropriate analgesic(s) when more than one is ordered.	2. More than one analgesic is often available. Which one does the nurse give? Two at the same time? Avoid one? This decision is based on pharmacological knowledge along with skills in assessment and evaluation.
3. Be alert to the possibility of certain side effects as a result of the analgesic.	3. Nurse plays key role in identifying life-threatening side effects, e.g., respiratory depression. Identifies constipation, which can seriously influence patient's comfort as much as pain itself.
4. Evaluate effectiveness of analgesic at regular frequent intervals following each administration, but especially the inital dose.	4. This is a vital step in ensuring effective pain control. Assessment and evaluation are continuous processes. A flow sheet is recommended.
5. Report promptly and accurately to the physician when a change is needed.	5. Every new prescription of analgesic for the individual patient is merely a guess that must be evaluated. Too small a dosage should be changed as quickly as too large a dosage.
6. Make suggestions for specific changes, e.g., drug, route, dosage, and interval.	6. The nurse has unique blend of knowledge: pharmacological information and direct observation of patient. The result is that nurse is in ideal position to make an educated guess about what may work better for the individual patient.
7. Advise the patient about the use of analgesics, both prescription and nonprescription.	7. Nurse has a key educational role about dosage, side effects, addressing misconceptions, preventive schedule, and how to talk with physician or nurse about questions or problems with drug.

Misconception: Injections are the most effective route of medication for severe pain.

Correction: PO route is the first choice and can control severe pain *if:*

- Patient can swallow.
- Nausea and vomiting is controlled.
- Use preventive approach.
- Use high enough dose.

Misconception: Pain medication taken regularly will result in Mrs. M. becoming addicted.

Correction: Addiction does not occur when people are taking pain medication to relieve pain. The majority of people stop taking pain medication when the pain stops.

5. *Never give up approaching physicians.* Although the ultimate power to change analgesic regimens lies legally with the physician, nurses must continue to suggest changes based on assessment, consistent evaluation of the patient's response, and knowledge of pharmacology, supported by current references from the literature. It is our responsibility as professionals to assure that the control of pain is a priority in health care. Re-education is difficult and frustrating. However, *persistence is the key,* with the ultimate goal being effective pain control through the appropriate use of analgesics and adjuvant medications.

KEY CONCEPTS IN ANALGESIC THERAPY

How an analgesic is used is probably more important than which one is used. The following three key concepts for effective analgesic therapy apply to both acute and chronic pain.

1. Use a Preventive Approach

Stay on top of the pain. This approach has been the mainstay for treatment of prolonged pain from cancer (Foley and Inturrisi, 1987; Levy, 1985). It is also recommended for acute pain, such as the control of postoperative pain (Rutter et al, 1980). A preventive approach means that the analgesic is given before pain occurs or before it increases, i.e.:

- ATC (Around The Clock at regularly scheduled intervals). If pain occurs consistently and predictably throughout a 24-hour period, then ATC is appropriate. This may mean waking the patient at night to take the analgesic if pain usually awakens him at night or if he awakens in the morning with pain out of control.
- PRN (as needed, requires nursing assessment and evaluation). PRN dosing should be used to prevent pain from occurring or increasing. Some pain cannot be predicted, so occasional dosing, rather than scheduled dosing may be appropriate, but it too should be used preventively *as soon as* pain begins and *before* it gets out of control.

If ongoing pain can be predicted, the analgesic that is

Benefits of a Preventive Approach with Analgesics

1. Patient spends less time in pain.
   Result: Can direct energy to restoring health, e.g., ambulation, physical therapy, immediate postoperative activities of turning, coughing, and deep breathing.
2. Doses of analgesic can be lower than if pain is allowed to increase or become severe.
3. Fewer side effects due to lower dose.
4. Decreased anxiety about return of pain, erases memory of pain and stops fearful anticipation of its return.
5. Decreased concern about obtaining relief when needed.
   Result: Decrease in craving the drug for pain relief, prevents "clockwatching" behavior.
6. Overall increase in activities.

---

prescribed PRN should be implemented around the clock.

Patient Example

Postoperative orders for Mrs. A. include pain medication every 3 to 4 hours PRN. By assessing Mrs. A.'s pain, the nurse establishes that it regularly returns about every 3 hours. Based on this information, the nurse gives the pain medication on a regular 3-hour schedule. To assure the safety and effectiveness of this regimen, assessment and evaluation of Mrs. A.'s pain and response continue.

KEY POINT: Teach patient to request pain medication as soon as pain occurs or *before* it increases.

Patient Example

Mr. S. is scheduled for total hip replacement. The nurse teaches Mr. S. the 0 to 10 scale (0 = no pain, 10 = worst pain) preoperatively so that he is familiar with the scale and can use it postoperatively to rate his pain. It is apparent that at a rating of 4, Mr. S.'s pain begins to escalate quickly. He asks for pain medication at this rating and finds he is able to stay comfortable. The nurse regularly evaluates this plan with Mr. S., thereby assuring continuous and effective pain control.

The box above summarizes the benefits of a preventive approach in the scheduling of analgesic medication.

2. Titrate to Effect

Adjust and individualize the analgesic for each patient. The effect desired is pain relief with the fewest side effects. This involves tailoring analgesics by adjusting the following.

Dose

Patient Example

After a dose of medication, Mrs. A. rates her pain at 8 on the 0 to 10 scale, and her respirations have remained stable between 18 and 20. The next time it is administered the narcotic dose is titrated up to obtain better pain control.

Interval between Doses

Patient Example

Mr. P. states that his pain is at about 3 on the 0 to 10 scale. He notices that after 3 hours the pain increases quickly, and by the time the 4-hour interval is up his pain is at 7. It takes him longer and longer each time to get comfortable again. The interval between narcotic doses is changed to q3h.

Route of Administration

Patient Example

Mr. B. is admitted to the hospital because his pain suddenly increases at home and PO oxycodone and aspirin (Percodan) did not relieve the pain below 9. For the past 2 days he has been unable to sleep because of the pain. The goal now is to get Mr. B. comfortable quickly with an IV continuous infusion (CI) of narcotic while diagnostic studies are being done. Allow him to get some sleep without pain, then titrate back onto an appropriate equivalent PO narcotic and nonnarcotic in preparation to discharge home.

Choice of Drug

Patient Example

Mr. F. states that meperidine 75 mg IM helps his post-operative pain, but it wears off in 2 hours. He also notices that he feels "jumpy" and that this same feeling resulted from the analgesic he got during his last surgery. Because of the short duration of analgesia felt by Mr. F. and the possible cumulative effects of an active metabolite of meperidine in his system (see p. 84), the meperidine was stopped. Using an equianalgesic chart, the physician prescribed a dose of morphine more effective than 75 mg meperidine, i.e., 15 mg morphine IM, and a nonnarcotic analgesic, acetaminophen 650 mg, was added.

KEY POINT: The only safe and effective way to administer analgesics is to watch the individual's response to the drug. Use a pain medication flow sheet to monitor these responses (see p. 27 for an example).

3. Patient Controlled Analgesia (PCA)

The person who feels the pain is the person who must have, to the extent possible, control of all measures to relieve it. It is essential to remember that pain can only be felt by the person who has it.

In its broadest sense, the key concept of PCA may be defined as the patient's self-administration of all forms of pain control by methods that consider safety, as well as the patient's ability and willingness to exercise control. The person with pain is not always able to understand or do much regarding pain control, but with guidance and safety precautions, the following aspects of pain control are determined by the patient as a result of his direct action, his directions to others, or carefully monitored indications of need:

• Start or stop a form of pain relief.
• Increase or decrease the amount of pain relief.

Patient Example

Mrs. F., age 62, is admitted for orthopedic surgery. She is a possible candidate for IV PCA postoperatively. The nurse explains that her analgesia will be administered IV after surgery, with a continuous amount of medication adjusted for ongoing pain relief and additional increases given as boluses for brief episodes of pain, such as may occur with movement. The nurse explains that she will be asked to rate her pain on a 0 to 10 scale so that the continuous infusion can be adjusted, but that she can give herself her own boluses when she needs them by simply pressing a button.

When the nurse asks the patient if she would like to administer her own boluses, the patient replies "No, I don't think so. I'm afraid I'll be drowsy or confused after the operation. I might give myself too much or forget what to do. I'll feel safer if the nurses give it." This patient chooses not to use the PCA machine, but her analgesic administration is still under her control. The nurse operates the machinery, so to speak, but the patient still identifies the need. The patient is in control of what the nurse does within the limits of safety. The nurse not only administers boluses when the patient requests them (if it is safe) but also monitors the patient carefully and asks for pain ratings rather than waiting for the patient to request medication.

Clinical Implementation and Patient Teaching

Although the key concepts of a preventive approach, individualizing the medication and enabling the patient to control his care, are used in virtually all health-illness situations, their application to pain control often sounds like a totally new idea. Unlike many other health care problems, pain is subjective—it cannot be objectively measured, touched, or seen. Further, people have exaggerated fears about one of the major methods of controlling pain—narcotics. For these reasons it is often difficult to implement concepts for pain control that are commonly used elsewhere.

An analogy is sometimes helpful in explaining to the health team the wisdom of prevention of pain and individualizing pain relief, especially with narcotics. Controlling diabetes may be compared with controlling pain. Health care professionals and most laymen are aware that diabetes may need to be controlled by daily doses of insulin. These doses are given preventively to avoid a return of the symptoms of diabetes. The dosage of insulin is carefully titrated in accordance with the individual's response. Hence, it would be insulting to approach health care professionals about the care of the diabetic by reminding them that insulin should be given before the patient develops diabetic coma and that the same dose of insulin should not be given to every diabetic. Equally absurd is the reminder that we do not tell the diabetic that no matter how high his blood sugar level is, he cannot receive any more insulin and he must handle this some other way.

What is done in the care of the person with diabetes is not very different from what is advocated in the care of the person with pain. We want to provide pain relief before pain returns and individualize the dosage. A reminder of the analogy of the diabetic is sometimes helpful when a preventive approach or titration of a drug fails to be implemented clinically. For example, when health care professionals are tempted to put an arbitrary limit on the dosage or frequency of narcotic, the analogy with insulin can be used. Telling a patient who is in severe pain but alert and breathing well that he cannot have any more narcotic is just as senseless as placing a limit on the insulin dosage regardless of the blood sugar level.

Another example of applying the diabetic analogy is in relation to using a preventive approach with narcotics. If the patient is on scheduled doses of narcotic ATC, the nurse giving the change of shift report may tell you that the last dose of narcotic due 2 hours previously was not given because the patient was not in pain. This nurse might be reminded of the diabetic analogy. You may add that just as we do not wait for the diabetic to feel poorly before giving insulin, we try not to wait until the patient is in pain before giving the narcotic. If the reason for not giving the narcotic is that the patient was sleeping, you may add that if the prescription had been for insulin (or antibiotics, digoxin), 2 hours would not have elapsed before giving the dose. The patient would have been awakened because we have a better appreciation of preventing the return of symptoms and maintaining a blood level with other drugs than we do with narcotics.

Some of the most common misunderstandings about the key concepts of prevention and titration are related to the high doses of narcotic that may occur and the reasons for ATC versus PRN dosing. These areas concern both the health team and the patient and his family. They are explained more fully below, along with patient/family teaching tools (see boxes on pp. 51 and 53).

Dosage of Narcotic—Is There a Limit?

Question: The authors are frequently asked "What is the highest dose of narcotic that I can give?"

Answer: There is no answer to that question in terms of milligrams, because there is no set optimal or maximal

---

Titrate to Effect: Dose and Interval

What is it? Titrating the analgesic dose and interval means finding the lowest dose and longest interval of a drug that relieves pain to the patient's satisfaction with minimal side effects.

How do you do it? Use a flow sheet and look at the following patient responses, in the following order:
- First, respiratory function, e.g., rate.
- Second, pain rating.
- Third, based on the above, determine what should be done with the number of milligrams of analgesic the patient is receiving. *The last thing you look at are the milligrams being given; look at effect first.*

Example of titrating up: If the patient is breathing well, e.g., 12/minute, with a pain rating of 8 on a 0 to 10 scale, the milligrams of analgesic should be increased probably by 50% to 100% (see p. 95 for discussion of percentages).

Example of titrating down due to problems with respiratory function: If the patient's respiratory rate has dropped from 12 to 6/minute during the hour following IV narcotic administration, the milligrams of analgesic should be decreased, probably by 50%, and possibly even discontinued until respiratory rate improves.

Example of titrating down due to excessive pain relief or side effects: If the patient's respiratory rate is 14/minute, he complains of sedation, i.e., he cannot continue a conversation without falling asleep, and he rates his pain at 0 to 1 on 0 to 10 scale, reduce the milligrams of analgesic, e.g., by 20%.

---

dosage of narcotic (Levy, 1985). The dosage that should be used is the one that controls the pain to the satisfaction of the patient with minimal side effects. For some patients this may be 10 mg PO morphine q4h, for others it may be 480 mg/hr IV morphine (Portenoy et al, 1986) or 50 mg/hr IV hydromorphone (Dilaudid) (Levy, 1985).

The fear behind this question on dose really concerns safety, i.e., "What is the highest dose of narcotic that I can *safely* give?" Again, because each patient reacts to medication differently, there is no maximal number of milligrams that will apply to every individual. The following points can, however, facilitate the safe administration of narcotics.

Use a pain flow sheet (p. 27) to monitor the patient's responses, specifically pain rating and side effects, e.g., respiratory rate. Nurses readily titrate down when a narcotic dosage is too high for the individual patient. All we are suggesting is that titration be in the upward direction when analgesia is inadequate, and it is safe for the individual. For example, if you give morphine 10 mg IM and the patient has complete pain relief, becomes sedated, and his respirations drop from 12 to 6, you would no doubt *lower* the next dose of morphine. Conversely, if you give

---

Patient/Family Teaching Point: Your Pain Medication Dose

TO: _____ (patient's name)   DATE: _____

Information about Pain Medication Dose

Your pain medication(s):

• _____

• _____

• _____

Other health care professionals may question the dosage of pain medication you are taking. This may leave you feeling that they doubt your pain or that you "should not be taking" that amount. Remember if your pain is controlled with this dosage, then it is the right one for you—one that you, your doctor, and nurse have adjusted and tailored just for you. Other people who question this dosage are not fully informed about your individual case and treatment.

Additional comments: _____

_____

If you have any questions about the above, contact:

_____ (RN or MD name)   Phone: _____

■ May be duplicated for use in clinical practice. From McCaffery, M, and Beebe, A: PAIN: CLINICAL MANUAL FOR NURSING PRACTICE, St. Louis, 1989, The CV Mosby Company.

---

that same dose of morphine 10 mg IM and the patient has minimal relief, is fully alert, and maintains his previous respiratory rate of 14, you should *increase* the next dose.

Specific aspects of "titrate to effect" are explained in the box on p. 50 and a tool for patient/family teaching is provided above.

ATC Dosing vs. PRN

Pain that continuously recurs requires analgesics on a regular schedule (see p. 48). The purpose is to stay on top of the pain, keeping the patient as comfortable as possible all of the time and preventing the pain from escalating out of control. A successful preventive approach breaks the cycle of pain and anxiety and eases the fearful anticipation of pain. Figures 4-1 and 4-2 illustrate the concept of a continuous level of analgesia vs. the peaks and valleys that can occur with PRN dosing. A tool for teaching the patient and his family is in the box on p. 53.

KEY POINT: (1) Patients are usually not aware that they must ask for pain medication. If PRN dosing is used, initiate teaching about this early in the course of treatment, e.g., preoperatively. (2) When narcotics

are withheld from people who need them for pain relief, the result is clock-watching behavior (see p. 69 for further discussion).

Taking medication on an "as needed" or PRN schedule may be appropriate in instances when the pain is incidental, intermittent, or unpredictable. However, even in this instance, education of patient and family is vital to effective analgesia. The individual must know to take or ask for the medication as soon as the pain begins and before the pain becomes severe. PRN medication may be used to supplement regular analgesic doses when a particular activity is known to cause pain. The following two examples illustrate this concept.

Patient Examples

1. During her hospitalization, Mrs. J. begins radiation therapy treatments. Although her pain is well controlled on morphine 30 mg PO q4h ATC, movement associated with the treatment increases her pain to 8 on a 0 to 10 scale (0 = no pain, 10 = worst pain). Morphine 15 mg IV PRN before radiation therapy treatment helped prevent pain on movement from increasing above 4. The IV route was chosen for PRN medication because treat-

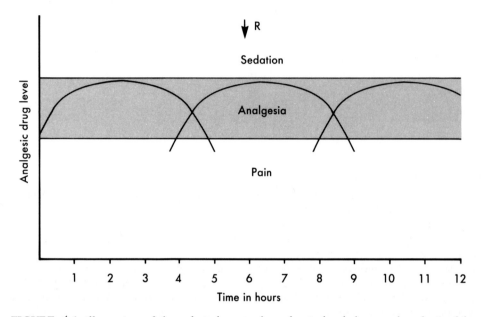

FIGURE 4-1 Illustration of the relatively smooth analgesic level that can be obtained by individualizing the dose and using an ATC approach with PO, IM, or SC analgesics. Analgesics are administered before the pain returns; ideally no noticeable peaks and valleys occur. That is, the drug level does not rise above what is required for analgesia, causing side effects such as sedation and respiratory depression; and the drug level does not fall below what is required for analgesia, causing increasing pain.

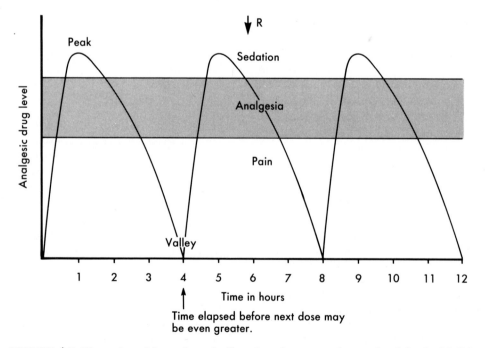

FIGURE 4-2 Illustration of the peaks and valleys that often occur when analgesia by the PO, IM, or SC route is given in the traditional PRN manner that requires the patient to wait for the return of pain before requesting or obtaining the next dose of analgesic.

Patient/Family Teaching Point: Preventive Approach with Pain Medication

---

TO: _____ (patient's name)   DATE: _____

Your Pain Medication(s):

• _____

• _____

• _____

Important Points about Pain Medication

• If you are in the hospital, you may have to ask the nurse for pain medication. Do not assume that it is included with your other pills and do not assume that the nurse knows when you hurt; you must tell her.
• Ask the doctor or nurse how your pain medication is ordered for you.
• Your pain medication may be scheduled to be given or taken regularly at certain hours. However, if it is not, ask for it, and let the nurse know when the pain *first starts*.
• If you are at home, take the medication when you first notice the pain.
• Do not wait until the pain is bad before you call for or take the pain medication. Trying to "wait a little longer" only allows the pain to get worse and means that it will take longer to control it and you may need higher doses of medication if it becomes severe.
• You may be holding off because you are worried about getting "hooked" on the medication. Remember you are taking the medication for a medical reason: pain relief. When the pain stops, the overwhelming majority of people stop taking the medication.
• Tell the nurse or doctor if the medicine does not help the pain so they can adjust it until you are comfortable.

Additional comments: _____

_____

If you have any questions about the above, contact:

_____ (RN or MD name)   Phone: _____

_____ (Nurse's signature)

■ May be duplicated for use in clinical practice. From McCaffery, M, and Beebe, A: PAIN: CLINICAL MANUAL FOR NURSING PRACTICE, St. Louis, 1989, The CV Mosby Company.

---

ment time changed each day and something was needed that started to work immediately.

2. Ambulation increases Mr. T.'s pain to 6 on the 0 to 10 scale. The home health nurse encouraged his wife to have him take an extra dose of oxycodone and acetaminophen (Percocet) about 1 hour before his daily walk. With further assessment, the additional Percocet dose was stopped because of dizziness during walking. Mr. T. had fewer side effects and the pain was well controlled by taking only plain acetaminophen 650 mg before his walk.

In the hospital setting, an analgesic is typically ordered "PRN for pain." Unfortunately this "as needed for pain" prescription allows many different interpretations, with the medication often given only when the pain becomes severe. Understanding and applying the preventive approach to pain control results in a consistent interpretation of PRN prescriptions and better analgesia for the patient.

Patient Example

Analgesics continue to be prescribed "PRN pain" on a surgical unit despite the nurses' attempt to educate physicians to change to ATC dosing for the first 48 hours postoperatively. Physicians' prescriptions for an analgesic q3h were *implemented* in the nursing care plan as ATC after assessment of each individual's response to the first dose.

To assure effective analgesia, the nurses used a pain medication flow sheet, consistent assessment, and concise documentation to support their administering PRN medication on an ATC schedule. For example, if pain relief was adequate but lasted no longer than 3 hours, the following was written in the nursing care plan:

Give analgesic q3h ATC to prevent severe pain for the next 24 hours: 9 AM-12 N-3 PM-6 PM-12 MN-3AM-6AM. Re-evaluate patient's pain rating at 9 AM.

Patient Teaching Regarding PCA

Not all patients are candidates for PCA, especially via IV, SC, or spinal route. Some patients are not able to understand instructions, and others do not feel confident handling their own analgesia or the technical aspects of the pump. However, our belief is that the patient should be given as much information as he can understand about his analgesic delivery system, even when it is not in his direct control.

Certainly when the patient is given direct control, e.g., to initiate boluses, the patient should be told how often he can administer the bolus, whether he will receive a dose each time he makes an attempt, what the drug is, and the dose. (Some pumps deliver a dose in proportion to the amount of time that has elapsed if the full lockout interval has not elapsed.) Bell tones or other noises that occur when a bolus is initiated should never be used to fool the patient into thinking he has received a dose when he has not.

In addition, explain the concept of prevention to the patient and instruct him to keep his pain under control by administering additional medication as soon as pain begins to return or increase or prior to a painful event, e.g., pain on ambulation. Leave instructions for whom to notify if the medication seems too much or if pain relief is not satisfactory.

PHARMACOLOGICAL INTERVENTIONS

This chapter discusses three main types of pharmacological interventions for pain relief: (1) nonnarcotic analgesics or nonsteroidal antiinflammatory drugs (NSAIDs), (2) narcotic analgesics or opioids, and (3) adjuvant analgesics. A summary of these three analgesic groups can be found in the box above. Certainly not all of these are appropriate for all patients with pain, and for each drug there are specific contraindications. However, general suggestions for situations or patients with painful problems most likely to benefit from various pharmacological approaches along with possible problems and limitations are listed at the beginning of the discussion of each of the three groups. These suggestions are based on the definitions and classifications of pain appearing in Chapter 2 on assessment (p. 19).

Nonnarcotic Analgesics (NSAIDs)
Indications for Nonnarcotics

Examples of situations in which nonnarcotics, especially NSAIDs, may help relieve pain are:

Three Main Groups of Analgesics

1. Nonnarcotics or nonsteroidal antiinflammatory drugs (NSAIDs) (pp. 54-66)—work primarily at the peripheral nervous system level:
   a. Over the counter (OTC)—mainly ASA, acetaminophen (e.g., Tylenol), and ibuprofen (Advil, Nuprin, 200 mg tablets).
   b. Prescription, e.g., ibuprofen (Motrin), naproxen (Naprosyn), and indomethacin (Indocin).
2. Narcotics or opioids (pp. 66-113)—work primarily at the CNS level:
   a. Narcotic agonists, e.g., morphine, meperidine (Demerol), hydromorphone (Dilaudid), levorphanol (Levo-Dromoran), oxymorphone (Numorphan), and codeine.
   b. Narcotic agonist-antagonists, e.g., pentazocine (Talwin), nalbuphine (Nubain), butorphanol (Stadol), and buprenorphine (Buprenex).
3. Adjuvant analgesics (pp. 113-123)—various mechanisms of action:
   a. Anticonvulsants, e.g., phenytoin (Dilantin) and carbamazepine (Tegretol).
   b. Antidepressants, e.g., amitryptyline (Elavil) and imipramine (Tofranil).
   c. Others, e.g., caffeine and dextroamphetamine.

- Highly inflammatory conditions such as rheumatoid arthritis.
- Mild to moderate acute or chronic pain of peripheral origin, e.g., low back pain caused by muscle strain, headache.
- As a coanalgesic providing a baseline of nonnarcotic analgesia in severe acute or chronic pain requiring narcotics.
- Conditions associated with excessive prostaglandin at the site of injury or pain, e.g., dysmenorrhea, certain malignant tumors, certain cancer therapies, bone metastasis, and postoperative pain.
- Desire by the patient to avoid drugs that affect thinking or emotions ("mind-altering" drugs) or the desire to be fully alert.

Disadvantages of Nonnarcotics

Examples of possible disadvantages or limitations of some nonnarcotic analgesics are:

- Undesirable side effects in certain patients (e.g., allergic response, increased bleeding time, fluid retention, tinnitis, GI upset) may occur, necessitating changing administration, dosage, or drug.
- Analgesic ceiling, i.e., beyond a certain dosage, increased analgesia will not occur.
- Impossibility of predicting to which nonnarcotic (especially those with a strong antiinflammatory effect) the

individual patient will respond best or tolerate. Matching patient to drug is done by trial and error.

- In most instances, if they are used alone, they relieve only mild to moderate pain, not severe pain.
- Daily use for months or longer of high doses or combinations of nonnarcotics could lead to organ damage.
- Route of administration is limited since many are only available orally and a few rectally (parenteral use is very limited in the United States).
- Although recommended dosing schedules are available, some patients will require careful titration to arrive at a safe and effective dosage.
- Some analgesia will usually occur within a few hours, but the full benefit may not be realized until days or weeks of regular administration.
- Effectiveness is underrated. Health team members tend not to be educated about uses of nonnarcotics, especially NSAIDs, for conditions other than arthritis.

Mechanisms Underlying Effects of NSAIDs

NSAIDs* are nonnarcotics that usually have three effects:
1. Antiinflammatory.
2. Analgesic.
3. Antipyretic.

However, the NSAIDs differ in the degree to which they produce these effects. For example, acetaminophen is effective as an analgesic for mild to moderate pain and as an antipyretic but has little antiinflammatory effect. On the other hand, diflunisal (Dolobid) has antiinflammatory and analgesic effects but minimal antipyretic effects.

Reasons for the important differences between these drugs is not clear but may be due in part to variation in the sensitivity of enzymes in the different tissues and the fact that different drugs have different modes of inhibiting the inflammatory process. Most likely the NSAIDs reduce inflammation and pain by inhibiting the synthesis of prostaglandin. The significance of this is obvious when one considers the following discoveries about *prostaglandins:*

- They have been detected in almost every body tissue and fluid.
- They are always released when cells are damaged.
- There are numerous prostaglandins, and they have diverse effects.
- Some are important contributors to the signs and symptoms of inflammation, e.g., swelling and redness.
- Some sensitize the afferent nerve endings to bradykinin (a pain substance) and other effects of chemical or mechanical stimuli, i.e., amplifying the system for producing pain.
- Even low concentrations can cause hyperalgesia, a state

in which pain is caused by stimulation (e.g., touch) that is normally painless.

Most NSAIDs probably prevent the synthesis of prostaglandins from arachidonic acid by inhibiting the cyclooxygenase enzyme that is necessary for the formation of the cyclic endoperoxides (Figure 4-3). When cyclooxygenase is inhibited, so is the synthesis of all products beyond this step in the pathway of inflammation. This accounts for some of the side effects of NSAIDs. The synthesis of thromboxane, an important factor in platelet aggregation, is blocked by many NSAIDs, and this leads to increased bleeding time.

Not all NSAIDs inhibit platelet aggregation, however. The nonacetylated salicylates apparently have little effect on platelet aggregation. For this reason and others, it is thought that they inhibit the synthesis of prostaglandin somewhere after the production of the endoperoxides but prior to the formation of the prostaglandins involved in pain. Blockage of prostaglandin formation and other possible modes of action of NSAIDs in inhibiting inflammation, relieving pain, and producing side effects are shown in Figure 4-3.

The exact mode of action for acetaminophen, which has weak antiinflammatory action, is not clear. Except for acetaminophen, NSAIDs probably should not be combined due to increased risk of side effects, especially gastric and renal damage.

Selection of an NSAID for Analgesia

Selecting an NSAID for use as an analgesic is certainly a more simple matter than selecting one for the long-term treatment of a highly inflammatory condition such as rheumatoid arthritis. Yet, using NSAIDs simply as analgesics, not necessarily for their antiinflammatory effects, is a relatively new idea. Aspirin and acetaminophen have been used as simple analgesics for many years but only recently have the other NSAIDs been studied as analgesics per se. Thus existing guidelines for selecting NSAIDs for the individual patient are primarily based on the need for an antiinflammatory effect and the need for a drug that would be tolerated over a long period. Such guidelines are not always relevant to the selection of an NSAID for analgesia alone.

Further, although the mechanism for analgesia may be separate from the antiinflammatory mechanism, these two effects may very well overlap when a drug is given to the individual patient. The analgesic effect usually occurs within 2 hours of the initial recommended dose, but the maximal antiinflammatory effect may not occur for a week or longer. When the antiinflammatory effect does occur, however, it may very well provide increased analgesia.

Thus the question of how much the antiinflammatory effect of the drug contributes to the analgesic effect complicates the issue. Add to this the fact that the effectiveness of NSAIDs in relieving pain depends on the type of pain, and the matter becomes fairly complex.

*Except where noted otherwise, the information on NSAIDs is obtained from Chapters 28 and 29 of *Goodman and Gilman's The Pharmacological Basis of Therapeutics,* ed 7, New York, 1985, Macmillan Publishing Co.

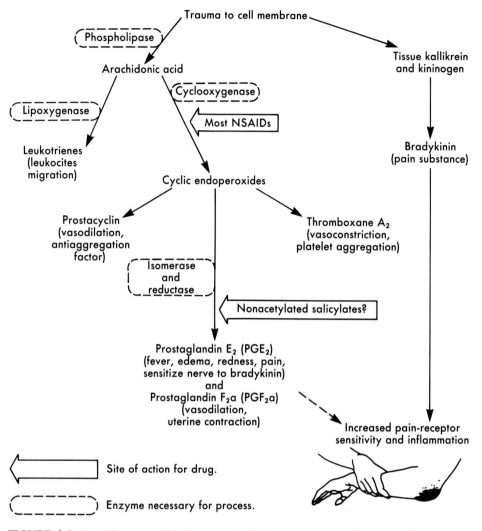

FIGURE 4-3 Possible points of blockage by the NSAIDs in the process leading to inflammation and pain.

It has been said that no NSAIDs are superior to aspirin, and this may well be true if the patient can tolerate high enough doses of aspirin. One distinct advantage that some other NSAIDs have over aspirin is simply that they are better tolerated in that they produce fewer or less intense side effects; some NSAIDs are easier for the patient to take and less dangerous than aspirin.

An overview of NSAIDs used as analgesics is presented in Table 4-2. Currently, numerous publications of research and clinical experience with the use of NSAIDs have resulted in vast and varied claims about the drugs as analgesics as well as antiinflammatory agents. In an attempt to provide as accurate and as simple a guide as possible, one basic reference was used—the well-respected *Goodman and Gilman's The Pharmacological Basis of Therapeutics,* ed 7, New York, 1985, Macmillan Publishing Co. Although it is tempting to add some recent

findings, we decided to limit the table to information that seems to have an acceptable level of proof rather than risk premature inclusion of new information. Thus although the table may lack information that will eventually prove to be useful, the information in the table is likely to stand the test of time.

Doses are omitted from Table 4-2 because recommendations for doses change fairly often. Usually new recommendations are for higher doses, but a current reference should be used to determine the dose. Also, in determining the dose, note that the recommended dose for analgesia is often lower than the dose recommended for an antiinflammatory effect.

Certain NSAIDs are omitted from Table 4-2 because current data indicate that they *would not be good initial choices* of analgesics, although they may be good choices for their antiinflammatory effect or as analgesics if other drugs are ineffective or intolerable. Those omitted along with the reasons are listed below:

- The pyrazolon derivatives, phenylbutazone (Butazolidin) and oxyphenbutazone (Tandearil), should not be used routinely as analgesics because of their severe toxicity, e.g., aplastic anemia.
- The pyrole acetic acid derivative, tolmetin (Tolectin), has been reported to cause severe anaphylactoid reactions in patients who are not sensitive to aspirin and other similar drugs.
- The fenamates, or anthranilic acid derivatives, meclofenamate (Meclomen) and mefenamic acid (Ponstel), are analgesic but cause side effects frequently, particularly severe diarrhea, and are felt to have no advantages over other NSAIDs. Since meclofenamate is not recommended as initial therapy in rheumatoid arthritis and osteoarthritis, it may not be a logical first choice as an analgesic either. Mefenamic acid is indicated only for analgesia and primary dysmenorrhea, but it is omitted because it should not be given for longer than 7 days. Thus mefenamic acid is probably a good choice for dysmenorrhea but not for pain that may last longer than a few days.

Based on the above reasoning, one may question the inclusion of indomethacin in Table 4-2. However, indomethacin is often used as a standard of comparison, in addition to aspirin. Further, pertinent to the use of NSAIDs as analgesics in acute pain, indomethacin is currently the only NSAID besides aspirin and acetaminophen that is available in rectal suppository and therefore appropriate for the patient who is unable to take oral medication. In addition, studies of its use rectally in the immediate postoperative period are very promising. Other NSAIDs given rectally may very well be as effective but are not yet available as rectal suppositories.

KEY POINT: A simple overall guideline to using NSAIDs as analgesics:

Acetaminophen is the easiest to take; it has fewer side effects than any, but may be a less effective analgesic for more than mild pain.

Aspirin is a good analgesic for mild to moderate pain but is one of the most difficult to take; it has many side effects that may be intense enough to limit its use in some individuals.

Some of the *other NSAIDs* are likely to be better analgesics than acetaminophen and at least equal to aspirin in analgesic ability, but they are usually easier to take than aspirin, i.e., have fewer or less intense side effects.

Adverse Side Effects

Comments on the side effects of NSAIDs are included in Table 4-2 and are discussed in the patient/family teaching form for home use of nonnarcotic analgesics on p. 65.

Because the side effects of NSAIDs include fluid retention, gastric ulceration, bleeding, nephritis, and decreased growth of new bone (Amadio and Cummings, 1986; Ritter and Gioe, 1982), these drugs should be used with extreme caution in patients with ulcers, bleeding problems, low platelet count, edema, high blood pressure, congestive heart failure, poor renal function, or joint replacement requiring generation of new bone. The presence of aspirin sensitivity or asthma in a patient also dictates caution, as the sensitivity may also apply to NSAIDs.

Combinations of aspirin with certain NSAIDs remain controversial and may not be recommended. However, documentation in a few patients shows that the combination of aspirin with Motrin or Naprosyn may result in better pain relief. The risk of peptic ulceration and GI bleeding is greater with this combination (Fisher and Schwinghammer, 1984).

Promising Uses of NSAIDs

Many times in clinical practice, NSAIDs are overlooked and underestimated as an effective analgesic choice. The following is an overview of selected painful conditions shown to be responsive to NSAIDs. With this information and specific references, nurses can be instrumental in suggesting these analgesics for the appropriate situation.

1. *Postoperative pain.* Research has shown that NSAIDs such as aspirin and ibuprofen are effective in the relief of pain following episiotomy, herniorrhaphy, orthopedic surgery, and tooth extraction (Dionne and Cooper, 1978; Slavic-Svircev et al, 1984).

In postorthopedic surgery patients, ibuprofen 400 mg was more effective, longer acting, and caused greater mood improvement than codeine 30 mg plus acetaminophen 300 mg (Heidrich et al, 1985).

In postthoracic surgery patients, indomethacin rectal suppository 100 mg every 8 hours provided analgesia allowing patients to move and effectively perform deep breathing and coughing exercises. Many patients required no additional pain medication (Tejada, 1986). Another study of patients after major abdominal surgery who received indomethacin rectal suppository 100 mg every 8 hours had less pain on each of the first 4 postoperative days than those who received intramuscular (IM) morphine (Reasbeck et al, 1982).

2. *Cancer pain.* Kantor (1984) estimates that of all patients with cancer, probably about 50% have pain that could be controlled with NSAIDs alone, i.e., without the addition of a narcotic. NSAIDs can be particularly effective for pain from bone tumors and bone metastasis. In addition to inhibition of prostaglandins in bone tumors, NSAIDs may actually inhibit the progress of bone tumors (Ventafridda et al, 1980). Many people with metastatic cancer may have hypercalcemia, which increases pain. The NSAIDs can reduce serum calcium levels and thereby decrease pain (Kantor, 1984).

TABLE 4-2 Selected NSAIDs Used for Analgesia*

Class/Medication	Formulations and Frequency†	Comments
ACETYLATED SALICYLATES		
Aspirin (e.g., Bayer)	Capsules, tablets, enteric-coated tablets, chewable tablets, sustained release, rectal suppository; every 4-6 hr initially.	Nonprescription. Tends to be the standard for comparison and evaluation of other NSAIDs. Platelets are especially susceptible to its acetylating action so that a single dose as low as 40 mg per day of aspirin will inhibit platelet cyclooxygenase for the life of the platelet (8-11 days); a single dose of 650 mg aspirin approximately doubles the mean bleeding time of normal persons for 4-7 days.
NONACETYLATED SALICYLATES		
(As a group they are much better tolerated than aspirin and have little, if any, effect on platelet aggregation and bleeding time.)		
Choline magnesium trisalicylate (Trilisate)	Tablets, liquid; every 12 hr.	Prescription.
Diflunisal (Dolobid)	Tablets; every 8-12 hr.	Prescription. Minimal antipyretic effect.
Salsalate (Disalcid)	Capsules, tablets; every 8-12 hr.	Prescription.
PARA-AMINOPHENOL DERIVATIVES		
Acetaminophen (e.g., Datril, Tylenol)	Capsules, tablets, chewable tablets, liquids, rectal suppository; every 4 hr.	Nonprescription. Effective analgesic and antipyretic but weak antiinflammatory. Well tolerated; lacks many of the side effects of aspirin, such as no gastric irritation and no effect on bleeding time. May be given with other NSAIDs. Total daily dose should not exceed 4000 mg.

Drug actions: All of the above are not only analgesic but also antiinflammatory and antipyretic, unless noted otherwise.

†If this is duplicated, add to this column the current recommended doses and date the entry.

General guide: The individual's response to these drugs is unpredictable. If a drug is ineffective or has intolerable side effects, it is often logical to try another. The drugs are grouped according to chemical categories to emphasize the point that they may share similar therapeutic actions and side effects but may be chemically unrelated. Significant differences exist even within a chemical category. Thus one should expect a large variation in response of individuals to the same drug and different drugs regarding pain relief and side effects.

Most of the data in this table are obtained from:

Flower, RJ, Moncada, S, and Vane, JR: Drug therapy of inflammation, pp 674-715. In Gilman, AG, et al, eds: Goodman and Gilman's the pharmacological basis of therapeutics, ed 7, New York, 1985, Macmillan Publishing Co.

Moncada, S, Flower, RJ, and Vane, JR: Prostaglandins, prostacyclin, thromboxane A_2, and leukotrienes, pp 660-673. In Gilman, AG, et al, eds: Goodman and Gilman's the pharmacological basis of therapeutics, ed 7, New York, 1985, Macmillan Publishing Co.

Reasbeck, PG, Rice, ML, and Reasbeck, JC: Double-blind controlled trial of indomethacin as an adjunct to narcotic analgesia after major abdominal surgery, *Lancet* 2:115-118, July 1982.

■ May be duplicated for use in clinical practice. From McCaffery, M, and Beebe, A: PAIN: CLINICAL MANUAL FOR NURSING PRACTICE, St. Louis, 1989, The CV Mosby Company.

If cancer pain progresses, combining a narcotic with an NSAID can produce significant analgesia (Beaver, 1984b). Ibuprofen 600 mg added to 2.5 or 5 mg of PO methadone significantly increased the analgesic effect of methadone alone without increased side effects. It was more effective with bone metastasis than tissue or visceral involvement (Ferrer-Brechner and Ganz, 1984).

Patient Example (Hill, 1986)

Forty-seven-year-old man with metastatic adenocarcinoma with extreme pain from subcutaneous lesions and edematous right leg. The following analgesics were tried with little success until a narcotic plus nonnarcotic combination was used:

- Meperidine 50 mg PO q4h. Result: no relief.
- Meperidine 100 to 150 mg PO q4h. Result: minimal relief.
- Morphine 30 mg PO q4h plus diazepam (Valium) 10 mg PO q6h. Result: side effects unacceptable to patient, i.e., a "wiped-out" feeling with confusion and nightmares.
- Meperidine 150 mg PO q4h. Result: no relief.
- Morphine 90 mg PO q4h plus methadone (Dolophine) 10 mg q8h. Result: controlled leg pain, not effective for subcutaneous lesions.
- Choline magnesium trisalicylate (Trilisate) 1500 mg PO bid plus morphine 90 mg PO q4h. Result: good pain control.

3. *Other conditions.* Many back disorders have no clearly or easily determined etiology but are thought to

TABLE 4-2 Selected NSAIDs Used for Analgesia—cont'd.

Class/Medication	Formulations and Frequency	Comments
PROPIONIC ACID DERIVATIVES		
(As a group they are usually better tolerated than aspirin or indomethacin; they have similar, although less intense, unwanted side effects.)		
Fenoprofen (Nalfon)	Capsules, tablets; every 4-8 hr.	Prescription.
Ibuprofen (e.g., Advil, Motrin)	Tablets; every 4-8 hr.	Nonprescription in doses of 200 mg/tablet; prescription in doses over 200 mg/tablet. More effective than aspirin for relief of dysmenorrhea.
Ketoprofen (Orudis)	Capsules; every 6-8 hr.	Prescription.
Naproxen (Naprosyn)	Tablets, liquid; every 6-12 hr.	Prescription. More effective than aspirin for relief of dysmenorrhea. Better tolerated than ibuprofen, fenoprofen, and indomethacin.
Naproxen sodium (Anaprox)	Tablets; every 6-8 hr.	Prescription. Similar to naproxen but more rapid onset of analgesia.
INDOLE ACETIC ACID DERIVATIVES		
Indomethacin (Indocin)	Capsules, sustained release, rectal suppositories; every 8-12 hr. (Available IV for treatment of patent ductus arteriosus in neonates.)	Prescription. Use as analgesic probably should be restricted to a few days, if possible, e.g., postoperative pain (use cautiously if the patient is at risk for postoperative bleeding). High risk of side effects is associated with chronic administration, i.e., weeks. For unknown reasons doses given at night are better tolerated. A useful way to employ the drug and avoid side effects is to give a large dose at night and use a better tolerated analgesic during the day. (NOTE: Currently is only NSAID, other than acetaminophen and aspirin, available rectally for administration to NPO patient.)
Sulindac (Clinoril)	Tablets; every 12 hr.	Prescription. Lower incidence of GI toxicity than indomethacin. Relative lack of effect on kidneys. Little or no placental transfer.
OXICAMS		
Piroxicam (Feldene)	Capsules; every 24 hr, but may be given twice a day.	Prescription. Long acting, e.g., 24 hr. Better tolerated than aspirin or indomethacin. Maximal antiinflammatory effect takes 2 weeks or longer.

■ May be duplicated for use in clinical practice. From McCaffery, M, and Beebe, A: PAIN: CLINICAL MANUAL FOR NURSING PRACTICE, St. Louis, 1989, The CV Mosby Company.

be associated with greater or lesser degrees of inflammation (Kantor, 1982). Clinicians working with patients who have low back pain have noted that NSAIDs are sometimes effective in relieving the pain (Brena, 1983).

Various research has shown that NSAIDs may be effective in relieving the pain of or as prophylaxis for migraine, but not all patients respond well (Bernstein, 1982). This may reflect differences in types of migraine headaches, as well as differences in patients. Varied responses of migraines to NSAIDs may be due to insufficient doses prescribed because of fear of side effects. For example, a migraine patient may require up to 150 mg of indomethacin daily.

Indomethacin in particular has been studied. It is thought to be 50 to 60 times more potent than aspirin in the inhibition of prostacyclin, a prostaglandin that causes cerebral vasodilation and plays a major role in inducing the pain of migraines. People with migraines seem to synthesize excessive amounts of prostacyclin. NSAIDs may also block the prostaglandin mediated platelet aggregation and serotonin release associated with migraine. In addition to indomethacin, other NSAIDs such as fenoprofen (Nalfon), mefenamic acid (Ponstel), and naproxen (Naprosyn) have been effective (Bernstein, 1982). NSAIDs also seem particularly effective in treating menstrual-related migraines.

Painful menstrual cramps afflict many women, resulting in some being unable to function for a day or more once a month. For many women, NSAIDs provide very effective relief and replace the need for narcotics for pain

TABLE 4-3 Common Considerations in Selection of NSAIDs as Analgesics

Factor	Consideration
1. Individual patient problem:	
a. History of ulcer disease	1. a. Consider propionic acid derivatives, non-acetylated salicylates or acetaminophen. Avoid Indocin, aspirin.
b. Poor renal function	b. Consider renal sparing NSAID, e.g., Dolobid, Clinoril.
c. Bleeding problems	c. Avoid pyrazolone derivatives. Consider nonacetylated salicy-lates or acetaminophen.
2. Prior experience	2. Prior use of NSAID and resulting problems or success can help with present selection.
3. Ease of dosing and route	3. Liquid form for patients with trouble swallowing, e.g., Trilisate; suppository form, e.g., Indocin, aspirin, Tylenol; IV, e.g., Indocin. Consider those which can be taken one or two times daily, e.g., Feldene, Trilisate, Dolobid, Naprosyn.
4. Cost	4. There is considerable variation in price between pharmacies and drugs. When this is an important factor, it may decide one drug over another.

control (Amadio and Cummings, 1986; Dingfelder, 1981; Wenzloff and Shrimp, 1984). Excessive concentrations of prostaglandins in the endometrium, menstrual fluid, and peripheral circulation is probably what leads to painful cramps, and prostaglandins can be decreased by NSAIDs (Anderson et al, 1978; Marx, 1979). Pretreatment before the onset of menstrual flow is not necessary (Dawood, 1981).

Which NSAID to Use

Unfortunately there is no absolute answer to this frequently asked question. It is impossible to predict which patient with a specific pain problem will respond favorably to NSAIDs and which patient will respond best to which NSAID. Factors considered in the selection of an NSAID are listed in Table 4-3.

Guidelines for Effective Use of Nonnarcotics (NSAIDs)

To obtain the maximal benefit from nonnarcotics, two general guidelines are:

1. If pain stays in the mild to moderate range of intensity, try a nonnarcotic first rather than a narcotic. Occasional mild to moderate pain is usually treated with single doses of OTC products such as two regular or two extra-strength aspirin or acetaminophen (approximately 650 to 1000 mg). If mild to moderate pain is continuous, e.g., 24 hours a day, day after day, it makes sense to give nonnarcotics on a regular ATC basis.
2. Even when pain relief requires narcotics because it is too severe to be relieved by nonnarcotics, continue nonnarcotics if possible. It is this guideline that is most commonly overlooked (implementation of this is discussed below).

Nonnarcotics Used Alone

One of the main reasons for emphasizing these guidelines is that nonnarcotics are more effective analgesics than most laymen and health care professionals realize. For example, how effective do you think a dose of 650 mg of aspirin or acetaminophen is compared with oral narcotics? A list of PO doses of narcotics that relieve no more pain than 650 mg of aspirin or acetaminophen are in the equianalgesic list in Table 4-4. Although there are individual differences in responses to medications, this table shows that in most people the following doses relieve only as much pain as two regular aspirin or acetaminophen—or, conversely, two regular aspirin or acetaminophen (650 mg) relieve as much pain as the following:

- Codeine 32 mg, PO.
- Meperidine 50 mg, PO.
- Propoxyphene hydrochloride (Darvon-N) 100 mg, PO.

Based on these findings it is evident that we underestimate ordinary aspirin and acetaminophen and overestimate the effectiveness of low doses of PO narcotics. Obviously, we can relieve more pain with plain aspirin and acetaminophen than most people realize.

Further, from a practical standpoint, nonnarcotics are generally easier to obtain than narcotics. Physicians more readily prescribe nonnarcotics than narcotics, providing the specific nonnarcotic is not contraindicated, and some nonnarcotics require no prescription.

In the home care setting, the nurse may teach the patient and family how to effectively and safely use OTC nonnarcotics to enhance pain relief. To facilitate patient/family teaching and to assist the nurse in identifying the ingredients of OTC analgesics the patient may have taken, Table 4-5 gives the ingredients of selected nonprescription nonnarcotics.

A view of the ingredients of combination products (Table 4-5) reveals that most rely on aspirin or acetaminophen or a combination of the two for pain relief. Since combination products are often more expensive than "straight" products, e.g., plain aspirin, the nurse may be able to help the patient who takes combination OTC analgesics analyze the ingredients and spend less money but obtain the same relief by using the less expensive

TABLE 4-4 Equianalgesic Chart: Approximate Equivalent Doses of PO Analgesics for Mild to Moderate Pain*

Analgesic	PO Dosage (mg)
Nonnarcotic Analgesics	
Acetaminophen (Datril, Tylenol)	650
Aspirin (ASA, acetylsalicylic acid)	650
Phenacetin	650
Sodium salicylate	1000
Narcotic Analgesics	
Codeine	32
Meperidine (Demerol)	50
Oxycodone	5 (probably much more effective than others listed, especially during first 2 hr)
Hydrocodone	5
Pentazocine (Talwin) (narcotic agonist-antagonist)	30 (available in 50 mg scored tablets)
Propoxyphene hydrochloride (Darvon)	65
Propoxyphene napsylate (Darvon-N)	100

*The equianalgesic doses in this chart are based primarily on recommendations of the Analgesic Study Section, Sloan-Kettering Institute for Cancer Research, New York, based on double-blind analgesic research (Houde, 1979).

Table references:

Houde, RW: Systemic analgesics and related drugs: narcotic analgesics. In Bonica, JJ, and Ventafridda, V, eds: Advances in pain research and therapy, vol 2, pp 263-273, New York, 1979, Raven Press (See p 266 for above list plus IM-PO list.)

Moertel, CG: Relief of pain with oral medications, *Aust NZJ Med* (suppl 1) 6:1-8, 1976 (This double-blind study of ambulatory cancer patients suggests that the above list may be a conservative estimate of the potency of nonnarcotics, e.g., Moertel found it may take more than 65 mg of codeine PO to equal 650 mg aspirin. He also found that 10 mg morphine PO was not as effective as 650 mg aspirin.)

Rogers, AG: Pharmacology of analgesics, *J Neurosurg Nurs* 10:180-184, Dec 1978

■ May be duplicated for use in clinical practice. From McCaffery, M, and Beebe, A: PAIN: CLINICAL MANUAL FOR NURSING PRACTICE, St. Louis, 1989, The CV Mosby Company.

"straight" products. For example, a substitute for the ingredients of two Anacin is simply 2½ regular, plain aspirin containing 325 mg each (any inexpensive brand) plus a cup of tea or coffee (if the caffeine is actually desirable). A substitute for 2 Anacin Maximum Strength Capsules is 3 regular aspirin containing 325 mg each plus a cup of tea or coffee.

KEY POINT: **Pain relieving effects of nonnarcotic analgesics are underestimated and underused.**

Regarding all NSAIDs, the degree of pain relief is variable, with some individuals with seemingly similar pathology being more responsive than others. NSAIDs in the same chemical class (Table 4-2) may affect individual patients differently. Several explanations have been suggested (Kantor, 1982):

1. There are probably differences in the way individuals absorb and metabolize these drugs.
2. There may be genetic differences in inflammatory responses of individuals.
3. Certain inflammatory pathways may be used preferentially over others at various stages of a disease process.

Although there is no research to verify this, some pain specialists suggest that when there is little analgesic response to one NSAID, it may be more helpful to *switch to another in a different chemical class* (Table 4-2) as opposed to selecting another from the same chemical class

(Amadio and Cummings, 1986; Portenoy, 1987b). Suggested guidelines for effective use of nonnarcotics are in Table 4-6.

Nonnarcotics in Combination with Narcotics

When pain cannot be relieved by NSAIDs alone, combine them with PO, IM, or IV narcotics. The rationale is:

- Nonnarcotics are more effective than most people realize.
- Nonnarcotic plus narcotic equals peripheral nervous system plus CNS attack.
- This combination produces an additive effect and reduces the narcotic dose needed, thereby decreasing narcotic side effects (Beaver, 1981).

Approaches to combining narcotics plus nonnarcotics are:

1. PO narcotics plus nonnarcotics.
   a. If the pain is continuous, consider ATC doses of nonnarcotic along with the narcotic, e.g., morphine 35 mg PO q4h ATC and Motrin 800 mg q8h ATC.
   b. Some PO narcotics are already compounded with nonnarcotics, but the nonnarcotic dose is inadequate. Use the optimal therapeutic dose for effective analgesia. Refer to Table 4-7 (p. 64) to identify the amount and type of nonnarcotic compounded with the narcotic in some commonly prescribed PO analgesics. For example:

TABLE 4-5 Common Nonprescription Analgesics

Brands	Ingredients per Tablet	Brands	Ingredients per Tablet
STRAIGHT		BC Powder	650 mg aspirin
Advil	200 mg ibuprofen		195 mg salicylamide
Aspergum Chewing Gum	228 mg aspirin		32 mg caffeine
Aspirin Free Anacin-3	500 mg acetaminophen	Bromo-Seltzer	325 mg acetaminophen/
Aspirin Suppositories	125, 300, or 600 mg aspirin		capful
Bayer, St. Joseph, and most	325 mg aspirin		2.85 g sodium citrate/capful
other plain aspirin		Bufferin	324 mg aspirin
Bayer Timed-Release Aspirin	650 mg aspirin		magnesium carbonate
Datril Extra Strength Capsule,	500 mg acetaminophen		aluminum glycinate
Tablet			(no dose listed for last two
Ecotrin	324 mg aspirin enteric		ingredients)
	coated	Extra Strength Bufferin Capsule	500 mg aspirin
Empirin	325 mg aspirin		calcium carbonate
Nuprin	200 mg ibuprofen		magnesium oxide
Tylenol Extra Strength Tablet,	500 mg acetaminophen		magnesium carbonate
Caplet			(no dose listed for last three
Tylenol Liquid	33.3 mg acetaminophen/ml		ingredients)
Tylenol Regular Strength Tablet	325 mg acetaminophen	Extra Strength Bufferin Tablet	500 mg aspirin
			aluminum glycinate
COMBINATION			magnesium carbonate
Alka-Seltzer Effervescent Pain	324 mg aspirin		(no dose listed for last two
Reliever and Antacid	1.916 g sodium bicarbonate		ingredients)
	1.0 g citric acid	Excedrin Extra Strength	250 mg aspirin
Anacin	400 mg aspirin	Capsule, Tablet	250 mg acetaminophen
	32.5 mg caffeine		65 mg caffeine
Anacin Maximum Strength	500 mg aspirin	Excedrin P.M.	500 mg acetaminophen
Tablets, Capsules	32 mg caffeine		38 mg diphenhydramine
Arthritis Pain Formula	486 mg aspirin		citrate
	(microniazed)	Momentum	500 mg aspirin
	20 mg aluminum hydroxide		15 mg phenyltoloxamine
	60 mg magnesium		citrate
	hydroxide	Trigesic	230 mg aspirin
Arthritis Strength Bufferin	486 mg aspirin		125 mg acetaminophen
	magnesium carbonate		30 mg caffeine
	aluminum glycinate	Vanquish Caplet	227 mg aspirin
	(no dose listed for last two		194 mg acetaminophen
	ingredients)		33 mg caffeine
Ascriptin	325 mg aspirin		50 mg magnesium
	75 mg magnesium		hydroxide
	hydroxide		25 mg aluminum hydroxide
	75 mg aluminum hydroxide		gel, dried
	gel, dried		
BC Tablet	325 mg aspirin		
	95 mg salicylamide		
	16 mg caffeine		

The specific analgesics included in the above list of nonprescription analgesics are either commonly used ones or are representative of the variety of combinations available. Reference: Van Tyle, WK: Internal analgesic products. In Handbook of nonprescription drugs, ed 8, pp 191-214, Washington, D.C., 1986, American Pharmaceutical Association.

- Empirin #3 and #4 contain only 325 mg aspirin and could logically be boosted with one tablet of aspirin 325 mg.
- Tylenol #3 and #4 contain only 300 mg acetaminophen and could be boosted with 325 mg to increase pain relief.
- If several doses of these combinations are given, be careful not to exceed the recommended total daily dose of ASA or acetaminophen.

2. IM, IV narcotics plus nonnarcotics.
   If the patient on IM and IV narcotics can take oral medication, it is logical to consider adding aspirin, acetaminophen, or one of the other NSAIDs ATC for ongoing pain, or at the time of the narcotic for incident pain. If given at the same time as the IM injection, peak effect of the nonnarcotic would begin after about 2 hours, the time the IM's effectiveness tends to decrease.

TABLE 4-6 Guidelines for Effective Use of Nonnarcotic Analgesics

Guideline	Comments
1. Weigh risk vs. benefits in selection.	1. E.g., aspirin: risk of GI upset but it is least expensive in this group. Acetaminophen: less antiinflammatory effect but generally fewer side effects.
2. Start with a low dose to determine patient's reaction, e.g., side effects. Increase gradually to a dose that relieves pain, not exceeding maximal daily dose.	2. May need to increase to 1-2 times the starting dose. Ineffective analgesia may be due to inadequate doses.
3. If maximal antiinflammatory effect is desired in addition to analgesia, allow adequate trial before discontinuing or switching.	3. An effective dose should provide pain relief within 2 hours. Maximal antiinflammatory effect occurs later as drug accumulates. With regular doses for 1 week or longer, pain relief may increase.
4. If one drug becomes ineffective, but the pain is about the same, try a drug from a different chemical class (see Table 4-2 on NSAIDs).	4. The inflammatory process may have changed. A different drug may attack this process in another way.
5. If they do not relieve pain when used alone, combine with PO, IM, or IV narcotics for added analgesic effect.	5. Rationale: nonnarcotic analgesics stop pain at peripheral nervous system (PNS) level, and narcotics stop pain at CNS level. Combination of PNS plus CNS attack will provide added analgesic effect.

Although the IV route may be used to give immediate relief and allow quick titration in dosage, many of these patients may still be able to take PO medication. ATC dosing of NSAIDs along with IV narcotics will boost analgesic effect.

If you are suggesting a nonnarcotic plus narcotic combination to the physician and other health team members, the following points and references will be helpful:

1. Many prescription analgesics already combine narcotic plus nonnarcotic, e.g., Tylenol #3 and Percodan. Table 4-7 lists these common combinations.
2. Combining an *optimal* therapeutic dose of aspirin or acetaminophen with a narcotic produces an additive analgesic effect (Beaver, 1981).
3. Research on cancer patients clearly indicates the benefit of combining narcotic and nonnarcotic analgesics.
   - A clinical research study using double-blind technique with people with cancer pain found that giving 600 mg of aspirin along with morphine 10 mg IM provided significantly greater pain relief than morphine alone (Houde et al, 1960).
   - 600 mg ibuprofen added to 2.5 or 5 mg PO methadone significantly increased the analgesic effect of methadone alone without increased side effects in cancer patients (Ferrer-Brechner and Ganz, 1984).
   - 400 mg ibuprofen four times per day in addition to the cancer patient's scheduled oral narcotic resulted in greater analgesia than the narcotic plus placebo combination and no increase in side effects (Weingart et al, 1985).

KEY POINT: Combining two classes of analgesics, narcotic and nonnarcotic, is a simple yet frequently overlooked strategy. This combination provides a safe and logical method of pain relief. They are two *different* analgesics:

- They relieve pain in two different ways.
- They have different side effects.
- Giving them at the same time poses no more danger than alternating them, e.g., q2h.

Patient Example

On the evening following surgical removal of rectal polyps, Ms. P., 74 years old, says her pain is poorly relieved with injections and she feels very drowsy. Her analgesic is nalbuphine (Nubain) 15 mg IM. One hour after the injection, her pain is reduced from 7 to 4 on a scale of 0 to 10, and she is arousable and slightly confused, with respirations at 14 per minute.

Since increasing the nalbuphine would probably increase the sedation, a nonnarcotic is added. Because of a history of ulcer disease, acetaminophen is chosen. PRN prescriptions are implemented ATC to prevent the return of pain. Attacking her pain centrally with the narcotic, Nubain 15 mg IM q6h, and peripherally with the nonnarcotic acetaminophen 650 mg q4h, her pain is reduced to 2 with no increase in sedation. She appears well oriented and says she feels more alert, probably because of better pain relief (Jain et al, 1986).

Patient/Family Teaching Point

The patient/family teaching point (p. 65) may be duplicated, completed, and given to the patient who will be taking NSAIDs (other than acetaminophen) as analgesics on an outpatient basis. When NSAIDs are used as analgesics in the hospital, some of the same points may need to be discussed with the patient, but unless the patient goes home with a prescription for them, use of the writ-

Text continued on p. 66.

TABLE 4-7 Common Combination Narcotic and Nonnarcotic Oral Analgesics*

Proprietary Name	Ingredients	Proprietary Name	Ingredients
Ascriptin with Codeine No. 2	15 mg codeine 325 mg aspirin 150 mg Maalox (magnesium-aluminum hydroxide)	Percodan	4.5 mg oxycodone hydro-chloride 0.38 mg oxycodone tereph-thalate 325 mg aspirin
Ascriptin with Codeine No. 3	30 mg codeine 325 mg aspirin 150 mg Maalox (magnesium-aluminum hydroxide)	Percodan-Demi	2.25 mg oxycodone hydro-chloride 0.19 mg oxycodone tereph-thalate 325 mg aspirin
Damacet-P	5 mg hydrocodone 500 mg acetaminophen	Phenaphen with Codeine No. 2	15 mg codeine 325 mg acetaminophen
Damason-P	5 mg hydrocodone 224 mg aspirin 32 mg caffeine	Phenaphen with Codeine No. 3	30 mg codeine 325 mg acetaminophen
Darvocet-N 50	50 mg propoxyphene napsylate 325 mg acetaminophen	Phenaphen with Codeine No. 4	60 mg codeine 325 mg acetaminophen
Darvocet-N 100	100 mg propoxyphene napsylate 600 mg acetaminophen	Phenaphen-650 with Codeine	30 mg codeine 650 mg acetaminophen
Darvon Compound	32 mg propoxyphene hydro-chloride 389 mg aspirin 32.4 mg caffeine	SK-Oxycodone with Acetaminophen	5 mg oxycodone hydro-chloride 325 mg acetaminophen
Darvon Compound-65	65 mg propoxyphene hydro-chloride 389 mg aspirin 32.4 mg caffeine	SK-Oxycodone with Aspirin	4.5 mg oxycodone hydro-chloride 0.38 mg oxycodone tereph-thalate 325 mg aspirin
Darvon with A.S.A.	65 mg propoxyphene hydro-chloride 325 mg aspirin	Synalgos-DC	16 mg dihydrocodeine 356.4 mg aspirin 30 mg caffeine
Empirin with Codeine No. 2	15 mg codeine 325 mg aspirin	Talwin Compound	12.5 mg pentazocine 325 mg aspirin
Empirin with Codeine No. 3	30 mg codeine 325 mg aspirin	Tylenol with Codeine No. 1	7.5 mg codeine 300 mg acetaminophen
Empirin with Codeine No. 4	60 mg codeine 325 mg aspirin	Tylenol with Codeine No. 2	15 mg codeine 300 mg acetaminophen
Empracet with Codeine No. 3	30 mg codeine 300 mg acetaminophen	Tylenol with Codeine No. 3	30 mg codeine 300 mg acetaminophen
Empracet with Codeine No. 4	60 mg codeine 300 mg acetaminophen	Tylenol with Codeine No. 4	60 mg codeine 300 mg acetaminophen
Fiorinal with Codeine No. 1	7.5 mg codeine 325 mg aspirin 50 mg butalbital 40 mg caffeine	Tylenol Elixir (each 5 ml)	12 mg codeine 120 mg acetaminophen 7% alcohol
Fiorinal with Codeine No. 2	15 mg codeine 325 mg aspirin 50 mg butalbital 40 mg caffeine	Tylox	5 mg oxycodone hydro-chloride 500 mg acetaminophen
Fiorinal with Codeine No. 3	30 mg codeine 325 mg aspirin 50 mg butalbital 40 mg caffeine	Vicodin	5 mg hydrocodone 500 mg acetaminophen
		Wygesic	65 mg propoxyphene hydro-chloride 650 mg acetaminophen
Percocet	5 mg oxycodone hydro-chloride 325 mg acetaminophen	Zydone	5 mg hydrocodone 500 mg acetaminophen

*Product information as given in Physicians' desk reference, ed 41, Oradell, NJ, 1987, Medical Economics Co.

Patient/Family Teaching Point: Instructions for Home Use of Nonnarcotic Analgesics

TO: _____ (patient's name)   DATE: _____

Facts about your pain reliever and how to take it. This nonnarcotic medicine is sometimes called a nonsteroidal antiinflammatory drug (NSAID) or an aspirin-like drug. It is commonly used for arthritis but also may be used to relieve many other types of pain. Pain relief is usually felt within 2 hours or less after taking it. In addition to relieving pain, it reduces inflammation and fever. This medicine does not, however, cure the cause of your pain. The advantages of this medicine over a narcotic are that it is not associated with addiction, you do not get tolerant to it and have to take more for the same amount of pain, and usually it does not cause constipation or drowsiness.

To relieve your discomfort or pain, you are taking the following nonnarcotic medicine:

Name of medicine: _____ (other names: _____)

Dose: _____ (number of pills per dose: _____)

How often: _____

The method checked below is the appropriate approach for relief of your pain:

_____ For ongoing pain, it is usually recommended that you take this on a regular daily basis, every day, without skipping a dose. This helps keep your pain under control.

_____ For occasional or unpredictable pain, you may be instructed to begin taking this at the onset of pain, and then take it on a regular basis, without skipping a dose, until the pain goes away.

Take this medicine with food or at least a full glass of water to avoid stomach upset. If this does not prevent stomach upset or indigestion, you may try an antacid. If stomach upset continues, notify your nurse or doctor. *Do not take it with alcohol* because stomach irritation can occur.

Never take this on an empty stomach. Even if it does not upset your stomach, it can still damage the stomach.

If you take two or more doses as prescribed and the medicine does not relieve your pain, notify your nurse or doctor. It may be necessary to increase the dose or change to another medicine.

Do not take any additional medicine known as a nonnarcotic or nonsteroidal antiinflammatory drug (NSAID) except for acetaminophen, unless it is recommended by a doctor who knows what you are taking now. Taking more than one nonnarcotic pain reliever can dramatically increase side effects and/or cause serious organ damage that you would not necessarily notice initially.

Watch for nonprescription products with "hidden aspirin." Many cold remedies and other patented medicines contain aspirin. The addition of aspirin could increase your risk for side effects. If you are already taking aspirin, this additional aspirin could raise your dose to a toxic level.

If you have any side effects from your medicine that you cannot control by trying the suggestions on this form, stop taking the medicine and notify your nurse or doctor. Some of the side effects that may occur with some of the NSAIDs are stomach upset or indigestion; dizziness; headache; blurred vision; ringing in the ears or hearing loss; swelling in legs, ankles, or neck; skin rash; shortness of breath; black bowel movements; diarrhea or constipation; unusual bleeding; onset of or increase in symptoms of asthma; depression; or confusion. Elderly patients should be especially alert to possible memory loss, inability to concentrate, or personality change.

Contraindications: Before you take this medicine, notify your nurse or doctor if you are pregnant; breast-feeding; taking blood thinners, antidiabetic drugs, or antiseizure drugs; have bleeding problems; heart disease; kidney problems; stomach ulcers; or allergy or sensitivity to aspirin. Also, notify your nurse or doctor if any of these occur while you are taking this medicine.

Additional comments: _____

_____

If you have any questions or problems with the above, contact:

_____ (RN or MD name)   Phone: _____

_____ (Nurse's signature)

■ May be duplicated for use in clinical practice. From McCaffery, M, and Beebe, A: PAIN: CLINICAL MANUAL FOR NURSING PRACTICE, St. Louis, 1989, The CV Mosby Company.

ten form is probably unnecessary. The drugs are given by the nurses, and the patient can be directly observed for side effects.

In the "Additional Comments" section of the patient/family teaching form for home use of nonnarcotic analgesics, the following should be included if the patient is on the particular drug:

Aspirin. Do not take if it has a strong vinegar smell. This means it has decomposed. Discard it and get a fresh supply.

Enteric-coated aspirin. Do not take with antacids or milk because the coating may be destroyed.

Diflunisal (Dolobid). Has very little ability to reduce a fever.

Indomethacin (Indocin). Urine or bowel movement may be green, but this is no cause for alarm. (If side effects are intolerable, consider the suppository form or a single oral dose at bedtime. Nighttime doses or the rectal route are better tolerated for unknown reasons. During the day, another better tolerated analgesic, such as acetaminophen, may be used.)

Naproxen (Naprosyn). It is particularly important to avoid alcohol because naproxen may cause drowsiness and alcohol will increase the drowsiness.

Narcotic (Opioid) Analgesics
Indications for Narcotics

Examples of situations in which narcotics may be appropriate for pain relief:

- Moderate to severe acute pain, e.g., orthopedic fractures, postoperative pain, cystoscopy.
- Recurrent, acute pain, e.g., sickle cell crisis, tanking for burn care.
- Prolonged, time-limited pain, e.g., terminal illness, cancer pain, burns.
- Desire for immediate relief of sudden, severe pain, e.g., renal colic, trauma. IV route provides relief in minutes.
- Desire for immediate, very brief, and reversible relief of moderate to severe pain, e.g., cystoscopy performed with IV narcotic and reversed with naloxone at the end of procedure.
- Selected patients with chronic nonmalignant pain who do not benefit from other pain relief methods but are able to function well on a stabilized dose of narcotic.

Disadvantages of Narcotics

A common misconception is that addiction will be a disadvantage in using narcotics; however, narcotic addiction as a result of treating pain with narcotics is very unlikely.

Examples of possible limitations or disadvantages of relieving pain with narcotics:

- Initial doses, changes in dosing, or a change in the patient's physical condition or pain require careful observation of the individual patient to arrive at a safe and effective dose.
- Failure to watch the individual's response to narcotic may lead to undertreating or overtreating pain. Needless suffering may occur that could be corrected by increasing the narcotic. Unnecessary side effects, such as respiratory depression or excessive sedation, may occur that need to be reversed with naloxone or eliminated by decreasing the dose.
- Even after careful titration, some patients will continue to experience undesirable side effects such as sedation, nausea, and vomiting, necessitating a change in narcotic or medication regimen or additional medication, e.g., an antiemetic.
- Re-education of health professionals, families, and patients is usually necessary if narcotics are to be used effectively. Underuse results from many misconceptions and exaggerated fears about narcotics.
- In certain chronic nonmalignant pain conditions that would be more successfully treated with other modalities such as active physical therapy or behavior modification, overuse of narcotics may result in increased sedation and depression along with decreased function.
- Inadequate relief may occur with neuropathic pain (e.g., lancinating nerve pain) or pain related to a highly inflammatory condition (e.g., rheumatoid arthritis).
- Prolonged use of narcotics may require an increase due to tolerance to analgesia and almost always requires measures to prevent constipation. This can be done safely and effectively, but it does require vigilance.
- Must be used with caution by persons engaged in potentially dangerous activities, such as driving a car, until degree of alteration of mood and level of consciousness is determined.
- Recovered substance abusers usually want to avoid narcotics since they do not want to be exposed to mind-altering drugs.

Mode of Action of Narcotics

Currently there are two types of narcotics available in the United States:

1. Narcotic agonists, pure agonists, e.g., codeine, oxycodone, morphine, dolophine (Methadone), hydromorphone (Dilaudid), meperidine (Demerol), levorphanol (Levodromeran), and oxymorphone (Numorphan).
2. Narcotic agonist-antagonists, e.g., buprenorphine (Buprenex), nalbuphine (Nubain), butorphanol (Stadol), and pentazocine (Talwin).

Narcotics, regardless of type, probably relieve pain at the level of the CNS by attaching to opioid receptor sites at the brain and spinal levels (Houde, 1979; Lim, 1967). In addition, the agonist-antagonists are also capable of blocking the analgesic effect of pure narcotics similar to the narcotic antagonist effect of naloxone (Narcan). (The theory underlying these various actions is discussed on pp. 38-40.)

Forms of Undertreatment with Narcotics

Even when narcotics are clearly indicated, undertreatment of pain continues to be a pattern in health care today. The problem of undertreatment of pain is even greater in children. The result is needless suffering.

It is generally estimated that 85% to 90% of patients with acute pain or prolonged pain from end-stage disease could be comfortable if narcotics alone were used properly. However, it is apparent that people continue in moderate to severe distress from pain even when narcotics are used.

Nurses can make a difference in changing this unacceptable practice in health care. Being aware of the following specific forms of undertreatment of pain is a beginning.

1. *Physicians underprescribe narcotics* (Angell, 1982; Charap, 1978; Grossman and Sheidler, 1985; Marks and Sachar, 1973; Sriwatanakul et al, 1983). This takes two forms:
a. Using less than the effective dosage of narcotic.
b. Allowing longer intervals between doses than the drug's duration of action.

Examples of underprescribing are prescriptions for 50 and 75 mg of meperidine q4h PRN pain. In fact for many people, especially younger patients, larger doses may be required for pain relief (Jaffee and Martin, 1985, p. 514). Although meperidine is cited as having a 2 to 4 hour duration of action (Jaffee and Martin, 1985, p. 505), in our experience, its duration is often only 2 to 3 hours.

2. *Nurses administer less* than what the patient could receive according to the physician's prescription (Cohen, 1980; Fox, 1982; Marks and Sachar, 1973). This takes two forms:
a. Administering narcotics at longer intervals than allowed.
b. Administering less than the prescribed dose of narcotic. Legally this is a questionable practice.

An example of this involved one patient's prescription for "Dilaudid q4h PRN." This drug was administered by the staff at 8- and 16-hour intervals despite repeated documentations of unrelieved pain (Fox, 1982). In another now classic study in the pain literature, a person with chronic cholecystitis suffered unrelieved pain but received only 150 mg of the 450 mg of meperidine available to him over a 24-hour period (Marks and Sachar, 1973).

3. *People experiencing pain do not request or take narcotics* (Cleeland, 1987; Frank, 1980; Sriwatanakul et al, 1983). This takes three forms:
a. Taking the medicine at longer intervals than the duration of action.
b. Taking less than the prescribed dose.
c. Not taking the drug at all.

KEY POINT: All groups, nurses, physicians, patients and families, tend to underuse narcotics and need to be re-educated.

Why do these forms of undertreatment of pain exist? The four factors that often contribute to the undertreatment of pain are summarized in Table 4-8 and are discussed in the following section.

Reasons for Undertreatment with Narcotics

Physicians, nurses, and patients and their family members have similar fears that result in the undertreatment of pain. Following are four common fears.

1. Fear of Addiction

This appears to be the major reason for undertreatment among both health professionals and the public (Aguwa and Olusanya, 1978; Angell, 1982; Charap, 1978; Cohen, 1980; Frank, 1980; Trotter et al, 1981). The fear that *appropriate* use of narcotics causes addiction is irrational and undocumented. Increasing recognition of this fact is evidenced by an article in a substance abuse journal on "opiophobia" defined as "the irrational and undocumented fear that appropriate use of narcotics causes addiction" (Morgan, 1985-1986, p. 163).

A factual and unemotional approach to addiction requires that the term be defined and distinguished from other conditions related to narcotic use. In recent years the term *addiction* has been redefined. Not too long ago it was thought that addiction was both psychological and physiological dependence. Now physiological changes from repeated use of narcotics are recognized and treated as separate entities. Definitions and important differences between addiction and physiological conditions appear in Table 4-9.

Important aspects of the definitions in Table 4-9 are (Jaffe, 1985):
- Narcotic addiction, physical dependence, and tolerance are separate conditions. Each may occur alone, any two may occur together, or all three may be present at the same time.
- Physiological changes from repeated doses of narcotic are not the same as psychological dependence, and physiological changes do not automatically lead to psychological dependence. A patient may develop tolerance and require a higher dose, but this is not addiction. He may experience withdrawal syndrome if the narcotic is suddenly stopped, but again, this is not addiction.
- If a person is taking narcotics for the purpose of relieving pain, it is inappropriate to refer to him as an addict, no matter how much narcotic he is taking, how long, or how often. Pain relief is a legal, medical reason for prescribing and using narcotics.
- Misuse of narcotics for pain relief is not the same as abuse or addiction. Some patients with pain may have narcotics misprescribed for them. For example, other forms of pain relief, such as physical therapy or nonnarcotics, may be more appropriate than narcotics. The patient with a mental illness such as endogenous de-

pression may need psychotropic medication, not narcotics, to increase his ability to cope with pain. However, if a patient misuses narcotics because the physician inadvertently misprescribes, labeling the patient an addict is entirely inappropriate.

• The term *addiction* should be used with extreme care, since, in our society, to be addicted is often viewed as being a "bad person." When use of a drug is labeled addiction, considerable social stigma is attached.
    Incidence of Addiction. The incidence of addiction as

TABLE 4-8 Common Reasons for Undertreatment of Pain with Narcotics

Misconceptions	Corrections
Health professionals, patients, and families fear causing: 1. Addiction (psychological dependence), e.g., relieving pain with narcotics, especially high doses or prolonged use, will automatically lead to compulsive use in a large percentage of persons.	1. *No evidence* supports fear of addiction as a reason for withholding narcotics when they are indicated for pain relief. All studies show that regardless of doses or length of time on narcotics, the incidence of addiction is *less than 1%*.
2. Physical dependence (withdrawal syndrome), e.g., hard to get the patient "off" narcotics, could be life-threatening.	2. Withdrawal syndrome from narcotics is *rarely life-threatening* (except in infants born to physically dependent mothers). Most patients can be easily treated by gradually reducing the dose over 7 to 10 days. *Clinically, it is rarely noticed* since pain usually subsides gradually with concomitant decrease in narcotic.
3. Tolerance to analgesia, e.g., if narcotics are started too soon or escalated too fast, pain relief will be impossible because doses will be fatal or a ceiling on analgesia will be reached.	3. Tolerance does not develop uniformly to all narcotic effects. Usually tolerance to analgesia is accompanied by even greater tolerance to respiratory depression and sedation. Hence, the *lethal dose is markedly elevated.* Further, there is *no ceiling on analgesia* of the strong narcotics, e.g., morphine.
4. Respiratory depression, e.g., large or frequent doses will be fatal, low doses are safe, or going beyond a certain dose in any patient is unsafe.	4. *No dose is automatically safe or fatal.* A low dose may be fatal for one patient, but 10 times that dose may be safe for another. *The only safe way to administer a narcotic is to watch the first doses* given to the individual. A safe dose usually continues to be safe unless the drug accumulates or the patient's condition changes. *No patient need die of narcotic-induced respiratory depression.* It can be completely reversed with naxalone. (An exception is respiratory depression from buprenorphine.)

Table references:
Hodding, GC, Jann, M, and Ackerman, IP: Drug withdrawal syndromes—a literature review, *West J Med* 133:383-391, Nov 1980.
Jaffe, JH: Drug addiction and drug abuse. In Gilman, AG, et al, eds: Goodman and Gilman's the pharmacological basis of therapeutics, ed 7, pp 532-581, New York, 1985, Macmillan Publishing Co.
Opiate abuse—Part I, *The Harvard Medical School Mental Health Letter* 3:1-4, Jan 1987.
Perry, S, and Heidrich, G: Management of pain during debridement: a survey of US burn units, *Pain* 13:267-280, Jul 1982.
Porter, J, and Jick, H: Addiction rare in patients treated with narcotics, *N Engl J Med* 302:123, 1980.
Twycross, RG: Clinical experience with diamorphine in advanced malignant disease, *Int J Clin Pharmacol* 9:184-198, 1974.

TABLE 4-9 Definitions of Addiction, Tolerance, and Physical Dependence*

Term	Definition	Differences
Addiction	*Behavior* of overwhelming involvement with obtaining and using a drug for its psychic effects, not for approved medical reasons. High tendency to relapse back to continuing the drug once the pain is gone.	*Behavior* that involves active, compulsive drug seeking and a tendency to relapse even after physical withdrawal subsides. Use of narcotics for pain relief is not addiction since pain relief is an approved medical use.
Tolerance	After repeated administration of a narcotic, a given dose begins to lose its effectiveness, resulting in the need for larger and larger doses. The first indication of tolerance is decreased duration, then decreased analgesia.	Involuntary behavior based on *physiological changes*. The presence of drug tolerance *does not* mean the patient is addicted.
Physical dependence	After repeated administration of a narcotic, withdrawal symptoms occur if the narcotic is abruptly stopped.	Involuntary behavior based on *physiological changes*. The presence of physical dependence *does not* mean the patient is addicted.

*Adapted from Jaffe, JH: Drug addiction and abuse. In Gilman, AG, et al, eds: Goodman and Gilman's the pharmacological basis of therapeutics, ed 7, p 533, New York, 1985, Macmillan Publishing Co.

a result of taking narcotics for pain relief is extremely overestimated. Addiction rarely occurs when a person takes narcotics for pain relief. Of major importance in dealing with exaggerated fears of addiction is to identify the following *research* about narcotic addiction:

1. Far less than 1% of hospitalized patients receiving meperidine 100 mg q4h regularly ever became addicted (Marks and Sachar, 1973).
2. Of almost 12,000 hospitalized medical inpatients who received at least one narcotic, only 4 patients could be reasonably well-documented as addicts (Porter and Jick, 1980).
3. The length of time a person is on narcotics does not increase the incidence of addiction (Foley and Rogers, 1981; Twycross, 1974).

Some people will disagree with these statements, but ask if they can supply studies with different findings. Common areas where laymen and health professionals lack knowledge about addiction are summarized in the box on the right. Corrections to frequently expressed misconceptions about indicators of addiction are addressed in Table 4-10.

KEY POINT: The overwhelming majority of people stop taking narcotics when pain stops.

Guidelines for Discussing Addiction. When addiction is discussed among health professionals, it is usually an emotional issue, and accurate discussions are often overshadowed by unclear definitions, lack of awareness of research, and inappropriate labeling of patients. The nurse can foster accurate and knowledgeable use of the term *addiction* by following these guidelines:

1. Ask "Do you believe the person has pain?"

Believing the patient is basic to the successful treatment of pain. If you do not believe the patient when he asks continually for pain medication, then it is understandable that you might conclude that the patient is addicted. The error in this line of reasoning begins when the patient is not believed.

Overview of Why Patients May Be Erroneously Labeled as Narcotic Addicts

Fact: Most people do not know the facts about narcotic addiction. When narcotic addiction is suspected, people react emotionally instead of factually.

Common reasons for erroneously suspecting addiction are *lack of knowledge* about the following:

- What is the current definition of narcotic addiction? (See Table 4-9.)
- What do studies show regarding the probable percentage of people who become addicted following treatment for pain with narcotics?
- Are the following indicators of addiction?
  1. Prolonged use of narcotics.
  2. Clock-watching.
  3. Prefers "needle" to pill.
  4. "Enjoys his Demerol" or other narcotic.
  5. Knows the name and dose of narcotic.
  6. "Orders" his narcotic in anticipation of the pain.
  7. Requires higher and higher doses given more frequently.

None of the above are reasons for suspecting addiction. Table 4-10 explains why.

TABLE 4-10 Misconceptions about Indications of Addiction

Misconceptions about Indicators of Addiction	Comments/Corrections
1. Prolonged use of narcotics	1. Some pain is prolonged or lasts longer than expected. Length of time on narcotics does not increase likelihood of addiction.
2. Clock-watching	2. This usually results from inadequate pain relief. Some narcotics are short acting; some patients metabolize narcotics rapidly. The pain returns before the designated interval elapses.
3. Prefers "needle" to the pill	3. This can be the result of not applying equianalgesic dosages when the route of narcotic is switched from injections to PO. The result is often undermedication. The effectiveness of a dose given IM may be 2 to 6 times greater than the same dose given PO.
4. "Enjoys his Demerol" (or other narcotic)	4. Why not? If a person has been in pain, he will probably be happy to get relief.
5. Knows the name and dose of narcotic	5. This knowledge should be encouraged. It can be helpful information in assessing effective analgesics at a future time.
6. "Orders" narcotic in anticipation of pain	6. This can be an indication that the interval between doses is not timed correctly for his individual pain. Reassess the pain and evaluate the interval; or, the patient may have been instructed appropriately in the use of a preventive approach.
7. Requires higher and higher doses given more frequently	7. The underlying reason for the pain could be advancing, e.g., cancer metastasis. The other possibility is the development of tolerance.

Patient/Family Teaching Point: Your Concerns about Addiction

TO: _____ (patient's name)   DATE: _____

The fears you or your family may have about addiction could:
• Prevent you from requesting or taking the pain medication.
• Result in your "holding off" as long as possible between doses.
• Result in your taking lower doses of medication even though pain is not controlled.

   Doing any of the above will only result in needless suffering. Talk to the nurses about your concerns and fears. They will help you learn the facts about addiction:
1. Addiction very rarely happens in people who are taking pain medication to relieve pain.
2. Being on narcotics a long time does not increase your chance of becoming addicted.
3. When the pain stops or is less, most people are able to stop or reduce their pain medication without any problem.

   Ask yourself "Is there any reason that I would want to take this narcotic when I no longer have pain?" If you can answer no, then you will be able to stop taking the medication when the pain stops.

Additional comments: _____

_____

If you have any questions or concerns about the above, contact:

_____ (RN or MD name)   Phone: _____

_____ (Nurse's signature)

■ May be duplicated for use in clinical practice. From McCaffery, M, and Beebe, A: PAIN: CLINICAL MANUAL FOR NURSING PRACTICE, St. Louis, 1989, The CV Mosby Company.

---

2. Define and use the terms *addiction, tolerance,* and *dependence* appropriately.

   Addiction is often used inappropriately to label patients with pain who have merely demonstrated withdrawal signs or an increased need for pain medication. Nurses can be instrumental in stopping this labeling.
3. Cite references to address facts about addiction when communicating with health team members.
   These articles specifically address the overestimation of addiction:
   • Marks and Sachar (1973) and Porter and Jick (1980) both cite research showing the incidence of addiction following use of narcotics for pain relief is *far less than 1%*.
   • Foley (1982) discusses the fact that the medical use of narcotics is rarely if ever associated with addiction and that chronic narcotic use for analgesia is *not* associated with high risk of addiction.

Patient Example

After exhaustive titration of Mrs. S.'s hydromorphone, her pain from end-stage ovarian cancer was finally at a pain rating that was satisfactory to her. Before she was discharged home, the resident cautioned her about increasing the dose, stating that he did not want her to become an addict. The nurse asked him to explain what he meant by addiction. The reply was that she was at risk for addiction because she needed higher and higher doses to control her pain. (In fact at home, Mrs. S. gradually decreased the narcotic dosage on her own.) The nurse pointed out that what he described was either drug tolerance or the result of progressive disease. These are not the same as addiction. The physician concluded that it was all just a lot of semantics!

But it was not just semantics to Mrs. S., who was terrified of becoming addicted. This label from a physician was devastating. Some experts claim that the issue does not matter for someone who does not have long to live. But because of social stigma, addiction does matter to the people who take pain medication—no matter what their life expectancy. Addiction is often a moral issue. In our society, addicts are not "good" people. It is unacceptable to be seen as one or to die with this label.

The nurse working with Mrs. S. approached the resident the next day with copies of the articles discussed above. She stated that she wanted to follow up their discussion on addiction with these articles.

For people taking narcotics and their families, fears about addiction may go unspoken. They may never use the word addiction but may make statements like "I don't want to take too much medication" or "Shouldn't I try to hold off as long as possible between doses of pain medication?" The nurse must explore the fears behind these statements. The patient/family teaching point on p. 70 helps clarify concerns about addiction.

KEY POINT: It is important for nurses to *initiate* discussions about addiction with patients and their families.

2. Fear of Physical Dependence (Withdrawal Syndrome)

This fear is related in part to the misconception that if withdrawal signs are present they are the result of addiction or will automatically lead to addiction. It is important to distinguish between physical dependence and addiction (Table 4-9). Other common misconceptions are that withdrawal from narcotics will be life-threatening, that the symptoms will be difficult to control, and that the occurrence of withdrawal symptoms will prevent decreases in doses as the pain subsides. However, as discussed below, physical dependence is rarely life-threatening, is easy to manage in most patients, and does not prevent decreases in narcotic doses as the pain decreases.

Incidence of Physical Dependence. The incidence of physical dependence is greater than most health care professionals realize (Charap, 1978; Marks and Sachar, 1973). However, development of physical dependence is somewhat unpredictable. It probably begins to develop with the first dose of narcotic; after therapeutic doses of narcotic several times a day for 1 or 2 weeks, mild withdrawal symptoms may occur when the narcotic is stopped (Jaffe, 1985). These symptoms are so mild they are not usually recognized as withdrawal and certainly require no treatment. Clinical observations have shown that some patients on narcotics for long periods of time may demonstrate no recognizable withdrawal symptoms when the narcotic is stopped.

Symptoms of Narcotic Withdrawal. The symptoms of narcotic withdrawal are variable, ranging from mild to severe, and are less of a problem to manage than health care professionals believe (Charap, 1978; Fox 1982). Symptoms of withdrawal and their severity depend on many factors, such as the particular narcotic used and the dose. In a survey of 72 hospital-based nurses, 83% erroneously feared that the hazard of withdrawal from morphine was as great or greater than withdrawal from barbiturates (Fox, 1982). However, even when symptoms of narcotic withdrawal are severe, they are rarely life-threatening (except in the newborn).

The following is a list of general characteristics of symptoms that may occur after abrupt discontinuation of a narcotic in a person who is physically dependent (Jaffe, 1985):

- *Approximately 8 to 12 hours* after last dose: yawning, lacrimation, rhinorrhea, and sweating.
- *Approximately 12 to 14 hours* after last dose: restlessness, irritability, tremors, dilated pupils, and anorexia.
- *Approximately 48 to 72 hours* after last dose: increasing irritability, violent yawning, severe sneezing, nausea and vomiting, diarrhea, chills alternating with excessive sweating, muscle spasms, and low back pain.
- *Within 7 to 10 days,* these symptoms subside.
- *Abrupt withdrawal of methadone* may result in symptoms that develop more slowly and are more prolonged.
- *Abrupt withdrawal of meperidine* can result in symptoms appearing within 3 hours after the last dose and subsiding after 4 to 5 days.

Treatment of Withdrawal Symptoms. The purpose of treatment is to suppress these symptoms and keep the person comfortable (exceptions are newborns of addicted mothers where the purpose is to maintain life). Treatment of withdrawal usually is not necessary because pain usually subsides gradually and narcotics are automatically gradually decreased.

If management of withdrawal symptoms is necessary, a formula to suppress withdrawal symptoms in a patient who does not need the narcotic for pain relief is (Foley and Inturrisi, 1987):

- Administer one fourth of the previous narcotic daily dose in four divided doses for 2 days.
- Then decrease by one half and continue to administer in four divided doses with 50% reductions every 2 days until a total daily dose of 10 to 15 mg of morphine is reached.
- After 2 days at this dose, the narcotic can be discontinued.

Another common formula used for preventing significant withdrawal symptoms while narcotics are being reduced is to reduce the total daily dose by 10% a day over a 10-day period or by 5% a day over a 20-day period. For acute opiate withdrawal symptoms, clonidine (Catapres) 5 μg/kg administered bid for 1 to 2 weeks may be used with caution (Gold et al, 1979).

Oddly, clinical experience suggests that sometimes the initial decreases are easier to tolerate than the final decreases. In other words, the patient may not feel any significant withdrawal symptoms during the first part of the detoxification process, but when low doses are reached, decreases may cause symptoms. The solution often is simply to maintain the patient on low doses for a bit longer before further decreases are made.

The reassuring facts about physical dependence are:
- It is rarely life-threatening.
- It does not prevent decreases in doses.
- Symptoms can usually be easily treated by gradually reducing the narcotic dose.
- It is not the same as addiction and does not result in addiction.

KEY POINT: The most frequent problem caused by withdrawal symptoms is misunderstanding their meaning. *Their presence is not to be interpreted as addiction.*

3. Fear of Tolerance to Narcotic Analgesia

This tends to be of special concern in patients with prolonged pain, e.g., cancer, burns, and life-threatening illness. The physician, nurse, patient, and family may be afraid to:

• Start narcotics "too soon" and/or
• Escalate the narcotic dose "too fast."

They fear, especially with patients in the end stages of a disease but with weeks or months to live, that if pain increases, pain relief will be impossible or lethal.

Reassurances for Patients, Families, and the Health Care Team. These include the following:

1. If tolerance does occur, it can usually be treated safely and effectively by increasing the narcotic dosage.
2. The analgesic dose in a patient who has become tolerant to a narcotic is *not lethal* because the person also develops tolerance to the life-threatening side effect of respiratory depression as well as to sedation (Catalano, 1987; Foley, 1986; Jaffe, 1985; Twycross, 1974).
3. There is no such thing as the body becoming "immune" to analgesics. An adequate increase in dose almost always results in increased pain relief.
4. There is *no ceiling* on the analgesic effects of strong narcotics such as morphine, methadone, levorphanol, and hydromorphone (Levy, 1985; McCaffery, 1981; Miser et al, 1980).

KEY POINT: The longer the person is on narcotics, the wider the margin of safety. Time works in favor of safety.

Treatment of Tolerance. Guidelines are:

1. Maintain the oral route as long as possible since tolerance develops slower than with the IM or IV route (Foley and Rogers, 1981).
2. Increase the dose and/or decrease the interval between doses.

Patient Example

Mr. R., 26 years old, has a history of sickle cell disease and painful crisis about once a year. In each of four admissions over 4 years, IV narcotics relieved pain and were titrated down after about 3 days using PO narcotics, and he was narcotic free after 7 days. However, a crisis 6 months ago led to continuous pain due to multiple complications and more painful crises.

Initially, the painful crisis was relieved with a regimen similar to previous ones, consisting of a total of 20 mg morphine IV bolused over 30 minutes followed by continuous hourly infusion at 10 mg/hr, titrated down to hydromorphone 8 mg PO q4h ATC for ongoing, less severe pain. The dose and frequency of narcotics increased over the 6 months in a manner typical of tolerance to narcotic analgesia. Hydromorphone increased to 20 mg PO q3h ATC. Sudden increases in pain required IV MS boluses totaling 50 to 70 mg over 30 minutes and 40 mg infused hourly. During his fourteenth hospitalization lasting 3 weeks, Mr. R.'s complications finally resolved and he was pain free. As his pain subsided his narcotic dose decreased to zero, and he was discharged with no evidence of narcotic addiction.

This example is typical of the aggressive treatment that is needed for pain relief in complicated sickle cell crisis. The following articles may be helpful in getting the health care team to be willing to treat crises adequately:

Brozovic, M, Davies, SC, Yardumian, A, et al: Pain relief in sickle cell crises, *Lancet* 2:624-625, Sept 13, 1986.

Cole, TB, Sprinkle, RH, Smith, SJ, and Buchanan, GR: Intravenous narcotic therapy for children with severe sickle cell crisis pain, *Am J Dis Child* 140:1255-1259, 1986.

Ives, T, and Guerra, M: Constant morphine infusion for severe sickle cell crisis pain, *Drug Intell Clin Pharm* 21:625-626, July-Aug, 1987.

KEY POINT: Drug tolerance and physical dependence (withdrawal syndrome) are involuntary behaviors involving physiological responses. The person has no control over these conditions developing. The presence of tolerance or withdrawal symptoms does not mean the person is addicted.

4. Fear of Respiratory Depression

All narcotics are capable of producing respiratory depression and in fact to some extent affect all phases of respiratory activity. This is not life-threatening or even clinically significant in most patients. This capability in no way should prevent narcotics from being used to the fullest extent to relieve pain in all age groups. Studies show that equianalgesic doses of narcotic agonists produce about the same degree of respiratory depression (Jaffe and Martin, 1985). There is a ceiling to respiratory depression with narcotic agonist-antagonists. If narcotic-induced respiratory depression does occur, and if the patient is conscious, he can breathe if instructed to do so (Jaffe and Martin, 1985). An exception to this occurs with the use of fentanyl, which causes muscular rigidity along with respiratory depression.

Occurrence of Respiratory Depression. It is impossible to know what dose will produce clinically significant respiratory depression in a given patient. *Low doses cannot be assumed safe for all patients.* In a study of 3263 hospitalized medical patients receiving meperidine IM in doses ranging from 25 to 100 mg, 3 patients had clinically significant respiratory depression. The doses were 50 mg in two patients and 25 mg in one patient (Miller and Jick, 1978).

KEY POINT: The only safe and effective way to administer a narcotic is to *watch the individual's response,* especially to the first dose.

FLOW SHEET—PAIN: For Mrs. D

Patient _Mrs. D_ _____ Date _____

Pain rating scale used _0-10 (0 = no pain, 10 = worst pain)_ _____

Purpose: To evaluate the safety and effectiveness of the analgesic(s).

Analgesic(s) prescribed: _Morphine 150 mg PO q4h ATC_ _____

Time	Pain rating	Analgesic	R	P	BP	Level of arousal	Other	Plan & comments
9 AM	3	Morphine 150 mg PO	18			Awake and alert		
10 AM	1		16			States she is comfortable		
11 AM	1		12			Sleeping easily awakened		↓ Resp. due to pt. sleeping
12 N	2		16					
1 PM	2	Morphine 150 mg PO	18			Awake and alert		
5 PM	2	Morphine 150 mg	16			Talking with family members		
9 PM	1	Morphine 150 mg PO	12			Sleeping. Quickly awakens when name called		

This flow sheet is an example of the data that are useful to a nurse who is unfamiliar with the patient. No matter how large or small the dose of narcotic prescribed, the patient's previous response is extremely helpful in determining the probable safety and effectiveness of the next dose. In this situation, if the nurse is fearful of administering the prescription for morphine 150 mg PO q4h ATC, the data on this flow sheet reassure her that it has been given safely and effectively. She is therefore more likely to administer it.

Reassurances for Patients, Families, and the Health Care Team. When people with severe pain and those who have developed tolerance need high doses of narcotic, respiratory depression usually is not a problem. High doses will usually be safe because:

- Severe pain appears to be nature's antidote since it counteracts the respiratory depressant effects of the narcotic.
- Tolerance to narcotic analgesia usually assures tolerance to respiratory depressant effects (Jaffe and Martin, 1985).

The pain flow sheet (p. 27) is a tool that allows quick and easy monitoring of respiratory status.

Patient Example

You are asked to administer Mrs. D.'s pain medication, 150 mg morphine PO ATC. You question the dosage because your main concern is that the high dosage will cause her to stop breathing. You gather some facts to help you make your decision about the safety of giving this dose. The pain flow sheet for Mrs. D. is shown above. By quickly scanning the respiratory column, the nurse sees that Mrs. D.'s respiratory rate has remained stable despite this dose. In reviewing her prescriptions, you also note that she has been on this present dose for the past 2 weeks. With this information, you can confidently give the medication while continuing to monitor Mrs. D.'s comfort level.

Treatment of Respiratory Depression. This is safe and effective (except in situations of overdose involving unknown quantities and substances). Many instances of narcotic-induced respiratory depression that occur in the clinical setting do not need any particular treatment other than decreasing the dose or frequency of narcotic. Following are guidelines for more aggressive treatment of respiratory depression, if required.

1. Naloxone is titrated slowly at 0.1 to 0.4 mg IV over 2 to 3 minutes or 0.4 mg in 10 ml of saline slow push until respirations are normal.

   The purpose in most cases is to reverse the side effects, *not* the analgesic effect, of the narcotic. The most effective way to do this is to titrate the naloxone slowly. If the patient is conscious he can be instructed every 5 to 10 seconds to breathe.

   In the hospitalized patient, it is rarely necessary or appropriate to push IV 0.4 mg (1 ml) or 0.8 mg (2 ml) of naloxone. This practice is likely to eliminate *all* narcotic so that the patient has an abrupt return to severe pain. The ideal is both adequate ventilation and pain relief. Antagonize enough narcotic so that the patient breathes well again, but leave enough of the narcotic in the system to control pain.

2. Continue to observe the patient. Naloxone may wear off before the respiratory depressant effects of the narcotic decrease. The duration of action from IV naloxone may be as short as 30 minutes.

Pain Relief for Narcotic Addicts

Substance abuse disorder related to narcotics is the preferred terminology, but the term addiction is more commonly used. The term *narcotic addict* may refer to either recovered addicts or active users. However, since it is essential to distinguish between the two, they are discussed separately. The concern here is mostly with *narcotic* substance abusers, both recovered and active, but most of the recommendations also apply to the care of persons with other forms of substance abuse, e.g., alcohol.

Approaches to the Recovered Narcotic Substance Abuser with Pain

With some patients who admit to former narcotic or other substance abuse, it may not always be clear to what extent they have recovered or are committed to remaining free of psychological dependence on narcotics or other drugs. However, when the patient receives health care for problems other than substance abuse, the patient's commitment to recovery from substance abuse is not questioned; it is respected and accepted.

Whether the patient has abused narcotics or other substances, the health team may be concerned that the use of narcotics for pain relief will have an adverse effect on the patient's recovery from substance abuse. This decision, however, is the patient's, not the health team's. It is helpful to remember that recovery from substance abuse requires the patient's voluntary and strong commitment. Recovery cannot be forced on him. Therefore when narcotics are required for pain relief in a person who has abused substances, the health team *consults with the patient* about how to accomplish pain relief and how to support his efforts to remain free of substance abuse.

KEY POINT: The patient is responsible for his recovery from narcotic addiction or any substance abuse. The health team supports the patient's efforts to remain drug free by consulting with the patient about the use of narcotics for pain relief.

Most substance abuse programs advocate abstinence not only from the specific drug that was abused, e.g., narcotics, alcohol, or cocaine, but also strict avoidance of any medications that affect consciousness, i.e., have an effect "from the neck up." Of course, this includes avoidance of narcotics. However, the intent is not to make the recovered substance abuser suffer pain needlessly. Most substance abuse programs suggest methods of handling a period during which narcotics are needed.

For example, a recovering alcoholic who participates in Alcoholics Anonymous usually has a sponsor, a person who is also a recovered alcoholic to whom he may turn for individual guidance to stay sober. The person with pain who is a recovered alcoholic probably will contact his sponsor for guidance. Thus the patient and the sponsor are responsible for handling any problems that might occur with the appropriate use of narcotics for pain relief. The patient and sponsor may decide to talk daily about the patient's use of narcotics for pain relief. Upon discharge, the patient may even decide to give his narcotic prescription to his sponsor who will then give him 1 day's supply at a time. This is, however, a decision made only by the patient and sponsor.

The recovered substance abuser has a high stake in remaining recovered. He may already have spent considerable time, effort, and sometimes money to remain drug free. Such efforts are admirable. Such a person deserves the respect of the health team. It is presumptuous of a health professional to try to take control of substance abuse in a person who has maintained control of it himself.

Important considerations in providing pain relief with narcotics for a person recovering from narcotic or other substance abuse are:

- Explain to the patient the intent to use narcotics and why, e.g., that his pain is usually most effectively and efficiently relieved with narcotics.
- Ask the patient if he has any concerns about using narcotics for this episode of pain.
- Ask the patient if he is now or has been involved with a substance abuse program.

   If so, suggest that he contact staff or members of the program for suggestions about narcotic use for pain relief. Offer to talk with people from the substance abuse program.

   If not, offer specific guidelines for use of narcotics, and alter them in accordance with the patient's suggestions. The specific choice of narcotic, dose, frequency, and duration of use may be outlined. Some patients will want to be free of narcotic at the time of discharge.

- If the patient is not satisfied with the above approaches, consider nonnarcotic alternatives, such as regional nerve blocks, TENS, NSAIDs, cold packs, acupuncture, or infiltration of the wound with a local anesthetic.
- If the person is on methadone maintenance, i.e., a daily dose of methadone, for narcotic substance abuse, this dose must be continued. If PO methadone is not possible, approximately half the PO dose may be given IM in divided doses. For pain relief, *additional* narcotic is needed.
- Anticipate the need for larger than usual narcotic doses in the recovered addict or one who is on methadone maintenance. Either person may have tolerance to narcotic analgesia. Even the person who has not taken narcotics for months or years may quickly develop tolerance again if he was tolerant to analgesia previously, requiring larger than usual doses for pain relief. This should not be interpreted as addiction—it is a physiological change.
- If the patient has taken naltrexone, a long-acting narcotic antagonist used in some programs to prevent impulsive return to narcotic abuse, it is useless to give narcotics for pain relief until the drug is out of his system. For moderate to severe pain, aggressive use of nonnarcotic alternatives mentioned above is required.

Approaches to the Active Narcotic Substance Abuser with Pain

It is, of course, essential to determine if narcotic substance abuse is an appropriate label and what goals are realistic (see the box on the right for suggested questions to guide planning care). When an active narcotic addict, or other substance abuser, develops a painful condition, helping this person with pain control can be difficult. Why? Because health care professionals may fear:
- Promoting the person's addiction by administering narcotics.
- Being manipulated by the addict to obtain additional narcotics.
- Lack of experience in dealing effectively with addicts.

KEY POINT: The narcotic addict has the same right to pain control as any other person. Narcotics should not be withheld as a punitive or rehabilitative measure. Treatment of the pain in this case requires different rules and expectations.

The goal is to deliver humane care to a person with pain who happens to be a narcotic addict by:
1. Relieving the pain.
2. Keeping the person out of withdrawal.

Remember that long-term use of narcotics may have caused marked tolerance to narcotic analgesia. Therefore the person may require very large doses of narcotic for pain relief.

Approaches that may be used when the person with pain is also a narcotic addict are:

The Patient with Pain Who is also Addicted to Narcotics: Questions to Ask before Formulating a Plan of Care

- What evidence is there to document that this patient has a substance abuse disorder related to narcotics?
- Has the patient voluntarily admitted himself to this facility for treatment of substance abuse?
- Is this a substance abuse unit?
- What is the goal of this hospitalization?
- Is rehabilitation from substance abuse a realistic goal during this hospitalization?
- How do we prevent withdrawal syndrome?
- How do we relieve pain and avoid punishment or judgmental actions?
- How do we plan to detoxify the patient before discharge?

---

1. Determine the accuracy of the label "addict." The term *addiction* is too often used loosely or confused with the physiological changes of tolerance to analgesia (high, more frequent doses) and physical dependence (withdrawal syndrome). Identify whether any drug screening tests were performed. Realize that false results do occur. Identify whether the patient has obvious physical signs of addiction such as multiple needle marks, or has verbally admitted that he is an addict. If the patient has been using narcotics for *pain relief,* he should not be called an addict.
- Dependence on narcotics (drug dependence) *for relief of pain* is not psychological dependence, because pain is not a psychological or emotional problem. People react emotionally to pain just as they do to other symptoms such as bleeding or vomiting. However, this reaction does not mean that the pain is psychological in origin.
- For the person with pain to depend on narcotics is comparable to the person who is diabetic depending on insulin.
- Encourage use of appropriate terminology. "Addiction" arouses negative reactions. Even if the patient is addicted to narcotics, the more appropriate terminology would be substance abuse disorder. If the patient is not addicted, consistently use the more appropriate terms, e.g., physical dependence, tolerance to analgesia, misuse due to misprescribing.

2. If your clinical area is not a substance abuse unit, remember that the goal is not rehabilitation—it is treatment of the condition for which the patient was admitted, prevention of withdrawal, and relief of the person's pain.

3. Patient's statement of pain is believed. As with any person with pain, there can be no arguments about the presence or absence of pain. The narcotic addict experiencing the pain is the authority about his pain. Admittedly,

however, when the patient is addicted to narcotics, the chance of exaggeration of pain increases. This possibility, however, does not alter the fact that the patient may have pain and is the only person who can feel that pain.

4. Suggest that the following approach be considered in an effort to avoid an adversarial relationship with the patient, assure humane and safe treatment, and provide an opportunity for rehabilitation from substance abuse. The patient may be told that:

- He will receive as much narcotic as he requests unless it jeopardizes his welfare, e.g., decreased respirations.
- Most narcotic addicts are very knowledgeable about narcotics and know that the higher the dose, the more difficult the withdrawal.
- Medication will be given on a regular schedule.
- He will be tapered off narcotics (detoxified) prior to discharge.
- Upon discharge, he will receive only nonnarcotics if analgesics are needed. However, there are exceptions to this. The desired result is for the patient to understand that once the pain is controlled, the addiction will not be maintained with prescriptions.
- Upon discharge, give the patient information on rehabilitation.
- It is helpful if one physician in the hospital or clinical area is responsible for prescribing analgesics for all substance abusers. It is unreasonable to expect all physicians to keep abreast of current substance abuse practices and how to handle them safely and effectively.

Questions that may be helpful in formulating the care for a person with pain who is said to be addicted to narcotics are summarized in the box on p. 75.

The following three annotated references may be helpful if you are caring for an active narcotic addict with pain:

1. Fultz, J, Senay, E, Pray, B, and Thornton, W: When a narcotic addict is hospitalized, *AJN* 80:478-481, March 1980. This article presents facts about medical complications, signs and symptoms of withdrawal, and doses for methadone maintenance. Extensive bibliography and factual presentation may be helpful to intellectually understand the process of controlling an addict's physical needs while hospitalized.
2. Leporati, NC, and Chychula, LH: How you can really help the drug-abusing patient, *Nursing* 12:46-49, June 1982. Five specific guidelines are suggested for interacting with a substance abuser who is in your care. Two scripts of nurse-patient dialogues to get the patient talking about his problem are included. A chart lists commonly abused drugs and their effects. This helpful article presents realistic and unrealistic goals for patient care.
3. Stimmel, B: Pain, analgesia and addiction: the pharmacologic treatment of pain, New York, 1983, Raven Press. Excellent guidelines for the care of narcotic-dependent populations are presented on pp. 294-297.

The management of pain in heroin addicts and in people on methadone maintenance programs is discussed.

Equianalgesic Doses of Narcotics

Unfortunately, one of the best kept secrets in all of pharmacology seems to be the equianalgesic doses of narcotics by various routes for relief of moderate to severe pain, particularly the dose of narcotic required PO to equal the analgesia obtained by an IM dose. Lack of specific knowledge about this contributes to undertreatment as well as inappropriate conclusions about possible abuse and addiction.

Patient Example

The analgesics prescribed are meperidine 50 mg IM or PO PRN pain. The patient refuses the meperidine pills, saying that only the shot brings the pain from 9 to 5 on a 0 to 10 scale (0 = no pain, 10 = worst pain). The outcome of this situation is that the patient is unjustifiably labeled as a drug abuser because he "prefers the needle to the pill."

Misconception: Patients who "prefer the needle to the pill" are abusers or potential addicts.

Correction: Narcotics given IM are two to six times more effective than the same dose given PO. The patient logically asks for the medication that effectively relieves the pain.

Using the same dose regardless of route in the above example is inappropriate and ignores the concept of equianalgesic dosing. Equianalgesic means approximately equal analgesia, i.e., doses of medication that provide about the same pain relief when:

- Switching from one route of administration to another, such as from IM to PO or IV to PO.
- Switching from one drug to another, such as meperidine to morphine.

KEY POINT: The most common cause of undermedication in people with pain is the lack of knowledge of equianalgesic doses of drug (Foley, 1985b).

Application of information about the equianalgesic doses in Table 4-11 is one of the important steps in tailoring an analgesic regimen for each individual patient.

To become familiar with the equianalgesic chart in Table 4-11, note that there are four columns. Each column is discussed below, beginning with the left column.

1. *Analgesic* column lists the analgesics with morphine first, since it is the usual standard of comparison. The remainder of the analgesics are listed in alphabetical order by generic name. Only those analgesics and formulations available for human use are listed. Some analgesics, e.g., heroin, and some formulations, e.g., sublingual buprenorphine, have been studied and are used in some countries, but they are not on this list because they are not now approved for use in the United States.

2. *IM Route (mg)* column lists the doses of analgesics by the IM or SC route that are approximately equal to each other in the ability to relieve pain. Any dose in this column would be a reasonable initial dose to use to substitute for any other dose of analgesic in this column or in the PO column.

For example, if the patient has a prescription for Demerol 75 mg IM, and if you wish to switch the patient to a dose of morphine IM or SC that will relieve the same amount of pain, you would follow these steps:

- Locate meperidine, the generic of Demerol, in the left column.
- Find the dose listed for meperidine for the IM column. In this case it is the dose you wish to change, 75 mg.
- Locate morphine in the left column.
- Find the dose listed for morphine in the IM column. The dose is 10 mg. Thus 10 mg of morphine IM is an educated guess about the initial dose of morphine IM that would provide the same relief as meperidine 75 mg IM.
- Check the list under "Important Characteristics of the Equianalgesic Chart" (see heading below) and Table 4-11 for any indications that this initial dose should be revised. For example, has the patient been on meperidine so long that it is not being absorbed entirely or has the patient become tolerant to it? If either of these is a possibility, you probably would want to lower the initial dose of morphine 10 mg to 7 or 8 mg.
- If an analgesic is listed but the dose you are looking for is not the same dose that appears in the IM column, you may still use the list to calculate the initial dose. For example, if a child is receiving meperidine 50 mg IM and you wish to switch to morphine IM, you calculate that 50 mg is two thirds of 75 mg and that you will need two thirds of any IM dose listed, e.g., approximately 6.5 mg of morphine IM. (NOTE: The IM doses listed in this column are also used for calculating IV doses when switching from one analgesic to another via the IV route or switching from IM to IV; some clinicians regard the IM and IV doses as approximately equal, others suggest that the IV dose equals one half the IM dose.)

3. *PO Route (mg)* column lists the doses of analgesics by the PO route that are approximately equal to each other in their ability to relieve pain. Any dose in this column would be a reasonable initial dose to use to substitute for any other dose of analgesic in this column or any dose in the IM column.

For example, if you wished to switch a patient from a dose of codeine 90 mg PO (1.5 grains, or the equivalent of codeine in three Tylenol #3 or Empirin #3, exclusive of the nonnarcotics acetaminophen or aspirin, respectively) to a PO dose of hydromorphone, you would follow these steps:

- Locate codeine in the left column.
- Find the dose listed for codeine in the PO column. In this case the dose listed is 200 mg, but you wish to switch from only 90 mg, approximately one half of the listed dose. Thus to substitute for the PO codeine, you will need only one half of whatever PO or IM dose you find in this table.
- Locate hydromorphone in the left column.
- Find the dose listed for hydromorphone in the PO column. The dose is 7.5 mg. Since you need only one half of this dose, your initial guess would be about 4 mg of hydromorphone PO.
- Check the list under "Important Characteristics of the Equianalgesic Chart" (see heading below) and Table 4-11 for any indications that this initial dose should be revised. For example, if the patient has been on several doses of codeine daily for several weeks, the patient may be tolerant to codeine. Since cross-tolerance is not complete, you probably would lower your initial guess for the hydromorphone dose to 2 to 3 mg PO.

As a further example, if you wished to switch a patient from meperidine 75 mg IM to a dose of hydromorphone PO that would relieve the same amount of pain, you would follow steps similar to those above and find that the initial dose of hydromorphone is 7.5 mg, which is 8 mg in practical terms because of how the drug is supplied, i.e., tablets of 1, 2, 3, or 4 mg.

4. The *Comments* column mentions various considerations pertinent to the specific analgesic, in particular any differences from the standard of comparison (morphine). Comments may include information about onset, duration of action, accumulation of the analgesic or its active metabolites, the ratio for converting IM to PO, and special formulations such as sustained release.

Important Characteristics of the Equianalgesic Chart

1. The doses in this chart are based on research and are the doses recommended by the Analgesic Study Section, Sloan Kettering Institute for Cancer Research, New York. Doses at variance with the Sloan-Kettering recommendations are in parentheses. It is important the health team realize that this information is based on double-blind analgesic studies from leaders in the field of analgesic research.

2. The table is to be used only as a guide when tailoring drug and dosage for individual patients. The individual patient's response must be observed. Dose, time interval, route, and choice of drug are then adjusted according to the individual's response.

3. The doses in the table are not necessarily starting doses. They suggest the *ratio* to use when calculating doses.

4. The conversion factor for calculating the PO dose needed to substitute for the IM dose is written where applicable in the comments column of each drug. For example, in the comments about hydromorphone, the statement "PO dose is 5 times the IM dose" allows an easy, quick reference for calculating route or dose changes.

TABLE 4-11 Equianalgesic Chart: Approximate Equivalent Doses of IM and PO Analgesics for Moderate and Severe Pain*

Analgesic	IM Route (mg)†	PO Route (mg)‡	Comments
Morphine	10	60 (30)§	Both IM and PO doses of morphine have a duration of action of about 4 to 6 hr. Sustained-release tablets, rectal suppositories, and preservative-free for spinal analgesia are also available. The PO dose is 3 to 6 times the IM dose. The lower PO dose is suggested by several clinicians (Lipman, 1980, 1982; Walsh, 1984) and is based on anecdotal evidence, not experimental research (Kaiko, 1986); it may be appropriate for some patients, especially elderly patients with chronic cancer pain. *All IM and PO doses in this chart are considered equivalent to 10 mg of IM morphine in analgesic effect.*
Buprenorphine (*Buprenex*)	0.4 (0.3)	—	A narcotic agonist-antagonist that may precipitate withdrawal in patients *very* physically dependent on narcotics. Dose for the sublingual form (not available in the US) is 0.8 mg. Compared with morphine, this drug is longer acting and more likely to produce nausea and vomiting (Bradley, 1984). Respiratory depression is rare but serious because it is not readily reversed by naloxone ("Buprenorphine," 1986). Not available in Canada.
Butorphanol (*Stadol*)	2	—	A narcotic agonist-antagonist that may produce withdrawal in patients physically dependent on narcotics. May also produce psychotomimetic effects such as hallucinations. Not available in Canada.

*The equianalgesic doses in this chart are based primarily on recommendations of the Analgesic Study Section, Sloan-Kettering Institute for Cancer Research, New York, based on double-blind analgesic research (Houde, 1979). This format is adapted from McCaffery, M: A practical, portable chart of equianalgesic doses, *Nursing* 17:56-57, Aug 1987.

†Based on clinical experience, many consider the IM and IV dose equianalgesic (Portenoy, 1987). However, some recommend using ½ the IM dose for the IV dose (American Pain Society, 1987).

‡Initial PO doses are usually lower than those listed here, especially for mild to moderate pain.

§Values in parentheses refer to differences of opinion among clinicians.

A guide to using the equianalgesic chart

• Equianalgesic means **approximately** the same pain relief. Onset, peak effect, and duration of analgesia for each drug often differ and may also vary with individual people.

• Variability among individuals may be due to differences in absorption, organ dysfunction, or tolerance to one narcotic and not to another.

• An equianalgesic chart is a *guideline*. The individual patient's response must be observed. Doses and intervals between doses are then titrated according to the individual's response.

• An equianalgesic chart is helpful when (1) switching from one drug to another or (2) switching from one route of administration to another.

• Dosages in this chart are *not* necessarily starting doses. They suggest the *ratio* for comparing the analgesia of one drug with another.

• Based on clinical experience, the IV dose is approximately the same as the IM dose. Dose adjustments are then made according to the individual's response. Some clinicians suggest approximately ½ the IM dose equals the IV dose.

Table references

American Pain Society: Principles of analgesic use in the treatment of acute pain and chronic cancer pain: a concise guide to medical practice, Washington, DC, 1987, The Society

Beaver, W: Management of cancer pain with parenteral medication, *JAMA* 244:2653-2657, Dec 12, 1980

Beaver, W, and Feise, G: A comparison of analgesic effect of oxymorphone by rectal suppository and intramuscular injection in patients with postoperative pain, *J Clin Pharmacol* 17:276-291, May/June 1977

Bradley, J: A comparison of morphine and buprenorphine for analgesia after abdominal surgery, *Anaesth Intens Care* 12:303-310, Nov 1984

Buprenorphine, *Med Lett Drugs Ther* 28:56, May 23, 1986

Houde, RW: Systemic analgesics and related drugs: narcotic analgesics. In Bonica, JJ, and Ventafridda, V, eds: Advances in pain research and therapy, vol 2, pp 263-273, New York, 1979, Raven Press

Jaffe, J, and Martin, W: Opioid analgesics and antagonists. In Gilman, A, et al, eds: The pharmacological basis of therapeutics, ed 7, pp 491-531, New York, 1985, Macmillan Publishing Co

Kaiko, R: Controversy in the management of chronic cancer pain: therapeutic equivalents of I.M. and P.O. morphine, *J Pain Sympt Manag* 1:42-45, Winter 1986

Kaiko, R, et al: Central nervous system excitatory effects of meperidine in cancer patients, *Ann Neurol* 13:180-185, Feb 1983

Kantor, T, et al: Adverse effects of commonly ordered oral narcotics, *J Clin Pharmacol* 21:1-8, Jan 1981

Lipman, A: Comment on pain cocktail article, *Drug Intell Clin Pharm* 16:332, Apr 1982

Lipman, A: Drug therapy in cancer pain, *Cancer Nursing* 3:39-46, Feb 1980

McGee, J, and Alexander, M: Phenothiazine analgesia—fact or fantasy? *Am J Hosp Pharm* 36:633-640, May 1979

Narcotic agonists and analgesics. In Facts and comparisons: drug information, 242b, Philadelphia, 1986, JB Lippincott Co

Portenoy, RK: Continuous intravenous infusion of opioid drugs, *Med Clin North Am* 71:233-241, Mar 1987

Romagnoli, A, and Keats, A: Ceiling effect for respiratory depression by nalbuphine, *Clin Pharmacol Ther* 27:478-485, Apr 1980

Vernier, V, and Schmidt, W: The preclinical pharmacology of nalbuphine. In Gomez, Q, ed: Nalbuphine as a component of surgical anesthesia, pp 1-9, Princeton, NJ, 1985, Excerpta Medica

Walsh, T: Oral morphine in chronic cancer pain, *Pain* 18:1-11, Jan 1984

TABLE 4-11 Equianalgesic Chart: Approximate Equivalent Doses of IM and PO Analgesics for Moderate and Severe Pain—cont'd.

Analgesic	IM Route (mg)	PO Route (mg)	Comments
Codeine	130	200	Relatively more toxic in high doses than morphine, causing more nausea and vomiting and considerable constipation. The PO dose is about 1.5 times the IM dose.
Fentanyl (*Sublimaze*)	0.05	—	Most common use is for anesthesia, given IV. Onset of action when given IM is about 15 min; duration of action, about 90 min. Analgesic effect is not significantly increased by droperidol (Jaffe and Martin, 1985). Has been used as a substitute for high-dose IV morphine in terminally ill patients when morphine caused excitation. Used IV in neonates and for brief procedures.
Hydromorphone (*Dilaudid*)	1.5	7.5	Somewhat shorter acting than morphine. Also available as rectal suppository and in high-potency injectable form (10 mg/ml). The PO dose is 5 times the IM dose.
Levorphanol (*Levo-Dromoran*)	2	4	Longer acting than morphine when given in repeated, regular doses. Useful alternative to PO methadone. Careful titration required because drug accumulates; both dose and interval must be adjusted. Onset of action with PO dose occurs within 1½ hr. Because drug accumulates, analgesic effect may increase with repeated doses. *Initial* PO dose is twice the injectable dose. (The SC route is recommended over the IM route.)
Meperidine (*Demerol*)	75	300	Shorter acting (2 to 4 hr) than morphine. Watch for toxic effects on the central nervous system (CNS) caused by accumulation of the active metabolite normeperidine, which produces neuroexcitability. Use with caution in patients with renal disease. *Because of the risk to the CNS, 300 mg PO is not recommended.* Since normeperidine has a long half-life (15 hr or longer), decreasing the dose in patients exhibiting a toxic reaction may increase CNS excitability, causing seizures. Effects of normeperidine are increased (not reversed) by naloxone (Kaiko et al, 1983). The PO dose is 4 times the IM dose.
Methadone (*Dolophine*)	10	20	Longer acting than morphine when given in repeated, regular doses. Careful titration required because drug accumulates; both dose and interval must be adjusted. Onset with PO dose occurs within 1 hr. Because drug accumulates, analgesic effect may increase with repeated doses. *Initial* PO dose is twice the IM dose.
Methotrimeprazine (*Levoprome*)	20	—	A phenothiazine (nonnarcotic) drug. Duration of action is 4 to 5 hr. Common adverse effect is hypotension; not recommended for ambulatory patients (McGee and Alexander, 1979).
Nalbuphine (*Nubain*)	10 (20)	—	A narcotic agonist-antagonist that may produce withdrawal in patients physically dependent on narcotics. Longer acting and less likely to cause hypotension than morphine. In doses above 10 mg/70 kg, it causes no additional respiratory depression (Romagnoli and Keats, 1980; Vernier and Schmidt, 1985), so patient may be started on a high dose.
Opium (*Pantopon*, opium tincture)	20 (13.3)	(6 ml)	Infrequently used. Pantopon is the injectable form; opium tincture, the oral form. Pantopon, 20 mg, equals 10 mg of IM morphine (Beaver, 1980) or 15 mg of IM morphine ("Narcotic Agonists and Analgesics," 1986). Opium tincture contains 1% morphine, that is, 0.6 ml equals 6 mg of PO morphine. Therefore 6 ml equals 60 mg of PO morphine (Jaffe and Martin, 1985).
Oxycodone	—	30 (15)	Has faster onset and higher peak effect than most PO narcotics; duration of action is up to 6 hr. In one study of postoperative pain, a preparation similar to the old formulation of Percodan (containing oxycodone, aspirin, phenacetin, and caffeine) was more effective and caused fewer adverse reactions than 90 mg of PO codeine or 75 mg of PO pentazocine, and was almost equivalent to 12.5 mg of IM morphine (Kantor, et al, 1981).
Oxymorphone (*Numorphan*)	1 (1.5)	—	Also available as rectal suppository; 10 mg given rectally equals 10 mg of IM morphine (Beaver and Feise, 1977). Up to 1.5 mg IM is now recommended as equal to 10 mg of IM morphine (Jaffe and Martin, 1985).
Pentazocine (*Talwin*)	60	180	Narcotic agonist-antagonist that may produce withdrawal in patients physically dependent on narcotics. Could produce psychotomimetic effects. The PO dose is 3 times the IM dose.
Propoxyphene HCl (*Darvon*)	—	500	The one recognized use is for mild to moderate pain unrelieved by nonnarcotics. *Never give as much as 500 mg PO*, only low PO doses (65 to 130 mg) are recommended. The IM form is not available in the US.

■ May be duplicated for use in clinical practice. From McCaffery, M, and Beebe, A: PAIN: CLINICAL MANUAL FOR NURSING PRACTICE, St. Louis, 1989, The CV Mosby Company.

5. Based on *clinical* experience an hourly equianalgesic IV drip narcotic dose is approximately the same as the IM dose (Portenoy, 1987a). If 10 mg morphine IM q4h controls pain and the patient is switched to IV morphine, the initial q4h dose would be 10 mg IV or 2.5 mg per hour. Other authors suggest that one half the IM dose gives an equivalent IV dose (Foley, 1982; Yasko, 1983). Controlled studies are needed for this route of administration.

6. All of the IM and PO doses listed in the chart are considered equivalent and are compared with the analgesic standard, 10 mg of IM morphine. For example, by referring to the PO and IM columns in the equianalgesic chart (Table 4-11), we see the following: hydromorphone 1.5 mg IM is equivalent to methadone 20 mg PO, and levorphanol 4 mg PO is equivalent to meperidine 75 mg IM. Further, these are all approximately equal to each other.

KEY POINT: The initial calculation of an analgesic dose is merely an educated guess. Individualizing the dose, time interval, route, choice of drug, and then monitoring the person's response are vital steps to the effective use of analgesics.

7. Two PO doses are listed as being equivalent to 10 mg morphine: 60 mg and 30 mg. The 30 mg PO dose is widely used in clinical practice; however, it is not supported by research (refer to comments column next to morphine in Table 4-11 for references). The lower dose of 30 mg may be especially appropriate for elderly patients with chronic cancer pain, while the higher dose of 60 mg may be more appropriate for children and young adults. Although it is disconcerting to see this degree of controversy regarding the PO dose of morphine, remember that all doses in the chart are merely educated guesses. When a dose is given, it is immediately titrated up or down according to the patient's response.

8. References are listed within the chart so that when nurses discuss this information with physicians and other health team members, their suggestions are supported by appropriate, accessible data.

9. Several factors are considered when changing drugs or route of administration. Although the equianalgesic chart serves as an accurate guideline, there are additional factors to consider when switching from one narcotic to another or when changing the route of medication, for example from IM to PO or PO to IV. Some of the potential problems that may alter the doses suggested in the equianalgesic chart include those listed in Table 4-12.

Suggestions for the Use of the Equianalgesic Chart

This information is of no use filed away in a desk drawer. Following are some effective ways to use the equianalgesic chart to re-educate the health team and encourage them to refer to it.

- Copy this chart directly from pp. 78-79. Post copies of it in the medication area and chart area where nurses and physicians can refer to it when prescriptions are dispensed and written. Send it to the pharmacy. For home care, mail it to the physician's office when requesting changes in analgesic orders. Suggested words to introduce the physician to the chart: "My analgesic suggestions and dosage changes are based on the enclosed equianalgesic chart. References are included in the comments column opposite the drugs."
- Carry with you the laminated pocket-size equianalgesic chart enclosed inside the front cover. For additional copies, duplicate and reduce the chart on pp. 78-79 to pocket-size and distribute it (include the pharmacy) as a handy guide with references within the table.
- Distribute the chart to nursing students, medical students, interns, and residents who rotate through your clinical area. Ask to be part of their introductory session to the area to explain the use of the chart. This is important for all areas where nurses administer or monitor narcotics.
- If the hospital, office, clinic, or agency uses computerized medication ordering systems, incorporate the chart into the system so that the health care team members can readily refer to it when writing prescriptions or evaluating analgesic regimens.

KEY POINT: Nurses have a leadership role in suggesting analgesic titration. Therefore it is important that they are active in educating health team members about the effective use of an equianalgesic chart.

Know the Pharmacology of the Specific Narcotics

Knowledge of basic pharmacology is essential if initial prescriptions and subsequent changes are to relieve pain as quickly, effectively, and safely as possible. Pharmacological facts that guide decision-making include knowing that there is no hierarchy among the four strong narcotics, but that differences between narcotics determine which one is selected. Following is a discussion of the characteristics of narcotics with a long duration of action, the problems encountered with meperidine, and possible interactions between narcotic agonists and agonist-antagonists.

No Hierarchy among the Four Strong Narcotics

Each of the four most commonly used strong narcotics, morphine, hydromorphone, levorphanol, and methadone, are equally capable of relieving pain. There are no data to support the misconception "save the morphine for the end" because it is the "strongest" drug available. If equianalgesic doses are selected and then individualized along with time intervals, each of these four strong narcotics will provide equal analgesia, and morphine or any strong narcotic may be begun early.

TABLE 4-12 Considerations when Switching Drugs or Routes

Potential Problems	Possible Solutions
1. Calculating PO dose if incomplete absorption of IM dose	Consider decreasing the amount of the PO dose needed for equal analgesia.
Example: Mrs. V.'s muscle mass no longer absorbed the regular doses of morphine 10 mg IM. Fluid leaked out the injection site.	*Approach:* Mrs. V. was able to swallow without problem, so she was switched to PO morphine. She was elderly and stated she was sensitive to drugs, so the equianalgesic PO morphine dose of 30 mg rather than 60 mg was used initially.
2. Differences in the absorption of PO dose	The initial dose may need to be adjusted up or down.
Example: Mr. P.'s first dose of morphine 30 mg PO resulted in sedation with pain relief.	*Approach:* Mr. P.'s dose of morphine was decreased by 5 mg PO. Pain rating remained between 2 and 3 on 0-10 scale, and sedation decreased. Patient observed for further adjustments.
3. Organ dysfunction	A shorter-acting narcotic or a lower dose may be needed. This may be especially true in the elderly or anyone with poor kidney and liver clearance. Methadone is poorly tolerated by many elderly patients since a general decrease in organ function may lead to a cumulative effect. Analgesia may increase with repeated doses, and metabolites causing side effects are not readily eliminated.
Example: On methadone PO, Mrs. A., 80 years old, was very sedated at the doses required for pain relief.	*Approach:* Mrs. A. was switched to morphine, a shorter-acting narcotic, and was alert at doses that relieved her pain.
4. Switching narcotics after tolerance to analgesia has developed	Tolerance often develops with repeated administration of a narcotic, but tolerance may not be present to the same extent with a new narcotic, i.e., cross-tolerance tends not to be complete. Therefore to avoid too many side effects, start with a lower equianalgesic dose and adjust up or down according to the patient's response.
Example: Mr. S. has taken 48 mg PO hydromorphone q3h ATC for the last month. Number of pills to swallow at each dose and cost became problems. He was switched to PO morphine.	*Approach:* To replace hydromorphone 48 mg PO, the equianalgesic PO morphine dose is 192 mg (calculated using 30 mg morphine equals 7.5 mg hydromorphone). Consider beginning with 150 mg to compensate for incomplete cross-tolerance. Then titrate up or down according to Mr. S.'s response.

Selection of a Narcotic

Morphine is the standard strong narcotic for severe acute pain and chronic cancer pain (American Pain Society, 1987). Reasons for choosing a narcotic other than morphine may include the following:

1. Patient or family member has had a good prior experience with another narcotic or insists on using previous narcotic.
2. The individual patient experiences unacceptable side effects from morphine. For example, some patients may have continued problems with nausea and vomiting despite an aggressive antiemetic regimen.
3. A strong narcotic is needed in a high concentration and limited volume. For example, parenteral administration may be needed for a cachectic patient. Hydromorphone can be prepared by the pharmacist in concentrations of more than 100 mg/ml and is commercially available in high potency (HP) of 10 mg/ml. This would be particularly useful for high doses of continuous SC infusions. The solubility of morphine is approximately 62.5 mg/ml (Drug Information, 1987) and is usually mixed in concentrations no greater than 50 mg/ml. Not only can more milligrams of hydromorphone than morphine be concentrated in each milli-

liter, each milligram of hydromorphone provides approximately 6 to 7 times more pain relief than each milligram of morphine. For example, the equianalgesic chart (Table 4-11, pp. 78-79) shows that 1.5 mg IM of hydromorphone equals 10 mg IM of morphine.

4. When rapid absorption and quicker onset of action are needed by the parenteral or spinal route. Methadone, meperidine, and fentanyl are more lipid soluble than morphine and are therefore more quickly absorbed into the spinal system. Fentanyl given IM or IV has a more rapid onset than other narcotics and it might be more desirable as premedication for a brief painful procedure, e.g., bone marrow aspiration.
5. The need for a drug of longer duration of action. Methadone, levorphanol, and sustained-release morphine provide a longer duration of action than morphine. A longer interval between doses may be desirable, e.g., to allow the patient to sleep through the night uninterrupted and for children and young adults who tend to metabolize narcotics rapidly. This group of drugs is discussed below.

Narcotics of Long Duration. Oral narcotics that provide a long duration of action are methadone, levorphanol, and sustained-release morphine (American Pain

TABLE 4-13 Oral Narcotics of Long Duration

Narcotic	Duration
Methadone	4 hours initially, sometimes 6 to 8 hours after accumulation. Carefully evaluate dose, interval, and patient's response because drug accumulates with regular, repeated doses.
Levorphanol (Levo-Dromoran)	4 hours initially, sometimes 6 to 8 hours after accumulation. Carefully evaluate dose, interval, and patient's response because drug accumulates with regular, repeated doses.
Sustained-release morphine (MS Contin, Roxanol SR)	12 hour dosing. In some instances 8 hour dosing may be needed.

Society, 1987). They may be especially appropriate for the person with chronic pain who is (1) inconvenienced by a 3 to 4 hour schedule with the short-acting narcotics, i.e., meperidine, morphine, and hydromorphone, or (2) overwhelmed by the numbers or frequency of pills prescribed.

Because their cumulative analgesic effect could be even more pronounced, methadone and levorphanol should be used with caution in the elderly (see Chapter 11 for elaboration) and in those patients with liver dysfunction.

Narcotics of long duration, i.e., methadone, levorphanol, and sustained-release morphine, should not be escalated rapidly. Therefore a short-acting narcotic, or "rescue" analgesic, is often given along with the long-acting narcotic, either on a regular basis while the long-acting narcotic is being gradually increased or PRN for sudden increases in pain (breakthrough pain). Table 4-13 lists the specific narcotics of long duration.

Specifics about Methadone PO. Methadone might be chosen because it is one of the least expensive narcotics. However, it is the most difficult to titrate because of its long and variable half-life of 15 to 30 hours (Foley and Inturrisi, 1987).* With regular, repeated doses of methadone, accumulation occurs over a 3 to 5 day period or longer, and the patient's response must be monitored carefully during this period. Therefore methadone is considered a second-line choice unless the patient is tolerant to narcotics (Foley and Inturrisi, 1987) or metabolizes narcotics rapidly, e.g., a child or young adult.

When switching a patient who is tolerant from one narcotic to a different one, it is usually recommended that the equianalgesic dose be reduced by 50%. However,

*Half-life is the time it takes a drug to fall to half of its concentration in the blood.

experience with methadone has resulted in some clinicians suggesting an even greater dose reduction, i.e., 75%, when switching to methadone in the patient who is tolerant (Rogers, 1988 a and b). Significant tolerance to narcotic analgesia may occur after regular administration of the narcotic for a week or longer. Indications that tolerance to narcotic analgesia has developed include the need to take the narcotic at more frequent intervals or the need to increase the dose to relieve the same amount of pain.

During the initial dosing period it may not be a good idea to give methadone at regular intervals. Until regular intervals can be established, a preventive PRN schedule is suggested, i.e., the dose is not given until pain begins to return or increase. *Remember that adjustment of dosage and interval according to each individual patient's response is the safest way to administer any narcotic.* With methadone this process of adjustment usually takes longer than with the shorter-acting narcotics such as morphine.

Methadone PO may be initiated in several ways. Following is an example of a fairly conservative approach:

1. Calculate the initial PO methadone *dose*. If the patient has not been on narcotics, start with a relatively low dose of methadone PO, e.g., 5 to 10 mg. If the patient is taking a narcotic that relieves his pain, use the equianalgesic chart to estimate the equianalgesic dose of methadone PO. If the patient is tolerant to narcotic analgesia, reduce this methadone dose by 75%.

2. Begin PO methadone on a *preventive PRN schedule*. Monitor the patient's response with a flow sheet. Use a quick-acting narcotic with a short duration (e.g., 25% of the previous narcotic dose, if applicable) as a rescue analgesic until pain is controlled with PO methadone. Decrease the methadone dose at once if sedation or respiratory depression occurs.

3. After 72 hours of administration, determine the interval and increase the dose if necessary. Since it usually takes about 72 hours or longer before the cumulative effects of methadone are known, wait about 72 hours before scheduling doses ATC or before increasing the methadone dose.

Specifics about Levorphanol PO. This drug is similar to methadone in its duration of action, but it has a shorter half-life, i.e., 12 to 16 hours, and may be better tolerated by some patients. It is a useful alternative for patients who are unable to tolerate morphine or methadone.

Initiating Methadone and Levorphanol PO in the Home. These analgesics may be particularly difficult to monitor in the home. Consider continuing the previous narcotic and start methadone 5 mg PO or levorphanol 1 mg PO q8h PRN while gradually decreasing the original narcotic. If long duration is desired and if there are no limiting side effects from morphine, then the authors suggest sustained-release morphine rather than methadone or levorphanol. The lack of cumulative properties in morphine makes this an easier drug to adjust in situations that do not allow constant monitoring.

Specifics about Sustained-Release Morphine Tablets. Sustained-release morphine formulations have a long duration of action, i.e., 8 to 12 hours, without the cumulative effects of methadone or levorphanol. Side effects are essentially the same as those seen with the regular immediate-release morphine.

Suggestions for Converting to Sustained-Release Morphine. Several approaches may be used. A common approach is to stabilize the patient's pain on PO immediate-release morphine *before* beginning the sustained-release preparation. To do this:

- Use an equianalgesic table to convert the present total 24 hour narcotic intake to an equianalgesic dose of PO immediate-release morphine. (See pp. 106-107 for guidelines for changing from IM or IV to PO.)
- Give immediate-release morphine q4h, adjusting dose and interval as needed according to the individual's response.
- When good pain control is achieved on immediate-release morphine, calculate the total 24 hour dose and divide into 2 doses q12h for sustained-release morphine. Although theoretically the initial calculation should work for most patients, it may not always. Be prepared to adjust the dose up or down depending on the individual patient's response. While 12 hour intervals are appropriate for many patients' pain, even after dose adjustments, some patients may need to take sustained-release morphine at 8 hour intervals.

Remember: With any change in narcotic the patient must be observed closely and changes made in dose and interval according to the individual's response.

Patient Example

Mrs. Z. was taking Percocet 2 tablets q4h and rating her pain at 8 on a 0 to 10 scale. In this situation it is inappropriate to switch directly to sustained-release morphine. Instead, pain was first controlled with immediate-release morphine, and then the switch was made to sustained-release morphine. Following are the calculations:

Each Percocet tablet = oxycodone 5 mg + acetaminophen 300 mg. At 12 tablets per 24 hours, the present 24 hour dose = 60 mg oxycodone + 3600 mg acetaminophen. Based on oxycodone 30 mg PO = morphine 60 mg PO (see equianalgesic chart in Table 4-11, pp. 78-79), 60 mg oxycodone/24 hours is equivalent to 120 mg PO morphine/24 hours. Morphine 20 mg PO + 650 acetaminophen was begun q4h. To provide increased pain relief, morphine was increased to 40 mg q4h, which reduced pain to 2. Then the switch was made to sustained-release morphine by calculating the total 24 hour dose of morphine, i.e., 40 mg × 6 = 240 mg/24 hours. Thus the dose of sustained-release morphine q12h = 120 mg, i.e., 240 mg ÷ 2.

Mrs. Z.'s pain rating was closely monitored using a flow sheet to make sure that her pain was controlled at 2 or less and that analgesia lasted for the 12 hour period.

Other important aspects of using sustained-release morphine are:

- Use a rescue analgesic, or short-acting narcotic, e.g., immediate-release morphine, for breakthrough pain, pain that occurs between dosing intervals. To calculate the rescue dose of immediate-release morphine, consider what the four hourly dose would be if the patient were using immediate-release morphine. For example, if the patient is taking sustained-release morphine 120 mg q12h, the four hourly dose is 40 mg. A rescue dose is usually 50% to 100% of this.
- Sustained-release morphine formulations are not appropriate for PRN dosing, incidental, or breakthrough pain. They have a slow onset and potentially longer duration of action than the incidental or breakthrough pain.
- A patient may initially receive only 8 hours of relief or may need additional doses of short-acting morphine in between. Increasing the dose may allow a 12 hour interval and no need for PRN rescue doses. However, do not escalate a long-acting narcotic rapidly. Use rescue doses of short duration while the sustained-release dose is gradually increased.
- Sustained-release morphine should not be given any more frequently than q8h.
- For patients who have difficulty swallowing, choose the formulation with the smaller size tablet. Presently Roxanol SR tablets are slightly larger than the typical aspirin tablet, while MS Contin is considerably smaller.
- Do not break, crush, or allow patient to chew sustained-release tablets. If patient has problems swallowing tablets or has an N-G tube, use a liquid morphine preparation.

Potential Problems with Meperidine

Although meperidine is one of the most frequently prescribed IM narcotics, several characteristics of this drug make its popularity questionable. Compared with other parenteral narcotics, meperidine is:

a. Shorter acting (Beaver, 1980). Although there are no studies to document how short acting meperidine is, the authors and many other clinicians find that it often lasts only 2 to 3 hours (Jaffe and Martin, 1985; Marks and Sachar, 1973; Westring, 1974). Others disagree (Foley, 1987). Research does show that duration of action may be even shorter in younger people, i.e., the younger the patient, the shorter the duration of action tends to be (Kaiko, 1980). Smokers may also experience a short duration of action (Jick, 1974).

b. Irritating to tissue with the potential for severe muscle tissue fibrosis with frequent injections (Beaver, 1980; Jaffe and Martin, 1985) and must be given IM, not SC.

c. Responsible for neuropsychiatric effects, such as disorientation, bizarre feelings, and hallucinations. These occur frequently with parenteral meperidine, while they occur less frequently with morphine (Miller and Jick, 1978).

d. More toxic, due to the accumulation of an active metabolite, normeperidine, which is a CNS stimulant (Kaiko et al, 1983; Szeto et al, 1977).

e. Prescribed in inadequate PO doses, resulting in poor analgesia. A PO dose of 300 mg is needed to provide the equianalgesic effect of 75 mg IM but is not recommended due to greater amounts of normeperidine that would result. *Remember that meperidine 50 mg PO is about equivalent to the analgesic effect of 650 mg aspirin* (refer to the equianalgesic chart, Table 4-4, p. 61). The result is often poor pain control with the PO route of administration.

Based on the above data, when meperidine IM is chosen to relieve pain the result is that a neurotoxic, irritating substance with neuropsychiatric effects must be administered frequently for analgesia. *Clearly there is limited use for this drug as an analgesic for ongoing pain.* In fact in two recent publications on analgesic drug therapy, meperidine is listed as "not recommended" in the equianalgesic charts (American Pain Society, 1987, p. 4; Foley and Inturrisi, 1987, p. 214).

Cause, Symptoms, and Treatment of Meperidine-Induced Toxicity. This discussion concerns *toxicity,* not side effects. The side effects of meperidine are those that occur with most other narcotics: respiratory depression, sedation, and hypotension. The probable cause of meperidine-induced toxicity is the accumulation of normeperidine, an active metabolite of meperidine. Normeperidine is a CNS stimulant, whereas meperidine is a CNS depressant. If normeperidine accumulates, symptoms of neurotoxicity occur and increase in the following order:

• Shaky feelings.
• Hand tremors.
• Twitches.
• Multifocal myoclonus (muscle jerks).
• Grand mal seizures (Kaiko et al, 1983).

Patients at Risk for Accumulating Normeperidine. Patients most at risk for accumulating normeperidine and developing toxic symptoms are probably those who are exposed to any *one* of the following:

• Six days or longer on meperidine with daily doses of 300 mg, e.g., 50 mg given six times in 24 hours, or 75 mg given four times in 24 hours, or more (Kaiko et al, 1983). However there are unpublished reports of seizures following one dose.

• High frequent doses to relieve pain of any type, e.g., sickle cell crisis, cancer, terminal illness, or pancreatitis. One study reported a total of 14 instances of grand mal seizures in 7 patients with sickle cell disease who received meperidine (Tang et al, 1980).

• Renal dysfunction (Kaiko et al, 1983; Szeto et al, 1977). However, patients with normal renal function are also at risk (Mauro et al, 1986). In one study of 67 patients, 5

patients who showed severe meperidine toxicity with myoclonus and seizures had no evidence of renal problems (Kaiko et al, 1983).

Nursing Interventions Related to Meperidine-Induced Toxicity. Unfortunately meperidine is the most frequently prescribed parenteral narcotic. Nursing responsibilities related to patients for whom meperidine is prescribed are outlined below.

1. Patients already receiving meperidine:

a. Be alert to early signs of neurotoxicity, e.g., tremors, twitching, or jerking, or patient's report of being awakened by involuntary jerking movements.

b. Inform physician of possible neurotoxicity from accumulation of normeperidine.

c. Obtain copy of the Kaiko et al 1983 article to document your concern.

d. Recommend basing decisions on the following facts:

• It takes about 5 half-lives for a drug to be eliminated from the body.

• Meperidine is a CNS depressant with a half-life of about 3 hours.

• Normeperidine is a CNS stimulant with a half-life of about 15 hours or more. Therefore avoid simply decreasing the meperidine since the CNS depressant will leave the body much sooner than the CNS stimulant, leaving the patient at risk for increasing neuroexcitation, including seizures.

• Naloxone, a narcotic antagonist, and narcotic agonist-antagonists (e.g., Nubain) will eliminate meperidine but not normeperidine. If these were given, symptoms of neuroexcitation would worsen and a seizure might occur.

e. Recommend changing to an equianalgesic dose of another pure narcotic agonist to be continued at the same dose for about 3 days to allow time for normeperidine to be eliminated from the body.

f. Suggest considering the addition of a CNS depressant to prevent seizures until normeperidine has been eliminated.

2. Patients who are at risk for accumulating normeperidine but have not yet received meperidine:

a. Be alert to those situations that place the patient at risk for accumulating normeperidine:

• High, frequent doses.
• Renal dysfunction.
• Prolonged narcotic treatment, e.g., 6 days or longer.

b. Obtain copy of the Kaiko et al 1983 article to document risk.

c. Recommend that meperidine *not* be given and that another narcotic agonist, e.g., morphine, or narcotic agonist-antagonist, e.g., nalbuphine, be used.

Alternatives to IM Meperidine. The following drugs are less irritating to the tissue, longer acting, and less toxic:

- Morphine IM or SC.
- Hydromorphone IM or SC. It is almost as short acting as meperidine; however, it is less toxic and less irritating to the tissue.
- Levorphanol SC.
- Methadone IM or SC. Accumulation of metabolites of methadone after parenteral administration may present the same problems as it does after PO doses.

If the physician is unfamiliar with equianalgesic doses of the above, use the chart, Table 4-11, pp. 78-79, to calculate the dose. For example, if the physician ordinarily prescribes Demerol 75 mg IM, he could prescribe Dilaudid 1.5 mg IM.

The box below lists annotated references concerning choice of narcotic which may promote effective communication.

Mixed Agonist-Antagonist Narcotics

This group of drugs is called "agonists" because they bind to opioid receptors to produce analgesia, and "antagonists" because they also partially reverse the effects of pure narcotic agonists (i.e., morphine, meperidine). Refer to Chapter 3, pp. 38-40, for discussion of these analgesics and the clinical application of the multiple opioid receptor theory.

Three agonist-antagonists will be discussed:

- Nalbuphine (Nubain) IM, IV.
- Butorphanol (Stadol) IM, IV.
- Pentazocine (Talwin) IM, IV, PO.

Buprenorphine (Buprenex) is also a narcotic agonist-antagonist, but it is unlike the others in this group. It does not antagonize at the mu site except at very high doses or in very physically dependent persons. Also, although respiratory depression is rare with this drug, it is the only one in which narcotic-induced respiratory depression cannot be completely reversed by naloxone.

Some confusion about the narcotic agonist-antagonists exists because government regulations often do not classify them as narcotics, or controlled substances. However, pharmacologically they are narcotics, or opioids.

Potential Problems with Narcotic Agonist-Antagonists. If the narcotic antagonist property of butorphanol, nalbuphine, and pentazocine is not understood, these drugs may cause the following difficulties.

They may precipitate withdrawal in a person who has been on pure narcotic agonists for a week or more. After a course of narcotic agonists, the person may become physically dependent, i.e., if the narcotic is abruptly discontinued, the person experiences withdrawal. Narcotics with an antagonist property may precipitate withdrawal by abruptly blocking the action of the pure agonist. Therefore the three above narcotic agonist-antagonists

---

References for Effective Communication Concerning Choice of Narcotic: Morphine as the Standard; Inappropriate Uses of Meperidine

Cancer pain relief, World Health Organization, 1986. A 74-page booklet discusses the prevalence of cancer pain, education and training, legislative factors, and specific methods for relief of cancer pain with medications. Order from: WHO Publications Center USA, 49 Sheridan Avenue, Albany, N.Y. 12210. $7.80 USD/copy.

Foley, KM: The treatment of pain in the patient with cancer, 1985. Available free as an American Cancer Society Professional Education Publication (PEP) #3308-PE. Originally published in *N Engl J Med* 313:84-95, July 11, 1985. A review of pharmacological, neurosurgical, and behavioral approaches to cancer pain by a recognized specialist in the field.

Inturrisi, CE, and Umans, JG: Pethidine and its active metabolite, norpethidine, *Clin Anaesthesiol* 1:123-138, Apr 1983. A review of the studies that relate to the mechanism of pethidine (meperidine) induced neurotoxicity.

Kaiko, RF, Foley, KM, Grabinski, PY, et al: Central nervous system excitatory effects of meperidine in cancer patients, *Ann Neurol* 13:180-185, 1983. In 67 patients with postoperative or chronic cancer pain treated with IM meperidine, 47 showed CNS excitatory effects. In 47 postoperative patients receiving meperidine, all had mild negative mood

changes. A key article that supports avoiding or discontinuing meperidine and switching to a different narcotic.

McCaffery, M: Giving meperidine for pain—should it be so mechanical? *Nursing 87* 17:61-64, 1987. Reviews the adverse effects of meperidine, inappropriate route and frequency, and discusses alternatives to this drug.

Principles of analgesic use in the treatment of acute pain and chronic cancer pain: a concise guide to medical practice, American Pain Society, 1989. A 29-page booklet authored by physicians who specialize in the pain control field and published by a national professional organization. It has an equianalgesic table and discusses guidelines for effective use of analgesics. Order by writing to: American Pain Society, 5700 Old Orchard Rd., 1st Floor, Skokie, IL 60077-1024, (708) 966-5595. $2/copy. It was also published as an article in *Clin Pharm* 6:523-532, July 1987.

Walsh, TD: Common misunderstandings about the use of morphine for chronic pain in advanced cancer. Available free as an American Cancer Society Professional Education Publication (PEP) #3312-PE. Originally published in *CA—Cancer J Clinic* 35:164-169, May-June 1985. A very useful article to share with those who are reluctant to use morphine.

must be used with caution after a person has been on pure narcotics for a week or longer. A physically dependent person may be carefully switched from a narcotic agonist to an agonist-antagonist, but it may take up to 10 days or longer of small, daily decreases in the agonist accompanied by small, daily additions of the agonist-antagonist.

Given along with pure narcotics, they may eventually antagonize analgesia from the pure narcotics. Initially, giving the two narcotic groups together may be additive, and it is difficult to predict when the agonist-antagonist will begin to reverse analgesia of the agonist. Early in narcotic therapy, a decision should be made about which group of narcotics will be used. A person can be switched from a narcotic agonist-antagonist to a narcotic agonist without much difficulty, except for some possible initial decrease in analgesia until the agonist-antagonist is excreted.

Benefits of the Narcotic Agonist-Antagonists. All four of the narcotic agonist-antagonists (buprenorphine, butorphanol, nalbuphine, and pentazocine) have a ceiling on the amount of respiratory depression they cause. Beyond a certain dose, additional respiratory depression does not occur. Therefore an increase in dose usually results in more pain relief without more respiratory depression.

However, nalbuphine appears to be the drug of choice if limited respiratory depression is desired when high doses are needed for pain relief. As mentioned above, buprenorphine-induced respiratory depression, although rare, is not completely reversed with naloxone. Further, high doses of butorphanol and pentazocine are likely to cause psychotomimetic effects. By contrast, respiratory depression from nalbuphine can be reversed by naloxone, and psychotomimetic effects are rare, although sedation occurs. Situations in which nalbuphine is recommended include the following:

- Emergency rooms in areas of high street drug activity. Nalbuphine discourages use of emergency room by well-documented narcotic street addicts who fake pain for narcotics, since nalbuphine can precipitate withdrawal in people who are physically dependent on narcotics.
- Postoperative narcotic-induced respiratory depression. The strong antagonist effect of nalbuphine can be used to reverse unwanted side effects of pure narcotics, particularly respiratory depression, without reducing analgesia. (The other narcotic agonist-antagonists do not seem to have a strong enough antagonist effect at the mu site to be used in this manner. For an explanation of the mu, kappa, and sigma opioid receptor sites, see pp. 38-40). To reverse respiratory depression from a pure narcotic agonist, the usual adult dose of nalbuphine is 2 to 3 mg IV every 2 to 3 minutes up to 9 mg (Magruder, Delaney, and Difazio, 1982).

Patient Example

Ms. M. is admitted to the recovery room following surgery, and IV morphine boluses are given to relieve her pain. Her respirations decrease from 14 to 4/minute. Rather than reverse the morphine-induced respiratory depression with naloxone, which also reverses analgesia, nalbuphine 3 mg IV is given twice. This reverses respiratory depression (at the mu site) and provides analgesia (at the kappa site). Five minutes after the last dose of nalbuphine 3 mg IV, Ms. M.'s respirations are 12/minute and she reports only slight pain. The patient was continued on nalbuphine 20 mg IM for postoperative analgesia.

- Childbirth (labor and delivery). Given IV, nalbuphine lasts only 1 hour and causes limited respiratory depression.
- Postoperative pain relief. There is a ceiling on the amount of respiratory depression beyond a dose of 10 to 20 mg IM, and it is supportive of blood pressure.
- Burn tanking or debridement. Up to 1 mg/kg can be given without significant risk of respiratory depression or psychotomimetic effects.

Patient Example

Mr. J., 20 years old, weighing 160 lb is admitted for second- and third-degree burns over 50% of his body. For the initial cleansing and debridement, he is given nalbuphine 15 mg IV, resulting in no clinically significant respiratory depression, but no pain relief. Nalbuphine 70 mg IV is given, resulting in no change in respiratory function, considerable sedation, and, according to the patient, "better relief."

- IV patient-controlled analgesia (PCA). The danger of accidental overdose due to mechanical malfunction or operator error is minimized since nalbuphine is supportive of blood pressure and has a ceiling on amount of respiratory depression. It is also safer *initially* than a pure narcotic agonist, such as morphine, when a patient requires especially high doses to relieve pain and is not yet tolerant to respiratory depression.

Patient Example

Following upper abdominal surgery, 25 patients with moderate to severe pain received IV nalbuphine via PCA. A maximum of 20 doses of 5 mg (100 mg maximum) was available per hour, and in some cases up to 200 mg in 1 hour was given with no clinically significant cardiovascular or respiratory problems (Kay and Krishnan, 1986).

Summary of Important Pharmacological Facts

Important pharmacological facts summarized here include reminders about choice of strong narcotic, avoidance of meperidine, and use of narcotic agonist-antagonists. These are reflected in the patient example on p. 87.

Although morphine, hydromorphone, methadone, and levorphanol are equally capable of relieving severe pain, morphine is usually the drug of choice. It is available for administration via more routes than the others, including IV, IM, rectal, PO, and spinal. It is also formulated in sustained-release tablets, permitting a long interval between doses without the potential problems posed by the cumulative effects of the longer-acting narcotics methadone and levorphanol. However, morphine is not always the drug of choice. For example, methadone or levorphanol are probably better choices than morphine for young patients who metabolize narcotics rapidly or for those who are very tolerant to narcotics. Hydromorphone may be a better choice than morphine when high doses are required SC or IV, since hydromorphone can be prepared in higher concentrations than morphine.

Unfortunately, the most frequently prescribed injectable narcotic is meperidine. However, there is great risk of toxicity from accumulation of its active metabolite, normeperidine.

Narcotic agonist-antagonists have the advantage of a ceiling on respiratory depression. Currently, four are marketed in the United States, buprenorphine, butorphanol, nalbuphine, and pentazocine. Of these, the latter three have a clinically significant antagonist effect against the pure narcotic agonists, such as morphine and meperidine. Because butorphanol, nalbuphine, and pentazocine partially antagonize the effects of pure narcotic agonists, they must be used with caution when pure narcotic agonists are being given. These three narcotic agonist-antagonists may reverse the analgesia of pure narcotic agonists, or they may precipitate withdrawal-like symptoms in the patient who has become physically dependent. Physical dependence may occur after a pure narcotic agonist has been administered for a week or longer.

The following patient example illustrates application of the above summary.

Patient Example

Mr. F., 61 years old, is terminally ill with metastatic cancer and is being cared for at home. Until yesterday his pain was well controlled with codeine 60 mg and acetaminophen 300 mg (Tylenol #4) plus 500 mg acetaminophen (Extra Strength Tylenol) q4h, with an occasional additional Tylenol #4, especially at bedtime so he could sleep through the night without awakening with pain. Increasing the codeine dose might relieve his pain, but there is usually a ceiling to the analgesia that can be obtained by increasing codeine doses, and at high doses codeine often causes nausea and is very constipating. He already takes daily medication to prevent constipation. Further, with progressive disease his pain probably will continue to escalate and soon require even stronger analgesia.

Now is the time to switch to a narcotic that may be used for the remainder of his life—a strong narcotic that can be given orally, with the flexibility of other routes if needed, and with at least a 4 hour duration of action. Following are the reasons for considering or eliminating specific narcotics:

- Meperidine is ruled out mainly because prolonged use increases the risk of meperidine-induced CNS excitability from accumulation of normeperidine. It is short acting and also irritating to the tissues if IM or SC routes must be used. For these reasons meperidine is not recommended for chronic cancer pain.
- Narcotic agonist-antagonists, e.g., nalbuphine, are ruled out since the patient probably has developed physical dependence from prolonged use of narcotics, and these drugs could precipitate withdrawal. Also, of this group of narcotics, only pentazocine is available PO and it tends to cause psychotomimetic effects, especially at high doses.
- Choice is narrowed to any of the following four strong narcotics: morphine, hydromorphone, methadone, or levorphanol.
- Methadone and levorphanol are longer acting than morphine and hydromorphone but are not available rectally, although they probably could be made into suppositories and given effectively by that route. The main reason for not selecting methadone and levorphanol is that their long duration of action is due to accumulation, and patients with organ dysfunction due to age or disease (both are possibilities with this patient) may have difficulty eliminating metabolites that cause side effects.
- Morphine and hydromorphone are available for all routes of administration and do not accumulate but are relatively short acting.
- Morphine is available in sustained-release oral formulation that results in a long duration of action without accumulation of metabolites. The sustained-release formulation is a significant reason for choosing morphine over hydromorphone.

Decision: Acetaminophen 1000 mg q4h is continued, and the patient is begun on MS Contin q12h. The initial dose is calculated by:
1. The total daily dose of codeine (6 to 7 doses/day × 60 mg = 360 to 420 mg/day),
2. Converted to morphine equivalent (200 mg codeine PO = 30 mg MS PO for elderly patient with cancer pain; 360 to 420 mg codeine PO = about 60 mg MS PO), and
3. Divided into two doses, i.e., 30 mg MS Contin q12h.

The rescue analgesic can be Tylenol #4 since the patient has some left and is familiar with its effects.

The patient starts at 6:00 P.M. with Tylenol #4 plus 500 mg acetaminophen as usual plus his first dose of MS Contin 30 mg. The reason for giving Tylenol #4 at the same time as the initial dose of MS Contin is that initial onset of analgesia for MS Contin is about 2 hours, so the Tylenol #4 will cover the patient until MS Contin takes effect. An NSAID with greater antiinflammatory ability than acetaminophen may be considered in the future.

The Appropriate Route of Administration

Adjust the route of drug administration according to the individual patient's needs. These needs would include such considerations as convenience, side effects, cost, and onset of analgesia.

It is also important to consider the method by which a route is delivered. Patient-controlled analgesia (PCA) is a method that usually refers to the patient's self-administration of IV boluses of narcotic using a special infusion pump. However, a broader and more useful definition includes all drug routes that allow the patient to be in control.

Therefore PCA evolves into a concept that includes the patient's self-administration of any analgesic drugs and other forms of pain relief by a method that considers safety as well as the patient's ability and willingness to control any or all of the following (McCaffery, 1987b):
- Stopping and starting an ongoing form of analgesia.
- Increasing or decreasing the ongoing amount.
- Initiating an occasional increase in relief above the ongoing amount.

The concept of PCA should be applied to all routes of administration, including oral, IV, SC, and spinal routes.

Oral Route

The oral (PO) route has these advantages:
- Convenient and easy to administer.
- Provides a steady state of analgesia.
- Allows mobility and independence.
- Less expensive than parenteral route.

Indications for the PO route. Unfortunately, many patients who are able to take PO medication are on parenteral narcotics. Indications for the PO route are:
- Mild to severe pain.
- If patient can swallow.
- If nausea and vomiting can be controlled.

Misconception: Moderate or severe pain will only be controlled with IM or IV routes of administration.

Correction: Oral narcotics can relieve severe pain if the doses are high enough and a preventive approach is used.

Guidelines and Recommendations for PO Route. Two *guidelines* for controlling moderate to severe pain with PO narcotics are:
1. Use a preventive approach to stay on top of the pain. This is especially important because the onset of oral analgesia is slower than that of IM or IV medication, with the peak effect normally occurring approximately 1.5 to 2 hours after dosing.
2. Use high enough doses (refer to equianalgesic chart on pp. 78-79). Typically health care professionals are accustomed to giving PO narcotics for the relief of mild or moderate pain; therefore they are afraid of the high PO doses needed for severe pain. Re-education is vital and must emphasize equianalgesic doses and the ratio of drug needed depending on the route.

If fear continues to be a barrier to adequate PO doses, one strategy might be to recommend an unfamiliar narcotic that has a relatively low number of milligrams and uses few tablets. It may be easier to get physicians to prescribe this and nurses to administer it. For example,

morphine 30 mg to 60 mg PO and levorphanol 4 mg PO are both equianalgesic to meperidine 75 mg IM. The levorphanol may be more acceptable to a fearful health care team because it is a lesser known narcotic; 4 mg "sounds less risky" than a 30 or 60 mg dose of morphine and requires only two pills of 2 mg each.

Recommendations for using the oral route include:
- Tablets are usually preferred because they are less expensive than liquid.
- Liquid may be considered if there is difficulty swallowing or if titration involves very small amounts, e.g., 1 to 4 mg.
- Use a flow sheet (discussed on pp. 26-29) to determine safety and effectiveness of analgesics. Adjust dose up or down depending on these findings.

Method of Administration: Oral PCA. In the home setting, the patient and family commonly control administration of oral narcotics and nonnarcotics. While patient control of oral analgesics in the hospital is far less common, it has been done with good results. For example, hospitalized patients 1 to 4 days postoperative were given their own supply of 25 capsules of acetaminophen and codeine (Tylox). They kept this medication at the bedside and charted what they self-administered on a hospital medication sheet. The 26 patients who agreed to self-administer experienced no loss of capsules, no overdosage, and no significant difference in number of Tylox taken compared with patients given medication by the nurses; all stated they would prefer to self-administer again (Jones, 1987).

In another report, patients and the health care team on a postpartum unit expressed satisfaction with a 5 year program of self-administered pain medication and other routinely prescribed drugs (Anderson and Poole, 1983).

Intramuscular Route

Although the intramuscular (IM) route is frequently used for most types of postoperative pain, it is often ineffective for these patients as well as others with severe acute pain such as sickle cell crisis.

Disadvantages of the IM route are:
- IM injections are painful to receive.
- Suitable injection sites may be lacking.
- The patient is usually dependent on someone else for pain relief.
- Preparation and administration are time-consuming. This may prolong the interval between doses, allowing pain to return.
- Repeated injections are impractical for prolonged pain.
- In the immediate postoperative period, absorption of IM narcotics may be especially poor. In one study, meperidine 100 mg IM given in the first 4 hours postoperatively provided no pain relief in 8 of 10 patients. Blood concentrations of meperidine showed that absorption was poor at this time, probably due to decreased peripheral circulation (Austin et al, 1980).

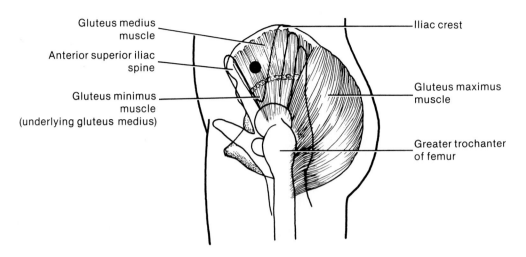

FIGURE 4-4 *Ventrogluteal site for IM injection.* To locate this site, the nurse palpates the greater trochanter of the femur with the heel of the hand. The index and middle fingers are spread to form a V from the anterior superior iliac spine to just below the iliac crest. The triangle formed between the index finger, the middle finger, and the crest of the ilium is the injection site. The injection is made in the center area of the triangle with the needle directed slightly toward the iliac crest or at a right angle to the muscle. This site is relatively free from major nerves and vessels and has a larger muscle mass and less subcutaneous tissue than the dorsogluteal site. It is recommended for adults and children over 3 years of age who have been walking.

From Pagliaro, AM, and Pagliaro, LA: Pharmacologic aspects of nursing, St. Louis, 1986, The C.V. Mosby Company.

Variability in absorption poses a specific danger in the postoperative period when an IM dose is repeated. For instance, as a result of poor absorption, the first IM dose may not provide pain relief for the patient. The dose may be repeated. As circulation improves, the initial dose may be absorbed just as the second dose is taking effect. The result may be a patient who is in pain just before the second dose, and afterwards is more likely to be sedated or have respiratory depression.

• On an ongoing basis, drug absorption is highly variable and dependent on the following factors: blood flow at the injection site, muscle activity, and the choice of site for injection (Lukacsko, 1987). To promote optimal absorption, the nurse should look for healthy muscle mass that is not painful to touch, e.g., abscesses, sloughing tissue, or degenerated tissue as in the inactive elderly or emaciated patient. Avoid paralyzed muscles, e.g., below level of spinal cord injury, or those that are not exercised, e.g., with bedridden patients.

Appropriate Site for Injections. The four choices of site for injections are the deltoid, ventrogluteal, dorsogluteal, and vastus lateralis muscles. The following specifics about each site may assist the nurse to select the appropriate site for the individual situation.

1. Absorption is more rapid after injections into the *deltoid* muscle than the gluteal muscle (Grabinski et al, 1983). However, because of the small size of the deltoid and the proximity of major nerves and blood vessels, this site is appropriate only for small volumes of medication—0.5 ml or less (Pagliaro, 1986). *The deltoid site is not recommended for children under 1½ years.* The deltoid may be the site of choice if the patient:

a. Needs a rapid degree of pain relief.
b. Is older than 1½ years.
c. Has well-developed deltoid muscles.
d. Receives a small volume IM, 0.5 ml or less.

In most patients, a ⅝ inch needle should be used to reach the deltoid.

2. For comfort and safety, the *ventrogluteal* site (Figure 4-4) seems to be the best choice (Farley et al, 1986; Feldman, 1987; Pagliaro, 1986); yet it is the site least used by nurses. Because this site is mostly free of major nerves and blood vessels, it is safer than the dorsogluteal site; it also has a larger muscle mass and less fat (Pagliaro, 1986).

The ventrogluteal is a good site for elderly, nonwalking, and emaciated patients. It is not recommended for children under 3 years of age.

When the ventrogluteal site is used with the patient in the prone position, the toes are pointed inward to relax the muscle. In a sidelying position, the top knee is flexed and in front of the lower leg to promote muscle relaxation (Pagliaro, 1986).

Usually a 1½ to 3 inch needle is needed to reach the ventrogluteal muscle. If a shorter needle (1¼ inch) is

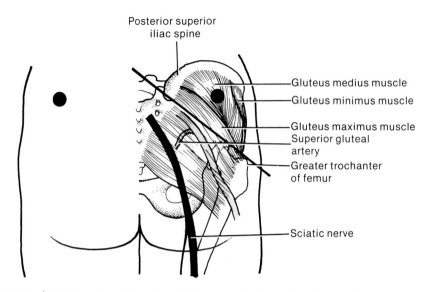

FIGURE 4-5 *Dorsogluteal site for IM injection.* To locate the site for injection, the nurse should draw an imaginary line from the posterior superior iliac spine to the greater trochanter of the femur. Because this line is lateral to and parallel to the sciatic nerve, a site selected laterally and superiorly will be away from the nerve as well as the superior gluteal artery. The injection is made into the gluteus medius muscle. To relax the muscle for injection and to reduce pain, the patient should toe-in. The needle should be inserted at right angles to the surface on which the patient is lying. The dorsogluteal site is *not* recommended for use in infants less than 18 months of age because the muscle mass is not well developed until the child has been walking for at least a year. Great care must be taken in mapping this site because of the proximity of the sciatic nerve and major vessels.

From Pagliaro, AM, and Pagliaro, LA: Pharmacologic aspects of nursing, St. Louis, 1986, The C.V. Mosby Company.

used, then the medication may be injected into fat instead of muscle, thereby interfering with adequate absorption.

3. The *dorsogluteal* site (Figure 4-5) is the most commonly used, even though this site requires careful mapping because of the proximity of the sciatic nerve and major blood vessels. This site is not appropriate for elderly or emaciated patients as the muscle in this area is likely to be degenerated; it is not recommended for infants less than 18 months because the muscle mass is not well-developed (Pagliaro, 1986).

Positioning the patient on the abdomen with toes pointed inward will relax the muscle and reduce pain (Kruszewski et al, 1979).

The biggest problem with this site is the use of needles that are too short. The result is that the muscle is not reached and there is pain and poor absorption. A 1¼ inch needle is too short. A needle 1½ or 2 inches long is needed to reach the muscle (Farley et al, 1986).

4. The *vastus lateralis* site (Figure 4-6) is recommended for giving large volumes, up to 5 ml in the adult, as it is a large muscle in healthy adults and is free from major nerves and blood vessels. It is also good for deep IM and Z-track injections (Pagliaro, 1986). It is the preferred IM site for children; however, it may be inap-

propriate in elderly or emaciated patients due to muscle wasting.

Recommendations Regarding the IM Route. As popular as the IM route is, it is not the ideal route. Recommendations concerning the IM route are:

1. IM is appropriate in the following situations, *only if* IV access is impractical or impossible:
- Premedication before painful procedures.
- Bolus dose to get quick control of the pain, before beginning or resuming scheduled PO doses.

2. Avoid IM route for postoperative pain control. Instead, use an IV continuous infusion (CI) of narcotic, which provides consistent absorption for the highest level of analgesia with the smallest amount of narcotic (Austin et al, 1980; Malhotra and Artusio, 1985; Rutter et al, 1980; Stapleton et al, 1979). For pain in the immediate postoperative period, continuous infusion is safer and probably provides a steadier level of analgesia than IM injections. Refer to the section on IV route (pp. 93-97) for specifics.

(Unlike IM injections, which can last up to 3 hours, IV bolus doses last only 45 minutes to 1 hour. Prescriptions for IV bolus dosing every 3 to 4 hours will be *ineffective* in the vast majority of patients.)

3. If the patient is NPO and the IV route is not an

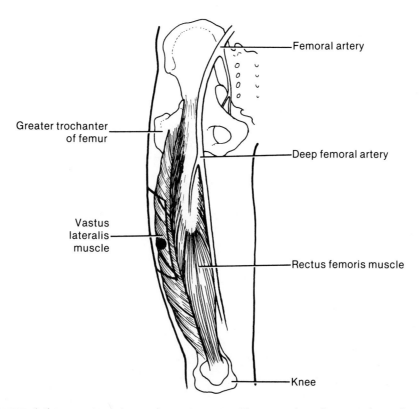

FIGURE 4-6 *Vastus lateralis site for IM injection.* The vastus lateralis site is located on the medial outer aspect in the center third portion of the thigh in children. The belly of the muscle is one-third the distance between the greater trochanter and the knee. It is the preferred site in children as it is well developed at birth. It is also recommended for adults because the muscle is large and can take up to 5 ml of medication per single injection. In the adult the site for injection is from one hand's breadth below the greater trochanter to a hand's breadth above the knee. The injection should be given at a right angle to the muscle or on an angle slightly toward the knee.
From Pagliaro, AM, and Pagliaro, LA: Pharmacologic aspects of nursing, St. Louis, 1986, The C.V. Mosby Company.

option as an alternative to IM injections in your setting, few good choices are left. However, the following suggestions may help maximize the effectiveness of the IM method of administration:

• For quicker absorption consider the deltoid instead of the gluteal sites. Even if the deltoid muscle is well developed enough to be an appropriate site, the volume or choice of medication may need to be changed.

Meperidine should not be given in the deltoid. It causes local irritation, and frequent injections can cause severe fibrosis of muscle tissue (Jaffe and Martin, 1985). If meperidine is used, request a change to an equianalgesic dose of morphine so that the deltoid may be used.

Antiemetics prescribed in combination with a narcotic may cause the volume to be too great to inject into the deltoid, as well as cause local irritation. If so, request that the IM antiemetic be changed to a suppository.

• If the deltoid muscle is not an appropriate site for an

individual patient and the pain continues to be uncontrolled, talk with the physician again about switching to the IV route, or consider the rectal, sublingual, or buccal route. Research has shown that postoperative pain can be well controlled with oxymorphone (Numorphan) 10 mg rectally (Beaver and Feise, 1977). Discuss and document with research (Austin et al, 1980) the variability of absorption with IM injections and the danger this may pose by original doses being absorbed much later when another dose is being given (see earlier discussion of this point on p. 89).

• Use Z-track to decrease discomfort. Although the Z-track method has primarily been used for irritating substances such as iron preparations, recent research suggests that this technique would be appropriate to reduce discomfort for all injections (Keen, 1986). The clinical implications are particularly important for the patient who receives frequent injections. Regardless of the medication, this technique might decrease discomfort.

Rectal Route

The rectal route is often overlooked, probably because it tends to be socially unacceptable. However, patients often prefer it to the IM route once they discover how much easier and less painful it is.

Indications for Rectal Route. The rectal route is desirable when PO or IM medication is not tolerated. Narcotic suppositories should be considered instead of IM, SC, or IV injections in patients with the following problems:

- Unable to take PO medication because of nausea, vomiting, or difficulty swallowing. In the home, the need to switch back and forth between PO and rectal route can be anticipated and planned for, thereby preventing readmission to the hospital.
- Unconscious with end-stage disease.
- Fear of injections, especially a child.

Limitations of Rectal Route. The usefulness of the rectal route is limited by:

- Physical conditions that would make this route inappropriate such as diarrhea, anal fissures, or low platelet count.
- The dose of narcotic available commercially. However, suppositories may be individually prepared by the pharmacist in whatever dosage is required or they may be made in the home (discussed later in this section). The nurse can be instrumental in arranging this, thereby preventing a hospital admission or promoting discharge home.

Patient Example

Mr. A.'s pain was well controlled on a continuous morphine infusion of 15 to 20 mg/hr. His discharge home was delayed because this route was inappropriate for his individual needs and family resources. The hospital pharmacist prepared 200 mg morphine suppositories, which the patient took q4h. Once this dose and interval proved to be successful, the nurse and hospital pharmacist then worked closely with the community pharmacist so that Mr. A. could obtain future prescriptions. This coordination of effort and use of rectal morphine allowed Mr. A. to be discharged home using a more convenient route than IV.

Calculation of Dosage for Rectal Route. There are limited studies on the absorption, distribution, metabolism, and excretion of rectally administered narcotics. The studies that have been done involved a limited number of patients and showed wide variations in absorption and plasma concentrations (Ellison and Lewis, 1984; Westerling et al, 1982).

Dosing for this route is mostly based on clinical experience, not on research. In fact there is a lack of controlled studies establishing the equianalgesic doses for PO and rectal routes. Oxymorphone suppositories are the only ones for which an equianalgesic ratio has been established (refer to Equianalgesic Chart on p. 79). Oxymorphone 10 mg (2 suppositories) equals 10 mg morphine IM (Beaver and Feise, 1977).

For the remaining narcotic suppositories, clinical experience suggests that the dose used by mouth is the same dose recommended for initial rectal administration (Twycross and Lack, 1983), e.g., morphine suppository 20 mg rectally q4h may be given initially for pain that was controlled with 20 mg PO morphine. Then watch the patient's response, increasing or decreasing the dose. The principle of careful titration and frequent observation of the individual's response is the only way to safely administer a narcotic, regardless of route or dose.

Recommendations for the Rectal Route

- Anticipate initial patient resistance to this route. Encourage patient to try this route at least once. Establish reason and spend time with patient exploring other options. Patient is usually willing to try it once the reasons have been explained.
- Use the rectal route as an alternative route when PO analgesics cannot be taken, e.g., because of vomiting. Explain to patient/family in the home how to switch temporarily from PO to the rectal route using narcotic pills (see Immediate Help: Patient in Home Care Setting Unexpectedly Unable to Take Oral Analgesics, p. 45). If necessary, narcotic pills can be crushed and administered rectally in one of the following ways:
  1. Put into cocoa butter and hardened in the refrigerator.
  2. Placed in empty gelatin capsule with holes punched in it (Brook-Williams, 1982).
  3. Dissolved in a small amount of water and inserted into the rectum through a rubber catheter attached to a syringe (Pannuti et al, 1982).
- Instruct patient/family in method of administering the suppository (Pagliaro, 1986):
  1. Position patient on left side with upper leg flexed.
  2. Insert suppository the length of the finger at an angle toward the umbilicus and place to the side against rectal wall for absorption. The suppository should not be just left in rectal canal or pushed into a mass of stool.
- Use a flow sheet to assess effectiveness and safety of the suppository.

Sublingual and Buccal Routes

Regarding these two routes there are mostly anecdotal reports (Hirsh, 1984; Pitorak and Kraus, 1987; Wallace, 1987; Whitman, 1984). Very little research is available (Bell et al, 1985; Ellis et al, 1982; Pannuti et al, 1982). Pending more research and clinical experience, we view the sublingual (SL) and buccal routes as temporary alternatives until the patient can be stabilized on another route.

Definition:
- Sublingual—Tablet or liquid is placed under the tongue.
- Buccal—Tablet is placed between:
  —Upper lip and gum, *or*
  —Cheek and gum.

Both routes have the potential advantage of avoiding

the "first-pass" effect seen with the oral route (Payne, 1987a), provided the patient does not inadvertently swallow. A drug taken orally passes from the GI tract to the liver where it can be extensively metabolized, leaving a minimal amount of active drug available to reach the general circulation. The result is that less of the drug circulates, and less of its effect is seen.

The buccal route does not stimulate salivation and may be better tolerated than the SL route (Bell et al, 1985).

Disadvantages of SL compared with buccal are that unpleasant taste may be a problem and salivation can be promoted causing swallowing of the drug, thereby defeating the purpose of this route.

Indications for SL and Buccal Routes. Both routes are suggested for chronic cancer pain (Pitorak and Kraus, 1987; Whitman, 1984) and in one study the buccal route effectively relieved postoperative pain (Bell et al, 1985). Indications for buccal or SL are:

- Oral route impossible:
  - —Difficulty swallowing.
  - —Vomiting.
  - —Bowel obstruction.
  - —NG tube.
- Parenteral route temporarily impractical.

Recommendations for SL and Buccal Routes. Although more controlled studies are needed for conclusive answers to the considerations listed below (Wilkie, 1987), experiences from anecdotal reports are presented here as guidelines:

- Which formulation—tablets or liquid?

  Some prefer tablets over the liquid pain medication because tablets are less expensive and there is less chance of swallowing them (Pitorak and Kraus, 1987).

  Others recommend liquid, i.e., morphine solution, as an effective and safe formulation for an SL analgesic (Wallace, 1987). To avoid aspiration in a comatose or semicomatose patient, a maximum of 1 ml at a time is given, with at least 3 minutes between doses.

  To date none of the pain medication available in the United States is marketed in an SL formulation. Further developments in availability may eventually promote the choice of SL or buccal route over PO.

- Which route—SL or buccal?

  Rate and extent of delivery to the general circulation (bioavailability) of buccal morphine is reported to be 40% to 50% greater that IM morphine (Bell et al, 1985). However, this was reported in only one study and this contrasts with the bioavailability of SL liquid morphine, which is less than 10% of that after IM injection (Payne, 1987a).

  Buccal route poses less of a problem with swallowing and unpleasant taste.

- Withhold other PO intake to ensure absorption.

  After SL administration, withhold food, fluids, or other medications for 5 to 15 minutes (Pitorak and Kraus, 1987; Wallace, 1987).

Continuous Narcotic Infusion: IV and SC Routes

The IV route provides the most rapid onset of analgesia with the shortest duration of action. Analgesic effects can be felt within 6 to 10 minutes, but the duration of analgesia from a bolus dose is often only 45 minutes to 1 hour. Therefore with an IV bolus the patient experiences immediate relief but it diminishes quickly. For the vast majority of patients, prescriptions for an IV bolus q3 to 4h will result in the return of pain long before the next dose is given.

KEY POINT: Duration of IV bolus is much shorter than the duration of IM injections. For ongoing pain a continuous infusion is needed, not bolus doses. Initially IV boluses may be given to establish the dose of narcotic for continuous infusion.

In contrast, a continuous infusion of narcotic, either SC or IV, maintains a constant level of pain relief by delivering a continuous dose into the bloodstream. Figure 4-7 illustrates this concept.

While it is common to administer single or separate injections of medication via the SC route, continuous infusion by this route seems to have been abandoned at the time the IV route became more accessible. Many years ago, the term *clysis* was loosely used to mean an SC infusion, and fluids were often administered in this manner to dehydrated children. Very recently, the SC route for continuous infusion of narcotics has once again become popular. It is often used for prolonged pain in ambulatory patients at home, in part because of the ease with which the route can be accessed. IV and SC continuous narcotic infusions will be discussed.

KEY POINT: IV boluses are appropriate for rapid control of severe pain and for establishing the hourly dose for IV continuous infusion. Continuous infusion is appropriate for a steady level of analgesia to maintain control of pain.

Indications for the Use of Continuous IV or SC Narcotic Infusion. For ongoing pain, continuous IV or SC infusion is almost always preferred over intermittent injections. Indications for the use of continuous IV or SC narcotic infusion are:

- PO route is impossible, i.e., nausea, GI obstruction, difficulty swallowing or breathing.
- ATC PO or rectal routes provide inadequate analgesia. *Note:* First be sure that doses by these routes are high enough and frequent enough.
- Immediate relief is needed. Extreme anxiety from unrelieved pain can increase a person's perception of pain or make pain intolerable, which in turn promotes a cycle of increased anxiety and pain. By providing analgesia *quickly,* continuous infusions break this cycle and eliminate the fearful anticipation of pain.

Misconceptions Associated with Continuous IV Narcotic Infusion. Fears and misconceptions associated with

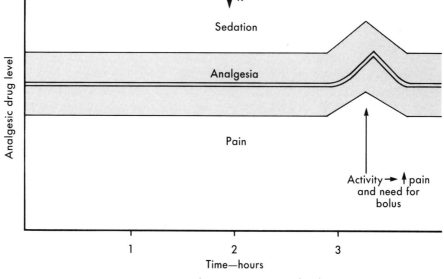

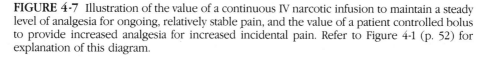

FIGURE 4-7 Illustration of the value of a continuous IV narcotic infusion to maintain a steady level of analgesia for ongoing, relatively stable pain, and the value of a patient controlled bolus to provide increased analgesia for increased incidental pain. Refer to Figure 4-1 (p. 52) for explanation of this diagram.

the administration of IV narcotics can prevent this route from being considered and used effectively.

Misconception: Continuous IV narcotic infusion is only to be used for the patient who is dying.

Correction: This route may be appropriate for postoperative pain (Rutter et al, 1980), pain in severe burns (Wermeling et al, 1986), sickle cell crisis (Cole et al, 1986; Ives and Guerra, 1987), and acute pancreatitis. Avoid limiting the use of IV continuous infusion to certain diseases or to only end-stage conditions. Instead assess each individual pain situation and apply "the indications for use" discussed above as guidelines.

Avoid statements in the continuous IV infusion policy that encourage the attitude that patients must convince health professionals that they are really hurting before a continuous narcotic infusion is used, e.g., avoid saying "The patient must exhibit intractable pain requiring injectable narcotics." Patients should not have to convince or exhibit anything to obtain pain relief: their statement of pain should be enough.

Misconception: Once the patient is on IV narcotics, a return to PO is difficult and unlikely.

Correction: Controlling a person's pain with continuous IV infusion does not interfere with switching back to the PO route when the pain is stabilized (Wright, 1981).

Not knowing how to change from IV continuous infusion to the PO route may be another reason why this route is not readily considered for situations where the pain will decrease.

Changing to another route can be successful if equi-analgesic doses are used and the person's individual response is assessed with a flow sheet. Guidelines for changing routes are discussed on pp. 106-107.

Misconception: Continuous IV infusion may enhance a patient's chance of becoming addicted.

Correction: There is no evidence to support this statement.

Research shows that addiction rarely occurs in people who are taking narcotics for the relief of pain (Porter and Jicks, 1980). In fact the overwhelming majority of patients stop taking narcotics when the pain stops (see pp. 67-71). For example, no evidence of addictive behavior was observed in 76 episodes of sickle cell vaso-occlusive crisis in 38 children and adolescents treated with continuous IV infusion (Cole et al, 1986).

Recommendations for Continuous IV or SC Infusion. Following are guidelines for safe and effective use of continuous infusion of narcotics IV or SC (Bruera et al, 1987a; Coyle et al, 1986; McGuire and Wright, 1984; Payne, 1987a; Portenoy, 1987a):

1. Choice of narcotic is usually morphine. However, hydromorphone (Dilaudid HP, high potency) may be used for continuous SC infusion when a high concentration of drug with little volume is needed.

At this time there are no studies comparing the effectiveness and side effects of various narcotics administered by continuous infusion. Other narcotics can be used; however, meperidine should be avoided especially in the SC route because of its irritation to tissue and its toxicity. Prolonged use or high doses of meperidine may result in

CNS excitation and dysphoria (Kaiko et al, 1983) (see pp. 83-85 for further discussion). This toxicity is particularly important to note for the treatment of sickle cell crisis pain for which meperidine is unfortunately frequently used (Tang et al, 1980).

It is suggested that infusions with drugs having a long half-life,* i.e., methadone or levorphanol may result in delayed side effects as plasma levels of the drug can continue to increase long after pain relief is reached. Therefore infusions with drugs of a short half-life, i.e., morphine or hydromorphone, are preferred especially for debilitated or elderly patients who have difficulty eliminating a drug (Bruera et al, 1987a; Portenoy, 1987a).

2. Use an infusion pump with an alarm for accurate delivery. For continuous SC infusion, a portable infusion pump encourages patient mobility and facilitates home care.

3. Calculate the appropriate concentration of drug to fluid. For continuous IV infusion, approximately 60 ml/hr of fluid or less is appropriate for most adults. For instance, 1 mg morphine per 5 ml may be appropriate if the patient is receiving 4 to 6 mg morphine/hr; this would be 20 to 30 ml/hr. However, this concentration would result in too much fluid, 500 ml/hr, for a patient receiving 100 mg morphine/hr.

For continuous SC infusion, the volume of fluid absorbed without irritation into the SC tissue is limited (Coyle et al, 1986). When a patient is cachectic and his tissue is unable to absorb much volume, increasing the narcotic concentration can provide small volumes of fluid for effective absorption. Although hydromorphone is available in a concentrated form (10 mg/ml), this may not be concentrated enough for some patients. Morphine and hydromorphone can both be reconstituted at even higher concentrations than those commercially available, e.g., instead of the usual 15 mg/ml, morphine can be reconstituted at 50 mg/ml; instead of 10 mg/ml, hydromorphone can be reconstituted in concentrations of more than 100 mg/ml. Refer to p. 99 for further discussion of fluid volume as it pertains to site irritation in continuous SC infusion.

4. Increases or decreases in dosage are made in terms of percentages (%) instead of a fixed number of milligrams. Percentages allow adjustments to be in proportion to the original dose and can be widely applied regardless of the dose.

For example, is an increase of 5 mg/hr of morphine appropriate? It may be appropriate for a patient receiving continuous infusion at 20 mg/hr. However, for the patient receiving an infusion at 150 mg/hr, this increase is only a small percentage of the dose and may have little analgesic effect. Instead, a guideline that suggests increasing mor-

phine by 20%, for example, is preferred to stating the number of milligrams. This promotes proportionate titrations regardless of the route.

5. Use a flow sheet (blank form on p. 27) to determine safety and effectiveness of dosage (example on p. 28). A flow sheet provides data in a format that allows quick scanning for the patient's respiratory function and pain rating. It can be a particularly helpful tool to all members of the health care team when fear and concern result in hesitancy to try a specific drug, route, or dosage.

Dosages may vary widely. Most of the time, patients with severe pain obtain relief from "usual" or initial, "recommended" doses, but the literature clearly shows that pain control in some patients requires titrating up to unusually high doses. Examples of high doses follow:

High doses for continuous IV infusions:
- 4 mg/hr to 480 morphine equivalent mg/hr (Portenoy et al, 1986).
- 440 mg/hr morphine (Lo and Coleman, 1986).
- 80 mg/hr morphine in a child (Miser et al, 1980).
- 1568 mg/hr morphine in teenager alert and talking with family (Miser et al, 1986).
- 50 mg/hr hydromorphone in alert and oriented patient (Levy, 1985).

High doses for continuous SC infusions:
- 3.5 mg/hr to 97 mg/hr morphine (Coyle et al, 1986).
- 15 mg/hr morphine (Campbell et al, 1983).

KEY POINT: Stop reacting to the number of milligrams in a dose. Instead, focus on the patient's response to that dose. Is his pain rating on the 0 to 10 scale satisfactory to him? Are there side effects? Are these side effects dangerous or unacceptable to the patient?

6. The actual amount by which a dose is increased or decreased is determined by finding a dose that relieves pain to the patient's satisfaction with minimal side effects. This is done by using a flow sheet and looking at the following patient responses in consecutive order:
- First, respiratory function, usually rate.
- Second, pain rating, e.g., on 0 to 10 scale (0 = no pain, 10 = worst pain).
- Third, based on the above information, determine whether to increase or decrease the number of milligrams of analgesic and at what percentage, e.g., 10%, 50%, 100%.

Because patients' responses to analgesics are so individual, there are no easy formulas that give the "right percentage." However general guidelines for increases might be 10% if pain is almost controlled, 50% if pain is partially controlled, 100% if there is no pain relief. No matter what percentage is chosen, it is vital to assess this adjustment immediately. Document the patient's response in the flow sheet so that further increases or decreases can be made without the patient enduring long painful periods between titrations. If a conservative dose increase is chosen, e.g., 10% to 20%, for a patient who is

---

*Half-life: The time it takes a drug to fall to half of its plasma concentration. It takes five half-lives for a drug to be completely eliminated from the body.

rating pain at 8 on 0 to 10 scale, realize that you will probably need to (1) increase at more frequent intervals than if you began with a more liberal dose, (2) anticipate that the total percentage increase may be 50% to 100%.

Patient Examples

These illustrate the different responses patients may have to drug titrations, and the differences from patient to patient in acceptable vs. unacceptable pain ratings.

A 23-year-old man with acute sickle cell crisis has been on a continuous IV infusion of morphine at 100 mg/hr for 2 hours. On a 0 to 10 scale, he rates pain at 8. Respirations are stable at 18/min; he is alert and oriented, but constantly shifting position because of the pain. Because of the severity of the pain rating, and no respiratory problems, a bolus of 75% of the hourly dosage, 75 mg, is given. Within 20 minutes his pain rating is 4, respirations remain at 18/min. Patient states that pain is at acceptable level right now. The continuous IV infusion is increased to 175 mg/hr, 75% increase over the previous hourly dose. With a flow sheet, the patient is assessed every hour, pain rating remains at 4, respirations are stable at 12 to 18/min, depending on whether he is sleeping.

A 56-year-old woman with metastatic cancer is on a continuous IV infusion of morphine at 20 mg/hr. The patient notices breakthrough pain that has increased her pain rating from an acceptable 1 to an unacceptable 3. Respirations have been 12 to 14/min. You know from her past history that she is sensitive to the slightest titration of analgesic. For this reason a conservative bolus of 10% of the hourly dose, 2 mg, is given. Twenty minutes after this bolus, her pain rating is 1, respirations are 10. She is sleepy, but easily awakens when her name is called.

One hour after the bolus, the pain has increased to 3, respirations are 12/min. The 2 mg bolus is repeated; the same response from the earlier bolus is noted. The infusion is increased to 22 mg/hr, and hourly assessments are recorded on the flow sheet. After 3 hours, her pain rating remains at 1, and respirations are between 10 to 12/min. Assessments are then done every 2 hours.

7. In the general guidelines or policy for continuous infusion, avoid a specific respiratory rate at which the infusion should be stopped or altered, e.g., do not specify "If respirations are below 14/min, stop the infusion."

Each patient's average respiratory rate is different, so it is not appropriate to state a set rate in a written procedure that applies to all patients. Instead the health care team decides for *each individual situation* at which respiratory rate the infusion rate is changed.

8. If possible, treat respiratory depression by decreasing the infusion flow rate instead of using naloxone. If not titrated slowly, naloxone reverses all analgesia and can result in total return of pain. Of course, treatment of respiratory depression must be individualized in every case.

9. Establish an alternate route and dose of medication in the original prescription, especially if the route is IV

and the patient is cared for at home. If IV or SC access is interrupted and cannot be resumed immediately, this allows analgesics via a different route to be given without the delay of contacting the physician for a new prescription. Loss of route access is a special problem with IV since it is much more difficult to enter a vein with a needle than to enter SC tissue. In fact, SC may be the alternate route for a patient on IV narcotics. Another likely alternative is rectal. SL or buccal may be used in an emergency.

Calculation of Initial Doses for Continuous IV Narcotic Infusion. Each individual patient's response to a dose of medication is highly variable. Therefore the guidelines below are suggested as a *starting point* to determine (1) hourly infusion rates and (2) bolus doses (Lukacsko, 1987; McCaffery, 1987b). Adjustments in both of these can then be made after the onset (within 10 minutes) or peak effect (within 20 minutes) based on the patient's pain rating and an evaluation of side effects.

1. **Determine the hourly infusion rate.** Use the equianalgesic chart Table 4-11 on pp. 78-79.

- **PO to IV using same narcotic.** For the patient who has been on a PO narcotic that can be used IV:
  a. Calculate the 24 hour PO narcotic dose.
  b. Convert this 24 hour dose to the equivalent IM dose using the equianalgesic chart. Based on clinical experience, many consider the IM and IV dose to be equianalgesic (Portenoy, 1987a). However, some recommend using ½ the IM dose for the IV dose (American Pain Society, 1987; Foley, 1982). To date there is no research comparing equivalencies of IV doses with other routes.
  c. Divide by 24 to arrive at the hourly IV continuous infusion dose and set the infusion accordingly.

  Note: This conversion method is intended to provide the *same analgesia* as the original narcotic. If the patient was not comfortable with the original dose, then increase the dose estimated for IV infusion. Remember, the equianalgesic chart is only a *guideline.* So the initial dose is always an educated guess. The vital step in this process is *consistent assessment* with titrations made up or down according to the patient's pain rating and respiratory status.

- **IM to IV using same narcotic.** If the patient has been on intermittent IM or SC narcotic and the same narcotic can be given IV:
  a. Calculate the 24 hour IM/SC dose.
  b. Divide by 24 to obtain the hourly IV continuous infusion dose and set the infusion accordingly.

- **PO, IM, SC to IV using a different narcotic.** If the patient is changed to a different narcotic when switching from PO, IM, SC to IV continuous infusion, use the equianalgesic chart to:
  a. Calculate the total 24 hour dose of the present narcotic and convert it to a 24 hour IV dose of the new narcotic.

b. Start with one half or two thirds of the calculated 24 hour IV dose. This is recommended because tolerance may have developed with the previous narcotic, but it may not be totally present when a new narcotic is started. This approach avoids possible overdose with the new narcotic. Be prepared to increase the dose quickly if this lower equianalgesic dose is not effective or decrease if it is too much.

- **Continuous IV infusion if no previous narcotic.** If the patient has not been on any narcotics:
  a. In an adult start with a bolus of morphine 2 to 5 mg IV or hydromorphone 0.5 to 1 mg IV. Repeat bolus every 10 minutes until pain is controlled unless respiratory rate drops to an unacceptable level.
  b. Calculate the cumulative bolus doses/hr and immediately start the hourly rate of infusion based on this number.

  2. **Give IV boluses as needed.**

- The dose of the bolus is usually equal to or one half of the hourly infusion, depending on the degree of uncontrolled pain that is likely to occur.

  As a rough guideline if the patient is on PCA, the total number of boluses allowed in 1 hour probably should not exceed the hourly infusion rate. For example, if the patient is receiving morphine 6 mg/hr by continuous IV infusion, a 2 mg bolus could be programmed at 20 minute lockout intervals, or a 1 mg bolus every 10 minutes.

- The minimal interval between boluses is based on the onset of pain relief for an IV dose. This is the period of time between the administration of a bolus and the onset of analgesia. The usual onset of relief for IV route is 6 to 10 minutes. However, individual assessment is crucial.

- Use the flow sheet to assess the patient's comfort following the bolus using the 0 to 10 pain rating scale. If repeated boluses are needed throughout the hour, recalculate the infusion rate based on the cumulative boluses per hour.

  Note: When first starting an infusion, a bolus IV dose may be given to achieve fast analgesia. Then the infusion is begun to continue a steady state of analgesia. Start the infusion immediately, certainly no longer than 30 minutes after the last bolus is given. Longer than that allows the blood level of narcotic to drop, the pain returns, and it will take longer to obtain pain control once the infusion starts.

  3. **If the degree of pain relief is not acceptable to the patient, there are the following choices:**

- Increase the bolus dose by a percentage, e.g., increase the bolus by 50% (see discussion of this on p. 95). Monitor the patient's responses and repeat the dose or continue increasing the dose until the patient is comfortable. Once the patient is comfortable, begin the infusion at the dose most consistently used (a flow sheet is helpful in tracking doses and responses).

Patient Example

Mrs. R. previously at home on 60 mg morphine PO had satisfactory pain relief until she experienced a sudden increase in pain along with nausea and vomiting. Upon admission to the hospital, the immediate goal is to reestablish pain control as quickly as possible. The box on p. 98 summarizes the approach used to relieve her pain. An IV bolus dose of one sixth the equianalgesic PO morphine dose, 10 mg, is given with poor results. An additional 50% of the bolus dose, 5 mg, was given at 8:15 AM and was repeated at 8:30 AM. Respirations remained stable. Pain rating of 4 was unacceptable to the patient, so 100% of the original bolus, 10 mg, was given at 8:45 AM. Although she exhibited some sedation (see comments in level of arousal column), her respirations remained stable at 12 to 18/min.

Finally, after a cumulative dose of 30 mg over 1 hour, Mrs. R. rated her pain at 2. This rating was acceptable to her; the IV continuous infusion was started immediately at the cumulative dose of 30 mg/hr. Continued assessments document an unchanged pain rating and stable respirations. The continuous IV infusion is started at this dose with continued assessment, probably hourly.

- Repeat the same bolus dose more frequently at whatever interval is needed for that particular patient until the pain is controlled. With this method, however, the patient may be exposed to extended periods of unrelieved pain and it will take longer to control the pain. Respirations, pain rating on 0 to 10 scale, and alertness are monitored and recorded on a flow sheet after each bolus.

Calculation of Initial Doses for Continuous SC Narcotic Infusion. Each individual patient's response to narcotics is highly variable; therefore the guidelines below are suggested as a starting point for SC continuous infusion.

- To calculate the initial doses for boluses and for continuous infusion, follow the same guidelines as for continuous IV infusion (see above). However, unlike the IV route there is no debate about SC doses being equianalgesic with IM doses. Also, some clinicians suggest an initial bolus dose equivalent to 2 hours of the infusion rate (Bruera et al, 1987a).

- To determine the interval between boluses, consider the time for onset of analgesia. The usual onset of pain relief for an SC injection is 30 to 60 minutes. Use the 30 to 60 minutes only as a guide, and assess the individual patient to determine how long it takes from the time the bolus is injected until the patient feels relief. Use that time interval to calculate the frequency with which boluses may be safely administered.

  Since the onset of analgesia is much longer for SC doses than for IV, escalating doses by the SC route takes considerably longer. For example, if morphine 5 mg is given IV, the analgesic effect will be known in about 10 minutes. If pain relief is inadequate, another IV dose can be administered at that time. However, if the same dose,

FLOW SHEET—PAIN: For Mrs. R.

Patient __Mrs. R._____ Date _____

Pain rating scale used __0-10 (0 = no pain, 10 = worst pain)_____

Purpose: To evaluate the safety and effectiveness of the analgesic(s).

Analgesic(s) prescribed: __Morphine IV bolus 10mg, ↑ or ↓ by 50% until pain is controlled, then calculate dose for continuous infusion.__

Time	Pain rating	Analgesic	R	P	BP	Level of arousal	Other	Plan & comments
Baseline 7:50 AM	9		20			Alert.		Establish continuous infusion dose
8 AM	9	Morphine 10mg IV bolus	20			Alert.		
8 15 AM	7	Morphine 5mg IV bolus	18			Alert.		
8 30 AM	4	Morphine 5mg IV bolus	16			Sleepy—awakens easily.	Pt. states first time she has slept in 3 days. States level of pain not acceptable.	Continue to decrease pain rating.
8 45 AM	4	Morphine 10 mg IV bolus	12			Eyes closed—but responds immediately when name is called.		Decrease pain rating.
9 AM	2	Continuous infusion began at 30 mg/hr.	12				Pt. states this pain rating is acceptable	Maintain "2" pain rating.
9 30 AM	2		16					
10 AM	2	Continues at 30 mg/hr.	12			Sleeping— awakens easily.		
11 AM	1		10					

This patient's flow sheet illustrates how IV boluses of morphine are used to control pain as quickly and safely as possible. The IV boluses are increased by 50% and given every 15 minutes until the pain rating is at an acceptable level for the patient. The patient's respiratory status and level of arousal are also noted every 15 minutes to assure that the dose is safe. Once the pain is controlled, a continuous IV narcotic infusion is begun.

morphine 5 mg, is given SC, the analgesic effect may not occur for 60 minutes or longer. Thus for 60 minutes or longer, there is no information available to help determine the need to repeat the dose or to increase the continuous infusion.

Special Considerations Regarding Continuous SC Narcotic Infusion. This route delivers a continuous infusion of narcotic into the SC tissue through a 27 gauge needle usually attached to a portable infusion pump (Figure 4-8). It offers an alternative to continuous IV infusion for ambulatory patients.

However, for *rapid* control of severe pain where frequent boluses and/or changes in dose are needed, SC continuous infusion may not be the route of choice. Instead, the IV route provides immediate onset of action and is ideal in this instance. SC continuous infusion is particularly useful for prolonged administration when a parenteral route other than IV is needed.

The *advantages* to using SC continuous infusion are (Bruera et al, 1987a; Coyle et al, 1986; Payne, 1987a):
- Avoids repetitive IM or SC injections.
- Avoids need for IV access. This is particularly helpful in home care situations, or for situations involving adults or children in whom it is difficult to maintain chronic IV access.
- Provides a continuous level of analgesia.
- Promotes patient mobility. A portable infusion pump allows patients to ambulate and go about their daily activities.
- Is less frightening for the health care team, patients, and families. Unlike IV continuous infusion, this route does not involve needles inserted directly into veins resulting in almost immediate absorption of the drug. Patients and families readily learn insertion of an SC needle.

Although one disadvantage may be the slower onset of

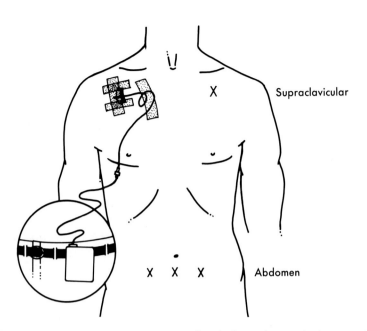

FIGURE 4-8 Suggested sites for SC infusion needle which may be attached to an ambulatory infusion pump. *X* marks sites which least interfere with mobility. Other sites to consider include upper arms and thighs.

action when compared with the IV route, the *primary disadvantage* is a limitation to the amount of fluid the SC tissue can absorb. If rapidly escalating doses are needed and require large volumes of fluid, this route is often discontinued because the tissue cannot absorb the volume. At this time there is no research that addresses the ideal volume of fluid to use for effective absorption. One clinical report noted local irritation when volumes greater than 1 ml/hr were used (Coyle et al, 1986). Another noted that a volume up to 10 ml/hr could be administered without irritation or pain at the site of infusion (Bruera et al, 1987a).

Following are *recommendations* for initiating and maintaining the SC continuous infusion route (Bruera et al, 1987a; Coyle et al, 1986):

- Selecting site for SC continuous infusion. Any SC site can be used on a rotating basis. The abdomen, subclavicular area, and the anterior chest wall are areas to consider first since they allow free movement of the patient's arms and legs. In one study of 17 children, the injection site was the thigh (Miser et al, 1983).
- Rotating sites for SC continuous infusion. The infusion site should be inspected at least twice a day for signs of irritation, i.e., swelling, redness, leakage from the site, and the site changed if needed. The patient or family member can be instructed to inspect the site in the morning before dressing and in the evening when undressing for bed.

One study of 45 patients with a total of 119 SC inser-

tions for continuous infusion of narcotics reported that the frequency with which sites needed to be changed varied from 1 to 29 days (Brenneis et al, 1986). Other than this there are no controlled studies examining frequency of site changes, but descriptive reports include site changes every 48 hours (Campbell et al, 1983; Sheehan and Sauerbier, 1986); every 24 to 48 hours (Miser et al, 1983); every 7 days unless symptomatic, then as often as needed (Coyle et al, 1986); and only when showing signs of irritation at the site (Moss, 1986).

Coyle et al (1986) reported increased irritation at the infusion site when the volume of fluid required was greater than 1 ml/hr. In those instances, changing the needle site daily to an opposite side of the body was an effective preventive measure.

- Handling breakthrough pain. If breakthrough pain occurs despite dose adjustments, poor absorption at that particular site may be the problem. Changing the infusion site may reestablish analgesia without increasing the dosage (Coyle et al, 1986).
- Increasing patient/family willingness to maintain SC continuous infusion. This is a vital factor to evaluate before considering the continuous SC route. Instructions on pump management and site care along with a contact person to call for help can ease some of the initial anxiety.
- Reassuring patient and family. Explain that another route can be substituted at any time if this one does not work.

Spinal Route*

Narcotics for spinal analgesia are presently administered in two ways: (1) into the epidural space and (2) into the subarachnoid space (Figure 4-9). In the past, these routes have most commonly been used to administer anesthetics for regional anesthesia, e.g., a spinal anesthetic.

Analgesia by the spinal route is the result of the drug's direct effect on the opioid receptors in the spinal cord, rather than supraspinally in the brain.

When systemic narcotics, i.e., oral or parenteral, are given, CNS side effects may be seen such as sedation and disorientation. The hope with spinal narcotic administration is that the drug will remain only at the spinal level and not ascend supraspinally (above the spine) to brain centers responsible for central side effects. Even though it is now known that small amounts of spinal narcotics do reach these supraspinal levels, fewer side effects are seen with this route than with the systemic administration of narcotics.

Purpose and Limitations of This Section on Spinal Route. "Few areas of clinical research have exploded into practice as rapidly as this method [spinal analgesia] of providing pain relief" (Rawal and Sjostrand, 1986, p. 43). Unfortunately, there are still many unanswered questions as to the role of spinal analgesia for acute and chronic pain. However, nurses everywhere are finding themselves monitoring these patients and in many instances administering the analgesic dose.

Because this route of administration is still in its developmental stages, there is simply not enough information to present specific guidelines similar to those presented for the other routes already discussed. We will present general findings to date that will enable the nurse to monitor a patient for safety and effectiveness of the spinal analgesic.

KEY POINT: The spinal route of administration is to be approached with caution. Many aspects about its safety and efficacy are not yet known. At this time, its role should be questioned for patients who obtain effective pain relief from systemic analgesics, e.g., PO, IV, SC.

Possible Indications for the Use of Spinal Route. It is vital to understand that more research is needed to define specific indications for using the spinal route to relieve pain. The spinal route has been used for both acute and chronic pain in the following situations:

- Postoperative pain following thoracic, orthopedic, and abdominal surgery (Leib and Hurtig, 1985; Ozuna and Snyder, 1987; Rawal and Sjostrand, 1986; Stenseth et al, 1985).
- Multiple trauma pain (Rawal and Tandon, 1985).
- Malignant pain (Moulin and Coyle, 1986; Payne, 1987 a and b; Penn and Paice, 1987).
- Chronic nonmalignant pain as a result of low back conditions, multiple sclerosis, arachnoiditis, herpes zoster, and severe osteoporosis (Auld et al, 1985; Dallas et al, 1987; Penn and Paice, 1987).

It is suggested that the spinal route may be particularly helpful for patients in the following circumstances:
- Acute pain *if:*
    —Mobility and full lung expansion immediately post-operatively is particularly important.
    —There is compromised pulmonary function.
    —There is a need to facilitate pulmonary hygiene.
- Chronic cancer pain *if* (Moulin and Coyle, 1986; Payne, 1987a):
    —Pain is unresponsive to pharmacologic approaches that have included aggressive titrations and combinations of narcotics, nonnarcotic analgesics, and adjuvant analgesics.
    —Pain is poorly controlled with systemic narcotics, e.g., PO, IV, because of dose limiting side effects, e.g., sedation.
    —Pain is located bilateral or midline below the mid-thoracic level, e.g., sacral or perineal pain.

The spinal route is *contraindicated* in the following situations:
- Bleeding disorder or clotting deficiency.
- Spinal abnormality or obstruction.
- Local skin infection or CNS infection.
- Lack of personnel to provide continual monitoring in hospital, or lack of patient/family willingness or resources to continue safe care for this route at home.

Analgesia by the spinal route has several potential *advantages* for postoperative and chronic cancer pain. For analgesia following orthopedic surgery, Lanz et al (1982) found that the spinal route had the following advantages:
- Pain was of shorter duration and less severe.
- Alertness was heightened.
- Postoperative feeling of well-being was noted.
- Additional need for analgesia and sedation was less.

For cancer pain, longer-lasting analgesia was seen without sedation in patients with dose-limiting responses to systemic drugs (Caballero et al, 1986; Coombs et al, 1984; Malone et al, 1985; Penn and Paice, 1987). The patients were:
- More alert.
- Less depressed.
- Able to resume daily activities when possible.
- Able to be cared for at home.

The long duration of analgesia, e.g., 16 hours or longer after spinal morphine, may also be an advantage. This is in comparison to a range of 3 to 12 hours for systemic administration, e.g., every 3 to 4 hours for most PO and

*The authors would like to thank Judith A. Paice, RN, MS, Assistant Professor and Acting Coordinator, Oncology Graduate Program, College of Nursing, Rush University; Oncology Clinical Nurse Specialist, Rush Presbyterian-St. Luke's Medical Center, Chicago, Illinois, for her review of the spinal route section, helpful comments, and for supplying the patient example.

IM narcotics and up to 12 hours for sustained-release PO morphine.

Important Considerations in Choosing Spinal Route. In spite of favorable results observed with spinal analgesia, it is still important to consider, is this an appropriate route? To answer this question, one must be aware that there is a critical lack of knowledge, research, and clinical experience concerning the spinal route. More information is needed to identify types of pain effectively treated by this route, which drug should be used, and whether it should be administered epidurally or intrathecally. In addition, use of the spinal route requires careful monitoring for an extended period of time after administration to detect potentially life-threatening respiratory depression. Other side effects also occur, but the incidence varies widely. Tolerance to analgesia may develop rapidly via this route, and contamination of the route is obviously extremely dangerous. Following is a discussion of problems and unanswered questions regarding the spinal route.

1. Knowledge about this route is still inadequate. Further clinical studies are needed to address the following controversial issues regarding appropriate selection of patients, drugs, and route (epidural or intrathecal).

a. Which patients and/or types of pain are appropriately treated? While numerous reports document the effectiveness of spinal analgesia for acute and chronic pain, criteria for patients most likely to benefit from this route have not been clearly identified.

In the treatment of labor and delivery pain, the spinal route is controversial (Rawal and Sjostrand, 1986). However, spinal analgesia following cesarean section appears to be effective (Cohen and Woods, 1983; Rimar, 1986). It seems especially appropriate for the breast-feeding mother so that analgesics in the breast milk are avoided.

In the treatment of cancer pain, few definitive criteria exist for patient selection. The spinal route appears to be successful in relieving pain from gynecological and colorectal tumors. Tumor infiltration of bone seems to be more likely to respond to spinal analgesics than deafferentation pain where there is tumor infiltration of nerve (Moulin and Coyle, 1986).

b. What is the most effective drug for spinal analgesia? Although many narcotics have been tried successfully, morphine is the most researched and the most widely used. However, its properties may not make it the ideal drug for spinal analgesia (Cousins and Mather, 1984; Moulin and Coyle, 1986).

The degree to which a drug is lipid soluble will directly affect its onset and duration of action. Morphine is the least lipid soluble; therefore it slowly moves into the spinal cord and blood vessels and may linger in the cerebrospinal fluid. The result is:

• A tendency for morphine to ascend to the brainstem centers responsible for central side effects (Moulin and Coyle, 1986). This may be less of a problem with very small doses given by continuous infusion.

• Delay in the onset of analgesia, 30 to 60 minutes, and a prolonged duration of action, 12 to 24 hours (Yaksh, 1981). Continuous infusions of spinal morphine circumvent the problem of delayed onset of analgesia.

The issue of ascension to the brainstem and delayed onset of action may not be as important for chronic continuous infusion via the spinal route. Very small doses of narcotic in a continuous spinal infusion do not appear to ascend supraspinally to the same degree as large doses.

Methadone and fentanyl are both highly lipid soluble; meperidine follows closely. Therefore each has a quick analgesic onset but a short duration if given by bolus. Methadone, for instance, begins to work in approximately 15 minutes and lasts for 4 to 6 hours (Jacobson, 1984).

Although the "best" drugs have not yet been identified, ideally they would have a segmental action of analgesia, without migration to the brainstem via the cerebrospinal fluid or systemic circulation (Moulin and Coyle, 1986; Payne, 1987b).

c. Which route is indicated? Intrathecal or epidural administration? Figure 4-9 shows the placement of the catheter tip in relation to the spinal cord for intrathecal and epidural analgesia. Understanding the very different process of distribution via the intrathecal or epidural approach helps explain the difference in the size of dose between the two routes. Although this process is not totally understood, the following pathways are suggested (Cousins and Mather, 1984; Moulin and Coyle, 1986):

• After intrathecal administration, and once in the cerebrospinal fluid, the drug moves gradually upward while diffusing into the spinal cord several centimeters away from the catheter tip. A small amount is also absorbed into surrounding blood vessels.

• After epidural administration, there are several factors that complicate drug distribution. The thick barrier of the dura mater may limit drug diffusion to the cerebrospinal fluid. At the same time, drug uptake into the general circulation and the cerebral venous system may be potentiated by the vast blood supply of the epidural space. Therefore it may be possible for a moderate to large portion of the drug to access the brainstem centers where central side effects are seen.

The variables in these two routes help to explain that the intrathecal dose is smaller than that needed for the epidural dose. Some suggest that the intrathecal route requires about one tenth of the epidural dose for comparable analgesia (Lukacsko, 1987; Moulin and Coyle, 1986). However, there are no studies to support this.

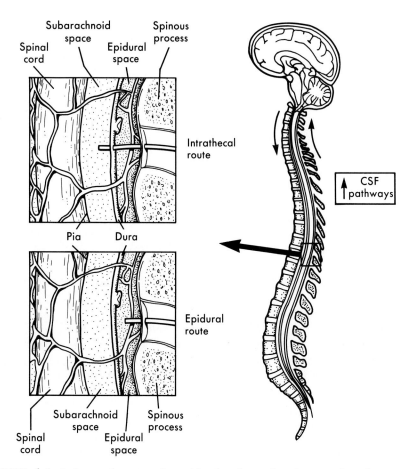

FIGURE 4-9 Catheter placement for epidural and intrathecal routes for administration of analgesia.

Adapted from Moulin, DE, and Coyle, N: Spinal opioid analgesics and local anesthetics in the management of chronic cancer pain, *J Pain Sympt Manag* 1:79-86, Spring 1986.

How this dose compares to the 24 hour equianalgesic dose systemically is also unknown. Some suggest that the 24 hour epidural dose is about one tenth that required IV or IM per 24 hours; the 24 hour intrathecal dose, about one one-hundredth that required IV or IM per 24 hours (Lukacsko, 1987). Again, while these ratios are cited in the literature, there are presently no controlled studies to support these figures.

The larger the volume of drug injected, the greater the chance of spread to the brainstem where central side effects can occur (Moulin and Coyle, 1986). Because the intrathecal route requires a smaller dose than the epidural route, this may be one reason for choosing the intrathecal route.

2. Careful monitoring is needed following spinal analgesia. Respiratory depression is a potentially life-threatening side effect of this route. Significant respiratory depression, however, has been reported mostly in acute postoperative pain and in patients who are narcotic naive, i.e., lacking tolerance because of no recent narcotic administration (see p. 105 for further discussion of respiratory depression following spinal analgesia).

3. The rapid development of tolerance may be a major limiting factor to the more widespread use of spinal analgesia for chronic pain. Although the mechanism of tolerance is not yet fully understood (see p. 72 for discussion of tolerance), there is some cross-tolerance between narcotics administered spinally and those administered systemically (Yaksh, 1981). In general, patients who require high doses of systemic narcotics will eventually require high spinal doses to achieve pain relief.

As the dose increases, central side effects may occur, thereby limiting the effectiveness of this route. With dose escalation, there is also the concern that eventually a dose too high in concentration or volume will be needed. Preservative-free solutions are highly recommended for the spinal route but are difficult to obtain commercially in high concentrations.

Further research is needed to clarify the extent and rate at which tolerance develops. In one study, 43 patients receiving intrathecal morphine by an implanted pump for 6 months or longer did not show evidence of rapid tolerance and its related problems. Of the 35 patients with cancer pain, the majority did need two or more times the initial spinal dose over the course of their treatment. This did not result in any central side effects that limited analgesic effectiveness. Only 2 of the 43 patients developed the need for drug dosages that were beyond the pump capabilities (Penn and Paice, 1987).

Another study involved 43 patients with nonmalignant pain receiving spinal morphine for up to 2 years. Tolerance appeared to develop, but in many patients the increased dose was due instead to technical problems with the catheter (Auld et al, 1985).

4. Incidence of side effects varies widely and may not occur in all patients. Pruritus, urinary retention, and nausea and vomiting are the most common and will be discussed here. Respiratory depression is also a side effect and is discussed on p. 105.

a. Although the mechanism is unknown, the characteristics of *pruritus* are that it (Payne, 1987b):
 - Is not dose related and occurs after acute and chronic spinal administration.
 - May occur after epidural or intrathecal route.
 - May continue for the duration of analgesia. However, some report that in patients receiving continuous morphine infusion, pruritus resolves in 48 to 72 hours (Penn et al, 1984).
 - Usually occurs in the face and palate.
 - Is not related to preservative in the drug solution.
 - Is frequent in pregnant women.
 - May worsen with coadministration of steroids.
 - May be severe enough to limit therapy.
 - May not be relieved with an antihistamine, i.e., diphenhydramine hydrochloride (Benadryl), although there is disagreement over this.
 - May be reversed with naloxone.

b. The characteristics of *urinary retention* are that it (Payne, 1987b):
 - May be a direct effect of the narcotic on the spinal cord which results in altered bladder tone.
 - Occurs mostly in elderly males or in people with preexisting bladder disorders.
 - Seems to have a higher incidence in the postoperative period and in pregnant women.
 - Has occurred as long as 18 hours after spinal administration and with epidural doses as low as 3 to 4 mg.

c. *Nausea and vomiting* may occur in patients with cancer, obstetrical, and postoperative pain treated with spinal analgesia. However, tolerance to this side effect develops rapidly (Yaksh, 1981).

5. Serious complications from contamination. While this is a problem with IM, IV, or SC routes, the complications are much more dangerous if the spinal route is contaminated. The potential for contamination is greater in chronic external catheter use than in implanted systems.

KEY POINT: In our enthusiasm to try a new method or initiate the latest trend in pain control, it is important to remember that this method may not be the most appropriate for a particular patient based on his individual situation.

Recommendations for the Spinal Route. As of this date (1989), research is lacking and clinical reports are varied and inconclusive regarding guidelines for the spinal route. Therefore this section will not discuss specific protocols and calculation of doses.

Instead, we will present recommendations that promote your effective delivery of spinal analgesia and safe monitoring of its effects. Use of the flow sheet (p. 27) is perhaps more essential when the route of drug administration is spinal than when other routes are used. Because of the direct access of the spinal route, the flow sheet is a vital tool to monitor the patient's safety and level of comfort.

General guidelines for nursing care of patients receiving narcotics via the spinal route are:

1. Identify the method of narcotic delivery by the spinal route. This varies for acute and chronic pain. Possibilities are:

a. Single bolus. To control acute postoperative pain, the patient may receive one bolus dose in the operating room, and there may be no further access to the spinal route since additional doses are not needed.

b. External catheter. For control of prolonged pain and sometimes for postoperative or brief pain, a catheter is placed intrathecally or epidurally to allow the administration of narcotics by:
 - Single or intermittent boluses. May be used to control acute or chronic pain. However, this method is not ideal. With intermittent injections, the patient may be subjected to peaks of potent analgesia followed by valleys of pain when the dose wears off.
 - Continuous infusion. This method avoids the peaks and valleys and provides a constant level of pain control. It is primarily used in chronic prolonged pain. However, it is certainly appropriate for acute pain because it not only avoids peaks and valleys, but also it limits the total volume delivered at one time. The larger the volume of drug injected, the greater the chance of spread to the brainstem where central side effects can occur.

c. Implanted port or reservoir. A catheter into the epidural or intrathecal space is tunneled under the skin and attaches to a port or reservoir which is implanted subcutaneously. These devices may be accessed for individual boluses or continuous infusion.

d. Implanted infusion pump. These devices are implanted in SC pockets in the abdomen and provide continuous infusion for a constant level of pain relief. However, because of the cost of the device and the need for a major surgical procedure, this method requires careful patient selection. Patients who might be considered appropriate candidates include those with (Paice, 1986 and 1987; Penn and Paice, 1987):

- Life expectancy of greater than a few months.
- Pain below the midcervical dermatome.
- Pain unsuccessfully treated with an aggressive regimen of analgesic therapy.
- Pain inappropriate for neurosurgical procedures.

2. Assess family/patient willingness and resources to care for chronic delivery of spinal analgesia. Each of the external delivery systems for spinal analgesia requires that the patient or family be willing and able to care for the system and administer the narcotic safely.

Careful consideration of family resources are also important factors in considering the appropriateness of the spinal route. The cost of a drug, e.g., preservative-free morphine, and some of the devices to deliver the drug, e.g., an implantable pump, are very expensive.

3. Taper systemic narcotics once spinal administration begins. If the patient has been receiving systemic narcotics, it is important to gradually reduce these while adjusting the dose needed for spinal analgesia. The number of days needed to taper systemic narcotics is variable and may depend on the length of time the patient has been taking the narcotic. Narcotic withdrawal syndrome may occur if narcotics are abruptly stopped by any of the following previous routes: IM, SL, IV, PO, rectal, or buccal (see p. 71 on physical dependence and treatment of withdrawal symptoms).

4. Limit the concentration of morphine. Morphine may be concentrated at no more than 50 mg/ml. If higher concentrations are used, morphine will not stay in solution and will precipitate. This may limit the dose of spinal morphine that can be given. Although there is controversy over the necessity of preservative-free morphine, many recommend it because some of the preservative agents are neurotoxic.

5. Increase or decrease the dose in terms of percentages instead of a fixed number of milligrams. Percentage adjustments keep dosage changes in proportion to the original dose and can be more widely applied regardless of the dose. See p. 95 for an example of this concept.

6. Use a flow sheet to determine safety and effectiveness of dosage (see form on p. 27). A flow sheet provides data in an easily read format that allows quick scanning for such responses as respiratory depression or unrelieved pain. This assessment form is particularly vital in assessing safety and efficacy of analgesia with spinal narcotics. It can be a helpful tool to all members of the health care team when fear and concern result in hesitancy to try a particular drug, route, or dosage.

Dosages for this route will vary depending on whether the patient is narcotic naive, e.g., a postoperative patient, or the patient has been on a long-term course of narcotics, e.g., a patient with cancer pain (see a discussion of tolerance to analgesia on p. 72).

- An initial bolus dose of morphine for the patient who is narcotic naive can range from 5 to 10 mg epidurally, 0.5 mg to 2 mg intrathecally.

- A total dosage range of epidural morphine 4 to 18 mg is reported following thoracic, abdominal, urological, or orthopedic surgery in over 1000 patients (Stenseth et al, 1985).
- For cancer pain:
  —Continuous intrathecal doses of up to 100 mg/day (Penn and Paice, 1987).
  —Continuous epidural doses of up to 90 mg/day (Caballero et al, 1986).

7. Be aware of the wide variety of analgesic onset and duration of spinal narcotics.

a. The usual onset of pain relief from a spinal narcotic varies greatly depending on what drug is used:
  - Approximately 5 minutes for lipophilic drugs, e.g., meperidine or methadone (Jacobson, 1984).
  - Approximately 30 to 60 minutes for morphine, a hydrophilic drug (Yaksh, 1981).

  Knowledge of these variations will serve as a guide to assess the individual patient for a repetition of bolus doses.

b. The interval between bolus doses involves considering the wide variability in duration of action among the spinal narcotics. The following have been reported (Yaksh, 1981):
  - For epidural analgesia: the duration can be from 4 to 36 hours with morphine administration, 4 to 18 hours with meperidine, and 4 hours with fentanyl.
  - For intrathecal analgesia: duration can be 12 to 24 hours following morphine and meperidine.

KEY POINT: For spinal analgesia, due to limited research and clinical experience, individual assessment of onset, duration, and side effects in each situation is mandatory.

8. The actual amount by which a dose is increased or decreased is determined by finding a dose that relieves pain to the patient's satisfaction with minimal side effects. This is done by using a flow sheet and looking at the following patient responses in consecutive order:

- First, respiratory function, usually rate.
- Second, pain rating on 0 to 10 scale.
- Third, based on the above information, determine whether to increase or decrease the number of milligrams of analgesic and at what percentage, e.g., 10%, 50%, or 100%.

Because patients' responses to analgesics are so individual, there are no easy formulas that give the "right percentage." No matter what percentage is chosen, it is vital to assess this adjustment based on the drug used and its onset of spinal analgesia. Document the patient's response on the flow sheet so that further increases or decreases can be made without the patient enduring long painful periods between titrations. If a conservative dose increase is chosen, e.g., 10% to 20%, for a patient who is rating pain at 8 on 0 to 10 scale, realize that you will probably need to go higher in percentage increases, e.g.,

50% to 100%, and at more frequent intervals than if you began with a more liberal percentage increase.

9. Close monitoring of respiratory depression is required.

a. Characteristics of respiratory depression include the following (Leib and Hurtig, 1985; Payne, 1987b):
   - Onset is variable. An *early* onset, within 1 to 2 hours, may be related to uptake of the drug by the systemic vasculature with shunting to the brain, *or a late* onset, within 4 to 24 hours, may be as a result of drug distribution in the cerebrospinal fluid with uptake by the receptors in the respiratory center.
   - It seems to be more common with hydrophilic (water-soluble) drugs, e.g., morphine, as opposed to lipophilic drugs, e.g., methadone and meperidine.
   - Life-threatening respiratory depression has been seen mostly in the postoperative setting with narcotic naive patients. It is rarely seen with treatment of chronic cancer pain since most of these patients have been on systemic narcotics long enough to develop tolerance to life-threatening side effects.

b. Factors for the nurse to be aware of that can predispose to respiratory depression include (Cousins and Mather, 1984):
   - Advanced age.
   - Hydrophilic (water-soluble) narcotics, e.g., morphine.
   - Marked changes in thoracic-abdominal pressure, including mechanical ventilation or "grunting" respiration associated with pain.
   - Narcotic naive or nontolerant patient.
   - Simultaneous administration of narcotics or other CNS depressants by systemic routes.

   Because of the increased chances of respiratory depression when additional systemic narcotics or sedatives are used, many protocols for short-term spinal therapy, e.g., in the postoperative period, state that these additional drugs will not be used unless approved in writing by the anesthesiologist. If they are used, extra careful monitoring is advised, e.g., assessment every 10 minutes.

   On the contrary, for chronic pain, e.g., cancer pain, concurrent drugs that contribute to analgesia are often administered systemically without the danger of decreased respirations.

c. In the acute care setting, there is current disagreement about the use of apnea monitors or ear oximeters vs. the nurse personally observing the patient's respiratory function every 30 minutes. However, no one disagrees with the importance of consistent, careful monitoring in whatever form for this patient population. Careful monitoring of respiratory function should not only include assessment of respiratory rate, but also assessment of (Leib and Hurtig, 1985):
   - Respiratory volume.
   - Quality of respiratory effort.
   - Skin color.
   - Auscultation of chest.
   - Arterial blood gas analysis.
   - Apneic spells.

   The health care team establishes acceptable limits to these respiratory functions for each patient. Documentation in the flow sheet under respirations would include additional categories to reflect this, e.g., blood gas results and duration of apnea.

   Naloxone IM or IV effectively reverses respiratory depression related to spinal analgesia. Because some of the spinal narcotic enters the general circulation and acts at the levels of the brain, naloxone will also reverse some analgesia. Reversal with naloxone may require multiple, repeated doses since its duration is shorter than the analgesic, i.e., duration of naloxone may be as short as 30 minutes.

10. Further research is needed before definitive recommendations for the spinal route can be made. Continuing research will offer the nurse new and more specific guidelines and will certainly explore the following unanswered questions (Moulin and Coyle, 1986; Payne, 1987a):
   - What are the optimal narcotics for spinal analgesia?
   - What are equianalgesic doses of epidural and intrathecal narcotics in comparison to oral and parenteral routes?
   - For chronic pain, what are appropriate indications for effective use of spinal route?
   - How can development of tolerance to analgesia be delayed or handled in chronic spinal administration of analgesics?
   - What is the role and approach to spinally administered nonnarcotics, e.g., clonidine, bupivacaine (Marcaine)?

Patient Example

A 45-year-old woman diagnosed with adenocarcinoma of the rectum was treated surgically with resection of the rectum and the formation of a colostomy. Due to the advanced stage of her disease at presentation, she was also treated with chemotherapy and radiotherapy. She received intermittent propoxyphene for mild pain.

After 6 months the patient developed severe pain in the rectal vault. Radiographic examination revealed a large tumor in that region as well as metastatic disease to the liver and abdomen. The patient was placed on trials of codeine, immediate-release morphine, sustained-release morphine, and levorphanol. She was unable to tolerate these agents due to severe nausea and sedation. Due to the midline nature of the pain, local blocks and neurosurgical procedures were not appropriate.

An epidural catheter was placed in the lumbar region and tunneled under the skin so that the exit site was several inches away from the midline of the back. An infusion was started at 2 cc/hr of 0.1 mg/cc preservative-free morphine via IMED pump. An apnea monitor was used for the first 24 hours after insertion, according to hospital policy. After titrating the dosage to 20 mg morphine/24 hr the patient received excellent analgesia. At this point an ambulatory infusion pump was attached and filled with 1.0 mg preservative-free morphine/ml. The patient and her family were taught how to manage the pump. A home health nurse was consulted to ensure pain management continued in the patient's home.

After receiving excellent relief for over 3 months the patient experienced severe pain one evening. Her daughter noticed that the catheter had become dislocated. The pain clinic staff reinserted the catheter, and the patient returned to her previous level of analgesia. After 1 month the husband noticed redness and drainage at the insertion site. The patient complained of pain upon palpation of the site. The physician ordered antibiotics, removed the catheter, cultured the tip, and re-inserted a new catheter after establishing that the infection was only superficial and had not extended into the CNS. However, after several weeks this catheter also became dislodged.

Due to these significant problems and the patient's excellent response on epidural narcotics, an implanted pump was inserted to provide continuous analgesia. Excellent relief was obtained with 35 mg morphine/day intrathecally. The device required refilling every 3 weeks. This was done either in the outpatient office or at home (Paice, 1988a).

Method of Administration: PCA by the IV, SC, or Spinal Route

The ideal way to administer IV, SC, spinal, or any form of analgesia is by a method that allows the patient control of his pain. For example, a patient-controlled pump that has the capacity to provide continuous infusion *in addition to* self-administration of bolus doses allows the patient to control sudden increases of pain, e.g., from movement or coughing, and/or breakthrough pain.

The technology of pumps is a constantly changing field. Examples of options or features that may need to be considered in choosing an appropriate pump for the individual patient or clinical setting are:
- Complexity and expense of operation, e.g., cost of pump, cost of any cartridges to reload, ease of operating and teaching patient, and ease of reloading.
- Alarms for malfunction, low battery, or low residual volume.
- Size and portability. For the ambulatory patient it is important to have a small, portable pump, a frequently desirable feature for patients with continuous SC narcotic infusion.
- Ability to convert easily from IV pole to wearable pump.
- Continuous hourly infusion.
- Boluses with or without a continuous infusion.
- Wide range of possible volume of bolus dose.
- Range of possible volume infused per hour, e.g., from 0.5 ml to 99 ml or more. Very large doses are sometimes needed for the IV route and very small doses for the SC and spinal routes.

- Range of possible lockout intervals, e.g., 5 to 90 minutes.
- Stored retrievable information, e.g., total dose per hour, per 4 hours, or per 24 hours, number of attempts to administer bolus vs. number of boluses given.
- Information on display panel, e.g., alarm messages, amount delivered.
- Allow patient various combinations of control, e.g., stop/start plus initiate bolus and with or without ability to change hourly infusion.

Changing from One Route to Another

Changing the route of narcotic administration has the biggest potential for undermedicating patients. To avoid problems and to make this transition as smooth as possible, the following guidelines are suggested:
1. Calculate the dose of narcotic for the new route using the equianalgesic chart (pp. 78-79). Remember this chart is a guideline for *initial* doses. The dose required varies from one patient to another. Use a flow sheet (p. 27) to assess the patient's comfort frequently and increase or decrease the dose according to the individual's response.
2. Educate the patient about the differences in this new route, especially when changing from IM or IV to PO. With PO narcotics, he will not experience the same fast onset of pain relief as with IM or IV route; however, the duration of PO medication is often longer. Explain that it may take a few days of adjustment to determine the most effective dose and interval.
3. Anticipate anxiety and possible doubts from the patient that the new route, especially the PO route, can control the severity of his pain. He may never have been given strong PO narcotics in adequate doses, or a previous attempt to switch routes may have failed. Reassure him that you will check with him frequently. If the route is PO, also reassure him that an IM or IV dose can always be given if immediate pain control is needed. Let him know he will not be abandoned on this new route and made to "tough it out."

Guidelines for Changing from IM or IV to PO. This change must be handled with care to prevent return of unnecessary pain, a loss of faith in the idea, abandonment of the attempt to titrate onto PO analgesics, and to minimize nausea and vomiting. Although it is possible to discontinue all IM or IV analgesics at once and give an amount orally that is estimated to be equianalgesic, there is significant potential for underdosing or overdosing. A more gradual changeover decreases the degree of potential error.

Use a flow sheet to implement the following guidelines for changing from IM or IV to PO narcotic/nonnarcotic analgesia:
1. Assess the pain relief obtained from the current IM or IV narcotic before making a change.

2. Select a nonnarcotic and administer it on a regular schedule.
3. Select a PO narcotic and use the equianalgesic chart (pp. 78-79) to calculate the approximate total dose needed to replace the current dose of IM or IV narcotic.* Consider a lower estimate if a nonnarcotic analgesic is added.
4. Decrease the IM or IV dose by a percentage, e.g., 10% to 30%, perhaps 50% in some cases. Calculate the percentage of the PO narcotic dose needed to replace this initial decrease in IM or IV narcotic dose. Give this PO narcotic dose along with the decreased IM or IV dose.
5. Assess the effectiveness of these analgesics, i.e., the nonnarcotic, the decreased dose of IM or IV narcotic, and the PO narcotic dose calculated to replace the amount omitted from the IM or IV dose.
6. Adjust the PO narcotic dose up or down depending on the person's response.
7. When pain relief is acceptable, decrease the parenteral narcotic again by the same dose, i.e., milligrams, and add the amount of PO narcotic required to replace this, as determined in step #6.
8. Continue to decrease the IM or IV narcotic dose by the same amount until the entire dose is converted to PO analgesics.

KEY POINT: In converting routes of medication, calculate equianalgesic doses using the chart as a guideline. Initial doses may not be effective. Therefore it is vital to consistently assess, titrate, and evaluate so that dose adjustments up or down can be made until the most effective dose is found.

Patient Example

The flow sheet on p. 108 summarizes how a patient may be changed from IM to PO. The following numbers refer to the numbers on the left side of the box.
1. Assess the effectiveness of the present analgesic, meperidine 75 mg IM, before changing it:
   • 8 AM—Patient's pain rating is 7 on 0 to 10 scale, meperidine is given.
   • At 1 and 2 hours later, pain rating is 3. This is the degree of relief the patient is accustomed to obtaining. The usual goal is to provide analgesia as good as or better than what the patient has been receiving.
2. Decrease IM by 33% (⅓) and replace this with PO narcotic and nonnarcotic.
   • Meperidine is reduced to 50 mg.
   • The equianalgesic chart (see pp. 78-79) is consulted. It suggests that either 60 mg or 30 mg morphine will be needed to replace meperidine 75 mg

IM. This is a young patient, 20 years old, so 60 mg is chosen.
   • An appropriate percentage of the PO narcotic is calculated. Roughly 33% of the 60 mg, i.e., 20 mg, is needed since the meperidine was decreased by 33%. However, we are also choosing a nonnarcotic, Trilisate 1500 mg PO. This added analgesia reduces the narcotic requirement, so we are estimating that morphine 15 mg will be enough.
   • 11 AM—all three medications are given.
3. Assess the effectiveness of the reduced IM meperidine plus the PO analgesics given as a replacement for the reduced meperidine dose.
   • 12 noon—pain rating is 3.
   • 1 PM—pain rating is 2.
   • 2 PM—pain rating is 1.
This is better pain relief than the patient had with meperidine IM. No side effects, e.g., depressed respirations, are noted.

We do not need to adjust the PO analgesic and can assume that a further reduction of 25 mg of meperidine IM can be replaced with the same PO dose, i.e., 15 mg morphine PO. The onset of Trilisate is about 2 hours, and it lasts about 12 hours on a bid dosing schedule (it can also be given in smaller doses tid). Thus because it is still having an effect it need not be given again now. However, the IM meperidine and PO morphine tend to wear off in 3 to 4 hours, so they need to be repeated at 3 PM.
4. Reduce the IM meperidine by another 25 mg and add another 15 mg morphine PO.
   • 3 PM—meperidine 25 mg plus morphine 30 mg PO are given.
   • 4 PM—pain rating is 1.
5. It is well established in this patient that each 25 mg of meperidine IM can be replaced with 15 mg morphine PO along with the nonnarcotic Trilisate. Therefore the final 25 mg of the IM meperidine can be omitted.
   • 7 PM—morphine 45 mg PO given.
   • 11 PM—Trilisate 1500 mg given again.
   NOTE: The patient is completely off injectable narcotic and on only PO narcotic plus nonnarcotic given on regular basis. Pain relief is better, and the switch was completed in only 11 hours.

Side Effects of Narcotics

Regardless of route, narcotics given regularly will result in side effects. The more common ones are constipation, nausea and vomiting, and sedation. They must be anticipated, and if they occur, they must be treated on a regular, preventive basis. However, these symptoms are not always due to narcotics. Assess patients for other causes. This is particularly important in the person with cancer in whom symptoms may be related to treatment, advancing disease, or a condition unrelated to the cancer.

Constipation Caused by Narcotics

The *mechanism* underlying constipation caused by narcotics is the binding of narcotics to receptor sites in the gastrointestinal tract. The result is decreased motility

---

*Based on clinical experience, many consider the IM and IV dose to be equianalgesic (Portenoy, 1987a). However, some recommend using one half the IM dose for the IV dose (American Pain Society, 1987; Foley, 1982).

FLOW SHEET—PAIN: From IM to PO

Patient ___Mr. T, age 20_____ Date _____

Pain rating scale used ___0-10 (0=no pain, 10=worst pain)_____

Purpose: To evaluate the safety and effectiveness of the analgesic(s) and to assist switch to PO morphine.

Analgesic(s) prescribed: __Demerol 25-75mg IM; Morphine PO 15-45mg q4h;__
__Trilisate 1500mg PO bid__

	Time	Pain rating	Analgesic	R	P	BP	Level of arousal	Other	Plan & comments
1.	8 AM	7	Demerol 75mg IM	18			Awake and alert		Assess effectiveness of Demerol
	9 AM	3		16			Drowsy		
	10 AM	3		14			Sleeping but easily awakens		
2.	11 AM	5	Demerol 50mg IM, Morphine 15mg PO, Trilisate 1500mg PO	16			Alert		1st part of switch. Assess effectiveness
3.	12 N	3		14			Alert—States feels "good"		
	1 PM	2		16			States pain is almost gone.		
	2 PM	1		16			Able to ambulate more this PM. "Very comfortable"		
4.	3 PM	3	Demerol 25mg IM, Morphine 30mg PO	18					2nd reduction in IM with Increase in PO
	4 PM	1		16			More comfortable than she's been in last 3 days.		
	5 PM	1		14			Sleeping		
5.	7 PM	2	Morphine 45mg PO	16			Alert — talking with family members		Totally converted to PO
	9 PM	1		14			Sleeping		
	11 PM	1	Trilisate 1500mg PO	12			Sleeping - but easily awakens—states still comfortable		

The flow sheet for this patient shows how hourly observations contributed to a safe and effective change from IM analgesics to PO analgesics. The numbered steps on the extreme left correspond to the discussion in the text. In summary, the IM analgesic was evaluated, and then the IM dose was decreased by about 33%. Analgesia from the IM was replaced with a sufficient amount of PO analgesics. The IM dose was decreased again by 33% of the original dose and then discontinued while at the same time the PO analgesics were increased to maintain satisfactory pain relief. No significant side effects were noted during this transition from IM to PO analgesics.

and delayed passage of gastric contents. Poor fluid intake, inadequate diet, and a lack of exercise intensify the problem.

The majority of people taking narcotics regularly will become constipated. Anticipate this and check prescriptions. If a narcotic is prescribed, a stool softener-stimulant should automatically be included. If constipation is not controlled, it can become as problematic as the pain itself.

KEY POINT: Use a *preventive, regular,* and *aggressive* **approach to avoid constipation. The need to treat constipation usually means a failure to prevent it.**

Points to remember in managing narcotic-induced constipation are:
• The goal is a bowel movement at least every 2 to 3 days,

except of course for the patient who is NPO or not taking fluids by mouth.
• Ask about the patient's usual bowel habits and methods used to control irregularity.
• Explain that the methods the patient usually uses probably will not be sufficient. A more aggressive approach is needed. However, the patient's preferences are incorporated into bowel care as much as possible.
• Frequent small liquid stools or fecal incontinence could mean impaction. Do a rectal examination to check.
• If fluid intake is decreased, avoid bulk laxatives, e.g., Metamucil, Perdiem, because their effectiveness depends on a sufficient intake of fluids.
• Encourage large intake (at least eight glasses) of water each day.

TABLE 4-14 Bowel Regimen to Prevent Narcotic-Induced Constipation*

Medication	Suggested Beginning Dose	Usual Range of Dosage
1. Begin with *one* of the combined stool softener and mild peristaltic stimulants:		
Diocytyl sodium sulfosuccinate, 100 mg plus casanthranol 30 mg (Pericolace)	1 capsule tid	1 capsule qd to 2 capsules tid
or		
Docusate sodium, 50 mg, plus senna 187 mg (Senokot-S)	1 tablet tid	1 tablet qd to 4 tablets tid
or		
Docusate calcium, 60 mg, plus danthron, 50 mg (Doxidan)	1 capsule bid	1 capsule qd to 2 capsules tid
2. If no bowel movement in any 48 hr period, add *one to two* of the following:		
Senna 187 mg (Senokot)	2-3 tablets hs	2 tablets hs to 4 tablets tid
Bisacodyl (Dulcolax)	10-15 mg PO hs	5 mg PO hs to 15 mg PO tid
Milk of Magnesia	30-60 ml hs	30-60 ml qd or bid
Lactulose (Chronulac: 10 g/15 ml)	30-45 ml hs	15-60 ml qd or bid
Per Diem (avoid if fluid intake is reduced)	2 teaspoons hs	1 teaspoon to 2 tablespoons qd
3. If no bowel movement by 72 hr, perform rectal examination to rule out impaction. If not impacted, go to #4. If impacted, go to #5.		
4. If not impacted, try *one* of the following:		
Bisacodyl (Dulcolax) suppository	10 mg	
Magnesium Citrate	8 oz PO	
Senna extract (X-prep liquid)	2½ oz PO	
Mineral Oil	30-60 ml PO	
Milk of Magnesia 25 ml and Cascara 5 ml suspension		
Fleet Enema		
5. If impacted:		
Manually disempact if stool is soft enough.		
If not, soften with glycerin suppository or oil retention enema, then disempact manually.		
Follow up with enema (tap water, soapsuds) until clear.		
Increase daily bowel regimen.		

*Adapted from Levy, MH: Pain management in advanced cancer, *Semin Oncol* **12**:404, 1985.

• Encourage foods and liquids that have helped the patient have bowel movements in the past. These might include foods rich in dietary fiber such as beans, carrots, bran-containing cereals and liquids such as prune juice or hot lemon water.

A suggested regimen to prevent and treat constipation is presented in Table 4-14.

Patient Example

Pain medication: Dilaudid 12 mg q4h. Preventive constipation medication: Senokot-S two capsules tid. Because of no bowel movement in 48 hours, Dulcolax 10 mg tid was added. Because this problem continued, Lactulose 45 ml HS was added to the Senokot-S and Dulcolax.

A fixed relationship between a narcotic dose and senna (Senokot tablet) has been suggested: one Senokot or Senokot-S tablet is needed to counteract the constipation from each dose of 120 mg of codeine PO, 4 mg of hydromorphone PO, 15 mg of morphine PO, or any other equianalgesic dose (Levy, 1985; Maguire et al, 1981).

New approaches to particularly difficult cases of constipation include the use of TENS and PO naloxone. TENS has been used to stimulate intestinal peristalsis, e.g., preventing and treating ileus, therefore it may be successful in preventing and treating constipation (refer to Chapter 5, p. 160 for further discussion).

In cases of unresponsive constipation, naloxone 3.6 mg PO q3h has been effective (Kreek et al, 1983). Naloxone given PO, as opposed to IV or IM, reverses little if any analgesia.

No magic formula exists for preventing or treating constipation. Each individual reacts differently. Monitoring the patient's initial response to medication and then making adjustments up or down accordingly is essential. See patient/family teaching point on p. 114 concerning constipation caused by narcotics.

Nausea and Vomiting Caused by Narcotics

The mechanism underlying narcotic-induced nausea and vomiting is complicated. Narcotics may cause nausea in three different ways:

1. Stimulation of the chemoreceptor trigger zone in the brain.

TABLE 4-15 A Sample Regimen for Narcotic-Induced Nausea

Antiemetics	Usual Range of Dosage
Start with:	
Prochlorperazine (Compazine)	PO 5 mg q4h to 20 mg q6h
or	IV 2 mg q4-6h
	Rectal 5-25 mg q6h
Thiethylperazine (Torecan)	PO 10 mg q8-12h
	Rectal 10 mg q8-12h
	IM 10 mg q8-12h
If there is component of motion sickness and patient is ambulatory, *add:*	
Dimenhydrate (Dramamine)	PO 50-100 mg q4-6h
	IM 50-100 mg q4-6h
If above is ineffective, *add:*	
Metoclopramide (Reglan)	PO 10-20 mg tid and hs
	IV Start with 10 mg q6h and increase as needed
Less commonly used antiemetics:	
Scopolamine	PO 0.6 mg q4h
	Transdermal patch, usually behind ear: replace q 3 days
Secobarbital (Seconal) (may be helpful with severe nausea especially from high dose IV morphine)	IV 50-150 mg q4-6h
	Rectal 120-200 mg

2. Inhibitory effect on GI motility.
3. Stimulation of the vestibular nerve (which carries the impulses for balance).

Points to remember in managing narcotic-induced nausea and vomiting are:

- Nausea may occur when a narcotic regimen is first begun, but it usually subsides after several days. If it does not subside or is not controlled with antiemetics, consider changing to a different narcotic.
- Nausea is often automatically blamed on narcotics. There may be other reasons, e.g., hypercalcemia, copious sputum, uncontrolled pain, or medications for conditions other than pain.
- The principle of good antinausea therapy is to *add* antiemetics that work at different levels. That is, continue the original antiemetic and add another that is effective at a different level.

KEY POINT: To treat narcotic-induced nausea, apply the same approach that is used to effectively treat pain, *preventive and regular.*

Examples of approaches to nausea and vomiting are summarized in Table 4-15 and Figure 4-10.

Patient Example

Mrs. M. is just back from surgery. After two doses of morphine 10 mg IM q3h, she rates her pain at 4 on a 0 to 10 scale (0 = no pain, 10 = worst pain). She states that she is feeling nauseated. The nurse notes that Mrs. M. becomes very anxious and holds her breath whenever she moves. Because postoperative nausea in the presence of pain should be treated with an increase in nar-

cotic first, morphine 15 mg is given. Pain is now rated at 2, however, some nausea is still present. Compazine 25 mg suppository is given and controls Mrs. M.'s nausea.

Sometimes phenothiazines are given parenterally as antiemetics. A common misconception is that they will provide added analgesia. In fact there are no data to support the frequent use of phenothiazines, e.g., promethazine (Phenergan) and chlorpromazine (Thorazine), solely as potentiators of the analgesia of narcotics (McGee and Alexander, 1979). See pp. 117-118 for more indepth discussion of "potentiators." They may, however, be useful additions to the narcotics if nausea and vomiting are present.

See patient/family teaching point on p. 115 concerning nausea and vomiting caused by narcotics.

Sedation Caused by Narcotics

The mechanism underlying narcotic-induced sedation is partly due to the narcotic's direct depressant effect on the CNS. However, total exhaustion from unrelieved pain is also a factor that can contribute to sedation once the pain is controlled.

Points to remember in managing narcotic-induced sedation are:

- Sleep deprivation resulting from unrelieved pain may be the main reason for signs of sedation. As long as respiratory function is stable and the person can be aroused, continue with the dosing schedule.
- Sedation may occur when a narcotic regimen is first begun or when there is a significant dosage increase. It usually decreases in 1 to 3 days, partly due to the patient developing tolerance to sedation.

DECISION PROCESS FOR NARCOTIC-INDUCED NAUSEA

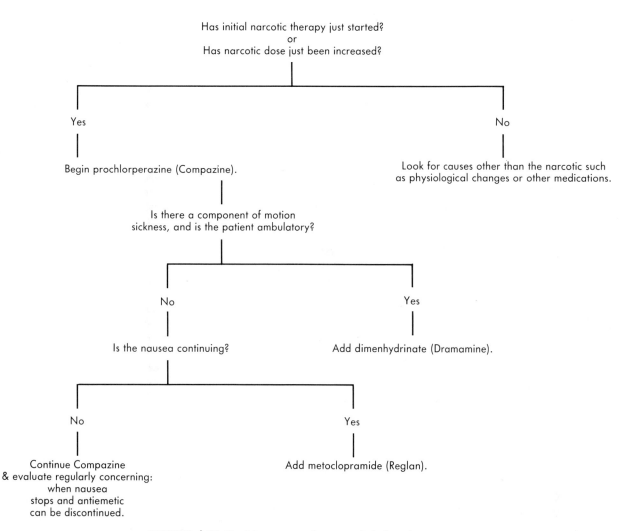

Has initial narcotic therapy just started?
or
Has narcotic dose just been increased?

Yes

Begin prochlorperazine (Compazine).

Is there a component of motion sickness, and is the patient ambulatory?

No

Is the nausea continuing?

No

Continue Compazine & evaluate regularly concerning: when nausea stops and antiemetic can be discontinued.

Yes

Add metoclopramide (Reglan).

Yes

Add dimenhydrinate (Dramamine).

No

Look for causes other than the narcotic such as physiological changes or other medications.

FIGURE 4-10 Decision process for narcotic-induced nausea.

- If sedation continues after 3 days and is unacceptable to the patient, consider lowering the narcotic dose and adding NSAIDs to boost analgesia without sedating side effects. The key here is to be able to *lower the dose without decreasing pain relief.* If this is not effective, consider changing to another narcotic.
- Dextroamphetamine PO or methylphenidate (Ritalin) PO may be used to increase alertness in patients when a narcotic dose reduction is unsuccessful (American Pain Society, 1987). The use of these stimulants should be short-term, as tolerance develops quickly. Refer to p. 120 for more discussion of stimulants.
- Sedation may be due to other factors: undiagnosed organic pathology, drugs other than narcotics, or psychological causes. Unfortunately the narcotic is often blamed before these other factors are explored.

- Sedation can occur without adequate pain relief. That is, a person might barely be able to stay awake while rating the pain at 8 on a 0 to 10 scale. *Do not doubt the patient in this situation.* Side effects of the narcotic have outweighed the beneficial analgesic effects. Alternatives to this must be explored, e.g., lowering the dose, changing to another narcotic, or changing to the spinal route of administration.

See patient/family teaching point on p. 115 concerning sedation caused by narcotics.

KEY POINT: A patient can be both sedated and in pain. Do not confuse sedation with analgesia.

Figure 4-11 provides an approach to narcotic-induced sedation.

DECISION PROCESS FOR NARCOTIC-INDUCED SEDATION

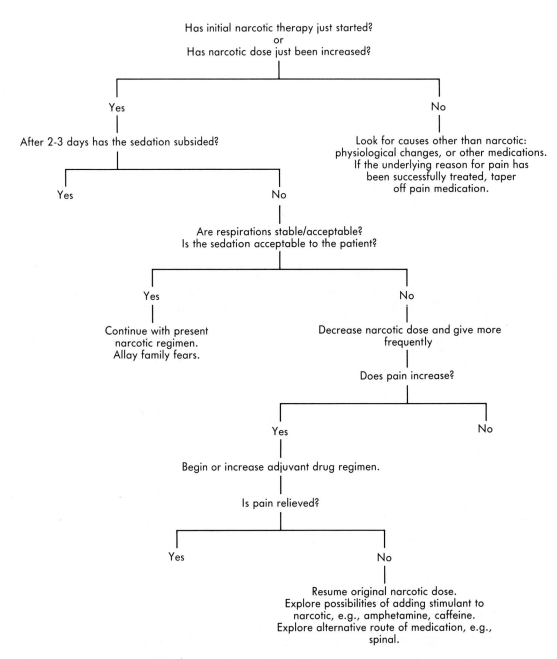

FIGURE 4-11 Decision process for narcotic-induced sedation.

The following two examples of sedation illustrate different causes and approaches.

Patient Example

Mrs. A. had widespread bone metastasis from end-stage breast cancer.

Pain medication: Morphine 120 mg PO q4h
Trilisate 1500 mg bid

Mrs. A. had been on this regimen for about 2 weeks with pain relief rated at 3 on a 0 to 10 scale. The family noticed that she became hard to arouse and would fall back to sleep immediately after speaking. The physician attributed the sedation to the morphine. However, the nurse could document on the flow sheet that although Mrs. A. was sedated, her respiratory rate remained stable at 18 to 20, so she was in no physiological danger. Further exploration showed that she had hypercalcemia. This was treated and the sedation subsided.

Patient Example

Mr. W., 22 years old, had hemophilia and was hospitalized to manage increased bleeding and to control severe pain from spontaneous hemorrhage into several muscles and joints. Upon admission he stated that his pain had been at 7 and 8 during the last 3 days in spite of PO codeine and acetaminophen and that he had not slept for at least 2 nights. Respirations were shallow at 20 to 24/min. Cold compresses were applied to the bleeding sites to help control both pain and bleeding. Hydromorphone IV was started with a 1 mg bolus and titrated up every 15 minutes to relieve pain. He was also receiving blood components IV. Within 1 hour he received a total of 4 mg of hydromorphone. After the last bolus his respirations were 12/min and deeper, he rated his pain at 2, and said he was comfortable. A continuous infusion of IV hydromorphone was started at 4 mg/hr. After 30 minutes the patient was sleeping and respirations remained about the same, 10 to 12/min. Sleep and inactivity tend to further lower respiratory rate, but this is not necessarily a concern if respirations are regular and deep and no cyanosis is noted. The patient slept for the next 8 hours, but he was coherent when he was aroused and continued to rate his pain at 2. When pain has been uncontrolled for a few days, it is not unusual for the patient to sleep for as long as 24 hours after pain is relieved. Sleep is not the same as sedation and is not an indication that the narcotic dose should be lowered. As long as the patient ventilates sufficiently, sleep does not indicate potential undesirable side effects.

KEY POINT: Be clear about who is the most concerned with a patient's sedation: the health team, patient, or family member? Probably no changes are needed if respirations are stable, indicating no physiological danger, and if the patient is satisfied.

Health professionals' and families' concerns can be addressed with re-education and the use of a flow sheet or daily diary (see pp. 27 and 30) to allay fears. On pp. 114-115 is a patient/family teaching point regarding narcotic side effects to be used with patients who have prolonged pain, e.g., prolonged cancer pain.

Adjuvant Analgesics and Medications

These drugs were originally intended for treatment of conditions other than pain. Most continue to be used in that manner, but they may also relieve pain in specific situations. Drugs that are not classified pharmacologically as analgesics but are used alone or in combination with narcotics to relieve pain are known as *adjuvant analgesics* or coanalgesics. Other medications often used to treat symptoms that commonly accompany pain, e.g., sleep disturbance, are referred to here simply as *adjuvant medications*. Table 4-16 summarizes some of the adjuvant analgesics and medications helpful for certain problems.

The appropriate use of these drugs is dependent on careful assessment of each individual person and his

symptoms. Specifically, adjuvant analgesics are appropriate when a pain syndrome does not respond to narcotics, e.g., phantom limb pain, causalgia, or postherpetic neuralgia. Adjuvant medications are appropriate when there is a component to the pain that analgesics alone cannot address, e.g., depression, sleeplessness, anxiety, or agitation. There may be considerable overlap with these drugs, i.e., one drug such as an antidepressant may serve dual purposes.

The use of an adjuvant drug in the following situation illustrates how a medication may not only relieve pain but also address a dimension of comfort that the narcotic alone could not relieve.

Patient Example

Mr. W. rates his pain at 4 on a 0 to 10 scale. Frequent awakenings during the night and a feeling of nervousness are what he describes as most bothersome right now. The narcotic and nonsteroidal antiinflammatory combination have been adjusted as carefully as possible. Mr. W. wants a better overall level of comfort. The nurse in this situation suggests adding a tricyclic antidepressant to help with the sleep disturbance. With amitriptyline 25 mg HS, the nervous feelings stop and Mr. W. sleeps through the night. He rates his general comfort at night at 1 to 2 on a 0 to 10 scale.

KEY POINT: Adjuvant analgesics and other medications are not a substitute for adequate doses of narcotic and nonnarcotic analgesics. Aggressive titration of analgesics to control pain comes first. Then, if additional symptoms remain, adjuvant analgesics or medications can be added.

Indications for Adjuvant Analgesics

Adjuvant analgesics characteristically do one of two things: enhance the effects of narcotics or nonnarcotic analgesics or have analgesic properties of their own. Examples of situations in which adjuvant analgesics may be appropriate are:

- Desire for analgesia in addition to or instead of narcotic or nonnarcotic analgesics, e.g., when narcotic or nonnarcotic use is limited by side effects or when they do not provide adequate relief, e.g., in neuropathic pain.
- Sleepless nights with increased anxiety and pain. These symptoms may improve with subtherapeutic doses (10 to 50 mg per day) of tricyclic antidepressants such as amitriptyline (Elavil) or doxepin (Sinequan).
- Sharp, shooting or lancinating pain, e.g., trigeminal neuralgia, may respond to anticonvulsants such as carbamazepine (Tegretol).
- Dull aching or burning pain, e.g., postherpetic neuralgia or diabetic neuropathy, may respond to tricyclic antidepressants such as amitriptyline (Elavil).
- Pain from bone metastasis or nerve compression may respond to corticosteroids, such as dexamethasone (Decadron) or prednisone.

Text continued on p. 117.

Patient/Family Teaching Point:
Common Narcotic Side Effects Related to Prolonged Narcotic Use

TO: _____ (patient's name) DATE: _____

Possible Side Effects Resulting from Narcotics

Constipation, drowsiness, and nausea are all possible effects from taking regular doses of narcotic medication for pain. Something can usually be done about each of these.

Constipation Caused by Narcotics: Important Points to Remember

- If you are taking pain medication regularly, you will become constipated.
- However, constipation is something that can be prevented; or if it occurs, it can be treated.
- It is unacceptable to be told that your pain medication cannot be increased because of constipation. Constipation can be prevented or controlled by careful assessment of your habits, and adjustments in your constipation medication and food and liquids.
- The usual methods you use to stay regular probably will not work well enough alone. Several approaches will be required and may be intensified as needed. We will try to incorporate your preferences for bowel care as much as possible.
- The usual goal is a bowel movement at least every 2 to 3 days.
- While medication to relieve and prevent constipation is important, combining this with nonmedicine methods can be even more effective. These include the following suggestions:
    1. Eat foods that help you have regular bowel movements. These include:

    _____.

    2. Drink as much water or other fluids as possible. Aim for _____ glasses each day of these fluids:

    _____.

    3. Exercise daily—such as walking. If you are in bed, exercises are important too. Your daily exercise routine will include:

    _____.

    4. Make a habit of going to the bathroom at regular times each day. Your time will be:

    _____.

    5. The urge to go to the bathroom is a natural message. Ignoring it can lead to constipation or make it worse.
    6. Take your time while having a bowel movement; hurrying can be as bad as delaying the urge to go.
    7. Do not strain or make a lot of effort to have a movement.
- If more than 2 days pass without a bowel movement, notify your nurse or physician immediately so that they can help you correct this problem.

Your daily medications for constipation are: _____

_____.

As long as you take narcotics, you must continue these measures to keep constipation under control. Do not stop any of these approaches simply because you have a bowel movement. You need to continue them in order to keep from being constipated.

Additional comments: _____

_____

■ May be duplicated for use in clinical practice. From McCaffery, M, and Beebe, A: PAIN: CLINICAL MANUAL FOR NURSING PRACTICE, St. Louis, 1989, The CV Mosby Company.

Continued.

Patient/Family Teaching Point:
Common Narcotic Side Effects Related to Prolonged Narcotic Use—cont'd

Nausea and Vomiting Caused by Narcotics: Important Points to Remember
- Some people become nauseated and vomit after first starting on pain medication.
- If this happens to you, let your nurse or doctor know so that you can begin on an antinausea medication (antiemetic).
- Nausea and vomiting should stop after several days. The dose of antinausea medication can then be decreased or stopped. However, some people need to continue on this medication as long as they are on narcotics.
- Sometimes there are causes of nausea other than the pain medication. Your doctor may look at other medications that you are taking or other things going on in your body.

Your medications for nausea are: _____

_____.

Additional comments: _____

_____

Drowsiness Caused by Narcotics: Important Points to Remember
- Some people feel drowsy after first starting on pain medication.
- This drowsiness usually goes away after several days. You may be able to stop the drowsiness with caffeine-containing beverages such as tea or coffee.
- You may have had no sleep because of the pain. When your body finally gets some relief, it is natural that you will probably sleep a lot at first because of total exhaustion.
- If you are sitting or lying in bed quietly, many people on pain medication find that they "catnap" throughout the day. This is normal and should not be seen as a bad effect. However, discuss this with your nurse or doctor if the drowsiness interferes with your ability to concentrate, talk with friends, or do the things that are important to you. They will work with you to try to correct this problem.
- If you are taking medication to control nausea, it may make you drowsy. Drowsiness from these medications will go away when you stop taking them.
- Other causes of drowsiness (other than the narcotic) may be explored by your doctor.

Additional comments: _____

_____

If you have any questions or concerns about the above, contact:

_____ (RN or MD name)   Phone: _____

_____ (Nurse's signature)

■ May be duplicated for use in clinical practice. From McCaffery, M, and Beebe, A: PAIN: CLINICAL MANUAL FOR NURSING PRACTICE, St. Louis, 1989, The CV Mosby Company.

TABLE 4-16 Selected Adjuvant Analgesics and Medications

Problem	Examples of Drugs Helpful for Problem	Usual Initial PO Dosage
Various types of pain, e.g., dull, aching neuropathic pain	*Tricyclic antidepressants:*	
	Amitriptyline (Elavil)	10-25 mg/day
	Doxepin (Sinequan)	10-25 mg/day
	Imipramine (Tofranil)	10-25 mg/day
	Desipramine (Norpramin)	10-25 mg/day
Lancinating neuropathic pain	*Anticonvulsants:*	
	Phenytoin (Dilantin)	300 mg/day
	Carbamazepine (Tegretol)	100 mg/day
	Valproic acid (Depakene)	15 mg/kg/day divided into bid or tid
Muscle spasm	*Antispastic agents:*	
	Baclofen (Lioresal)	5 mg tid
	Carisoprodol (Soma)	350 mg tid and hs
	Methocarbamol (Robaxin)	1.5 gm qid
	Cyclobenzaprine (Flexeril)	10 mg tid—not recommended for use beyond 2-3 wks
	Orphenadrine (Norflex)	100 mg bid
Pain resulting from:	*Corticosteroids:*	
Spinal cord compression	Dexamethasone (Decadron)	100 mg IV followed by maintenance PO dose
Tumor infiltration of peripheral nerve or plexus	Dexamethasone (Decadron)	4-24 mg/day
Incapacitating sedation related to narcotics	*Stimulants:*	
	Dextroamphetamine	2.5 mg bid
	Methylphenidate (Ritalin)	2.5-5 mg bid
Sleep disturbance	*Tricyclic antidepressants:*	
	Amitriptyline (Elavil)	25 mg qd
	Doxepin (Sinequan)	50 mg qd
	Antihistamine:	
	Hydroxyzine (Vistaril, Atarax)	50 mg qd
Anxiety	*Benzodiazepines:*	
	Alprazolam (Xanax)	0.25-0.5 mg tid
	Lorezapam (Ativan)	0.5-2 mg tid
	Oxazepam (Serax)	10-15 mg tid
	Antihistamine (when there is a component of pain and nausea in addition to anxiety):	
	Hydroxyzine (Vistaril, Atarax)	25-100 mg qid
	Tricyclic antidepressants (when there are signs of agitation, insomnia, and depression in addition to anxiety):	
	Amitriptyline (Elavil)	25 mg hs
	Doxepin (Sinequan)	50 mg hs
Psychosis (euphoria, paranoia, hallucinations) or delirium (acute onset of agitation, altered attention span, fluctuating level of consciousness)	*Antipsychotic medication:* Haloperidol (Haldol)	0.5-1 mg (0.25-0.5 mg IM)
Depression not caused by unrelieved pain	Various antidepressants including tricyclics	Higher than that required to relieve pain

Table references:

American Pain Society: Principles of analgesic use in the treatment of acute pain and chronic cancer pain: a concise guide to medical practice, Washington D.C., The Society, 1987.

Foley, KM: Adjuvant analgesic drugs in cancer pain management. In Aronoff, GM, ed: Evaluation and treatment of chronic pain, pp 425-434, Baltimore, 1985, Urban and Schwartzenberg.

Holland, JC: Managing depression in the patient with cancer, *CA—Cancer J Clinic* 37:366-371, Nov-Dec 1987.

Massie, MJ, and Holland, JC: The cancer patient with pain: psychiatric complications and their management, *Med Clin North Am* 71:243-258, Mar 1987.

Pagliaro, AM, and Pagliaro, LA: Pharmacologic aspects of nursing, St. Louis, 1986, The CV Mosby Company.

Plezia, PM, and Linford, J: Innovative approaches to refractory pain, *Hosp Ther* 10:25-42, Oct 1985.

- Various pains may respond to the analgesic effects of hydroxyzine (Vistaril) parenterally, dextroamphetamine, or diphenhydramine (Benadryl).

Disadvantages of Adjuvant Analgesics

While adjuvant analgesics are a logical consideration in the management of pain, it is important to realize that their role and guidelines for use are still being established. For drugs such as phenytoin (Dilantin) and carbamazepine (Tegretol), clinical trials have documented their analgesic effect in the treatment of trigeminal neuralgia (Swerdlow, 1984). However, for the use of antidepressants in cancer pain, clinical experience rather than research provides the guidelines.

Examples of possible limitations or disadvantages of relieving pain with adjuvant analgesics are:

- Very little research has been done on these drugs, so guidelines are minimal and results are unpredictable.
- Health team members tend to be undereducated about the new uses of these drugs for pain relief, and they are misinformed about so-called "potentiators" of narcotic analgesia, which often only sedate without contributing to pain relief.
- All have the potential for causing various undesirable side effects.
- Pain relief is not always immediate, and full effect of some of these drugs may not occur until after days or weeks of regular administration.
- Patient may fail to have prescriptions filled or to adhere to a medication schedule because pain relief is not immediate or because of a misunderstanding about why the drug is prescribed. Many of the adjuvant analgesics are called tranquilizers or antidepressants, and this may cause the patient to believe his pain is discounted and that he is being treated only for anxiety or depression.

Questionable Use of Potentiators

A potentiator of narcotic analgesic is a drug that is given along with the narcotic to increase the analgesia of the narcotic. Most health care professionals in the United States are taught that certain drugs are potentiators in spite of there being little evidence to support this belief. The term "potentiator" tends to be used loosely even by those who know differently, and this perpetuates the misconception that specific drugs are potentiators.

Misconception: When a patient's statement of unrelieved pain persists despite a dose of narcotic, a "potentiator" is often added and sometimes the narcotic dose is decreased. It is assumed that this "potentiator" will increase the degree or duration of narcotic analgesia.

Correction: There are few potentiators; most are additives, i.e., they add whatever primary effect they have to the action of the narcotic. In some cases the result is sedation with poor pain relief.

Phenothiazines, particularly promethazine (Phener-

gan), are among the most frequently prescribed of those erroneously thought to be potentiators (McGee and Alexander, 1979). Far from being a potentiator, promethazine may increase the perceived intensity of pain. According to some research, a dose as low as 12 mg IM may increase pain for an hour or longer (Dundee and Moore, 1961; Moore and Dundee, 1961). With higher doses the increased perception of pain lasts for 3 hours and is accompanied by a high incidence of restlessness in the second hour. Use of promethazine as an antiemetic is also questionable since research has not shown it to be effective (Keats, Telford, and Kurosu, 1961).

Chlorpromazine (Thorazine) is another phenothiazine that has not been shown to be effective in combination with narcotics. In one clinical study chlorpromazine 25 mg IM plus morphine 10 mg IM was no better than morphine 10 mg alone. Further, adding 600 mg of aspirin PO to morphine 10 mg IM was more effective than adding chlorpromazine (Houde et al, 1960).

Further, phenothiazines *do* potentiate narcotic-related sedation, hypotension, and respiratory depression. They also lower seizure threshold (Jaffe and Martin, 1985). Their use with narcotics for the sole purpose of pain relief is both questionable and potentially dangerous (McGee and Alexander, 1979). What confuses most health team members is that phenothiazines sedate, and this is mistaken for pain relief. Phenothiazines such as promethazine, chlorpromazine, and promazine are *not appropriate choices as additives to increase analgesia* (American Pain Society, 1987; McGee and Alexander, 1979).

KEY POINT: *Sedation does not equal pain relief.* **A person can be sedated but still tell you that he hurts.**

When both a narcotic and promethazine are prescribed for pain relief, one approach to avoiding increased pain and undesirable side effects is to ask that the prescriptions be separated so that they can be given alone *or* in combination. Since it is very difficult to convince most health professionals of the possibility that promethazine may in fact increase pain, not relieve it, the two most acceptable reasons for asking that the prescriptions be separated are: (1) promethazine sedates and sometimes patients are oversedated, so it is important at times to be able to give the narcotic without the promethazine, and (2) promethazine has a duration of action of about 6 hours, much longer than most narcotics, e.g., meperidine's duration of action is often 2 to 3 hours. To give the promethazine every time the meperidine is needed may very well oversedate the patient.

With the orders for the narcotic and promethazine separated, the nurse may use a flow sheet to record and compare the results of giving the narcotic plus the promethazine and then giving the narcotic in the same dose without the promethazine. Research suggests that in some patients the combination will result in incomplete pain relief and sedation, while the narcotic alone will result in better pain relief and less sedation. However, whichever works best for the patient can be noted and then recorded in the nursing care plan. In this manner the patient receives what is most effective for him, but the health team is not debating the relative merits of promethazine.

Another popular so-called potentiator is hydroxyzine (Vistaril). However, this drug is analgesic, adding analgesia when it is given with a narcotic. A dose of 50 mg or more of hydroxyzine given IM by itself relieves about as much pain as 5 mg of morphine IM (Beaver and Feise, 1976; Forrest, 1977; Stambaugh and Sarajian, 1978). The analgesic, antiemetic, and antianxiety effects of hydroxyzine make it particularly useful in the postoperative period (Beaver and Feise, 1976; Bellvile et al, 1979; Rumore and Schlichting, 1986). However, the injection itself is very painful and capable of causing tissue damage. Oral doses of hydroxyzine are preferable, although orally it may not have the analgesic effects noted with the IM route.

If hydroxyzine must be given IM, follow these guidelines to decrease potential pain and tissue damage:
- Give hydroxyzine IM in an area that contains large muscle mass such as the ventrogluteal or vastus lateralis site (see pp. 89-90).
- Use a needle long enough to reach the muscle, e.g., usually a 1½ to 3 inch needle to reach the ventrogluteal muscle. If a shorter needle (1¼ inch) is used, hydroxyzine may not reach the muscle. The result may be poor absorption and an increased chance of pain, and tissue damage.
- Use the Z-track method to give IM hydroxyzine (Keen, 1986).
- *As soon as the PO route is appropriate,* switch from IM to PO hydroxyzine. Be particularly watchful for this so that as few IM doses as possible are given.

Types of Adjuvant Analgesics
Antidepressants for Relief of Various Types of Pain

Antidepressants can affect the perception of pain and mood. The antidepressants most widely used as analgesics seem to be the tricyclics: amitriptyline (Elavil), doxepin (Sinequan), imipramine (Tofranil), and desipramine (Norpramin) (Stauffer, 1987). These drugs appear to have analgesic activity that is thought to be separate from their antidepressant actions (Spiegel et al, 1983). Although the exact mechanisms are still not known, it is thought that they (1) block the reuptake of brain serotonin, thereby increasing the availability of serotonin and blocking pain transmission; and (2) decrease the perception of pain by inhibiting the enzyme which breaks down enkephalin (Hendler, 1984).

KEY POINT: Anxiety and depression rarely cause pain. Anxiety and depression do make pain more difficult to handle. Brief pain often causes anxiety. Prolonged pain often causes depression. When anxiety or depression is caused by pain, it should be treated by relieving the pain, usually with narcotics and nonnarcotics.

When antidepressants are not needed in patients with pain for the sole purpose of decreasing depression, they may be used at subtherapeutic doses for:
- Relief of anxiety.
- Bedtime sedation.
- Analgesia.

The first two effects are discussed later in the adjuvant medication section. The analgesic effects can be seen in the following pain syndromes which have all responded to antidepressants: headache, arthritis, low back pain, diabetic neuropathy, postherpetic neuralgia, and cancer pain (Max et al, 1987; Stauffer, 1987). Usually the analgesic effects are seen at lower doses (often 25 to 150 mg/day for amitriptyline) than the antidepressant effects (American Pain Society, 1987).

Enhancement of the analgesia of morphine postoperatively has been noted with the tricyclic desipramine (Norpramin), if taken for 1 week prior to surgery (Levine, 1986). Also there is evidence that amitriptyline may increase the bioavailability (the rate and extent of delivery of drug to the general circulation) of morphine in cancer patients (Ventafridda et al, 1987).

Doses must be titrated to effect, starting low and increasing upward. For depression and chronic nonmalignant pain, doses tend to begin at 50 mg/day and can increase up to 200 mg/day. However, patients with chronic cancer pain require much lower doses beginning with 25 mg/day and increasing by 25 mg every 1 to 2 days until the desired effect is reached (Massie and Holland, 1987). Starting with an even lower dose of 10 mg/day may be wise if the patient is elderly, severely ill, or has a cardiac problem.

Many patients may not fill their prescriptions or may take it only a few times. The primary reasons are:
1. The assumption that a prescription for an antidepressant means that their pain is being discounted or that it is due mainly to depression.
2. The delay in feeling the benefits from the medication: sometimes 7 to 10 days for analgesia; 14 to 21 days for antidepressant effects. However, the sedative effect occurs within 1 to 2 hours, and insomnia may be relieved with the first dose if it is high enough.

Guidelines for titrating tricyclic antidepressants for analgesia include:
- Give the total daily dose 1 to 3 hours before bedtime.
- Start with a low dose, e.g., 10 to 25 mg.
- Increase gradually, e.g., by 10 to 25 mg every other night.
- Final dose for analgesia is usually 75 to 150 mg or less if patient cannot tolerate a higher dose.
- Encourage patient to continue at this dose for 1 to 3 weeks before deciding whether it works.

Patient/Family Teaching Point: Antidepressant Medications to Help with Pain Control

---

TO: _____ (patient's name)   DATE: _____

You are taking _____, a medication called an antidepressant. Although this drug at higher doses may help depression, you are taking it at lower doses for other reasons. These are:

• Relief of pain.
• Relief of sleep problems.
• Relief of anxiety.

   This drug can be very effective along with your pain medication. However, you may not notice the effects for 7 to 14 days. Do not give up and stop taking it! With regular doses you will feel a difference, but it does take time.

   One effect that you may notice right away is a really good night's sleep after one or two doses. Another effect that you may have is a dry mouth.

   Let your doctor or nurse know if you experience an excessively dry mouth, inability to urinate, extreme drowsiness, or dizziness when standing. These are possible side effects which need attention if they occur.

Additional comments: _____

_____

If you have any questions or problems with the above information, contact:

_____ (RN or MD name)   Phone: _____

_____ (Nurse's signature)

■ May be duplicated for use in clinical practice. From McCaffery, M, and Beebe, A: PAIN: CLINICAL MANUAL FOR NURSING PRACTICE, St. Louis, 1989, The CV Mosby Company.

The patient teaching form above may be helpful to explain these important points about antidepressant medication for pain.

Anticonvulsants for Relief of Lancinating Pain

Typically this kind of pain begins and ends suddenly and repeatedly occurs in the same area. It is described by patients as "shocklike," "shooting," or "like lightning" and may be accompanied by muscle spasm. These are descriptions of neuropathic pain, i.e., pain that is a result of injury to the nerve tissue. This pain is characteristic of trigeminal neuralgia, postherpetic neuralgia, diabetic neuropathy, and traumatic neuralgias.

Anticonvulsant drugs, phenytoin (Dilantin) and carbamazepine (Tegretol), are particularly useful for lancinating pain (Swerdlow, 1984). Their mechanism of action is suppression of abnormal nerve firings that occur as a result of nerve tissue injury (Plezia and Linford, 1985). For a detailed review of anticonvulsants see Swerdlow (1984); for a detailed review of treatment of neuropathic pain see Maciewicz et al (1985).

While it is generally agreed that carbamazepine is the drug of choice for trigeminal neuralgia pain (American Pain Society, 1987; Swerdlow, 1984), there are conflicting opinions about the choice of drugs for other neuropathic pain syndromes. For many patients, the shooting pain has an additional dimension of burning or aching. Some have found that anticonvulsant therapy is not effective in controlling this component of the pain (Foley, 1985a; Swerdlow, 1984).

Muscle Relaxants for Relief of Muscle Spasm

These can occur as a result of anxiety-related muscle tension, arthritis, vertebral disc protrusions, or a pain-producing process such as a compressed nerve, or bone metastasis.

Muscle relaxants may be helpful in this situation. Baclofen (Lioresal) and diazepam are two effective antispastic agents. Although baclofen and diazepam are considered comparable in effect, baclofen is preferred due to its fewer sedative effects. Further it may be more helpful for intermittent, painful flexor spasms (Aronoff and Evans, 1985). It is also being used successfully alone and in combination with carbamazepine (Tegretol) in the treatment of neuralgias (Fromm et al, 1984). Abrupt withdrawal of baclofen should be avoided because it can result in temporary hallucinations and a rebound in the number and severity of spasms (Aronoff and Evans, 1985).

Muscle relaxants such as carisoprodol (Soma), methocarbamol (Robaxin), cyclobenzaprine (Flexeril), and orphenadrine (Norflex) are commonly used by some pain specialists. They produce depression in neuronal activity affecting muscle stretch reflexes and also tend to cause mild sedation. These medications are for temporary use and should be combined with physical therapy that stretches and strengthens muscles. When physical therapy exercises are well tolerated, the muscle relaxant may be stopped.

Corticosteroids for Relief of Various Types of Cancer Pain

For many years corticosteroids have been widely recognized as effective in relieving cancer pain, particularly bone pain or pain related to nerve or spinal cord compression. Many anecdotal reports suggest that steroids relieve this type of pain and reduce the amount of narcotic needed (American Pain Society, 1987; Ettinger and Portenoy, 1988; Foley 1985a).

However, as of 1988, only one controlled study was reported regarding the analgesic effects of steroids in cancer pain. A randomized double-blind crossover study compared placebo with methylprednisolone 16 mg PO twice daily to establish its ability to relieve pain in patients with end-stage cancer. Those patients who received methylprednisolone for 5 days demonstrated a significant reduction in both pain and analgesic use (Bruera et al, 1985). Additional research is needed to explore the effective dose, the consequences of long-term use, and the differences among the various steroids.

Available data suggest that even with chronic administration of steroids the incidence of serious toxicity is low (Ettinger and Portenoy, 1988). Although possible side effects include peptic ulcer, GI hemorrhage, systemic edema, and weight gain, in most cases, the effects of providing comfort for patients with a short life expectancy outweigh the potential risks.

Other Possible Adjuvant Analgesics

Dextroamphetamine or Methylphenidate (Ritalin). These stimulants can be useful to counteract the sedative effects of narcotics. Some pain specialists find them useful in chronic cancer pain when there is effective analgesia but incapacitating sedation (American Pain Society, 1987; Foley, 1985a). Others maintain that their usefulness remains controversial (Levy, 1985).

Initially 2.5 mg PO or more of dextroamphetamine may be given after breakfast and lunch for a few days to counteract particularly bothersome side effects of the narcotic such as sedation, hypotension, and nausea. Dextroamphetamine IM was noted to produce additive analgesia in postoperative pain when combined with morphine, and it counteracted morphine's sedation and respiratory depression (Forrest et al, 1977). Dextroamphetamine 2.5 mg q_{AM} significantly reduced sedation in a 22-month-old toddler receiving morphine by continuous IV infusion (McManus and Panzarella, 1986).

In a randomized double-blind crossover study, 28 patients with pain from advanced cancer received 10 mg PO methylphenidate (Ritalin) at breakfast and 5 mg PO at lunch. Methylphenidate increased the analgesic effect of narcotics, decreased the drowsiness caused by narcotics, and significantly increased patients' activity. At these doses, it did not significantly impair hours of sleep or result in toxicity (Bruera et al, 1987b).

Caffeine. Adding doses of caffeine to aspirin or acetaminophen seems to increase analgesia for conditions such as postpartum uterine cramping, episiotomy pain, dental pain, and headaches. When aspirin or acetaminophen was given without caffeine, the doses had to be about 40% larger to obtain the same degree of pain relief as was obtained when the analgesics were given in combination with caffeine (Laska et al, 1984; Beaver, 1984a). On a long-term basis, adding caffeine to each 650 mg daily dose of aspirin or acetaminophen is felt to be safer than repeatedly giving larger doses without the caffeine.

An effective dose must contain 100 to 200 mg of caffeine. Examples of sources of caffeine are tea, coffee, cola, and No Doz. A 6 ounce cup of automatic drip coffee contains 181 mg of caffeine; percolated coffee, 125 mg; instant coffee 75 mg; and strong tea, 80 mg (National Headache Foundation, 1987-1988).

Alcohol. Researchers have found that alcohol in nonintoxicating quantities may be an effective adjunct to other analgesic modalities. Apparently the increase in pain tolerance that results from two ordinary cocktails (ethyl alcohol 100% 2 mg/kg) is comparable to that obtained from about 10 mg morphine SC (0.17 mg/kg) (Woodrow and Eltherington, 1988).

Beverages containing ethyl alcohol are actually nonprescription medications. Rarely do people consider that they are taking a drug when they drink alcohol socially, but in fact alcohol is usually consumed for its drug effects, not because of its taste or nutritional value.

Of all the effects that alcohol may have, those most relevant to the patient with pain usually are its tranquilizing, sedating, and/or analgesic effects. Many pain-afflicted working-class bar drinkers consciously and unconsciously use alcohol as a folk analgesic (Kotarba, 1983). Years ago, alcohol in 5% to 10% solution was administered IV drip to relieve mild to moderate pain. Taken orally it may have a similar analgesic effect in some people (Cutter, O'Farrell, Whitehouse, and Dentch, 1986). A moderate amount of alcohol, well below that causing inebriation, does not cause respiratory depression and has been recommended for pain relief in patients in whom respiratory depression from narcotics may be a problem, e.g., the elderly (Halpern and Bonica, 1976).

In selected patients, alcohol may be safely combined with narcotics and nonnarcotics. Caution the patient about the probability of an additive sedative effect when it is given with narcotics and about the possibility of alcohol increasing gastrointestinal upset or irritation.

Adjuvant Medications for Symptoms Accompanying Pain

Adjuvant medications that are effective for patients with pain are listed in Table 4-16. Clinical signs and symptoms that the nurse might assess as part of a patient's pain are listed below with a discussion of the corresponding adjuvant medication that is indicated.

Sleep Disturbance

This can include not being able to fall asleep, frequent awakenings throughout the night, early morning awakenings without being able to go back to sleep, or simply not feeling well rested after a night's sleep.

Important questions to ask before adding medication for sleep:

1. Is the pain controlled? Unrelieved pain can interrupt every part of a person's life. If the pain is not controlled, refer to the previous sections in this chapter on narcotics and nonnarcotic analgesics and Chapters 5 through 8 for nonpharmacological approaches.
2. Is the sleep disturbance a problem that began with the pain or has it been a lifelong occurrence? Other issues may need to be assessed if this has been a lifelong problem. It may not be possible to change these now.
3. Does the patient consider the sleep disturbance to be a problem?

Sleep disturbance is a common symptom in patients with pain. If the pain is controlled and the sleep disturbance continues, one of the following three groups of drugs might be helpful: tricyclic antidepressant, antihistamine, or temporary use of a short-acting hypnotic. These are discussed below (refer to Table 4-16, for specific pharmacological information).

1. Tricyclic antidepressant. The sedative effects of an antidepressant have a useful hypnotic effect if the total daily dose is given 1 to 3 hours before bedtime. The initial drugs of choice are amitriptyline (Elavil) and doxepin (Sinequan) at dosages of 10 to 75 mg per day to normalize sleep patterns and possibly provide pain relief. Begin with a low dose and increase gradually by 10 to 25 mg every 2 to 3 days. These dosages are much lower than those used to treat depression.

One pain specialist suggests amitriptyline as the first-line sleeping medication in patients with cancer pain (Foley, 1985a).

2. Antihistamine. Hydroxyzine (Vistaril, Atarax) PO has a mild sedative activity which could be effective at bedtime or on a regular schedule throughout the day when anxiety is an additional dimension to the pain.

3. Short-acting hypnotic. Although a hypnotic agent can relieve "simple" insomnia, the routine use of this class of drugs is not recommended (American Pain Society, 1987; Foley, 1985a). If a hypnotic is used, one with a short half-life is suggested,* e.g., triazolam (Halcion) with a half-life of 1.5 to 3 hours as opposed to flurazepam (Dalmane) with a half-life of 50 to 100 hours.

NOTE: It is all right to give a sleeping pill or antidepressant *at the same time* as the usual dose of narcotic. As with any medication, the individual's response must consistently be evaluated and adjustments made accordingly.

Anxiety

Anxiety is a common symptom in patients with pain. Efforts to deal with this symptom should focus first on relieving the pain with analgesics. When this is accomplished, the anxiety often subsides.

Anxiety may be acute or chronic. Acute anxiety may relate to the treatment of an underlying condition, e.g., procedures or surgery, while awaiting diagnosis or test results. Chronic anxiety may have existed before the medical condition and may be exacerbated by it. Relaxation therapy (Chapter 7) and distraction techniques (Chapter 6) can be helpful.

If the pain is controlled but anxiety still remains, the classes of drugs that can be useful are the benzodiazepines, antipsychotics, antihistamines, and antidepressants (Massie and Holland, 1987). Refer to Table 4-16 for pharmacological specifics.

1. Benzodiazepines. This class of drugs has no analgesic properties and does not result in additive analgesia when combined with a narcotic (Foley, 1985a). It is suggested that their usefulness in patients with pain is limited to situations in which severe anxiety is the principal and disabling symptom.

Diazepam (Valium) and clorazepate (Tranxene) used to be the drugs of choice for acute anxiety. However, alprazolam (Xanax), lorezapam (Ativan), and oxazepam (Serax) are now preferred (Massie and Holland, 1987). These drugs are shorter-acting, rapidly metabolized, and better tolerated by patients with impaired liver function and those taking other medications with sedative effects such as narcotics. Alprazolam has been shown to be an effective antidepressant in addition to having antianxiety properties (Feighner et al, 1983; Rickels et al, 1985). This dual action is particularly useful in cancer patients with symptoms of anxiety and depression (Massie and Holland, 1987).

The severity of the anxiety, the patient's hepatic and respiratory status, and the use of other medications are all factors in determining the starting dose. Refer to Table 4-16 for a listing of initial dosages.

2. Antipsychotic medication. Haloperidol (Haldol) can be beneficial for patients showing signs of psychosis (euphoria, fears, paranoia, or hallucinations) or delirium (acute onset of agitation, impaired cognitive function,

---

*Half-life is the time it takes the drug to fall to one half its concentration in the bloodstream. The longer the half-life, the longer the effects from the drug.

INDIVIDUALIZED NURSING CARE PLAN*

Patient Who May Benefit from Individualized Pharmacological Approach for Pain Control

Patient Description: Mrs. C., 53 years old, is bedridden at home due to extensive bone metastasis in the thoracic and cervical spine, and right and left ribs from breast cancer. During the initial home visit, the nurse reports to the physician the following pain assessment so that they can plan an effective analgesic regimen: Mrs. C. rates her neck, back, and rib pain at 9 on a 0 to 10 scale (0 = no pain; 10 = worst pain). When she tries to turn in bed, pain becomes "unbearable." The best the pain has been in the last 2 days is 7, when she lies totally still. She takes morphine 10 mg PO irregularly and tries to hold off as long as possible between doses. She has been unable to sleep for the past 2 nights because of the pain, and she insists on remaining at home. Her husband supports her decision. The nurse requests a 50% to 100% increase in morphine every 2 hours until Mrs. C. is comfortable. Then she suggests an around the clock (ATC) schedule of morphine, a nonsteroidal antiinflammatory medication, and in anticipation of constipation, a stool softener/stimulant combination. The physician agrees with this plan and prescribes Trilisate 1500 mg PO q12h and Pericolace two capsules PO bid.

Assessment	Potential Nursing Diagnoses	Planning/Intervention	Evaluation/ Expected Outcomes
• Complete Initial Pain Assessment tool (p. 21) and give priority to determining: location of pain, pain intensity, what helps pain or makes it worse. • Determine ability to use 0-10 scale to rate pain. • Establish what number on 0-10 scale is acceptable. • Determine pain rating and duration of pain relief after PO morphine. • Determine knowledge about use of nonnarcotic analgesics in combination with narcotics for added effectiveness.	Pain in back, neck, and ribs related to bone metastasis as a result of breast cancer	• Use a preventive approach: Trilisate q12h ATC and morphine probably q4h ATC. • Begin with 100% increase in PO morphine and one dose of PO Trilisate. • Monitor and document pain rating and side effects on Pain Flow Sheet (p. 27) (using 0-10 scale at least every 2 hr) by phone call or home visit during the first 24 hr. If pain is uncontrolled, calculate additional 50% increases every 2 hr and instruct patient/husband on administration. Then if pain is controlled, monitor and document at least twice a day for 48 hr, then at every home visit. • When pain is controlled, calculate dose of PO morphine from increases and implement this dose on ATC schedule. • Teach patient/husband how to use Daily Diary (p. 30) and to document every 2 hr during first 24 hr, then about every 4 hr: patient's pain rating on 0-10 scale, analgesics given, and any difficulty arousing patient. • Report to physician if analgesic regimen does not decrease pain rating to an acceptable level for patient.	Patient reports her pain is at or below the acceptable number for her pain with side effects absent or acceptable. Patient/husband maintains Daily Diary and shares this with nurse via telephone or during home visit.
• Determine patient/ husband's fears or misconceptions about addiction or narcotics losing their effectiveness.		• Initiate discussion about fears concerning narcotics, e.g., fears about addiction. If needed, review following patient/family teaching points: —Your Pain Medication Dose (p. 51) —Preventive Approach with Pain Medication (p. 53) —Instructions for Home Use of Nonnarcotic Analgesics (p. 65) —Your Concerns about Addiction (p. 70)	Patient/husband demonstrate understanding of importance of preventive, ATC dosing of narcotic and nonnarcotic analgesic by documenting their administration in Daily Diary.
• Sleep assessed above in relation to pain.	Sleep pattern disturbance related to unrelieved pain	Implement the above measures for pain relief which will ultimately help sleep disturbance.	As pain decreases, sleep increases.

*Although there are many additional diagnoses and interventions for this patient situation, the care plan is limited to the nurse's initial active role in multidisciplinary approach to pharmacological control of pain.

INDIVIDUALIZED NURSING CARE PLAN—cont'd.

Patient Who May Benefit from Individualized Pharmacological Approach for Pain Control—cont'd.

Assessment	Potential Nursing Diagnoses	Planning/Intervention	Evaluation/Expected Outcomes
• Determine measures that have helped constipation in the past, i.e., laxatives, foods, liquids.	Constipation related to regular narcotic regimen and no physical activity	• Use preventive approach: begin with Pericolace two capsules bid. • If no bowel movement in any 48 hr period, obtain prescription for laxative and add to Pericolace every day. • Monitor and document frequency of bowel movements at each home visit. • Review following patient/family teaching point: Common Narcotic Side Effects Related to Prolonged Narcotic Use: Constipation Caused by Narcotics (pp. 114-115).	Patient reports daily use of bowel regimen with a bowel movement at least every 2 days.

altered attention span, or a fluctuating level of consciousness).

Although it has been suggested that haloperidol is useful as an adjuvant analgesic in cancer pain (Breivik and Rennemo, 1982), presently its main role in cancer pain is the management of acute psychosis (Massie and Holland, 1987).

Haloperidol is chosen over other antipsychotics because of its low incidence of orthostatic hypotension and anticholinergic effects.

3. Antihistamines. Although not as effective for severe anxiety as the other classes of drugs mentioned in this section, hydroxyzine can be helpful when there are additional dimensions to anxiety such as pain and nausea (Foley, 1985a).

4. Antidepressants. Usually these are not used for symptoms of anxiety alone. However, when there are signs of depression, agitation, and insomnia, tricyclic antidepressants with sedating effects, e.g., amitriptyline or doxepin, can be helpful (Massie and Holland, 1987).

Depression

Depression can affect a person's ability to handle pain. The clinical picture of depression includes insomnia, anorexia, fatigue, and weight loss. In the person with cancer or other prolonged illnesses these may be signs of pain or the disease process itself. Therefore the identification of depression in these patients must depend on psychological symptoms such as feelings of sadness, anxiety, helplessness, worthlessness, guilt, loss of self-esteem, and thoughts of "wishing for death" (Massie and Holland, 1987).

Differentiating between the cause and effect within the cycle of pain-depression-insomnia-anxiety is difficult. The important point for the nurse to realize is that early as-

sessment of the presence of this cycle is vital so that active treatment can begin. If depression has been a prolonged symptom predating the pain or medical problem, then a psychiatrist or psychologist may be helpful to consult for a supportive plan of care or appropriate psychotropic medication.

REFERENCES AND SELECTED READINGS

Aguwa, CN, and Olusanya, OA: Analgesic prescribing for severe pain studied, *Drug Intell Clin Pharm* 12:556, Sept 1978

Amadio, P, and Cummings, DM: Nonsteroidal anti-inflammatory agents: an update, *Am Fam Physic* 34:147-154, 1986

American Pain Society: Principles of analgesic use in the treatment of acute pain and chronic cancer pain: a concise guide to medical practice, Washington D.C., The Society, 1987

Anderson, AB, Haynes, PJ, Fraser, IS, and Turnbull, AC: Trial of prostaglandin-synthetase inhibitors in primary dysmenorrhea, *Lancet* 1:345-348, 1978

Anderson, K, and Poole, C: Self-administered medication on a postpartum unit, *Am J Nurs* 83:1178-1180, Aug 1983

Angell, J: The quality of mercy, *N Engl J Med* 306:98-99, Jan 14, 1982

Aronoff, GM, and Evans, WO: Pharmacological management of chronic pain. In Aronoff, GM, ed: Evaluation and treatment of chronic pain, pp 435-449, Baltimore, 1985, Urban and Schwartzenberg

Auld, AW, Maki-Jokela, A, and Murdock, DM: Intraspinal narcotic analgesia in the treatment of chronic pain, *Spine* 10:777-781, 1985

Austin, KL, Stapleton, JV, and Mather, LE: Multiple intramuscular injections: a major source of variability in analgesic response to meperidine, *Pain* 8:47-62, 1980

Baggerly, J: Epidural catheters for pain management: the nurse's role, *J Neurosci Nurs* 18:290-295, Oct 1986

Ballantyne, J, Loach, AB, and Carr, DB: Itching after epidural and spinal opiates, *Pain* 33:149-160, 1988

Barkas, G, and Duafala, M: Advances in cancer pain management: a review of patient-controlled analgesia, *J Pain Sympt Manag* 3:150-160, Summer 1988

Beaver, WT: Management of cancer pain with parenteral medication, *JAMA* 244:2653-2657, Dec 12, 1980

Beaver, WT: Aspirin and acetaminophen as constituents of analgesic combinations, *Arch Intern Med* 141:293-300, Feb 23, 1981

Beaver, WT: Caffeine revisited, *JAMA* 251:1732-1733, 1984a

Beaver, WT: Combination analgesics, *Am J Med* 77(3A):38-53, Sept 10, 1984b

Beaver, WT, and Feise, GA: Comparison of the analgesic effects of morphine, hydroxyzine, and their combination in patients with postoperative pain. In Bonica, JJ, and Albe-Fessard, D, eds: Advances in pain research and therapy, pp 553-557, vol 1, New York, 1976, Raven Press

Beaver, WT, and Feise, GA: Comparison of the analgesic effect of oxymorphone by rectal suppository and intramuscular injection in patients with postoperative pain, *J Clin Pharmacol* 17:276-291, May-June 1977

Bell, MDD, Mishra, P, Waldon, BD, et al: Buccal morphine—a new route for analgesia? *Lancet* 1:71-73, Jan 12, 1985

Belville, JW, Dorey, F, Capparell, D, et al: Analgesic effects of hydroxyzine compared to morphine in man, *J Clin Pharmacol* 19:290-296, May-June 1979

Bernstein, J: Anti-inflammatories for migraine, *Aches & Pains* 3:32-37, Mar 1982

Blumenkopf, B: Combination analgesic-antispasmodic therapy in postoperative pain, *Spine* 12:384-387, May 1987

Botney, M, and Fields, HL: Amitriptyline potentiates morphine analgesia by a direct action on the central nervous system, *Ann Neurol* 13:160-164, Feb 1983

Breivik, H, and Rennemo, F: Clinical evaluation of combined treatment with methadone and psychotropic drugs in cancer patients, *Acta Anaesthesiol Scand* (Suppl) 74:135-140, 1982

Brena, SF: Drugs and pain: use and misuse. In Brena, SF, and Chapman, SL, eds: Management of patients with chronic pain, pp 121-310, New York, 1983, Raven Press

Brenneis, C, Michaud, M, Bruera, E, et al: Local toxicity during subcutaneous infusion of narcotics: a prospective study. In Proceedings of the VI World Congress on the Care of the Terminally Ill, Montreal, Sept 1986

Brook-Williams, P: Morphine suppositories for intractable pain, *Can Med Assoc J* 126:14, Jan 1982

Brozovic, M, Davies, SC, and Yardumian, A: Pain relief in sickle cell crises, *Lancet* 2:624-625, 1986

Bruera, E, Brennels, C, and MacDonald, RN: Continuous SC infusion of narcotics for the treatment of cancer pain: an update, *Cancer Treat Rep* 71:953-957, Oct 1987a

Bruera, E, Chadwick, S, Brennels, C, et al: Methylphenidate associated with narcotics for the treatment of cancer pain, *Cancer Treat Rep* 71:67-70, Jan 1987b

Bruera, E, Roca, E, Cedaro, L, et al: Action of oral methylprednisolone in terminal cancer patients: a prospective randomized double blind study, *Cancer Treat Rep* 69:751-754, 1985

Burns Stewart, SM: Controlling pain with epidural narcotics: nursing implications, *Crit Care Nurs* 6:50-56, May-June 1986

Caballero, GA, Ausman, RK, and Himes, J: Epidural morphine by continuous infusion with an external pump for pain management in oncology patients, *Am Surg* 52:402-405, 1986

Cancer Pain Relief, Geneva, World Health Organization, 1986

Campbell, CF, Mason, JB, and Weiler, JM: Continuous subcutaneous infusion of morphine for the pain of terminal malignancy, *Ann Intern Med* 98:51-52, 1983

Catalano, RB: Pharmacologic management in the treatment of cancer pain. In McGuire, DB, and Yarboro, CH, eds: Cancer pain management, pp 151-201, Orlando, 1987, Grune & Stratton

Charap, AD: The knowledge, attitudes and experience of medical personnel treating pain in the terminally ill, *Mt Sinai J Med* 45:561-580, July-Aug 1978

Clark, BE: Considerations in pain management of the hospice patient, *Am J Hospice Care* 1:23-27, Fall 1984

Cleeland, CS: Barriers to the management of cancer pain, *Oncology* (Suppl) 1:19-26, Apr 1987

Cohen, F: Postsurgical pain relief: patient's status and nurses' medication choices, *Pain* 9:265-274, 1980

Cohen, SE, and Woods, WA: The role of epidural morphine in the post-cesarean patient: efficacy and effects of bonding, *Anesthesiology* 58:500-504, 1983

Cole, T, Sprinkle, R, Smith, S, and Buchanan, G: Intravenous narcotic therapy for children with severe sickle cell pain crisis, *Am J Dis Child* 140:1255-1259, Dec 1986

Coombs, DW, Maurer, LH, Saunders, RL, and Gaylor, M: Outcomes and complications for continuous intraspinal narcotic analgesia for cancer pain control, *J Clin Oncol* 2:1414-1420, Dec 1984

Cousins, MJ, and Mather, LE: Intrathecal and epidural administration of opioids, *Anesthesiology* 61:276-310, 1984

Coyle, N, Mauskop, A, Maggard, J, and Foley, KM: Continuous subcutaneous infusions of opiates in cancer patients with pain, *Oncol Nurs Forum* 13:53-57, July-Aug 1986

Cutter, HSG, O'Farrell, TJ, Whitehouse, J, and Dentch, GM: Pain changes among men from before to after drinking: effects of expectancy set and dose manipulations with alcohol and tonic as mediated by prior experience with alcohol, *Int J Addict* 21:937-945, 1986

Dallas, TL, Lin, RL, Wu, W, and Wolskee, P: Epidural morphine and methylprednisolone for low-back pain, *Anesthesiology* 67:408-411, Sept 1987

Dawood, MY: Dysmenorrhea and prostaglandins: pharmacological and therapeutic consideration, *Drugs* 22:42-56, 1981

Dingfelder, JR: Primary dysmenorrhea treatment with prostaglandin inhibitors: a review, *Am J Obstet Gynecol* 140:874-879, 1981

Dionne, RA, and Cooper, SA: Evaluation of preoperative ibuprofen for post-operative pain after removal of third molars, *Oral Surg* 45:851-856, June 1978

Drug Information, American Hospital Formulary Service, p 979, Maryland, American Society of Hospital Pharmacists, 1987

Dundee, JW, Love, WJ, and Moore, J: Alterations in response to somatic pain associated with XV: further studies with phenothiazine derivatives and similar drugs, *Br J Anaesthesiol* 35:597-609, 1963

Dundee, JW, and Moore, J: The myth of phenothiazine potentiation, *Anaesthesiology* 16:95-96, 1961

Enck, RE: The role of continuous intravenous and subcutaneous narcotic infusions in pain management, *Am J Hospice Care* 4:43-45, Nov-Dec 1987

Ellis, R, Haines, D, Shah, R, et al: Pain relief after abdominal surgery—a comparison of IM morphine, sublingual buprenorphine and self-administered IV pethidine, *Br J Anaesthesiol* 54:421-427, 1982

Ellison, NM, and Lewis, GO: Plasma concentrations following

single doses of morphine sulfate in oral solution and rectal suppository, *Clin Pharm* 3:614-617, Nov-Dec 1984

Ettinger, AB, and Portenoy, RK: The use of corticosteroids in the treatment of symptoms associated with cancer, *J Pain Sympt Manag* 3:99-103, Spring 1988

Farley, HF, Joyce, N, Long, B, and Roberts, R: Will that IM needle reach the muscle? *Am J Nurs* 86:1327-1331, Dec 1986

Feighner, JP, Aden, GC, Fabre, LF, et al: Comparison of alprazolam, imipramine, and placebo in the treatment of depression, *JAMA* 249:3057-3064, 1983

Feldman, HR: Practice makes perfect but research makes a difference, *Nursing* 17:47, Mar 1987

Ferrel, BR, and Schneider, C: Experience and management of cancer pain at home, *Cancer Nurs* 11:84-90, 1988

Ferrel, BR, Wenzl, C, and Wisdom, C: Evolution and evaluation of a pain management team, *Oncol Nurs Forum* 15:285-289, 1988

Ferrer-Brechner, T, and Ganz, P: Combination therapy with ibuprofen and methadone for chronic cancer pain, *Am J Med* 77:78-83, July 1984

Fisher, J, and Schwinghammer, T: Should patients taking nonsteroidal anti-inflammatory (NSAIDs) be routinely warned to avoid the concurrent use of aspirin?, *US Pharmacist* 9:8-10, Oct 1984

Flower, RJ, Moncada, S, and Vane, JR: Drug therapy of inflammation, pp 674-715. In Gilman, AG, et al, eds: Goodman and Gilman's the pharmacological basis of therapeutics, ed 7, New York, 1985, Macmillan Publishing Co

Foley, KM: The practical use of narcotic analgesics, *Med Clin North Am* 66:1091-1104, 1982

Foley, KM: Adjuvant analgesic drugs in cancer pain management. In Aronoff, GM, ed: Evaluation and treatment of chronic pain, pp 425-434, Baltimore, 1985a, Urban and Schwartzenberg

Foley, KM: The treatment of cancer pain, *N Engl J Med* 313:84-95, July 11, 1985b

Foley, KM: Current controversies in opioid therapy. In Foley, K, and Inturrisi, C, eds: Advances in pain research and therapy, vol 8, Opioid analgesics in the management of clinical pain, pp 3-11, New York, 1986, Raven Press

Foley, KM: Author's reply, *CA- Cancer J Clinic* 37:376-377, Nov 1987

Foley, KM, and Inturrisi, CE: Analgesic drug therapy in cancer pain: principles and practice, *Med Clin North Am* 71:207-232, Mar 1987

Foley, KM, and Rogers, A: The management of cancer pain. The rational use of analgesics in the management of cancer pain, vol 2, Nutley, NJ, 1981, Hoffmann-La Roche, Inc

Forrest, WH: Tranquilizer-narcotic combinations in management of acute pain: rationale and history. In Considerations in management of acute pain, pp 14-16, New York, 1977, HP Publishing Co

Forrest, WH, Brown, BW, Brown, CR, et al: Dextroamphetamine with morphine for treatment of postoperative pain, *N Engl J Med* 296:712-715, 1977

Fox, LS: Pain management in the terminally ill cancer patient: an investigation of nurses' attitudes, knowledge, and clinical practice, *Milit Med* 147:455-460, 1982

Frank, RM: Pain management and the appropriate use of analgesics, *Cancer Nurs* 3:155-157, Apr 1980

Fromm, GH, Terrence, CF, and Chatha, AS: Baclofen in the treatment of trigeminal neuralgia: double-blind study and long-term follow up, *Ann Neurol* 15:240-244, 1984

Fultz, J, Senay, E, Pray, B, and Thornton, W: When a narcotic addict is hospitalized, *Am J Nurs* 80:478-481, Mar 1980

Gold, MS, Redmond, E, and Kleber, HD: Noradrenergic hyperactivity in opiate withdrawal, *Am J Psychiatry* 136:100-102, Jan 1979

Goudie, TA, Allan, MWB, Longsdale, M, et al: Continuous subcutaneous infusion of morphine for postoperative pain relief, *Anaesthesia* 40:1086-1092, 1985

Grabinski, PY, Kaiko, RF, Rogers, AG, and Houde, RW: Plasma levels and analgesia following deltoid and gluteal injections of methadone and morphine, *J Clin Pharmacol* 23:48-55, 1983

Greenberg, HS, Taren, J, Ensminger, WD, et al: Benefit from and tolerance to continuous intrathecal infusion of morphine for intractable cancer pain, *J Neurosurg* 57:360-364, 1982

Grossman, SA, and Sheidler, VR: Skills of medical students and house officers in prescribing narcotic medication, *J Med Ed* 60:552-557, July 1985

Grossman, SA, Sheidler, VR: An aid to prescribing narcotics for the relief of cancer pain, *World Health Forum* 8:525-529, 1987

Halpern, LM, and Bonica, JJ: Analgesics. In Modell, W, ed: Drugs of choice, pp 195-232, St. Louis, 1976, The CV Mosby Co

Heidrich, G, Slavic-S*rcev, V, Kaiko, R: Efficacy and quality of ibuprofen and acetaminophen and codeine analgesia, *Pain* 22:385-397, 1985

Hendler, N: Depression caused by chronic pain, *J Clin Psychiatry* 45 (3, sec 2):30-36, 1984

Hill, CS: Patients in pain—case reports, *Primary Care & Cancer* 6:43-48, Sept 1986

Hill, CS, Jr: Don't be 'spooked' into giving naloxone inappropriately, *Primary Care & Cancer* 7:31-34, March 1987

Hirsh, JD: Sublingual morphine sulfate in chronic pain management, *Clin Pharm* 3:585-586 (letter), Nov-Dec 1984

Houde, RW: Analgesic effectiveness of the narcotic agonist-antagonist, *Br J Clin Pharmacol* 7:2975-3085, 1979

Houde, RW, Wallenstein, SL, and Rogers, A: Clinical pharmacology of analgesics: a method of assaying analgesic effect, *Clin Pharmacol Ther* 1:163-174, 1960

Inturrisi, CE: Role of opioid analgesics, *Am J Med* 77:27-37, Sept 10, 1984

Inturrisi, CE, and Umans, JG: Pethidine and its active metabolite, norpethidine, *Clin Anaesthesiol* 1:123-138, Apr 1983

Ives, TJ, and Guerra, MF: Constant morphine infusion for severe sickle cell crisis pain, *Drug Intell Clin Pharm* 21:625-626, July-Aug 1987

Jacobson, L: Intrathecal and extradural narcotics. In Benedetti, C, Chapman, CR, and Moricca, G, eds: Advances in pain research and therapy, vol 7, pp 199-346, 1984, Raven Press

Jaffe, JH: Drug addiction and drug abuse. In Gillman, AG, Goodman, LS, Rall, TW, and Murad, F, eds: Goodman and Gillman's the pharmacological basis of therapeutics, ed 7, New York, 1985, Macmillan Publishing Co

Jaffe, JH, and Martin, WR: Opioid analgesics and antagonists. In Gillman, AG, Goodman, LS, Rall, TW, and Murad, F, eds: The pharmacological basis of therapeutics, ed 7, pp 532-581, New York, 1985, Macmillan Publishing Co

Jain, AK, Ryan, JR, McMahon, FG, and Smith, G: Comparison of oral nalbuphine, acetaminophen, and their combination in postoperative pain, *Clin Pharmacol Ther* 39:295-299, Mar 1986

Jick, H: Smoking and clinical drug effects, *Med Clin North Am* 58:1143-1149, Sept 1974

Jones, L: Patient-controlled oral analgesia, *Orthoped Nurs* 6: 38-41, Jan-Feb 1987

Kaiko, RF: Age and morphine analgesia in cancer patients with postoperative pain, *Clin Pharmacol Ther* 28:823-826, Dec 1980

Kaiko, RF, Foley, KM, Grabinski, PY, et al: Central nervous system excitatory effects of meperidine in cancer patients, *Ann Neurol* 13:180-185, 1983

Kane, NE, Lehman, ME, Dugger, R, Hansen, L, and Jackson, D: Use of patient-controlled analgesia in surgical oncology patients, *Oncol Nurs Forum* 15:29-32, Jan-Feb 1988

Kantor, TG: Anti-inflammatory drug therapy for low back pain. In Stanton-Hicks, M, and Boas, R, eds: Chronic low back pain, pp 157-169, New York, 1982, Raven Press

Kantor, TG: Nonsteroidal anti-inflammatory analgesic agents in management of cancer pain. In The management of cancer pain (Monograph), pp 30-34, Hospital Practice, Summer 1984

Kay, B, and Krishnan, A: On-demand nalbuphine for post-operative pain relief, *Acta Anaesthesiol Belg* 37:33-37, 1986

Keats, AS, Telford, J, and Kurosu, Y: "Potentiation" of meperidine by promethazine, *Anesthesiology* 22:34-41, Jan-Feb 1961

Keen, MF: Comparison of intramuscular injection techniques to reduce site discomfort and lesions, *Nurs Res* 35:207-210, July-Aug 1986

Kleiman, RL, Lipman, AG, Hare, BD, et al: A comparison of morphine administered by patient-controlled analgesia and regularly scheduled intramuscular injection in severe, postoperative pain, *J Pain Sympt Manag* 3:15-22, Winter 1988

Kotarba, JA: Chronic pain: its social dimensions, Beverly Hills, 1983, Sage Publications

Kreek, MJ, Hahn, EF, Schaefer, RA, and Fishman, J: Naloxone, a specific opioid antagonist reverses chronic idiopathic constipation, *Lancet* 1:261, 1983

Kruszewski, A, Lang, S, and Johnson, J: Effects of positioning on discomfort from intramuscular injections in the dorsogluteal site, *Nurs Res* 28:103-105, 1979

Lanz, E, Theiss, D, Reiss, W, and Sommer, U: Epidural morphine for postoperative analgesia: a double-blind study, *Anesthesiol Analg* 61:236-240, Mar 1982

Laska, E, Sunshine, A, Mueller, F, et al: Caffeine as an analgesic adjuvant, *JAMA* 251:1711-1718, 1984

Leib, RA, and Hurtig, JB: Epidural and intrathecal narcotics for pain management, *Heart Lung* 14:164-174, Mar 1985

Leporati, NC, Chychula, LH, Lo, SL, and Coleman, RR: How you can really help the drug-abusing patient, *Nursing* 12:46-49, June 1982

Levine, JD, Gordon, NC, Smith, R, and McBryde, R: Desipramine enhances opiate postoperative analgesia, *Pain* 27:45-49, 1986

Levy, MH: Pain management in advanced cancer, *Semin Oncol* 12:394-410, Dec 1985

Lim, RKS: Pain mechanisms, *Anesthesiology* 28:106-110, Jan-Feb 1967

Lo, SL, and Coleman, RR: Exceptionally high narcotic analgesic requirements in a terminally ill cancer patient, *Clin Pharm* 5:828-832, Oct 1986

Lukacsko, P: A guide to the parenteral management of moderate to severe pain, *Hospital Pharm* 22:361-412, Apr 1987

Maciewicz, R, Bouckoms, A, and Martin, JB: Drug therapy of neuropathic pain, *Clin J Pain* 1:39-49, 1985

Magruder, MR, Delaney, RD, and Difazio, CA: Reversal of narcotic-induced respiratory depression with nalbuphine hydrochloride, *Anesthesiol Rev* 9:34-37, Apr 1982

Maguire, LC, Yon, JL, and Miller, E: Prevention of narcotic induced constipation, *N Engl J Med* 305:1651, 1981

Malhotra, V, and Artusio, JF: Management of postoperative pain, *Semin Urol* 3:204-215, Aug 1985

Malone, BT, Beye, R, and Walker, J: Management of pain in the terminally ill by administration of epidural narcotics, *Cancer* 55:438-440, Jan 15, 1985

Marks, RM, and Sachar, EJ: Undertreatment of medical inpatients with narcotic analgesics, *Ann Intern Med* 78:173-181, 1973

Marx, J: Dysmenorrhea: basic research leads to a rational therapy, *Science* 205:175-176, July 1979

Massie, MJ, and Holland, J: The cancer patient with pain: psychiatric complications and their management, *Med Clin North Am* 71:243-258, Mar 1987

Mauro, VF, Bonfiglio, MF, and Spunt, AL: Meperidine-induced seizure in a patient without renal dysfunction or sickle cell anemia, *Clin Pharmacol* 5:837-839, 1986

Max, MB, Culnane, M, Schafer, SC, et al: Amitriptyline relieves diabetic neuropathy pain in patients with normal or depressed mood, *Neurology* 37:589-596, Apr 1987

McCaffery, M: Nursing management of the patient with pain, ed 2, New York, 1979, JB Lippincott

McCaffery, M: Large doses are safer than you think, *Nurs Life* 1:41-42, Nov-Dec 1981

McCaffery, M: Problems with meperidine, *Am J Nurs* 84:525, Apr 1984

McCaffery, M: Giving meperidine for pain—should it be so mechanical? *Nursing* 17:61-64, Apr 1987a

McCaffery, M: Patient-controlled analgesia: more than a machine, *Nursing* 17:62-64, Nov 1987b

McGee, JL, and Alexander, MR: Phenothiazine analgesia—fact or fantasy? *Am J Hosp Pharm* 36:633-640, May 1979

McGuire, DB, Barbour, L, Boxler, J, et al: Fixed-interval v. as-needed analgesics in cancer outpatients, *J Pain Sympt Manag* 2:199-205, Fall 1987

McGuire, L, and Wright, A: Continuous narcotic infusion: it's not just for cancer patients, *Nursing 84* 14:50-55, Dec 1984

McManus, M, and Panzarella, C: The use of dextroamphetamine to counteract sedation for patients on a morphine drip, *J Assoc Pediatr Oncol Nurs* 3:28-29, 1986

Miller, RR, and Jick, H: Clinical effects of meperidine in hospitalized medical patients, *J Clin Pharm* 18:180-189, Apr 1978

Miser, A, Moore, L, Greene, R, et al: Prospective study of continuous intravenous and subcutaneous morphine infusions for therapy-related or cancer-related pain in children and young adults with cancer, *Clin J Pain* 2:101-106, 1986

Miser, AW, Ayesh, D, Broda, E, et al: Use of a patient-controlled device for nitrous oxide administration to control procedure related pain in children and young adults with cancer, *Clin J Pain* 4:5-10, 1988

Miser, AW, Davis, DM, Hughes, CS, et al: Continuous subcutaneous infusion of morphine in children with cancer, *Am J Dis Child* 137:383-385, 1983

Miser, AW, Miser, JS, and Clark, BS: Continuous intravenous infusion of morphine sulfate for control of severe pain in children with terminal malignancy, *J Pediatr* 96:930-932, 1980

Moore, J, and Dundee, JW: Alterations in response to somatic pain associated with anaesthesia v. the effect of promethazine, *Br J Anaesthesiol* 33:3-8, 1961

Morgan, JP: American opiophobia: customary underutilization of opioid analgesics, *Adv Alcohol Subst Abuse* **5**:163-173, Fall 1985-Winter 1986

Moss, H: Subcutaneous continuous infusion narcotics at home, *Oncol Nurs Forum* (suppl) **13**:128, 1986 (abstract)

Moulin, DE, and Coyle, N: Spinal opioid analgesics and local anesthetics in the management of chronic cancer pain, *J Pain Sympt Manag* **1**:79-86, Spring 1986

National Headache Foundation Newsletter, no. **63**:12, Winter 1987-88

Ozuna, J, and Snyder, G: An experience with epidural morphine in lumbar surgery patients, *J Neurosci Nurs* **19**:235-239, Oct 1987

Pagliaro, AM: Preparation, administration, and monitoring of medications. In Pagliaro, AM, and Pagliaro, LA, eds: Pharmacologic aspects of nursing, pp 30-67, St. Louis, 1986, The CV Mosby Co

Paice, JA: Intrathecal morphine infusion for intractable cancer pain: a new use for implanted pumps, *Oncol Nurs Forum* **13**:41-47, May-June 1986

Paice, JA: New delivery systems in pain management, *Nurs Clin North Am* **22**:715-726, 1987

Paice, JA: Personal communication, 1988a. This clinical example was given to us by Judy Paice, RN, MS, Assistant Professor and Acting Coordinator, Oncology Graduate Program, College of Nursing, Rush University and a doctoral student at the University of Illinois at Chicago. We appreciate her willingness to share this example.

Paice, JA: The phenomenon of analgesic tolerance in cancer pain management, *Oncol Nurs Forum* **15**:455-460, July-Aug 1988b

Pannuti, F, Rossi, AP, Iafelice, G, et al: Control of chronic pain in very advanced cancer patients with morphine administered by oral, rectal, and sublingual route, *Pharmacol Res Commun* **14**:369-380, 1982

Parish, K, and Thompson, G: Epidural 'port-a-cath', *Austral Nurs J* **17**:44-47, Sept 1987

Pasternak, GW: Multiple morphine and enkephalin receptors and the relief of pain, *JAMA* **259**:1362-1367, Mar 4, 1988

Payne, R: Novel routes of opioid administration in the management of cancer pain, *Oncology* **1** (special suppl):10-18, Apr 1987a. Free copies available from Roxanne Laboratories—makers of Roxanol and Roxanol SR.

Payne, R: Role of epidural and intrathecal narcotics and peptides in the management of cancer pain, *Med Clin North Am* **71**:313-327, Mar 1987b

Penn, RD, and Paice, JA: Chronic intrathecal morphine for intractable pain, *J Neurosurg* **67**:182-186, 1987

Penn, RD, Paice, JA, Gottschalk, W, and Ivankovich, AD: Cancer pain relief using chronic morphine infusion, *J Neurosurg* **61**:302-306, 1984

Pfeiffer, FG: Nonsteroidal antiinflammatory drugs. In Pagliaro, AM, and Pagliaro, LA, eds: Pharmacologic aspects of nursing, pp 1319-1345, St Louis, 1986, The CV Mosby Co

Pitorak, EF, and Kraus, JC: Pain control with sublingual morphine, *Am J Hosp Care* **4**:39-41, Mar-Apr 1987

Plezia, PM, and Linford, J: Innovative approaches to refractory pain, *Hospital Ther* **10**:25-42, Oct 1985

Portenoy, RK: Continuous infusion of opioid drugs in the treatment of cancer pain: guidelines for use, *J Pain Sympt Manag* **1**:223-228, 1986

Portenoy, RK: Continuous intravenous infusion of opioid drugs, *Med Clin North Am* **71**:233-241, Mar 1987a

Portenoy, RK: Drug treatment of pain syndromes, *Semin Neurol* **7**:139-149, June 1987b

Portenoy, R, Moulin, DE, Rogers, A, et al: Intravenous infusion of opioids in cancer pain: clinical review and guidelines for use, *Cancer Treat Rep* **70**:575-581, 1986

Porter, J, and Jick, H: Addiction rare in patients treated with narcotics, *N Engl J Med* **302**:123, 1980

Rawal, N, and Sjostrand, UH: Clinical application of epidural and intrathecal opioids for pain management, *Int Anesthesiol Clin* **24**:43-57, Summer 1986

Rawal, N, and Tandon, B: Epidural and intrathecal morphine in intensive care units, *Intens Care Med* **11**:129-133, 1985

Reasbeck, PG, Rice, ML, and Reasbeck, JC: Double-blind controlled trial of indomethacin as an adjunct to narcotic analgesia after major abdominal surgery, *Lancet* **2**:115-118, 1982

Rickels, A, Feighner, JP, and Smith, WT: Alprazolam, amitriptyline, doxepin, and placebo in the treatment of depression, *Arch Gen Psychiatr* **42**:134-141, 1985

Rimar, J: Epidural morphine for analgesia following a cesarean, *Matern Child Nurs* **11**:345, Sept-Oct 1985

Ritter, MA, and Gioe, TJ: The effect of indomethacin on para-articular ectopic ossification following total hip arthroplasty, *Clin Orthop Rel Res* **167**:113-117, July 1982

Rogers, A: Analgesic consultation: the use of methadone in opioid-tolerant patients, *J Pain Sympt Manag* **3**:45, 1988a

Rogers, A: Analgesic consultation, *Am J Nurs* **88**:100, Jan 1988b

Rumore, MM, and Schlicting, DA: Clinical efficacy of antihistaminics as analgesics, *Pain* **25**:7-22, 1986

Rutter, PC, Murphy, F, and Dudley, HAF: Morphine: controlled trial of different methods of administration for postoperative pain relief, *Brit Med J* **280**:12-13, Jan 5, 1980

Sheehan, AP, and Sauerbier, GA: Continuous subcutaneous infusion of morphine, *Oncol Nurs Forum* **13**:92, 1986

Slavic-Svircev, V, Kaiko, G, Heidrich, RF, and Rusy, BF: Ibuprofen in the treatment of postoperative pain, *Am J Med* **77**:84-86, July 13, 1984

Smith, KA: Teaching family members intrathecal morphine administration, *J Neurosci Nurs* **18**:95-97, Apr 1986

Spiegel, K, Kalb, R, and Pasternak, GW: Analgesic activity of tricyclic antidepressants, *Ann Neurol* **13**:462-465, 1983

Sriwatanakul, K, Weis, OF, Alloza, JL, Kelvie, W, Weintraub, M, and Lasagna, L: Analysis of narcotic analgesic usage in the treatment of postoperative pain, *JAMA* **250**:926-929, 1983

St. Marie, B, and Henrickson, K: Intraspinal narcotic infusions for terminal cancer pain, *J Intravenous Nurs* **11**:161-163, May-June 1988

Stambaugh, JE, and Sarajian, C: Evaluation of hydroxyzine versus meperidine in the relief of chronic pain due to malignancy. In Pain abstracts, vol 1, p 203, International Association for the Study of Pain, Seattle, 1978

Stambaugh, JE, Jr, and Wainer, IW: Drug interaction: meperidine and chlorpromazine, a toxic combination, *J Clin Pharmacol* **21**:140-146, 1981

Stapleton, JV, Austin, KL, and Mather, LE: A pharmacokinetic approach to postoperative pain: continuous infusion of pethidine, *Anaesth Intens Care* **7**:25-32, Feb 1979

Stauffer, JD: Antidepressants and chronic pain, *J Fam Pract* **25**:167-170, Aug 1987

Stenseth, R, Sellevold, O, and Breivik, H: Epidural morphine for postoperative pain: experience with 1085 patients, *Acta Anaesthesiol Scand* 29:148-156, 1985

Stimmel, B: Pain, analgesia and addiction: the pharmacologic treatment of pain, pp 294-297, New York, 1983, Raven Press

Stuart, GJ, Davey, EB, and Wight, SE: Continuous intravenous morphine infusions for terminal pain control: a retrospective review, *Drug Intell Clin Pharm* 20:968-972, Dec 1986

Swerdlow, M: Anticonvulsant drugs and chronic pain, *Clin Neuropharmacol* 7:51-82, 1984

Szeto, H, Inturrisi, C, Houde, R, et al: Accumulation of normeperidine, an active metabolite of meperidine, in patients with renal failure or cancer, *Ann Intern Med* 86:738-741, 1977

Tang, R, Shimomura, SK, and Rotblatt, M: Meperidine-induced seizures in sickle cell patients, *Hosp Formul* 15:764-772, Oct 1980

Tejada, IM: Indocin suppository for control of pain in postthoracic surgery patient, *Oncol Nurs Forum* 13:87, May-June 1986

Trotter, JM, Scott, R, Macbeth, FR, et al: Problems of the oncology outpatient: role of the liaison health visitor, *Br Med J* 282:122-124, Jan 10, 1981

Twycross, RG: Clinical experience with diamorphine in advanced malignant disease, *Int J Clin Pharmacol* 9:184-198, 1974

Twycross, RG, and Lack, SA: Symptom control in far advanced cancer, London, 1983, Pitman

Twycross, RG: The management of pain in cancer: a guide to drugs and dosages, *Primary Care & Cancer* 8:15-23, May 1988

Ventafridda, V, Fochi, C, DeConno, D, et al: Use of non-steroidal anti-inflammatory drugs in the treatment of pain in cancer, *Br J Clin Pharmacol* 10:3435-3465, 1980

Ventafridda, V, Ripamonti, C, DeConno, F, et al: Antidepressants increase bioavailability of morphine in cancer patients (letter) *Lancet* 1:1204, May 23, 1987

Wallace, J: Morphine sulfate administered sublingually to control chronic pain, *Oncol Nurs Forum* (Practice Corner) 14:66, Mar-Apr 1987

Walsh, TD: Common misunderstandings about the use of morphine for chronic pain in advanced cancer, *CA—Cancer J Clinic* 35:164-169, May-June 1985

Ward, NG: Tricyclic antidepressants for chronic low-back pain, *Spine* 11:661-665, Sept 1982.

Watt-Watson, JH: Nurses' knowledge of pain issues: a survey, *J Pain Sympt Manag* 2:207-211, Fall 1987

Weingart, WA, Sorkness, CA, and Earhart, RH: Analgesia with oral narcotics and added ibuprofen in cancer patients, *Clin Pharm* 4:53-58, Jan-Feb 1985

Weinstock, M, et al: Effect of physostigmine on morphine-induced postoperative pain and somnolence, *Br J Anaesthesiol* 54:429-432, 1982

Wenzloff, NJ, and Shrimp, L: Therapeutic management of primary dysmenorrhea, *Drug Intell Clin Pharm* 18:22-26, 1984

Wermeling, DP, Record, KE, and Foster, TS: Patient-controlled high dose morphine therapy in a patient with electrical burns, *Clin Pharm* 5:832-835, Oct 1986

Westerling, D, et al: Absorption and bioavailability of rectally administered morphine in women, *Eur J Clin Pharmacol* 23:5964, 1982

Westring, EW: Meperidine vs morphine, *JAMA* 230:1512, Dec 16, 1974

White, PF: Use of patient-controlled analgesia for management of acute pain, *JAMA* 259:243-247, Jan 8, 1988

Whitman, HH: Sublingual morphine, *Am J Nurs* 84:939, July 1984

Wilkie, D: Sublingual efficacy challenged, *Oncol Nurs Forum* 14:13 (letter) Sept-Oct 1987

Woodrow, KM, and Eltherington, LG: Feeling no pain, alcohol as an analgesic, *Pain* 32:159-163, 1988

Wright, Z: From IV to PO: titrating your patient's pain medication, *Nursing 81* 11:39-43, July 1981

Yaksh, TL: Spinal opiate analgesia: characteristics and principles of action, *Pain* 11:293-346, 1981

Yasko, JM: Guidelines for cancer care: symptom management, pp 73-93, Virginia, 1983, Reston Publishing Co

CHAPTER

5

Cutaneous Stimulation

The warmth of the sun, massage by a human hand, and ice or snow (in those climates where it was available) may well have been among the very first pain relief methods used by primitive man. But today if you had pain somewhere between your lower trunk and upper thighs, would you seek relief by sitting in a basin of cold water or warm water? Research shows that some people tried both with varying results. These and other methods of stimulating the skin, such as vibrators and electric impulses, continue to be widely used in pain control. In fact, some methods of pain relief consist of inflicting pain to relieve pain. But what works for some people and some types of pain does not work for others. To each his own device.

DEFINITION OF CUTANEOUS STIMULATION

In this chapter the term *cutaneous stimulation* is defined quite simply as *stimulating the skin for the purpose of relieving pain*. The techniques selected, however, will be limited to those that meet the following criteria:
- Noninjurious or very low risk when used properly.
- Usually readily available in the home or hospital setting.
- Require very little expertise to use safely and effectively.

To increase patient acceptance and to avoid the complication of tissue damage, the directions will be to use the techniques at levels of stimulation that are either *comfortable to the patient or only moderately uncomfortable* for a brief time.

The methods of cutaneous stimulation discussed in this chapter are the *mild or superficial forms* of the following that are readily accessible to the nurse and do not require special educational preparation beyond the simple directions given in this chapter.

- Superficial massage.
- Pressure/massage.
- Vibration.
- Superficial heat and cold.
- Ice application/massage.
- Menthol application to skin.
- TENS (transcutaneous electrical nerve stimulation).

All of the above may be used by skilled, prepared nurses or other health professionals, such as physical therapists, for reasons other than those covered in this chapter. For example, a physical therapist may use ice massage to facilitate stretching a painful muscle or mobilizing a painful joint, but that use of ice massage is not included here.

In this chapter discussion of cutaneous stimulation will be *limited to methods that the nurse in general practice may use for palliative pain relief*. Methods that have only a superficial effect on skin and subcutaneous tissues will be covered. Thus superficial heating and cooling will be discussed, but vigorous or deep heating such as ultrasound or diathermy to heat a joint will not be. Nevertheless, remember that even superficial use of cutaneous stimulation has indirect effects on deep, striated muscles and on smooth muscles of visceral organs.

BENEFITS AND LIMITS OF CUTANEOUS STIMULATION

The cutaneous stimulation methods as discussed in this chapter are *not therapeutic or curative;* rather they are palliative, for the purpose of pain relief.

The *effects* of cutaneous stimulation are variable and unpredictable, but in general the expectation is that pain will be eliminated or the intensity of pain will be decreased, during and/or after stimulation. Sometimes cutaneous stimulation is briefly painful, and then pain relief

IMMEDIATE HELP FOR CUTANEOUS STIMULATION

Time involved: Reading time, 5 to 10 minutes; implementation time, 5 to 10 minutes.

Sample situation: The patient is in agony with sudden, unexpected, but fairly well-localized pain. This could be in an emergency room, in the home, or on a clinical unit in the hospital. The physician is notified and does not want to order analgesics until the patient is evaluated. How can you relieve at least some of the pain without the risk of masking symptoms?

Possible solution: Ask the physician for an order to use local application of heat, cold, or ice until diagnostic procedures begin or evaluation is complete. These methods of cutaneous stimulation are almost always available. If the physician says these might be contraindicated or if there is an open wound, suggest that heat, cold, or ice can be used at a site distant to the pain (see *Do's* below), e.g., on the opposite side of the body. Explain that this may partially override or mask the sensation of pain temporarily and will reassure the patient that something is being done. NOTE: Cold application is not the same as ice application. Cold is applied at a comfortable level of intensity, usually wrapped. In ice application a frozen substance is in direct contact with the skin.

Expected outcome: Patient temporarily experiences partial or complete pain relief.

Don'ts

1. Do not expect or suggest that this will relieve all of the patient's pain.
2. Do not tell the patient he simply must endure the pain until the doctor finds out what is causing it.
3. Do not tell the patient that he is merely frightened or that his pain is not as bad as it seems.
4. Do not tell the patient nothing else can be done to help him.
5. Do not apply heat to a site where there is bleeding or swelling.
6. Do not apply ice for longer than 10 minutes (to avoid tissue damage).
7. If cold completely relieves the pain, do not apply cold for longer than 30 minutes because pain returns much more slowly following cold than heat. You want to avoid pain relief that long outlasts the application of cold since the return of pain may be important in making a medical diagnosis.

Dos

1. Assure the patient you know he hurts as much as he says he does, and explain why medications cannot be used right now to relieve the pain.
2. Tell the patient what options you have for providing pain relief, e.g., heat, cold, or ice.
3. If there is a choice, tell the patient he can try whichever one has helped him before, but that cold or ice probably has a better chance than heat of relieving the pain.
4. Apply heat, cold, or ice to the site of pain if possible.

5. If the site of pain cannot be used for application, explain that heat, cold, or ice need not be applied to the site of pain. Acknowledge that it probably sounds unlikely but that clinical experience and research have shown the application of heat, cold, or ice to sites distant from the pain sometimes relieves pain, perhaps by distraction. The simple possibilities for sites distant from the pain are:
   - Between pain and the brain.
   - On the other side of, beyond, the pain (e.g., use the hand if the forearm is injured).
   - On the opposite side of the body corresponding to the site of the pain.
   NOTE: More than one of the above sites can be used at one time. (For further information regarding sites for application of cold, heat, or ice, see Figure 5-1 for general recommendations, Figures 5-2 to 5-12 for trigger points for musculoskeletal injuries, and Figure 5-13 for acupuncture points at a distance from the pain site.)
6. If heat or cold is used, encourage the patient to use intermittent stimulation, developing his own rhythm of on and off, perhaps every 5 seconds or every 1 to 2 minutes.
7. If heat and cold are both allowed, alternate them every few seconds or minutes.
8. If increased sensation of heat or cold is desired, use a moist cloth next to the skin.
9. If ice massage is used, remember:
   - Warn the patient that the sensations are not very comfortable and generally progress from extreme cold to burning, aching, and finally numbness.
   - Ice should be in direct contact with the skin (do not cover with anything waterproof).
   - Ice may be rubbed gently on the skin, avoiding pressure over boney prominences.
   - Provide a cloth to wipe up the water as the ice melts.
   - Discontinue application of ice after 10 minutes or whenever there is shivering, numbness, or skin irritation; skin color alternates between white and red; or the patient says it is intolerable. If ice must be discontinued at that site, another site may be tried. (For further information, refer to "Ice Application or Massage for Pain Relief," p. 156.)
10. Allow the patient or family to participate as much as they wish.
11. After 5 to 10 minutes, ask the patient if this has helped. If not, try one or more of the following:
    - Changing sites or using an additional site.
    - Switching to another form of stimulation if it is allowed (e.g., switch from warm to cold application).
    - Use intermittent stimulation. If this has been done, vary the rhythm.
12. Reassure the patient that more effective pain relief probably will be provided once the diagnosis is made.

occurs following the stimulation. In some instances the character of the pain may simply change to a sensation that is more acceptable, e.g., a change from sharp to dull.

Some methods of cutaneous stimulation undoubtedly have relaxing or distracting effects in addition to activating mechanisms that actually reduce the intensity of pain. Since cutaneous stimulation involves touching the patient in some way with the intent of helping the patient, it is also possible that the effectiveness of a method may be related to therapeutic touch.

KEY POINT: The major effect of cutaneous stimulation is usually a reduced intensity of pain during stimulation and/or for a period afterwards.

The underlying *mechanisms* of pain relief from cutaneous stimulation are usually unknown. Broadly speaking, the gate control theory suggests that stimulation of the skin may activate the large diameter fibers. In turn, that activation may provoke an inhibition of the pain messages carried by the smaller fibers, i.e., close the gate to the transmission of impulses felt as painful. Another possibility is that certain types of cutaneous stimulation may increase endorphins, the body's natural morphine. Some types of cutaneous stimulation, such as vibration or cold application, may cause decreased sensitivity to pain, such as partial or complete anesthesia or numbness of the skin.

When pharmacologically active substances are applied topically, pain may be relieved because an analgesic or anesthetic is absorbed through the skin and depresses cutaneous receptors, or because stimulation of cutaneous receptors causes distraction from pain by inducing sensations such as warmth.

Hyperstimulation analgesia, or *counterirritation,* is one type of cutaneous stimulation. These terms usually apply to various types of moderate to intense sensory stimulation, such as with cold, heat, rubbing, or pressure. Obviously, at intense levels these stimuli are often painful. This is an example of the phenomenon of one painful stimulus reducing pain caused by another painful stimulus—producing pain to abolish pain. A woman who bites her lip during a labor contraction may explain that biting relieves discomfort from the contraction by acting as a distraction, but the pain relief is very likely due to more complicated events. Brief, moderate pain seems to produce nerve impulses that act as a complex neural inhibitory mechanism leading to relief of more intense, prolonged pain at near or distant sites.

The *potential benefits* of cutaneous stimulation methods can be summarized as:

1. Decreases intensity of pain, sometimes eliminates pain. In some instances the sensation of pain may be changed to a more acceptable sensation, e.g., a change from sharp pain to a feeling of warmth.
2. Relieves muscle spasms secondary to underlying skeletal and joint pathology or nerve root irritation, i.e., interrupts the vicious cycle of muscle spasm, ischemia, pain, and more muscle spasm.
3. Increases physical activity and ability to engage in therapeutic exercises due to relief of muscle spasm and/or decreased perception of pain.
4. Some patients may report that the cutaneous stimulation distracts them from pain, promotes general relaxation, or decreases anxiety.
5. The onset and duration of pain relief may include the period during stimulation and/or a period following stimulation.
6. Strengthens the nurse-patient relationship and conveys caring through socially acceptable physical contact, e.g., touching, especially valuable for someone who is uncomfortable with physical demonstrations of affection or concern.
7. Physical contacts may improve body image, especially for a person who has undergone recent body image disturbances, e.g., mastectomy or amputation of a limb, or long periods of pain. Perception of a comfortable sensation such as warmth may be in marked contrast to constant awareness of pain.
8. Most methods require very little patient participation/activity and are therefore especially appropriate for patients with limited physical or mental energy or for use at bedtime.
9. Some methods, e.g., massage or simply application of heat or cold packs, are ideal ways to involve family and friends who feel helpless or want to do something for the patient.
10. Some methods, e.g., application of menthol or pressure on a trigger point, are quickly and easily done by the patient, providing him with a sense of control and independence while he continues other activities.

Some *possible limitations or disadvantages* of cutaneous stimulation for pain relief are:

1. Successful cutaneous stimulation may be misunderstood by the patient as meaning that the condition is cured.
2. Some methods may be unacceptable to certain patients because of inherent characteristics of the methods, e.g., the confusing or visible equipment associated with TENS, the odor of topical agents containing menthol, or the discomfort of ice massage.
3. Massage/pressure, vibration, cold, heat, ice, and menthol are so ordinary and commonplace that their effectiveness is usually underestimated by both patients and health professionals.
4. In spite of appropriate precautions, tissue damage may accidently occur, e.g., blistering from heat or cold applications.
5. Mild forms of cutaneous stimulation, such as those covered in this chapter, usually produce milder, more superficial, and less prolonged effects than vigorous

types of cutaneous stimulation such as kneading massage (squeezing and movement of deep tissues) or ultrasound for deep heating, e.g., to joint.

NURSING CARE GUIDELINES FOR SELECTING, DEVELOPING, AND USING CUTANEOUS STIMULATION FOR PAIN RELIEF

These general suggestions are intended to point you in the right direction. You will need to read further in this chapter for specific guidelines about the method selected. The following includes general information about the practical aspects of:
- Selecting the most appropriate type of cutaneous stimulation for the patient and the condition.
- Choosing a site for application.
- Determining duration and frequency of use.
- Modifying the method, e.g., to achieve greater relief or patient acceptability.

For all of the above, the basic approach is trial and error. Because these are physical modalities with well-defined parameters, e.g., measurable temperature ranges, it is tempting to think that we possess fairly precise knowledge about which conditions certain methods should and should not be used for, how often, how long, and where. However, ideas about uses of heat, cold, and other methods are more likely to be derived from our culture and personal experiences than from well-tested, scientific information. In fact, well-controlled research on cutaneous stimulation is scarce.

KEY POINT: Determining which method to use for the patient, at which site, when, and for how long is mostly a matter of trial and error.

Selection of method:
1. Keep in mind availability of method, cost, amount of time required of patient or caregivers, safety and possible side effects, potential effectiveness, contraindications, and patient acceptability. See the box below for a brief overview of these points for each method, including pages for further reading.
2. To the extent possible, give the patient a choice, especially initially. But keep in mind the following.
3. For many types of pain cutaneous stimulation methods can be used interchangeably unless there are contraindications. For example, contrary to popular opinion, heat and cold can be used interchangeably for many conditions, and cold is often more effective than heat.
4. Potentially effective methods may be disregarded because of preconceived ideas about which method can be used for specific types of pain.

Pointers on Selecting a Method of Cutaneous Stimulation

- Massage (p. 141). Minimal side effects and contraindications. Backrubs or body massage can be time consuming and may relieve only mild pain, but pain need not be localized and most patients enjoy it. Modest patients may object to touch or disrobing. Massage of feet and hands may be more accessible, acceptable, and even more effective.
- Pressure, sometimes with massage (pp. 141-143). Massage/pressure to trigger points or acupuncture points may be very effective but is briefly uncomfortable. Initially it requires time to locate the points. But then the patient can learn to work on some trigger points on his own.
- Vibration (pp. 143-145). A more vigorous form of massage that may be more effective. Low risk of tissue damage. Check on availability or cost of a vibrator. May be used for trigger points. May be unacceptable due to noise or intensity of stimulation if vibrator is not adjustable. Sometimes this is a less expensive substitute for TENS.
- Heat and cold (pp. 145-152). Probably works best for well-localized pain. Both may be done with a minimum of equipment and both should be applied at a comfortable level of intensity. Cold has more advantages than heat. Unwanted side effects, e.g., burns, and contraindications, e.g., bleeding and swelling, are more frequent with heat-

ing than with cooling. When cold relieves pain, it tends to be more effective than heat. However, patients usually prefer heat to cold, and use of cold often requires some persuasion.
- Ice application/massage (pp. 152-155). A frozen substance applied to the skin is uncomfortable, but only for a few minutes before numbness occurs. Continuous use for 10 minutes or less. Pain must be well localized. May relieve severe pain. Simple, low-risk technique for brief, painful procedures. Especially effective in obliterating needle stick pain. May be used on trigger points. Sometimes this is a very inexpensive substitute for TENS.
- Menthol (pp. 155-158). Refers to menthol-containing substances for application to skin. Intensity increases with amount of menthol; may be uncomfortable at higher concentrations. Odor offensive to some people. Use influenced by culture; more restricted use by Americans than other cultures, e.g., Asians. Inexpensive. Once it is applied, it provides continuous stimulation without additional effort. Well-suited for nighttime use.
- TENS (pp. 158-164). Compared with above methods, much more expensive, less available, and more time needed to teach nurse and patient, but supported by more research and regarded by many as more "scientific."

5. Sensations produced by cutaneous stimulation may be uncomfortable or unacceptable in the absence of pain, but they may be preferable or helpful in the presence of pain.

KEY POINT: Although massage, heat, cold, ice, and menthol products seem ordinary, they may be used to provide very effective pain relief and one may work as well as the other.

Selection of site. Trial and error combined with open-mindedness are needed. Following are groups of sites that may be stimulated in an effort to relieve pain (see the box below for definitions of terms used in this section; see Figures 5-1 to 5-14 for examples):
- Directly over or around pain. This is usually, but not always, the best site.
- Proximal to pain—"between pain and brain."
- Distal to pain.
- Contralateral to pain.
- Acupuncture point.
- Trigger point.
- Any site distant to the pain.

The *mechanisms* underlying pain relief produced by stimulation of sites distant to pain are not fully understood. Stimulation at one site may produce at least mild effects at distant sites in the body, called the *consensual response.* For example, heat applied to one site increases blood flow in other parts of the body such as the contralateral limb.

Terms Related to Site Selection

Acupuncture point: a point or spot on the body associated with a conceptual (not anatomical) system of meridians. Between 500 and 800 points were identified centuries ago by cultures of the Far East. Some are related to pain syndromes, but others are not. Those related to pain are often located near or in the same place as trigger points.

Contralateral: on the opposite side of the body; opposed to ipsilateral.

Distal: farthest from the center of the body; opposed to proximal.

Ipsilateral: on the same side of the body; opposed to contralateral.

Proximal: nearest the center of the body; opposed to distal. May be referred to here as "between pain and the brain."

Trigger point: a point or area of hyperirritability in tissue such as myofascial (skeletal muscle and its fascia). When compressed it is tender and may give rise to referred pain, but after stimulation, e.g., with ischemic pressure, pain may be relieved. They are often located near or in the same place as acupuncture points.

Still another explanation for pain relief at a site distant from stimulation is *counterirritation,* which is thought to produce nerve impulses that act as a complex neural inhibitory mechanism leading to relief of another pain. Surprisingly, spraying ethyl chloride (ice sensation) on the skin of the leg to the point of causing pain significantly reduced pain from electrical stimulation of a tooth filling (Parsons and Goetzl, 1945)—truly a case of inflicting pain to relieve pain, and it demonstrates that stimulation of sites very distant from the inflicted pain can affect pain.

It has also been theorized that the area of the brain responsible for exerting inhibitory control over pain signals may not have an anatomically correct representation of the human body. Not only may certain areas of the body be larger or smaller in the brain's representation than in reality, but also some areas may be close to each other in the brain but not on the actual body. Thus when one area of the body is stimulated, this may be perceived in the brain at a point near a representation of an area anatomically unrelated. However, the strength of the stimulation may spill over into the nearby area and send inhibitory signals to the anatomically unrelated body part.

Stimulation of *acupuncture points and trigger points,* within the area of pain or at a distance from the pain, have long been known to produce pain relief, but the underlying reason is unclear. Perhaps stimulation of an acupuncture point balances energy along the meridian, or stimulation of a trigger point reduces its irritability.

What is interesting and of great practical significance is that the locations of acupuncture points for pain and trigger points are similar. Further, both can often be found simply by using the balls of the fingers and thumbs to probe areas within and around the site of pain, asking the patient to identify which areas beneath the skin are the most sensitive. These sensitive areas are likely to be acupuncture points or trigger points. Sometimes pressure on the area produces or increases the pain. Hopefully, pain will decrease following stimulation of the point with one of the cutaneous stimulation methods, e.g., pressure or moist heat.

Since it is beyond the scope of this book to explain the location of all trigger points or acupuncture points, a few of each have been selected. Figures 5-2 to 5-12 illustrate trigger points associated with some common pain problems in the head, neck, and back. Trigger point sites vary from person to person, more so than acupuncture points are often thought to do. Therefore the trigger point illustrations are to be considered as a guide for where to start looking.

Some acupuncture points that are distant from the site of pain are illustrated in Figure 5-13. Traditionally, these points were needled to relieve pain. However, there are more practical approaches to finding and using acupuncture points. Not only can they often be located by probing with the fingers, but research has shown that the site of at least some points is not necessarily a discrete point but is a large area. For example, stimulation of the Hoku point (Figure 5-14) often relieves dental pain, but so does immersing the entire hand in ice water or stimulating between the fourth and fifth fingers. In this instance the site that can be effectively stimulated may be any point on the entire hand. In other words, stimulation of an acupuncture point may be effective even when the stimulation is not exactly where the point is supposed to be.

KEY POINT: Experiment to find the most effective stimulation site for the patient. It may be at some distance from the pain.

Duration and frequency. Again, this is determined by trial and error in addition to what is convenient and practical. Consider the following:
1. The most frequent period of time suggested for all cutaneous stimulation techniques, except ice application/massage, is 20 to 30 minutes.

2. To a certain extent, the longer stimulation is used, the longer pain relief will last after the stimulation is stopped.
3. Whenever possible, use the method before pain occurs or increases.
4. If any of the following occur, it is almost always advisable to discontinue the method:
   • Increased pain.
   • Skin irritation.

Modification of method that fails to relieve pain is certainly indicated since the lack of specific guidelines makes cutaneous stimulation largely a matter of trial and error. Modification may include the following considerations:
1. A single, initial failure need not be cause for discarding the technique. Several trials may be warranted.
2. Try changing some characteristics of the specific technique selected, e.g., switch from dry to moist, or re-

Text continued on p. 141.

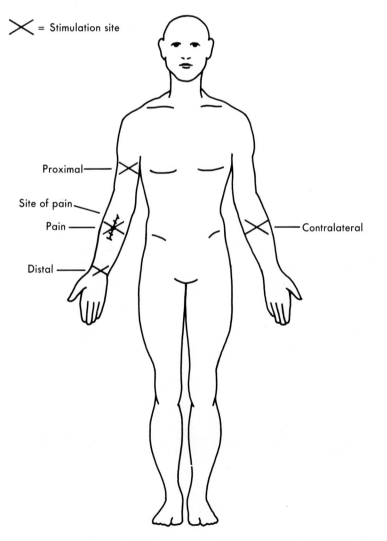

FIGURE 5-1 Illustration of sites for cutaneous stimulation. This figure gives examples of four possible sites: site of pain, proximal to pain, distal to pain, and contralateral.

FIGURES 5-2 TO 5-12 Trigger points and related areas of pain. *X,* Trigger point; *solid,* region of pain present in almost every patient; *stippling,* region where some but not all patients experience pain. Stimulation of the trigger point(s), e.g., by pressure, should produce the pain pattern shown. The major muscle involved is noted, and comments are made about names given the conditions and certain characteristics of the pain.

NOTE: Appropriate therapy should be used to treat the condition and reduce the pain, but techniques such as spraying the area with a vapocoolant and stretching the muscle are beyond the scope of this book. Temporary relief can be obtained by using the various cutaneous stimulation techniques described in this chapter. Moist heat and ischemic pressure are most often recommended. Experiment with what works best for the patient.

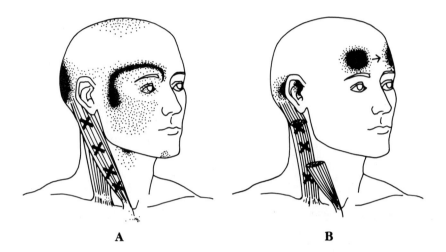

A   B

FIGURE 5-2 Muscle: sternocleidomastoid. *A,* Sternal (superficial) division; *B,* clavicular (deep) division. Comment: tension headache, atypical facial neuralgia, sometimes accompanied by ipsilateral sweating of forehead, tearing and reddening of eye, rhinitis, or visual disturbances; some soreness in neck but no stiffness. Called "whiplash" when muscles are bilaterally involved.

Adapted from Travel, JG, and Simmons, DG: Myofascial pain and dysfunction: the trigger point manual, Baltimore, 1983, Williams & Wilkins.

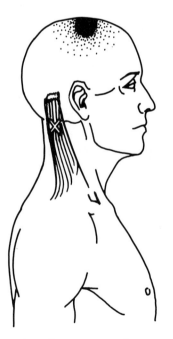

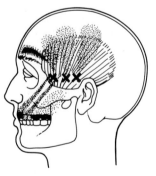

FIGURE 5-3 Muscle: splenius capitis. Comment: ache inside the top of the head.

Adapted from Travel, JG, and Simmons, DG: Myofascial pain and dysfunction: the trigger point manual, Baltimore, 1983, Williams & Wilkins.

FIGURE 5-4 Muscle: temporalis. Comment: temporal headache with intermittent toothache or a sense that "teeth don't meet right."

Adapted from Travel, JG, and Simmons, DG: Myofascial pain and dysfunction: the trigger point manual, Baltimore, 1983, Williams & Wilkins.

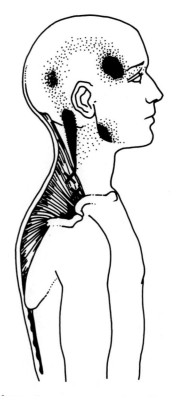

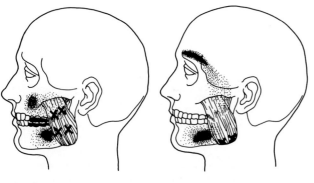

FIGURE 5-5 Muscle: masseter. Comment: patient may describe the maxillary pain as sinusitis.

Adapted from Travel, JG, and Simmons, DG: Myofascial pain and dysfunction: the trigger point manual, Baltimore, 1983, Williams & Wilkins.

FIGURE 5-6 Muscle: upper trapezius. Comment: tension headache and neck pain, or tension neckache; pain is usually unilateral; pain on motion usually occurs only when head and neck are almost fully rotated to the opposite side; may be misdiagnosed as cervical radiculopathy or atypical facial neuralgia.

Redrawn with permission from Travel, JG, and Simmons, DG: Myofascial pain and dysfunction: the trigger point manual, p. 184, Baltimore, 1983, Williams & Wilkins.

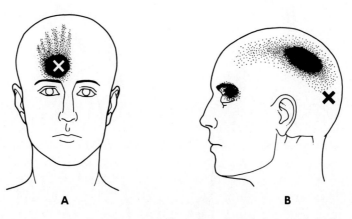

FIGURE 5-7 Muscle: occipitofrontalis. *A,* Right frontalis belly; *B,* left occipitalis belly. Comment: headache; these trigger points respond well to ischemic pressure easily applied by patient.

Redrawn with permission from Travel, JG, and Simmons, DG: Myofascial pain and dysfunction: the trigger point manual, p. 291, Baltimore, 1983, Williams & Wilkins.

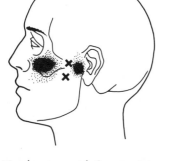

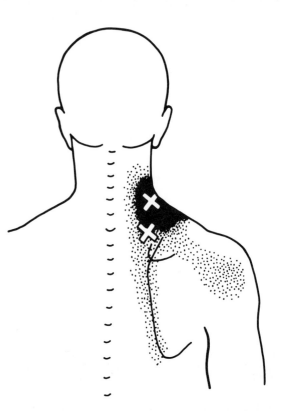

FIGURE 5-8 Muscle: pterygoid. Comment: temporomandibular joint (TMJ) dysfunction; chewing may cause pain. May be misdiagnosed as sinusitis or treatment may be misdirected to teeth or joint.

Redrawn with permission from Travel, JG, and Simmons, DG: Myofascial pain and dysfunction: the trigger point manual, p. 261, Baltimore, 1983, Williams & Wilkins.

FIGURE 5-9 Muscle: levator scapulae. Comment: stiff neck (limited neck rotation due to pain on movement); patient tends to hold neck rigid; head may be slightly tilted toward involved side.

Redrawn with permission from Travel, JG, and Simmons, DG: Myofascial pain and dysfunction: the trigger point manual, p. 335, Baltimore, 1983, Williams & Wilkins.

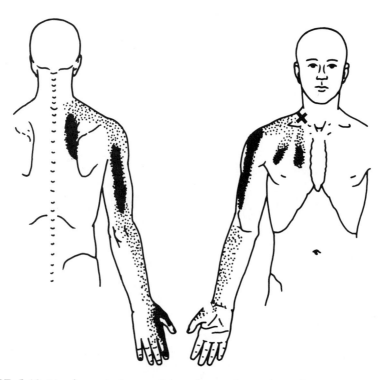

FIGURE 5-10 Muscles: anterior, medial, and posterior scalene. Comment: very common; muscle is tender to palpation.

Redrawn with permission from Travel, JG, and Simmons, DG: Myofascial pain and dysfunction: the trigger point manual, p. 345, Baltimore, 1983, Williams & Wilkins.

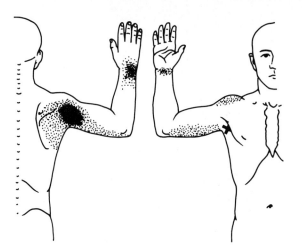

FIGURE 5-11 Muscle: subscapularis. Comment: frozen shoulder; severe pain both at rest and on motion; progressive limitation of arm movement.

Redrawn with permission from Travel, JG, and Simmons, DG: Myofascial pain and dysfunction: the trigger point manual, p. 411, Baltimore, 1983, Williams & Wilkins.

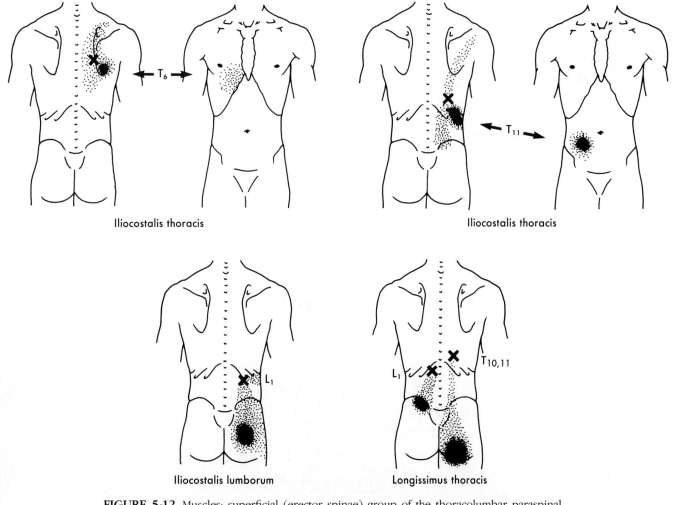

FIGURE 5-12 Muscles: superficial (erector spinae) group of the thoracolumbar paraspinal muscles consisting of iliocostalis thoracis, iliocostalis lumborum, and longissimus thoracis. *T,* Thoracic vertebra; *L,* lumbar vertebra. Comment: back pain or "lumbago"; markedly restricts activity; usually caused by sudden or sustained overload, e.g., as when lifting. The patient can learn to apply ischemic compression to the trigger points in these superficial back muscles by lying on a tennis ball on the floor, moving around until the ball presses on the sensitive point and gradually applying increasing body weight for 1 minute or longer. Moist heat may be applied afterward.

Redrawn with permission from Travel, JG, and Simmons, DG: Myofascial pain and dysfunction: the trigger point manual, p. 638, Baltimore, 1983, Williams & Wilkins.

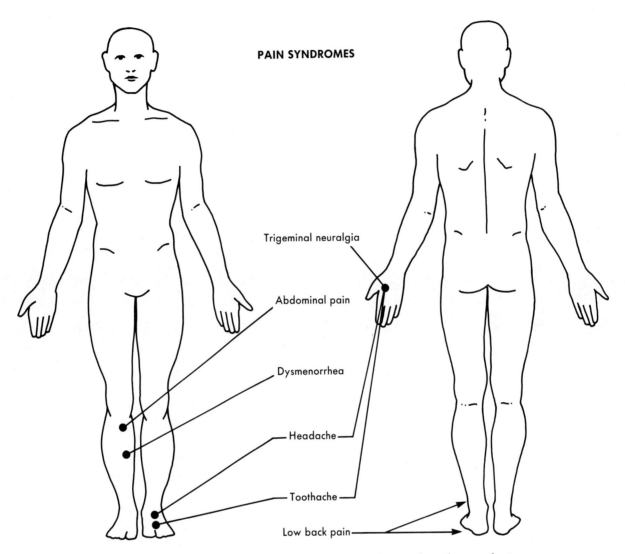

FIGURE 5-13 Basic acupuncture points that are at a distance from the site of pain.
Adapted from Melzack, Stillwell and Fox, 1977, p. 19.

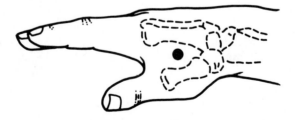

FIGURE 5-14 Hoku point, an acupuncture point, stimulated to relieve a variety of conditions, particularly those from the neck up, e.g., headaches and tooth pain. It may be stimulated sufficiently either with ice massage to the skin over the point or by pressure with the thumb against the second metacarpal bone.

duce pressure or weight of anything touching the skin.

3. Increasing the intensity of stimulation is especially likely to be effective.

4. If modifications of the originally selected technique are not successful, change from one type of cutaneous stimulation to another type, e.g., change from heat to cold or cold to ice. Each cutaneous stimulation technique produces a different sensation from the others.

5. Alternate methods of cutaneous stimulation. This may prevent adaptation to the sensation. Cutaneous stimulation methods may be alternated in several ways:
   - Choose two or more different methods and use each at different times, e.g., moist heat in the morning and menthol at night.
   - Rhythmically alternating between two different methods every few seconds or minutes can be very effective, e.g., pressure to a trigger point for 15 seconds followed by moist heat for 5 minutes, repeating this for about 20 minutes.
   - Rhythmically alternating between applying and withdrawing a method may also be very effective, e.g., 30 seconds of heat application and 30 seconds without.

KEY POINT: Although it takes more time and energy, much more pain relief may be achieved by alternating or interrupting cutaneous stimulation techniques every few seconds or minutes.

6. Use more than one method at the same time, e.g., apply a cold pack over menthol, or try heat at one site and cold at another site at the same time.

7. Remember to continue to include other appropriate forms of pain relief, e.g., analgesics.

SUPERFICIAL MASSAGE

The *effects* of superficial body massage are usually soothing and relaxing, both physically and mentally. Massage may decrease pain, perhaps mainly by relaxing muscles. It increases capillary circulation and ultimately improves general circulation. Some practitioners feel that massage has such negligible physical effects that its use is a waste of time and energy. However, a massage is enjoyed by almost all who receive it.

Probably the most common *areas of the body* to be massaged are the back and shoulders—the usual back rub. Extremities may be added. When it is inconvenient to do a back rub, massage of both hands or both feet may be equally or more effective.

Appropriate/Inappropriate Situations for Massage

Appropriate uses of massage include:
- A patient restricted to bed or a chair, especially if he lies on his back much of the time (massage improves circulation and decreases skin breakdown).
- Assist with sleep disturbance.

- Create an acceptable method of touch for a patient who experiences limited physical contact with others, e.g., a patient isolated from family.
- Pain of any type—the comfort of touch is reassuring and provides a welcome contrast to the feeling of pain.
- Create an opportunity to be with and/or talk with the patient.
- A method of communicating care and concern when verbal communication is limited or impossible, e.g., patient speaks another language or has impaired hearing.

Inappropriate uses or possible contraindications for massage include:
- A patient who says he does not want a massage—attempts to persuade the patient to accept a massage should be avoided. Massage involves a degree of intimacy (physical contact and exposure) that is uncomfortable for some patients. The nurse should not insist that the patient receive a massage.
- Situations in which there is limited time to spend with the patient—other nursing care activities might be a higher priority.
- Open lesions or skin areas that are tender to touch.
- A patient inclined to make inappropriate sexual advances.
- Whenever it causes pain.

Nursing Care Guidelines and Patient/Family Teaching Points for Using Massage

The patient/family teaching point on massage (p. 142) contains information and guidelines that are useful to the nurse as well as the patient and family. It is written in the exact words that might be spoken to the patient or duplicated and given to a patient or family member who can read.

PRESSURE/MASSAGE

Acupuncture points or trigger points that are related to the patient's pain may be massaged with pressure, or ischemic pressure may be applied to them. Pain relief may occur at the time pressure is applied because of numbness resulting from ischemia. Or, if tender acupuncture points or trigger points are stimulated, pain relief may occur after pressure is released. The exact mechanism underlying this type of pain relief is unclear in relation to acupuncture points, but pressure is thought to somehow decrease irritability of trigger points.

Appropriate/Inappropriate Situations for Pressure/Massage

Appropriate uses of pressure and/or massage are:
- Patients in whom acupuncture points or trigger points related to pain can be identified. Use Figures 5-2 to 5-14 as a guide to finding these sites and apply ischemic pressure, explained in the next section, p. 143.

Patient/Family Teaching Point: Massage of Body, Hands, or Feet

TO: _____ (patient's name)   DATE: _____

Almost everybody likes to receive a massage. You and the person who will be giving the massage, referred to as massager, may consider the following tips on making it as good as it can be.

1. What area is best? Most people think of the traditional back rub that includes the area from the lower back to the shoulders. Arms and legs can be added. However, if these areas are inconvenient, try massage of both hands or both feet.
2. When should it be done? You may enjoy it most when you're tired, when your pain increases, when you get anxious, or just before you go to sleep. If possible, you may want to set aside a specific time each day for a massage, perhaps the same time every day. This will give you something to look forward to.
3. How long should it last? This depends a lot on how much time is available to you and your massager. You'll have a better idea of what seems best for you after you've had a massage. Note the time massage begins and then note how long it takes for you to feel the benefits. Some people benefit from only a few minutes of massage. You may want to establish an exact period of time so you can enjoy the massage without wondering how long it will last or if you should give the massager permission to stop.
4. Bare hands or lotion? Do what feels best. If your skin is dry, you may want a moisturizing lotion. Warm the lotion in a microwave oven or by placing the bottle in a sink of hot water. Or, you may want to try powder. Either keeps the movement slippery, preventing uncomfortable friction on the skin or pulling tiny hairs.
5. What position? Both you and your massager should be in relaxed positions.
6. How is the rubbing done? Massage over the trunk and extremities is usually done with the palms of both hands, conforming to the body contours and using long strokes with firm enough pressure not to be ticklish. For massage of the feet or hands the massager usually uses the fingers of both hands. The entire foot or hand is massaged, including separate massage for each toe or finger. Initially, you need to tell your massager what feels good to you. Regardless of the type or area of massage, the movements should almost always be continuous, even, and rhythmical.
7. Should you talk during a massage? Probably not. Let your massager know this so neither of you will feel obligated to talk. Just concentrate on how good the massage feels.

As a reminder, you may wish to complete the following:

Date: _____   Massager: _____

Area to be massaged: _____   Warm lotion, oil, or powder? _____

Time of day: _____   Length of time for massage: _____

Special considerations: _____

From: _____ (nurse's name)   Phone: _____

■ May be duplicated for use in clinical practice. From McCaffery, M, and Beebe, A: PAIN: CLINICAL MANUAL FOR NURSING PRACTICE, St. Louis, 1989, The CV Mosby Company.

Pinch-Grasp Technique for IM Injection in Deltoid Muscle

For a painful IM injection, such as streptomycin sulfate 1 g in 2 ml water, the following technique has been shown to decrease pain (Locsin, 1985):

1. Grasp the deltoid muscle with the fingers on one side of the muscle and the thumb on the other side.
2. Pull the deltoid muscle about 1½ inches toward you.
3. Exert pinching pressure hard enough to cause some discomfort, making the muscle bulge and the skin tense.
4. With the other hand, administer the injection at a 90-degree angle, inserting the needle about 1½ inches into the deltoid.
5. Continue to pinch-grasp the muscle until the needle is removed and a cotton pledget is pressed over the injection site.
6. With the cotton pledget, rub the site with light pressure for 5 to 10 seconds.

- Muscle spasms or aching, sore muscles, especially muscles not suitable for spray and stretch, i.e., spraying a coolant on the skin over the muscle and stretching the muscle.
- Sharp pain from an acute injury, e.g., a cut. Pressure may relieve pain and reduce bleeding.
- "Back labor," occiput of baby's head pressing on coccyx (apply pressure to lower back, e.g., with fist, especially during contraction).
- IM at deltoid site (see the box above for pinch-grasp technique).

  Inappropriate uses of pressure and/or massage are:
- Patients with increased bleeding time or who bleed or bruise easily.
- Sites where skin has been injured, e.g., burned or cut.
- Areas of thrombophlebitis.

Patient/Family Teaching Points and Nursing Care Guidelines for Applying Pressure/Massage

Following are points to consider and possibly discuss with the patient regarding use of pressure/massage:

1. *Acupressure.* When a possible acupuncture point is located (see Figures 5-13 and 5-14), it can be stimulated with pressure and/or massage, referred to as acupressure. Basically this is acupuncture without needles. Pressure may be applied with the thumb, tip of the index finger, or sometimes the palm of the hand or the fingernail or thumbnail. Pressure is applied as firmly as the patient can tolerate. If massage is done, it is in tiny circles at the rate of about 2 to 3 circles per second. Pressure is firm enough that contact is maintained with the same area of skin but the tissues beneath are massaged.

For someone untrained in acupressure techniques, it is probably safest to try this for a few seconds to examine the results and then continue it, if desired, for up to 1 minute. The patient can learn to do this for himself if he can reach the site.

2. *Ischemic compression of trigger point* (also referred to as myotherapy or pain erasure). The goal is to apply sustained pressure to a trigger point (Figures 5-2 to 5-12) with sufficient force and for a long enough time to inactivate it. Since acupuncture points and trigger points are often in the same site, this will frequently be almost the same thing as acupressure.

The patient is told to relax his muscle; he must not tense his muscle to resist the pressure. Pressure is then applied over the trigger point with the ball of the thumb or finger and with as much force as the patient can tolerate, up to 20 to 30 lb of pressure. Pressure is continued for up to 1 minute. This may be repeated once after a hot pack has been applied for about 10 minutes or more. Briefer pressure of only 7 to 10 seconds may be used and repeated several times a day.

Explain to the patient that the force of the compression will be uncomfortable, but pain relief is expected afterward or may begin during the compression. However, excessive pain during compression may lead to failure of the technique, so explain to the patient the importance of letting you know how tolerable the pressure is. Pressure can be increased gradually with feedback from the patient.

Massage may be combined with pressure only if it does not cause a marked increase in pain. This combination is similar to the technique of Rolfing, or skin rolling. Upon release of the compression the skin is white (blanched) at first, then red.

For some trigger points, pressure may need to be applied with a knuckle or elbow, depending on the thickness and depth of the muscle.

For hard to reach trigger points on the patient's back, the patient can be taught to use a *tennis ball.* Instruct the patient to lie on the floor on his back with the tennis ball under his back. He can move around until the ball presses directly on the sensitive trigger point. Body weight can be used to gradually apply increasing pressure for up to a minute.

VIBRATION

Vibration is a form of electric massage or vigorous massage. It is not widely used for pain relief, but research suggests it may be very effective, possibly a substitute for TENS for some patients.

One mechanism underlying pain relief from vibration is that some types, especially from a hand-held vibrator applied with moderate pressure, cause numbness, paresthesia, and/or anesthesia of the area stimulated. Thus pain relief may occur during vibration. If this type of vibration is continued for 25 minutes or longer, pain relief may last for several hours after stimulation. If vibration is effective at trigger points or acupuncture points, it may also relieve pain following stimulation. Vibration may also change the character of the sensation, e.g., from sharp to dull.

A number of different *types of vibrating devices* are available commercially, and many have adjustable speeds. Common types are:

Hand-held vibrators, using batteries or house current. Pressure and movement are provided by the operator. Frequencies and amplitudes vary widely, coarser movement oscillating at 10 to 50 Hz and finer movements at 100 to 200 Hz, the latter probably being more common and comfortable. Many have interchangeable applicators of different shapes and sizes made of plastic or rubber. Those with the rounded tips, e.g., shaped like a phallus, are particularly good for getting at certain acupuncture or trigger points. Battery-operated ones are also convenient to use. However, they may be embarrassing to the patient. Some small vibrators are strapped to the dorsum of the hand, allowing the human hand to be in contact with the patient's skin. This type allows better adaptation to the contours of the body.

Stationary vibrators. Vibrating pads may resemble a seat cushion or be incorporated in an armchair or bed mattress. These are probably best suited to provide superficial massage. The body part, such as the back, is placed against the surface. Some are constructed especially for massaging the feet. Some have heating elements incorporated.

Appropriate/Inappropriate Situations for Using Vibration

Appropriate situations for use of vibration may include:
- Muscle pain or spasm, acute or chronic, e.g., back pain or neck pain.
- Tension headache (see Figure 5-15).
- Itch (either to site or contralateral).
- Near injection site, e.g., during IM injection.
- Neuropathic pain, e.g., postherpetic neuralgia (surround the area if site of pain is too sensitive) or other pain of a neuralgic nature in the thoracic regions radiating along the course of an intercostal nerve.
- Phantom limb pain.
- Rheumatoid arthritis.
- Orofacial pain, acute or chronic (use at the Hoku point or at the site of pain), e.g., dental pain.
- Acute tendinitis.
- As a substitute for TENS.
- Many types of chronic nonmalignant pain not listed above, as long as they are well-localized and can be covered with the vibrator.

Inappropriate uses of vibration usually include:

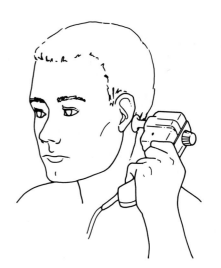

FIGURE 5-15 A vibrator, or electric massager, applied to the suboccipital region. Various attachments may be used. This may relieve neck pain or headache.

- Patients who bruise easily.
- Areas of thrombophlebitis.
- Sites where skin has been injured, e.g., burned or cut.
- Causalgia or other conditions that cause hypersensitivity to mechanical stimulation.
- Migraine headache or any headache that worsens with movement or sound.
- Marked increase in pain.

Nursing Care Guidelines and Patient/Family Teaching Points for Using Vibration

The following points may be discussed with the patient who is willing to try vibration for pain relief:
1. Be open-minded about the uses and possible effectiveness of vibration for pain relief. It tends to be underused.
2. In the hospital, obtain a physician's prescription for the use of vibration.
3. Experiment with vibration applied for 1 minute to various sites to determine which site results in the best pain relief. Since one of the main immediate effects of vibration is partial loss of sensation, the best site for stimulation with vibration is often in the area of pain. However, some success has been achieved with application to areas surrounding the pain, especially distal to the pain, and stimulation of acupuncture points or trigger points.
4. A hand-held vibrator applied with moderate pressure may provide the best relief.
5. The length of time for using a vibrator commonly varies from 20 seconds to 15 minutes, but there tends

to be very little poststimulation pain relief. However, vibration for 25 to 45 minutes may provide up to several hours of pain relief. Intermittent use may be the most effective approach, applying and withdrawing every few seconds.

6. After 45 minutes of vibration, a common skin reaction is redness and a feeling of warmth along with some loss of sensation. Itching may also occur.
7. High-frequency vibration, as opposed to slow, coarse vibration, tends to be the most effective.
8. Vibration should be nonpainful.
9. For chronic pain, use of vibration for as long as 30 to 45 minutes may best be limited to twice a day. Over a period of months, using it four times a day or more may lead to shorter periods of pain relief after vibration.
10. When pain relief extends beyond the period of vibration, warn the patient to be careful of injury afterward. Care should be taken not to perform physical activities that would injure the muscles, but supervised therapeutic exercises may be appropriate.
11. Vibration is easily self-administered and very suitable for home use.

Patient Example

Mr. L., 65 years old, has chronic low back pain that began 6 years ago following an injury to his back while he was lifting a heavy object. He is retired and lives with his wife. For many years their favorite outing was an evening of dinner and dancing. Since his injury, Mr. L. is only able to sit for a brief time, so dining out has become a short affair. The nurse suggested that prior to an evening out he could try vibration to the painful area of his back for as long as 45 minutes. The couple borrowed a hand-held vibrator and Mrs. L. applied it with moderate pressure for 45 minutes. Mr. L. reported 3 hours of pain relief following this, enough to enable him to enjoy a complete night of dining and dancing for the first time in 6 years.

SUPERFICIAL HEAT AND COLD APPLICATIONS

For centuries heat and cold have been used for pain relief, but surprisingly, the effects of superficial heating and cooling and the mechanisms that underlie the effects are still largely a matter of speculation. Possible mechanisms by which heat and cold may relieve pain are listed in the box on p. 146. Some of the effects of heat and cold may be similar, but the mechanisms underlying the effects may be different.

Also, interestingly, the effects of heat and cold are not always limited to the direct local effects; there may be distant effects. The mechanisms underlying this are poorly understood.

Superficial heating methods, with a temperature of approximately 40° to 45° C (104° to 113° F)* at point of contact with skin, usually warm only the skin; the muscles and other deeper tissues usually are not affected because they are insulated by the subcutaneous fat. Methods of applying superficial heat that are convenient and commonly available in the home or hospital setting include the following:

1. Packs
   - Rubber hot water bottle (wrap in towels to prevent burns).
   - Electric heating pad, dry or moist (avoid burns by not falling asleep on top of pad since heat output tends to increase; avoid electric shock by proper insulation and following instructions).
   - Hot moist compresses.
   - Hydrocollator (inconvenient to prepare; avoid burns by not lying on pack and by wrapping with towels).
   - Chemical pack (least desirable, until improvements are made; expensive, temperature poorly controlled, ingredients are irritating or harmful).
2. Immersion in water
   - Tub.
   - Basin or sitz bath.
   - Whirlpool.
3. Radiant heat with 40 watt bulb at a minimum of 18 inches (this method of heating avoids touching the area and keeps it dry).
4. Retention of body heat with plastic wrap, e.g., Saran wrap or plastic dry cleaner bag taped to itself.

Patient Example

Ms. S., 65 years old, with arthritic knees, had pain and stiffness, especially in the morning, and a significant increase in pain when she went to work on days that were cold and damp. Both of the incidents of increased pain were partially relieved by using plastic wrap. At night she wrapped both knees separately in plastic bags from the dry cleaners, taping the bag to itself. When she went to work she wore slacks to hide the plastic and further warm her legs. Apparently the plastic bags helped retain body heat and moisture, providing moist heat. (Of course, good skin care, such as regular bathing, is necessary to prevent a skin rash.)

Superficial cooling, around 15° C (59° F) at skin contact, usually cools the skin and, if applied long enough, the muscles. Cold application drops the muscle temperature in slender people after about 10 minutes; in obese

---

*The temperature ranges cited for methods of superficial heating and cooling are merely guidelines in case it becomes necessary to measure the temperature of a heating or cooling method, e.g., in a research project or in a situation where the patient cannot communicate easily regarding the comfort of an application of heat or cold. In daily clinical practice it is rarely necessary to actually use a thermometer since the patient's reported comfort along with close attention to skin reactions are sufficient and maybe better guidelines.

people, after about 30 minutes. The effect of cooling on the muscle lasts much longer than the effect of heat on muscle. After heat applications are removed, the muscle rapidly resumes its normal temperature. However, after cold application is discontinued, the fat layer insulates the muscle, and rewarming takes longer depending on the thickness of the fat layer.

Ideally, cold packs should be *sealed* to prevent dripping, *flexible* to conform to body contours, and applied in a manner that produces a *comfortable and safe intensity of cold.* Convenient and readily available, commercially or homemade, *methods of cold application* are:

1. Waterproof bags, e.g., rubber or plastic, filled with ice melting in water.
2. Terry cloth dipped in water with ice shavings, wrung out, and applied repeatedly (frequency of application is an inconvenience).
3. Frozen gel packs. These may be more convenient and may reduce temperature more quickly than the traditional ice bag. (See Figure 5-16 for uses of flexible cold packs.)
4. Chemical ice envelope (chemical is broken within package to produce cold; expensive; if leaks, contents are irritating to skin).

Heat and Cold: Possible Mechanisms of Pain Relief

The following lists of possible effects pertain only to *superficial* heating and cooling:
- Direct effect is limited to the skin and subcutaneous tissues and to the muscle to a limited extent.
- Any deeper effects or effects at a distance are indirect and are probably due to reflex activity.
- In some cases similar effects are obtained from heat and cold.
- In other cases, they achieve opposite effects.

Superficial Heating May Relieve Pain Because of the Following:

1. Reduces striated muscle spasm, possibly by relieving ischemia, cooling the muscles by increased blood flow, reducing muscle spindle excitability, or reducing the tension in muscle trigger points. However, if the muscle is inactive, blood flow may remain the same or be reduced.
2. Assists in resolution of superficial, localized infections or inflammations (e.g., thrombophlebitis), partly by increased blood flow.
3. Reduces sensitivity to pain (physiological basis unknown).
4. Reduces joint stiffness.
5. Relaxes smooth muscle, reduces peristalsis, and reduces gastric acidity, possibly by reflex reduction in blood flow to mucous membranes of stomach and intestines (occurs within 5 to 10 minutes when heat is applied to the abdomen).
6. Vasodilatation in skin and increased blood flow to skin.
7. Distant reactions, milder than those at the site of heating. The same reactions that occur at the site of heating may also occur at distant sites, such as contralaterally, but the distant reactions will be milder. For example, if heat is applied to the right leg, vasodilatation there will be greater than the vasodilatation that occurs at distant sites such as the left leg. (These distant reactions are reflexogenic and are referred to as consensual reactions.) Distant reactions are in proportion to the input at

the site of heating. Thus distant reactions are greater if the local heat application is more vigorous. That is, if the intensity of heat is greater, if the area of skin heated is larger, or if the rate of temperature rise is faster, the distant reactions will be greater.
8. Effects of heating do not last as long as effects of cold because the increased blood flow rapidly cools the tissues to normal temperature.

Superficial Cooling May Relieve Pain Because of the Following:

1. When the cold penetrates deep enough to lower the muscle temperature, it reduces muscle spasm by reducing the muscle spindle response or inactivating trigger points in muscles.
2. Reduces or prevents bleeding and edema through reflex vasoconstriction. Vasodilatation in response to cold occurs only if the temperature is low enough to be potentially destructive to the tissues.
3. Reduces sensitivity of skin by temperature reduction (cooling) of nerve fibers and receptors.
4. Effects of cold last longer than the effects of heat because the vessels remain constricted after cold application is removed, and rewarming of tissue from inside is delayed accordingly along with delayed warming from the outside. When cold penetrates deep enough to cool the muscle, rewarming of the muscle is further prolonged due to the insulating fat layer.
5. Reduces inflammation, possibly through destruction of enzyme activity.
6. Reduces joint stiffness or perception of stiffness if cooled sufficiently.
7. Increases peristalsis of the stomach, small bowel, and colon if cold is applied to the abdomen.
8. Relieves pain at a distance, possibly because it is placed on a superficial nerve innervating the painful area, an acupuncture point or a trigger point, or because it produces mild but similar effects contralaterally.

5. Homemade cold packs that are comfortable, quick, and inexpensive:
   - Sealed plastic container (e.g., plastic bag) with one-third alcohol and two-thirds water placed in freezer produces a flexible, unfrozen slush.
   - Sealed plastic container with damp cloth or towel placed in freezer produces flexible cold pack.
   - One lb bag of frozen green peas or kernels of corn—hit gently to separate peas or corn.

All containers of cold, e.g., plastic bags with gel or alcohol and water, should be *wrapped with cloth* to prevent tissue damage and to provide a comfortable intensity of cold. This slows down the cooling and helps prevent discomfort and tissue damage. A moist cloth allows for faster cooling, if desired.

A convenient *method of controlled, continuous heat or cold application* is now available, "Hot/Ice Dual Function Equipment." An electrically operated unit is attached

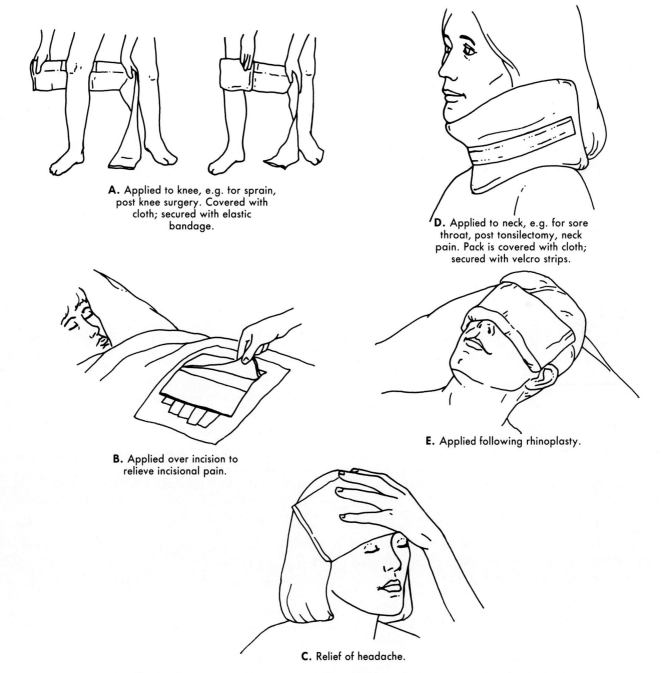

A. Applied to knee, e.g. tor sprain, post knee surgery. Covered with cloth; secured with elastic bandage.

B. Applied over incision to relieve incisional pain.

C. Relief of headache.

D. Applied to neck, e.g. for sore throat, post tonsilectomy, neck pain. Pack is covered with cloth; secured with velcro strips.

E. Applied following rhinoplasty.

FIGURE 5-16 Uses of flexible cold gel packs. Some may also be used for heat by warming them in water. Notice that the pack is covered with cloth.

to a small blanket, available in several shapes and sizes and set to operate at 4° to 40° C (40° to 105° F) in 1° increments. This is a consistent and efficient way to provide superficial heat or cold to a localized area if the patient is not very active. The unit is somewhat portable but relatively large and weighs about 22 lb. The unit is especially useful for acute musculoskeletal injuries and postoperative pain. Its main advantages are maintaining a constant temperature and ease of switching from heat to cold. (For product information and additional clinical suggestions, write: Hot/Ice Dual Function Equipment, Thermotemp, Inc., 1923 Tampa East Blvd., Tampa, FL 33619.)

Appropriate/Inappropriate Situations for Heat and Cold

Guidelines for when to use heat or cold are not as clear-cut as originally thought. Conflicting opinions and research results are probably due in part to differences in the methods of applying heat and cold. Although this section is limited to application of heat and cold for superficial, not deep, cooling or warming, there are still considerable differences in the temperatures that may be achieved, the depth of cooling or warming, and the amount of time it takes to achieve this.

For example, water is an excellent conductor of heat. Thus the effects of moist heat are likely to be much greater than the effects of dry heat. Also, since burns are caused by a high rate of heat transmission to the skin, water or moisture must be used cautiously along with heating because of the increased risk of burns. Dry towels, a poor conductor of heat, may be used over skin to reduce intensity of heat and risk of burn.

The following lists of indications and contraindications for using heat or cold are not rigid rules. They are merely suggestions or guidelines. Clearly both heat and cold may be used successfully in the same conditions.

Either heat or cold applied superficially usually relieves the following types of pain, although some exceptions exist and are noted in the separate lists for heat and cold:

- Muscle spasms secondary to underlying pathology.
- Joint stiffness.
- Low back pain.
- Myofibrositis (roughly defined as aching muscles of several months duration).

KEY POINT: **Use what works best for the individual patient unless it is contraindicated.**

Both heat and cold may be applied whenever heat and cold may be used interchangeably. One technique, contrast bathing, involves alternating immersion of a limb in hot and cold water (see the box above for instructions). Similar results might be obtained by substituting hot and cold packs. Alternating heat and cold or simply intermittent heat has been extremely effective for even severe

---

Contrast Bathing: Combined Heat and Cold

Uses: on extremities with severe pain, pain that responds to both heat and cold, or joint stiffness (results in increased blood flow).

Supplies: 2 containers of water.
- Cold water at approximately 15° C (59° F).
- Hot water at approximately 40° C (104° F).

Method: Immerse the limb for a total of 30 minutes, alternating as follows:

Time (min) in Hot Water	Time (min) in Cold Water
10	
	1
4	
	1
4	
	1
4	
	1
4	
(Total of 30 min)	

---

pain.* Suggestions to the patient regarding timing may be similar to those in the box above, or the patient may simply develop his own rhythm. Intervals may be very short, e.g., 5 to 40 seconds.

Obviously intermittent heat or alternating heat and cold is more time consuming and therefore inconvenient than constant application of heat or cold. Hence, it is usually reserved for severe pain.

KEY POINT: **Severe pain is likely to be relieved best by intermittent heat applications or by alternating heat and cold. The patient may develop his own rhythm or timing for the intervals.**

Appropriate uses of superficial heat to relieve pain include the following conditions:

- Muscle spasms secondary to underlying skeletal or neurological pathology, e.g , degenerative joint disease, intervertebral disc disease, nerve root irritation.
- Following trigger point stimulation, e.g., with pressure.
- Painful joint stiffness in arthritis.
- Superficial boils.
- Decubiti (pressure sores), especially immersion in warm water.
- Superficial thrombophlebitis.
- Low back pain, especially acute.

*Intermittent cold does not seem to provide the same contrast of sensations as does intermittent heat, probably because the sensation of cold lasts longer after the removal of a cold pack than does the sensation of heat after the removal of a heating device.

- Gastrointestinal upset with cramping, e.g., viral enteritis.
- Menstrual cramps.
- Reflex sympathetic dystrophy, e.g., shoulder-hand syndrome.
- Tennis elbow during recovery stage, not acute stage.
- During the healing phase of an acute injury after bleeding and edema have subsided.
- Anorectal pain (especially warm sitz baths).
- Superficial skin breakdown in tissue folds, e.g., perineal or inguinal areas—use radiant heat, e.g., light bulb; avoid higher temperatures that cause cyanosis and pain.
- Myofibrositis.
- Rheumatoid arthritis after the acute state.
- Itching from mosquito bites and poison ivy.
- Hematoma resolution after acute phase to increase rate of absorption—controversial.

Patient Example

Mr. L. had prolonged muscle spasm associated with a temporomandibular joint (TMJ; jaw) problem. His nurse suggested that when he took his morning shower he might try standing for awhile with the warm water aimed at his jaw area. He reported that 5 minutes of this relieved his pain for 1 hour or more.

Inappropriate uses of or possible contraindications for superficial heat to relieve pain may include the following conditions:

- Acute trauma (sometimes mild heating is acceptable if injury is minor).
- Bleeding or swelling (almost always contraindicated for these conditions).
- Impaired sensation or anesthetic areas.
- Unconscious patient—possible tissue damage because patient cannot report when it is too hot.
- Bursitis (unless cold is poorly tolerated).
- Acute state of rheumatoid arthritis (temperatures about $37°$ C tend to increase cartilage degeneration).
- Acute and subacute stages of muscle injury when active therapeutic exercise is being used—may increase edema.
- Tissues with irreversible inadequate vascular supply (heat may increase metabolic demand and cause necrosis).
- Superficial malignancies (may accelerate tumor growth).
- Person prone to orthostatic hypotension should be cautious if heat is applied to large parts of body or if total body is immersed in warm water.
- Person with light sensitivity should avoid radiant heat sources, e.g., light bulb.
- Over topical application of menthol-containing products.
- Sensitive persons such as those with adrenal suppression, systemic lupus erythematosus, multiple sclerosis, and possibly pregnant women should avoid or be cautious about total body immersion, e.g., hydrotherapy, with temperature maintained at $37.8°$ C $(100°$ F). For pregnancy, monitor oral temperature and discontinue if increases above $37.8°$ C.

Appropriate uses of superficial cold to relieve pain may include the following conditions:

- Muscle spasm secondary to underlying skeletal or neurological pathology, e.g., degenerative joint disease, intervertebral disc disease, nerve root irritation.
- Acute, but not severe, injury, e.g., acute surgical trauma such as episiotomy, minor sports injuries such as sprains (especially combined with compression). Recommended during the first 4 to 48 hours following injury.
- Following surgical procedures requiring casting, e.g., knee surgery, tendon repair, bone grafts, or fractures, to prevent pain from surgery or potential swelling.
- Joint stiffness in arthritis (*if* cooled enough; sometimes cold aggravates painful joint stiffness); especially effective for acute stage of rheumatoid arthritis.
- Bursitis.
- Low back pain, especially chronic.
- "Back labor" during childbirth.
- Therapeutic exercise in subacute stages of muscle injury, especially sports injuries (used with compression prior to and sometimes after therapeutic exercise to reduce edema).
- Headache, especially migraine, cluster, or mixed headache (migraine plus muscle contraction).
- Myofibrositis.
- Minor burns.
- Itching.

Inappropriate uses of or possible contraindications for superficial cold for pain relief may include the following conditions:

- Severe acute trauma.
- During the healing phase when bleeding and swelling have subsided following an acute injury (may retard healing).
- Peptic ulcer—application of cold to abdomen may increase gastric acidity.
- Peripheral vascular diseases with arterial insufficiency, e.g., Raynaud's disease.
- Stomach or intestinal cramping—cold packs to abdomen may increase peristalsis.
- Hypersensitivity or cold allergy (rare)—includes wheals, itching, puffiness of eyelids, respiratory distress, and very rarely the severe symptoms of cold anaphylaxis such as shock.
- Occurrence of "hunting reaction" after application of cold. The skin alternately blanches and turns red, signifying vasodilatation. Occurs only if temperature is low enough to be potentially destructive to tissues.

KEY POINT: For some conditions, heat and cold may be used interchangeably. In other conditions, one may be contraindicated or ineffective.

Patient/Family Teaching Point: Pain Relief with Heat? Cold? Both?

TO: _____ (patient's name)   DATE: _____

You've probably used heat and cold before for relief of discomfort. Maybe you used a heating pad for a backache or a cold pack for a black eye. You may have been taught to use cold on a new injury for the first 24 to 48 hours to reduce bleeding and swelling, and then switch to heat. But cold relieves pain too, long after the initial injury. Sometimes heat and cold can be used interchangeably. But did you know that sometimes cold relieves pain better than heat? Even for arthritis!

If you're thinking about using *either heat or cold,* consider the following:

1. Is either one contraindicated? In general, heat is contraindicated the first 12 to 24 hours after an injury or if there is swelling or bleeding. Cold is usually contraindicated if it increases pain. Otherwise there are not many common conditions for which cold is contraindicated. If you have questions, talk with your nurse or physician.

2. Use what has worked for you before, or simply follow your hunches. You can always change to the other. What works for one person or one type of pain will not necessarily work for another person or another type of pain. Heat and cold work differently for different people and different pains.

3. Intensity. Heat or cold should be applied at a comfortable level of intensity, not too hot or cold. It should not be painful or uncomfortable. Containers of heat or cold can be wrapped to make them less hot or cold. Moist cloth makes them feel hotter or colder.

4. Precautions with heating. To prevent burns it is safer not to lie on heating devices. Also, use a towel or cloth to soak up sweat beads (moisture) that could increase the temperature, and remove jewelry or other metal objects that come in contact with the heat.

5. Length of time. Heat or cold is usually applied for 20 to 30 minutes. It can be left on longer. The minimal effective time is about 5 to 10 minutes.

6. For better pain relief that lasts longer after the removal of heat or cold, try applying it for a longer period of time, e.g., up to 1 hour. But remember, heat and cold numb the skin to some extent and you won't be as sensitive to the heat or cold. Continuing with heat or applying fresh cold packs must be done carefully to avoid temperatures so cold or hot that skin damage occurs.

7. Site. Heat or cold is usually applied to the site of pain, but if you can't get to the pain site or if it is too tender to touch, heat or cold may be applied in other areas such as:
   - Around the pain site.
   - Between pain and the brain.
   - Beyond the pain, i.e., pain is between the brain and the heat or cold.
   - Opposite side of body corresponding to the pain site (contralaterally).
   - Acupuncture or trigger points. (Your nurse may be able to give you a diagram of these or help you find them.)
   To find the most effective site, experiment with different sites for about 5 minutes each.

8. Many people are reluctant to try cold, but remember:
   - A cold pack, not ice, will be applied.
   - The cold pack can be wrapped sufficiently to prevent an uncomfortable degree of cold. It can be wrapped so well that the first sensation is merely cool, not cold. Then unwrap gradually over a period of minutes, but avoid skin irritation, e.g., redness.
   - If cold causes generalized chilling, be sure to wrap yourself well, e.g., sweater, electric blanket, or cuddle up with a heating pad.
   - Changes in the weather, e.g., cold weather, and dampness often increase pain, but increased pain does not necessarily occur with the local application of cold, i.e., application of cold to a small area.
   - Research shows that cold may be very effective for conditions that are traditionally treated with heat, e.g., low back pain, arthritis.
   - If cold relieves the pain, cold probably will work better than heat because
        It relieves pain faster.
        It relieves more pain.
        Pain relief lasts longer after cold is removed.

9. If pain is severe or if you desire more relief:
   - Interrupt the application. Heat may be taken on and off, or heat and cold may be alternated. Intervals as frequent as 5 seconds or as long as several minutes may be used. Experiment to find your own rhythm.
   - Increase the intensity of heat or cold, but be careful not to cause pain or tissue damage.

■ May be duplicated for use in clinical practice. From McCaffery, M, and Beebe, A: PAIN: CLINICAL MANUAL FOR NURSING PRACTICE, St. Louis, 1989, The CV Mosby Company.

Continued.

===

Patient/Family Teaching Point: Pain Relief with Heat? Cold? Both?—cont'd.

===

10. If you have a muscle or joint injury and if you experience pain relief following use of heat or cold (most likely with cold), be careful not to perform any activities that would cause further injury. However, with proper supervision, therapeutic exercises are commonly recommended following heat or cold.
11. Heat and especially cold decrease skin sensitivity after removal. Be cautious to avoid injuries to the skin after use, since the skin is less able to feel pain and act as a warning signal of impending damage.
12. Oil- or menthol-containing substances may be applied to the skin along with cold, but not with heat since burns can result.
13. Water or moisture with heating is often recommended but must be used cautiously because of the increased risk of burns. (Burns are caused by a high rate of heat transmission to the skin, and water is an excellent conductor of heat.) Dry towels, a poor conductor of heat, may be used over skin to reduce intensity of heat and risk of burn.
14. Whenever possible, use heat or cold before pain occurs or becomes severe.
15. Discontinue use if increased pain or skin irritation occurs.
16. If cold causes chilling or shivering, discontinue.

As a reminder to yourself or those assisting you, fill in the following blanks.

Type of heat or cold: _____

Keep it from being too hot or too cold by: _____

Body site for application: _____

When should it be applied? _____

How long? _____

Precautions: _____

Keep a record of what happened, e.g., when you used it, how well it relieved pain, and any changes you made in how you used it. (For results, you may use a pain rating scale of 0 = no pain and 10 = worst pain, recording pain rating before and after use of heat or cold.)

Date	Time	Results	Any changes?

Instead of the above, you may ask your nurse for the "Daily Diary" form.*

From: _____ (nurse's name)   Phone: _____

*"Daily Diary" form is on p. 30, Chapter 2.

■ May be duplicated for use in clinical practice. From McCaffery, M, and Beebe, A: PAIN: CLINICAL MANUAL FOR NURSING PRACTICE, St. Louis, 1989, The CV Mosby Company.

Nursing Care Guidelines for Selecting and Using Superficial Heat and Cold Applications

The following guidelines along with the patient/family teaching point on pp. 150-151 summarize important aspects of using heat and cold for pain relief.

1. Be open-minded about the possible uses of heat and cold. Preconceived ideas based on experience or education may unnecessarily limit the possible choices considered. Remember also that research on heat and cold is limited and some results are conflicting.

2. Consider possible contraindications before using heat or cold. (The remainder of the guidelines assume that this has been done and, if necessary, discussed with the physician.)

3. In the hospital setting a physician's prescription for heat or cold applications is necessary.

4. As a general rule, for every patient admitted to the hospital it is wise to ask for a prescription for "application of heat or cold anywhere on the body as needed for relief of discomfort." This enables the nurse to respond immediately to any report of pain. Even if other pain relief measures are needed, heat or cold may provide at least some relief in the meantime or provide relief in addition to other methods.

5. Ask the patient if he prefers heat or cold. Prior use and results probably heavily influence this choice. Usually the patient's preference is used initially.

6. Help the patient select a method of heating or cooling that is appropriate, practical, and available (see methods listed on pp. 145-148).

7. If heat has not been effective, encourage the patient to *try cold*. Use the points under Patient/Family Teaching Point: Pain Relief with Heat? Cold? Both? (pp. 150-151).

8. For severe pain suggest intermittent heat or alternating heat and cold.

9. Most methods of applying heat and cold require wrapping with cloth to prevent tissue damage.
   - Moisture or water increase the intensity of the sensation more than dry wrappings (may or may not be desirable).
   - For added convenience, especially for the active or ambulatory patient, applications of heat or cold can be secured in place with plastic bandages or cloth pocket-holders with velcro straps.

Patient Example

About 4 hours following labor and delivery, Ms. M. reported moderate, very bothersome pain from her episiotomy. Otherwise she felt comfortable, energetic, and wanted to go home, but she was concerned about caring for herself and the baby since the discomfort made walking very difficult. She was breast-feeding and did not want to take medication. To secure a cold pack in place and provide sufficient covering to keep it from being uncomfortably cold, a disposable plastic glove was filled with ice and inserted through an opening torn in a small disposable diaper, placing the absorbent side of the dia-

per next to the mother. Panties and a sanitary belt held it in place. For increased comfort and convenience, the nurse suggested to the mother that she purchase two gel packs (about 3 by 10 inches) to keep in the freezer so one would always be ready for use. Ms. M. reported significant pain relief and was ready to be discharged early.

Patient/Family Teaching Points for Use of Heat and Cold

When the patient uses heat or cold or both for pain relief, the considerations covered in the patient/family teaching point in the box on pp. 150-151 should be discussed with him. It is stated in the exact words that may be spoken to the patient, or the list may be duplicated and given to the patient/family who can read.

ICE APPLICATION/MASSAGE

Ice application/massage rapidly relieves pain. The mechanisms underlying the effects of ice application are summarized in the box below.

Methods of ice application/massage. The numerous types and sources of ice make it easy to use. Most methods of applying it or massaging with it are inexpensive. Following are common examples of ways to apply ice:
- *Ice cubes/blocks.* Applied directly to skin, *not* through the barrier of a container. The melting of ice when it is used in direct contact with skin is a safety factor against overchilling. For added safety, use a small surface area

---

Icing:
Possible Mechanisms Underlying Effects

1. *Numbness* or anesthesia of skin may be caused by decrease in nerve conduction velocity.

2. The discomfort of burning and aching may act as *counterirritant,* activating areas in the brainstem which exert inhibitory influences on nerve impulses felt as painful.

3. Pain relief from brief, intense input, such as ice, may *disrupt memory-like processes* caused by prolonged pain, causing pain relief to far outlast the direct effects of ice.

4. *Trigger points* in muscles may be inactivated, resulting in relief of muscle pain or spasm.

5. *Acupuncture points* may be stimulated by ice instead of needling or pressure.

6. Sensation of ice may be felt more strongly by the patient than the pain. Feeling extreme cold may be a distraction or a *"trade-off"* for the pain, perhaps a form of perceptual dominance.

of ice, e.g., the corner of a small ice cube rather than the flat surface of the ice cube. Figures 5-17 and 5-18 show how ice may be made and handled conveniently to avoid chilling the hands.

- *Immersion in water* (useful for buttocks, perineal area, hand, foot, elbow). A container with water and melting ice assures a steady temperature of 0° C.
- *Terry cloth* dipped in water with ice shavings, then rung out and applied rapidly may work for large areas of the body, but must be repeated frequently to maintain freezing temperature.

Caution: the above methods result in an almost instantaneous drop in skin temperature and can cause tissue damage. Muscle temperature drops more slowly, taking longer with thicker layers of fat. In a slender person, muscle temperature may drop after 10 minutes but hardly falls at all in an obese person.

Appropriate/Inappropriate Situations for Ice Application/Massage

Usually the appropriate and inappropriate uses or contraindications for superficial cold also apply to the use of

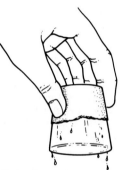

A. Ordinary ice cube in gauze. Anything cloth will work.

B. Ice frozen in paper medicine cup. Peel back paper to expose ice; grasp ice through remaining paper cup.

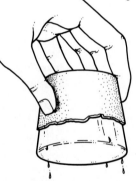

C. Ice frozen in styrofoam cup. Peel back styrofoam to expose ice; grasp ice through remaining styrofoam cup.

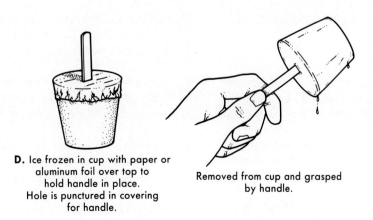

D. Ice frozen in cup with paper or aluminum foil over top to hold handle in place. Hole is punctured in covering for handle.

Removed from cup and grasped by handle.

FIGURE 5-17 Convenient and simple methods of making ice for massage.

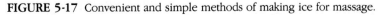

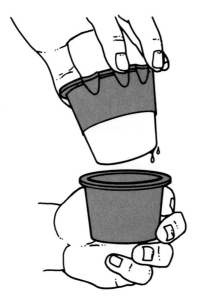

FIGURE 5-18 Cryocup, made of plastic, is an inexpensive, convenient method of using ice for massage. It has several advantages over the usual homemade devices: handle is sturdy enough not to tear in midmassage; handle is thick enough to protect fingers from cold; protrusions inside handle prevent it from falling out as it melts. (Available for about $1.98 from Cryo Therapy, Box 415, Monticello MN 55362-0415.)

ice (see p. 149). When the ice is used for only a few seconds, e.g., immediately prior to an injection, there are essentially no contraindications.

Appropriate uses of ice application/massage:
- Stimulation of trigger points for muscle spasm (see Figures 5-2 to 5-12).
- Stimulation of acupuncture points.
- Acute, but not severe, injuries to reduce bleeding and swelling, e.g., in emergency rooms.
- Myofascial (muscle) pain.
- Stretching muscles that are in spasm, especially using a fluoromethane spray, called "spray and stretch." Consult a physical therapist to determine the correct method for the individual patient.
- Myofibrositis.
- Joint stiffness. (Some studies have shown ice aggravates stiffness; but it may reduce the activity of destructive enzymes such as collagenase, a possible but questionable therapeutic effect for diseases such as rheumatoid arthritis.)
- Tendinitis (ice massage is often considered the treatment of choice).
- Needle sticks, e.g., IM injections, venipuncture (ice at a distance from the needle puncture site or ice pressed into the skin for 15 to 20 seconds immediately before cleaning area).

- Tennis elbow.
- Sports injuries such as sprains and strains.
- Chronic low back pain.
- Acute bursitis.
- Herpes lesions.
- A substitute for TENS or acupuncture, especially for low back pain.
- Tooth pain, and possibly pain anywhere from the neck up. Ice is applied to the hand by immersing the hand in water with melting ice or using ice massage on back of hand at web between thumb and index finger (Hoku point, see Figure 5-14) or between the fourth and fifth fingers.
- Headache. The application site can be the area of localized headache, trigger points (see Figures 5-2, 5-3, 5-4, and 5-6), or an ice cube pressed to the roof of the mouth with the tongue.
- Itching.
- Any painful but brief procedure, especially those lasting 10 minutes or less (see the box on p. 155).

Inappropriate uses of or possible contraindications for ice are:
- Anterior neck (ice on the vagus nerve can slow the heart).
- Newborns up to about age 3 months (ice can coagulate fatty tissue).
- Injuries to the skin, e.g., burn areas.
- Cardiac patient. (Although research on healthy volunteers showed no changes in blood pressure or pulse with use of ice massage, it is wise to check with the physician.)

Nursing Care Guidelines for Ice Application/ Massage

1. Many patients are very reluctant to try ice. Express understanding of the patient's view.
2. Explain carefully why ice may be effective. (See reasons listed in the patient/family teaching point regarding "Ice Application or Massage for Pain Relief," p. 156.)
3. Suggest an appropriate method of ice application, e.g., basin of water with melting ice for immersion of hand.
4. Determine if the patient can use the ice by himself. He may need help in preparing it or applying it, especially if he cannot reach the site.
5. Explain that the initial appearance of skin is *erythema* (redness). This is due to a histamine reaction in the skin and should not be mistaken for skin irritation. Interestingly, vasoconstriction does not cause blanching until later.
6. Stress the importance of avoiding tissue damage by discontinuing ice after 10 minutes or when there is numbness, alternating blanching and dilatation of vessels, or shivering.
7. If the patient desires to use ice massage for longer than 10 minutes, e.g., to get longer lasting relief for low back

---

Ice Massage for Painful Procedures

Any brief but painful procedure, especially one that lasts 10 minutes or less, may be felt as less painful or be better tolerated if ice massage is used.

Examples of procedures are:
Biopsy under local anesthesia.
Bone marrow aspiration.
Catheterization.
Chest tube removal.
Injection into joints.
Lumbar puncture.
Suture removal.

Technique of ice massage for procedures:
1. Begin 1 to 5 minutes prior to the procedure.
2. Apply the ice directly to the skin or through a porous covering.
3. Have a cloth available to wipe up melting ice.
4. Immediately prior to the procedure, if it can be timed appropriately, numb the site of the procedure with ice. Then move to a distant point.
5. Massage with ice at a distance from the site of the procedure, e.g., contralaterally.
6. If the procedure unexpectedly lasts longer than 10 minutes or if ice must be discontinued to prevent tissue damage, try a completely different distant site.
7. If the procedure can be predicted to last longer than 10 minutes, try intermittent ice massage, e.g., 2 minutes of massage followed by a rest period that allows skin to begin to return to normal color. Or, divide the area into several sites and change massage sites every few minutes.

---

pain, suggest dividing the painful area into several sites, massaging each site for 7 minutes, with a 3-minute waiting period between sites, for a total of 30 minutes.

8. Encourage the patient to try various sites distant to the pain, and explain that the brain's picture of the body is not the same as what we see. For example, a point distant from the pain on the surface of the body may be in the area of pain according to the brain's picture of the body.

Patient Examples

At the suggestion of her nurse, one patient with trigeminal neuralgia tried ice cube massage to the web on the back of her hand between the thumb and forefinger and experienced significant relief during her attacks. Two months later she was still successfully using this method. In one research study, a patient who had tried ice cube massage to the opposite hip during a bone marrow aspiration surprisingly found that ice massage to the hip successfully relieved rectal pain from fistulas (Collins,

1985). These are unusual findings, but they point out the wisdom of continuing to search for seemingly unrelated sites that might relieve pain when they are stimulated.

Patient/Family Teaching Points for Use of Ice

When the patient uses ice, discuss with him the patient/family teaching point on p. 156. It is stated in the exact words that may be spoken to the patient, or it may be duplicated and given to the patient or family member who can read.

MENTHOL APPLICATION TO SKIN

A topically applied substance containing menthol is one type of external analgesic and is commonly referred to as a counterirritant. The intent of an external analgesic is not to have an analgesic absorbed through the skin but rather to create a cutaneous sensation, such as warmth or coolness, that may relieve pain by distraction or simply by decreased perception of pain.

Menthol-containing preparations are often used with sports injuries in the United States and are popular home remedies in many cultures throughout the world. Interestingly, very little research has been done on the usefulness of such products.

People are remarkably different in their response to menthol. Menthol probably does not change the skin temperature, but it does produce sensations of temperature change. Some people feel warmth, others feel coolness or cold. Some experience warmth, quickly followed by coolness; others experience the reverse. Increased blood flow may occur to the skin and possibly to the muscles.

Further, menthol products come in different concentrations and in different vehicles (e.g., gels, lotions), both of which influence sensations. Naturally, the more concentrated, the greater the perceived sensations. Usually greater sensations are felt from gels than lotions or ointments. However, strength of the menthol odor is fairly positively correlated with strength of sensation. For a comparison of ingredients, vehicles, and concentrations of menthol, see Table 5-1.

Tiger Balm, not listed in Table 5-1, is a menthol-containing product imported from Singapore. The list of ingredients is extensive and the portions are unclear, but it does have a different odor and sensation than American-made menthol products and is sometimes preferred by Americans. The red variety is stronger than the white. It is popular among those of Asian descent and is available in their specialty stores. Tiger Balm is also available in many health food stores.

Appropriate/Inappropriate Situations for Menthol Application to Skin

Menthol-containing products are nonprescription, and the label usually states that they should be used for the

---

Patient/Family Teaching Point: Ice Application or Massage for Pain Relief

---

TO: _____ (patient's name)   DATE: _____

Using ice to relieve pain may sound questionable at best. It doesn't feel good at the time. In fact, it often hurts briefly. **So why should you try ice for pain relief?** Because:
- Ice may work better and longer than other methods of stimulating the skin.
- Pain relief usually lasts for 1 hour or longer after ice is used. It almost always relieves pain for longer than heat or cold.
- Research has shown that in some conditions pain relief from ice is equal to or better than relief from acupuncture or TENS (transcutaneous electrical nerve stimulation, a relatively expensive, new technique that uses electrodes on the skin to transmit mild electrical impulses).
- Acupuncture and TENS sometimes hurt too.
- The sensations from the ice may override other sensations. The discomfort of the ice may be better than feeling the discomfort of the other pain.

If use of ice is intolerable or ineffective the first time, consider trying it again. It may take several attempts before you find a way to tolerate the cold or before ice produces pain relief.

Two easy and inexpensive ways to apply ice are:
1. Immerse the painful part, e.g., hand, in water with melting ice.
2. Ice cubes or frozen water in cups that can be thrown away, e.g., paper or plastic cup.

Technique of ice massage:
- Ice should be in contact with the skin. Do not cover the ice with anything waterproof. The melting of the ice as it comes in contact with the skin is a safety factor that prevents tissue damage.
- Use a cloth to wipe up melting ice.
- Gently rub the ice on the skin, using circular or back-and-forth motions. Avoid pressure, especially over boney prominences.

How does ice feel? Ice application or massage is uncomfortable. Within 5 to 10 minutes, the sequence of sensations usually felt is: cold, burning, occasionally itching, aching, and numbness. Sometimes the feeling of cold proceeds directly to numbness.

What is the normal skin reaction? Usual changes in skin appearance begin with redness. This may proceed to blanching (white or pale), but at this point icing should not be allowed to proceed much longer.

When should icing be stopped? Discontinue ice if any of the following occur:
- After 10 minutes of constant application.
- Sensation is intolerable.
- Muscle chilling.
- Shivering.
- Numbness.
- "Hunting reaction," alternating blanching and dilatation of vessels (occurs several minutes after blanching). This is called an end-point; further icing may injure the skin.

Avoid injuries after use. The skin is at least partially numb and is unable to send a warning signal of impending damage. Also, underlying muscles may be relieved of pain and care should be taken not to perform physical activities that would injure the muscles. Therapeutic exercises under supervision are, however, frequently recommended.

Apply a hand lotion after ice massage to prevent skin dryness.

From: _____ (nurse's name)   Phone: _____

■ May be duplicated for use in clinical practice. From McCaffery, M, and Beebe, A: PAIN: CLINICAL MANUAL FOR NURSING PRACTICE, St. Louis, 1989, The CV Mosby Company.

TABLE 5-1 Counterirritants: Nonprescription External Analgesic Products

Product and Application Form	Counterirritant Ingredients
Analgesic Balm (ointment)	Methyl salicylate 15% Menthol 15%
Ben-Gay (lotion, greaseless base)	Methyl salicylate 15% Menthol 7%
Ben-Gay Extra Strength Balm (ointment, greaseless base)	Methyl salicylate 30% Menthol 8%
Ben-Gay Gel (hydroalcoholic gel base)	Methyl salicylate 15% Menthol 7%
Ben-Gay Greaseless/Stainless Ointment	Methyl salicylate 15% Menthol 10%
Ben-Gay Original (ointment, oleaginous base)	Methyl salicylate 18.3% Menthol 15%
Icy Hot (balm, lanolin)	Methyl salicylate 29% Menthol 8%
Icy Hot (rub)	Methyl salicylate 12% Menthol 9%
Mentholatum (rub, cream)	Camphor 9% Menthol 1.35%
Mentholatum Deep Heating (rub, greaseless)	Methyl salicylate 12.7% Menthol 6% Eucalyptus oil Turpentine oil
Mentholatum Deep Heating (lotion, greaseless)	Methyl salicylate 20% Menthol 6%

"temporary relief of minor aches and pain of muscles and joints," including simple backache, strains, and sprains. Following is a list of more varied uses.

Appropriate uses of menthol preparations include:
- Arthritis.
- Various pains of muscles, joints, and tendons, e.g., low back pain, tension headache, neck pain, and sports injuries.
- Application to appropriately related acupuncture points or trigger points.
- Visceral pain of various origins, e.g., gas pain, menstrual cramps (there may be some reflex dilatation of visceral vessels).
- Sore throat.
- Itch.

Inappropriate uses of menthol:
- Open wounds.
- Most mucous membranes, especially with high concentration of menthol.
- Over irritated skin.
- If it increases pain.

Patient Example

Mr. F., 67 years old, was terminally ill from cancer but was able to care for himself at home with the assistance of weekly visits from the hospice nurse. He was alert and ambulatory. By adjusting his doses of oral morphine and adding acetaminophen, he was usually comfortable with pain ratings of 0 to 3 on a scale of 0 to 10 (0 = no pain, 10 = worst possible pain). Two types of pain occurred briefly at intervals: (1) low back pain for a few hours in the evening if he had been more active than usual, and (2) mouth pain, about 15 minutes several times a day, from mucositis when he ate and drank certain things. Mr. F. said he had had back pain prior to his current illness and was able to handle it. When the nurse asked how, he looked a little embarrassed as he admitted that he had used Ben-Gay, was using it now, and that it worked very well. The nurse encouraged him to continue this. For the mouth pain, several suggestions were made, including ice cube massage to the web of both hands (see p. 154). The nurse and patient tried it together, each rubbing a web of one hand, but the patient said it didn't seem to work. However, he said he wanted to try it a few more times. On the next home visit, the patient reported trying ice cube massage several times without success, but he proudly said he had found an answer—rubbing Ben-Gay under his chin and over his neck. He said that this worked better than any medications that had been prescribed. (This illustrates that menthol agents may relieve pain in conditions for which they are not ordinarily used and that an open-minded nurse who was willing to encourage Ben-Gay and try the uncommonly used ice cube massage seemed to encourage open-mindedness and a sense of control in the patient.)

Nursing Care Guidelines and Patient/Family Teaching Points for Application of Menthol

The labels of menthol-containing products are required to have appropriate warnings, so most of the time the nurse can use the label for patient teaching purposes. Following are points to consider and discuss with the patient/family regarding use of menthol-containing products:

1. Initiate conversation with the patient about menthol products. Many people tend to regard them as unscientific and may hesitate to ask about using them, especially in the hospital.
2. Ask the patient if he has ever used a menthol product, naming a popular one as an example (e.g., Ben-Gay) so the patient knows what you mean. In particular, ask if he used any menthol product as a child. For many adults the mere odor evokes comforting childhood memories of the mother rubbing a menthol product on the chest and throat for upper respiratory infections.
3. If the patient has never tried the particular brand of menthol or has not tried it for this particular pain, test the skin first to determine what the patient feels and how the skin responds. Simply rub a small amount into a small area and wait a few minutes. Point out that the sensation lasts for an hour or more.
4. If the patient experiences an unpleasant burning sensation, avoid gels, massage, excessive quantities, high concentrations, and application after heating the skin,

e.g., after a hot shower. On the other hand, if increased sensation is desired, one or more of these methods may be used.

5. Avoid contact with eyes and be cautious of using high concentrations of menthol on any mucous membrane.

6. Menthol is usually applied three to four times a day. If the patient fears others will object to the odor, suggest use at nighttime or whenever the patient is alone.

7. If aspirin is contraindicated, e.g., due to allergy or bleeding problems, avoid preparations containing salicylate.

8. Do not apply a tight bandage over menthol; this could produce skin irritation.

9. Extreme caution is advised if menthol preparations are used along with heating devices. Severe burning or blistering of the skin may occur. Cold, however, is often applied over menthol, especially for sports injuries.

10. If allergy or skin irritation occurs, try a greaseless preparation—some people are allergic to lanolin.

11. Discontinue if a rash, blister, or excessive skin irritation occurs.

TRANSCUTANEOUS ELECTRICAL NERVE STIMULATION (TENS)

Transcutaneous electrical nerve stimulation is commonly referred to as TENS (pronounced like the number ten with an "s" for the plural). TENS is a method of applying controlled, low-voltage electricity to the body via electrodes placed on the skin. Most TENS units are small, portable, and battery operated, consisting of three major parts: (1) box with energy source, (2) lead wires, and (3) electrodes (two or more electrodes may be used). These three components with two electrodes placed on an adult body are illustrated in Figure 5-19.

The sensation felt by the patient from TENS is usually described as tingling or vibrating; however, some settings produce discomfort. TENS stimulation may be constant or intermittent.

The primary purpose of TENS is to relieve pain, either while natural healing takes place, e.g., postoperatively, or to enable appropriate therapy to be used, e.g., stretching and strengthening muscles to alleviate the source of chronic low back pain. It is a safe, noninvasive method of pain relief that is easy to use under the guidance of specially trained health professionals. The success rate of TENS varies. For relief of chronic nonmalignant pain, estimates of good results range from 20% to 40%; for relief of postoperative incisional pain, 70% to 90%.

TENS must be prescribed by a physician, but treatment with TENS is usually administered by physical therapists or registered nurses who have had special education in the use of TENS. The success of TENS is strongly dependent upon the skill of the person administering it. The administration of TENS, regardless of which health team member does it, is now a specialty area. Thus it is highly

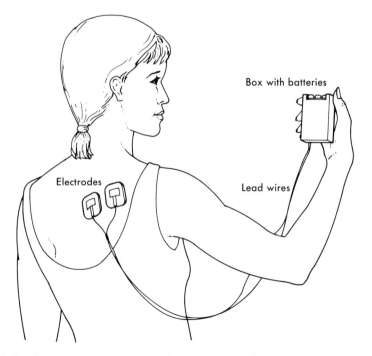

FIGURE 5-19 Three major components of a TENS unit with two electrodes placed on the upper back of the patient to relieve shoulder pain. This shows the size of the TENS unit in relation to an adult body, illustrating that it is small and portable.

recommended that the person administering TENS have specific education and experience in the complexities of this treatment, such as electrode placement, stimulation modes, and appropriate adjunctive therapies. It is beyond the scope of this book to provide such instruction. For a comprehensive guide to the use of TENS, the reader is referred to Mannheimer and Lampe, 1984.

The purpose of this section on TENS is limited to assisting the nurse to obtain sufficient knowledge to do the following:

- Know when it is appropriate to *recommend* TENS for pain relief.
- *Discuss its use, limits, and potential problems* with health team members and patients/families.
- Suggest *resources for assisting* the health team and patient/family with TENS.

The *mechanisms* underlying the effectiveness of TENS in relieving pain are unclear. Since there are several distinctly different electrical stimulation modes and many different methods of electrode placement, it is likely that different methods of TENS provide pain relief by different mechanisms. Some types of TENS, but not all, appear to relieve pain at least in part by increasing the patient's endorphin, or natural morphine. Another explanation is that TENS acts as a counterirritant, masking the pain or activating a complex neural inhibitory system that alleviates more intense or prolonged pain at near or distant sites.

Appropriate/Inappropriate Uses of TENS

Although TENS is no panacea, the indications for TENS are almost limitless as long as the pain is reasonably well localized. This makes it virtually impossible to list all the painful conditions that might be relieved by TENS. However, TENS is not an alternative to the diagnosis and appropriate treatment of the underlying cause of pain, nor does it usually replace all other methods of pain relief. *Common appropriate uses of TENS* may be divided into the three following but somewhat overlapping categories, accompanied by examples that are also somewhat overlapping:

1. *TENS along with physical therapy,* i.e., TENS as one part of a comprehensive program of pain management aimed at rehabilitation of the patient with musculoskeletal problems. TENS is usually used to prevent or break the three-part pain cycle, consisting of pain (#1) leading to muscle spasm and guarding (#2), leading to dysfunction (#3), leading to more pain (#1), as shown in Figure 5-20. TENS relieves pain so that muscles can receive appropriate therapy, e.g., stretching and strengthening exercises, and so that function can be restored automatically or with assistance, e.g., proper body mechanics. Examples of conditions in which TENS is used for pain relief along with appropriate physical therapy are:

- Stimulation of trigger points or acupuncture points related to musculoskeletal problems.
- Back pain, chronic or acute.
- Sciatic pain.
- Arthritis, e.g., wrist pain of rheumatoid arthritis.
- Temporomandibular joint (TMJ) syndrome.
- Cervical spine pain postlaminectomy.
- Neck pain, e.g., chronic cervical strain, whiplash.

2. *Analgesia for acute pain in which the underlying disorder will more or less spontaneously resolve,* e.g., healing of postoperative incisional pain or periodic migraine. These are often conditions that ordinarily require analgesics such as aspirin or a narcotic. TENS may be used to provide part or all of the pain relief. Examples include:
- Postoperative pain.
- Trauma typically seen in emergency rooms, especially when medications are withheld pending medical evaluation.
- Fractured ribs.
- Under the cast covering a fractured bone.

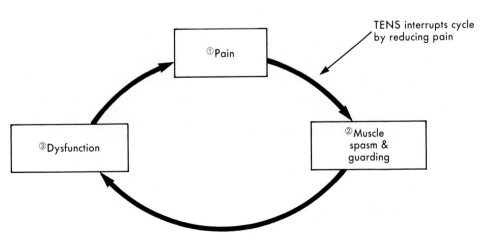

FIGURE 5-20 The three-part pain cycle. TENS interrupts this cycle by relieving pain.

- Prior to painful dressing changes.
- Thrombophlebitis.
- Pancreatitis.
- Phantom limb pain.
- Cancer pain (research is very limited in this area, but if pain is localized, even if the patient is on narcotics, TENS may be helpful).
- Headache due to tension, fever, hangover, or sinus conditions; possibly migraine and cluster headaches.
- Dysmenorrhea (menstrual pain).
- When narcotics are contraindicated, e.g., allergy to narcotics, desire of recovering substance abuser to abstain, during pregnancy or childbirth, a nursing mother following cesarean section.
- Itch.

3. *Prevention and treatment of ileus,* e.g., following surgery or spinal cord injury, and possibly related problems such as delayed or sluggish gut activity following surgery or constipation from various causes, including narcotics. Placement of electrodes is usually over the anterior abdominal wall, e.g., the ascending or descending colon (Figure 5-21). The stimulation mode is often the same as that for postoperative pain, and it is continued

until the patient expels flatus (see Richardson, Meyer, and Raimondi, 1979, in annotated reference section).

Possibly inappropriate uses of TENS, or situations in which precautions are warranted, include:

- In the presence of a cardiac pacemaker, especially a demand pacemaker.
- Over the carotid sinuses (front and sides of the throat) because of a possible hypotensive effect secondary to a vasovagal reflex.
- Over the eyes. However, electrodes may be placed on the boney orbit of the eye.
- Head and neck regions in patients with vascular or seizure disorders. These patients should at least be monitored carefully.
- Over burns or open wounds (electrodes can, of course, be placed nearby).
- Over skin that is already irritated, e.g., dryness or rash.
- Internal use, e.g., mouth or vagina. Mucosal linings probably would not tolerate the electrical stimulation.
- Anterior chest wall in cardiac problems (until more is known about the effects of this).
- Pregnancy, possibly. However, TENS has been used successfully without complications for pain during labor and delivery and in pregnant women for back pain resulting from a fall.
- As a substitute for appropriate medication or other therapy.
- Incompetent patient. The patient should at least be carefully monitored and safety precautions taken, e.g., securing the settings for electrical output.

Special attention needs to be directed toward the appropriateness of TENS for a *patient who is already taking narcotics.* Some studies have revealed that postoperative use of TENS significantly reduces the narcotic intake of patients who have not used narcotics preoperatively but does not reduce postoperative narcotic intake of those who used narcotics preoperatively (Solomon, Viernstein, and Long, 1980). However, not only are there few studies on this subject, but the studies of postoperative TENS are not well controlled enough to be considered conclusive.

One major flaw in some studies of postoperative TENS is that the measure of effectiveness of TENS is not based on patients' ratings of pain but is based on the amount of narcotic required or given. This does not accurately reflect the amount of pain the patient may have had. Patients with significant pain may not request narcotics, and those who request them may not receive them. Thus it is possible that patients who used narcotics prior to surgery are more comfortable or assertive about requesting narcotics, while those who have not taken narcotics may fail to request them due to exaggerated and unrealistic fears about the dangers of narcotics.

Further, several studies have been done using postoperative TENS on patients who more than likely took narcotics preoperatively, e.g., patients who had low back surgery, knee surgery, and hip replacement (a procedure

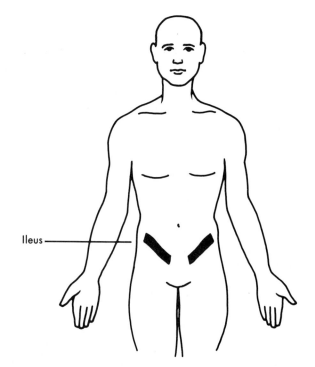

FIGURE 5-21 Treatment of ileus with TENS. Electrodes are placed over the ascending or descending colon.

Redrawn with permission from Mannheimer, JS, and Lampe, GN: Clinical transcutaneous electrical nerve stimulation, p. 520, Philadelphia, 1984, F.A. Davis Co.

almost always done solely for pain relief). These studies have shown that TENS reduced postoperative narcotic intake compared to control groups who did not have TENS (Pike, 1978; Schuster and Infante, 1980; Stabile and Mallory, 1978). Further, several clinical reports state that TENS is helpful for cancer pain (Mannheimer and Lampe, 1984), and these patients also are likely to have received narcotics prior to TENS use.

KEY POINT: There is insufficient evidence to automatically conclude that TENS will be ineffective for a patient who is or has been taking narcotics. A trial of TENS is warranted.

One final point in rebuttal to avoiding TENS if the patient is taking narcotics is that not all TENS relieves pain by increasing endorphins. Patients taking narcotics may develop tolerance to narcotic analgesia. Some have argued that if TENS relieves pain by increasing endorphins, the patient on narcotics may be tolerant to this analgesia as well. However, in some studies pain relief from TENS is not reversible by naloxone, a narcotic antagonist (Hansson, Ekblom, Thomsson, and Fjellner, 1986). Some types of TENS apparently relieve pain by mechanisms other than increasing endorphins, and therefore it is at least theoretically possible for TENS to provide effective pain relief for patients who are tolerant to narcotics.

Nursing Care Guidelines for General Use of TENS

1. Recommend TENS as early as possible, e.g., preoperatively for postoperative pain, or immediately following a musculoskeletal injury before pain becomes chronic.
2. A physician's prescription is necessary for the use of TENS.
3. Identify an "expert" resource person who can assist the health team and patient/family. One or more of the following may be appropriate:
   - Within the hospital, one person or one department, e.g., physical therapy or pain management, is usually responsible for TENS units and treatment.
   - For use in any setting, especially outpatient, contact the manufacturer of the TENS unit. Most major manufacturers have specially trained people, e.g., nurses or physical therapists, who will assist health team members or patient/families by coming to the physician's office, the hospital, an outpatient clinic, or the patient's home. They will provide initial instruction and follow-up. Currently, three major manufacturers of TENS who offer these services, only a phone call away, are:
     Dynex
     La Jolla Technology, Inc.
     11558 Sorrento Valley Rd.
     San Diego, CA 92121
     (619) 481-9488; outside California (800) 854-1915; inside California (800) 233-4899.

Medtronic, Inc.
6951 Central Ave. N.E.
P.O. Box 1250
Minneapolis, MN 55440
(612) 572-5000 or (800) 328-0810.
3M Medical-Surgical Division
Bldg. 225-5S
3M Center
St. Paul, MN 55144-1000
In Minnesota (800) 742-5685, ext. 8938; outside Minnesota (800) 328-5727, ext. 8938.

4. Thorough patient/family teaching is essential to the success of TENS. When the patient receives a TENS unit, be sure to request that the patient also be given written instructions, whether the patient is in or out of the hospital.
5. The most common, although not frequent, complication of TENS is an adverse skin reaction. This may be caused by a variety of factors such as electrical reactions or irritation from electrode gels or adhesive tape. Simple measures, such as altering electrode sites or using cortisone cream, usually alleviate the problem.
6. If the patient has problems using the TENS unit, all of the following are logical options:
   - Contact the resource person from the hospital or manufacturer.
   - Consult the written instructions. Most patients who are using TENS units have received written instructions developed by the resource person or the manufacturer. Ask the patient for these instructions, suggest that he review them, and offer to go over them with the patient/family, if time permits.
   - If all efforts to resolve the problem fail, suggest that TENS be discontinued until assistance is found.
7. If the patient asks about the cost of TENS, investigate the specific situation, keeping in mind the following:
   - The hospitalized patient will be billed separately for use of TENS.
   - When TENS is used on an outpatient basis for chronic pain, the usual recommendation is that a unit not be purchased until treatment has been successful for 30 to 60 days. Most third-party providers reimburse about 80% of the rental and purchase cost.

Nursing Care Guidelines for Use of TENS Postoperatively

The use of TENS is now so sophisticated that it has become a specialty area. However, one type of TENS use that the nurse needs to be very familiar with, if it is used in her clinical area, is postoperative TENS. Operating room nurses are involved in application of TENS, and recovery room nurses usually connect and turn on the unit. On the clinical unit the nurse is the only health team member immediately available to the patient 24 hours a day as he uses the TENS unit during his recovery.

Instructions about the particular TENS unit and guidelines for its use from the preoperative through the postoperative period usually can be obtained either from the inhouse person/department resource or the manufacturer. The nurse may not be responsible for preoperative teaching, but she should be knowledgeable enough to answer the patient's questions about TENS, be supportive of its use, and check to see that appropriate preoperative teaching has been done. Postoperatively, the nurse may need to remind the patient to use TENS or increase stimulation for painful events and be able to troubleshoot common problems.

Following is an overview of how TENS is initiated and used for postoperative pain, including nursing responsibilities in the operating room and recovery room.*

Contraindications

1. Cardiac pacemakers.
2. Application over a pregnant uterus.
3. Senility.
4. Application over the carotid sinus.

Preoperative Procedure

1. Provide a written information/education form for the patient relative to the postoperative use of TENS.
2. Surgical shave prep should be done with extreme caution to avoid any skin abrasions or irritation that could eliminate the patient as a candidate for the TENS program.
3. Explain the TENS program to the patient as it relates to his or her surgery.
4. Instruct the patient in the operation of the TENS unit, and give the patient the appropriate operational manual.
5. Inform the patient that TENS will be used for approximately 3 to 5 days unless otherwise ordered by the physician.
6. Note the parameter settings that are comfortable to the patient, and record them on the postoperative data sheet in the chart.

Operating Room Procedure

1. The circulating nurse should observe the patient's skin very carefully before and after the surgical scrub prep. Scrubbing with a stiff-bristled brush is not recommended.
2. If an iodine-based prep is used, the skin must be thoroughly rinsed prior to the application of the sterile postoperative electrodes.

*The material about postoperative use of TENS is copyrighted as Lampe, J, and Meyer, D: Postoperative T.E.N.S. analgesia: protocol, methods, results, and benefit, Kansas City, 1978, Pain Control Services, Inc. Recently the material, along with additional information, was published in Mannheimer, JS, and Lampe, GN: Clinical transcutaneous electrical nerve stimulation, pp 514-515, Philadelphia, 1984, FA Davis Company. It is reprinted here with permission from Gerald N. Lampe.

3. The circulating nurse will peel the outer package open so that the scrub nurse can receive the sterile inner package, which contains two sterile electrodes with attached lead wires.
4. The physician or the scrub nurse will place the self-adhesive electrodes parallel to the incision approximately 2 to 3 inches away from the sutures. *The electrodes should not touch each other.* Press gently around the border of pregelled electrodes to establish skin adhesion and avoid pressure on the center of the electrode. Karaya and polymer electrodes should be pressed from center to border to ensure total electrode contact and adhesion.
5. Wound dressings should be applied allowing the electrode lead wires to protrude from under the dressing.

Recovery Room Procedure

1. Plug the lead wires into the adapter, or appropriate receptacle, which is then attached to the TENS unit.
2. Adjust the amplitude, rate, and/or pulse width (some units may have only one or two external, independent variables) to the predetermined settings indicated on the postoperative data sheet in the chart.
3. When the patient is awake and alert, readjust the amplitude within the patient's tolerance and comfort.
4. Keep the TENS unit on continuously, unless otherwise ordered.
5. Check the settings on the generator frequently in the event they might have been inadvertently adjusted.
6. Within 8 to 12 hours, the patient's skin should be checked for rash or irritation (slight redness is normal). This is done by lifting a corner of the electrode and looking under the pad.
7. The patient should be encouraged to vary the TENS output amplitude since the level of discomfort varies.

Postoperative Surgical Floor Procedure

1. The physician should leave a standing order for TENS to be discontinued immediately if any complications develop.
2. Normal length of usage is 3 to 5 days.
3. The skin should be checked every 12 hours for rash or irritation. This is done by lifting a corner of the electrode and looking under the pad.
4. Depending on the sterile electrode materials employed and the conditions of the patient's skin or incision, electrodes may require replacement during recovery. If the conducting medium should dry out or the electrodes come loose, stimulation will be uncomfortable, indicating a need to secure or change the electrodes.
5. If replacing the electrodes is necessary, place each one parallel to the incision, approximately 2 to 3 inches from the sutures. If any skin irritation is present and stimulation is to be continued, place the electrodes at alternate sites parallel to the suture line to avoid the irritation.

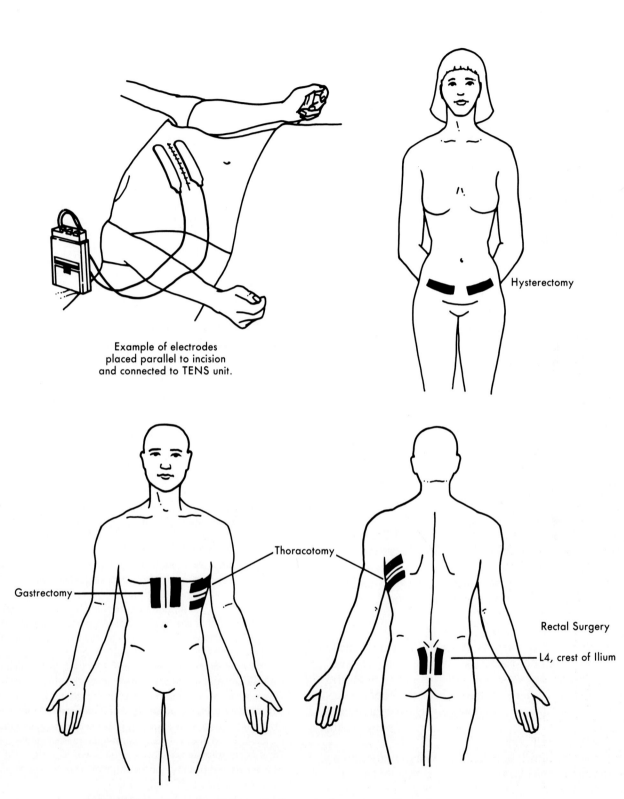

Example of electrodes
placed parallel to incision
and connected to TENS unit.

Hysterectomy

Gastrectomy

Thoracotomy

Rectal Surgery

L4, crest of Ilium

FIGURE 5-22 Examples of electrode placement for postoperative pain.
Redrawn with permission from Mannheimer, JS, and Lampe, GN: Clinical transcutaneous electrical nerve stimulation, pp.
518-522, Philadelphia, 1984, F.A. Davis Co.

6. The patient should reset the amplitude knob to a comfortable effective setting.
7. Increase generator output prior to coughing and increased physical activity, which may increase noxious input.
8. Chart on the postoperative analgesia record all pertinent information relative to the use of TENS throughout the recovery period.

The flow sheet on p. 27 may be used to record hourly pain ratings given by the patient, along with analgesic requirements and any problems. This can serve as the postoperative analgesia record referred to above.

Placement of electrodes for postoperative pain varies somewhat, but electrodes are often placed parallel to the incision, about 1 inch or more from the incision (Figure 5-22).

Nursing Care Guidelines and Patient/Family Teaching Points for Use of TENS in the Home

TENS is most often used on an outpatient basis for chronic pain problems, especially chronic nonmalignant pain such as back or neck pain. Sometimes TENS is used for chronic cancer pain.

Once again, unless the nurse has had specialized education in the use of TENS, the nurse is not expected to instruct the patient or provide follow-up in the home for the use of TENS. However, if the nurse is caring for a patient in or out of the hospital who is using TENS on an outpatient basis or is a candidate for this, the nurse will need to know enough about TENS to identify the patient's needs and obtain appropriate assistance.

If TENS is not relieving the patient's pain, probably the most important nursing actions are:

• Help the patient obtain assistance from a TENS specialist/resource person associated with the hospital or the manufacturer.
• Offer to review with the patient his written home instructions. These instructions usually provide the following information:
  Basic operation and care of the unit.
  Sites for electrode placement. Figure drawings usually show electrode placement, and often alternate sites for electrode placement (alternate sites might be used when other sites do not provide relief).
  Stimulation modes. TENS units usually have three dials that can be adjusted: (1) pulse rate, (2) pulse width, and (3) amplitude.
• If for any reason it is difficult to obtain written home instructions, refer to pp. 239-244 of Mannheimer and Lampe's 1984 book, and ask the TENS specialist if these can be adapted for the patient.
• Encourage the patient to continue to try, under supervision, various stimulation modes and electrode placements. For some patients, numerous attempts may be necessary before an effective approach is found.
  Stimulation modes and electrode placement for

chronic pain are extremely complicated and should be carefully determined by a health professional with special education in this. To illustrate the complexity of electrode placement, chronic low back pain may be treated with four or more electrodes connected to two different channels originating from the same battery-operated power source, placed on the site of pain as well as distant sites.

SELECTED ANNOTATED REFERENCES THAT CITE RESEARCH OR GIVE CLINICAL SUPPORT

Many of the noninvasive pain relief measures, such as cutaneous stimulation, have not yet been adequately researched. This sometimes makes it difficult to document or justify the use of these techniques. The following brief, annotated list provides some clinical or research support for use of cutaneous stimulation techniques as discussed in this chapter.

Bini, G, Cruccu, K-EH, Schady, W, and Torebjork, E: Analgesic effect of vibration and cooling on pain induced by intraneural electrical stimulation, *Pain* 18:239-248, 1984. Moderate or intense pain was experimentally produced by electrical stimulation in volunteers to examine the pain relieving effects of 20 to 60 seconds of vibration, pressure, cooling, or warming within or near the painful area of skin. The most effective results were obtained for moderate pain when vibration was applied within the area of pain. Pressure and cooling provided some pain relief, but mild warming produced inconsistent results. Vibration was applied contralaterally in only four subjects and was not effective. Sometimes vibration used for intense pain merely changed the sensation from sharp to dull.

Collins, PM: Contralateral ice massage during bone marrow aspiration, Masters thesis, University of Miami, June 1985. Ten patients received contralateral ice massage during one bone marrow aspiration (BMA) and a control treatment of an EKG patch during another BMA. Ice wrapped in a piece of gauze was gently massaged on the contralateral iliac crest beginning 5 minutes prior to the injection of the local anesthetic and continued until the completion of the procedure. Six of the ten patients had less pain with ice massage than with the EKG patch; one said both the ice and the patch helped; two said neither helped; one replied that the patch helped. An incidental finding was that one patient with a very painful rectal fistula said the ice massage decreased this pain, and he continued ice massage to the hip periodically on his own for his rectal pain.

Cooling more effective, *Aches & Pains* 3:37, 1982. In 100 patients with rheumatoid arthritis and knee pain, a heating or cooling device was placed around one knee for 20 minutes twice a day. Patients preferred heat, probably because of the initial discomfort of cold, but cooling produced more pain relief.

Ekblom, A, and Hansson, P: Extrasegmental transcutaneous electrical nerve stimulation and mechanical vibratory stimulation as compared to placebo for the relief of acute oro-facial pain, *Pain* 23:223-229, 1985. Only 10 of the 30 patients receiving actual stimulation (low frequency TENS of 2 Hz, high frequency TENS of 100 Hz, or 100 Hz vibration) to the Hoku point reported pain relief. However, several patients spontaneously reported paresthesia and/or anesthesia from the stimulated hand area. Vibration showed a slight tendency toward relieving orofacial pain in a larger number of patients than did either form of TENS.

INDIVIDUALIZED NURSING CARE PLAN

Patient Who May Benefit from Cutaneous Stimulation

Patient Description: Ms. B., age 26 years, an assembly-line worker at a toy factory, sees the industrial nurse about 45 minutes after reporting to work that morning. She says she awoke today with severe neck pain on the right side, radiating down the right arm and increasing with neck movement. These are the same symptoms she had 2 years ago following a work-related injury. With daily exercises under the supervision of a physical therapist she has continued work without medication. She thinks the current episode is due to a new work assignment in which her neck is bent forward for longer periods of time. She took acetaminophen 1000 mg and ibuprofen 800 mg 1½ hours ago and has only slight relief. Ms. B. is afraid the pain will worsen and is very upset about missing work. She has an appointment to see her physician that afternoon. Before she sends Ms. B. home for the remainder of the day, the nurse wants to help her obtain better pain relief and reduce some of her anxiety about her pain. The nurse checks with the physician who says cutaneous stimulation in the form of heat, cold, or ice may be used as needed until he sees Ms. B.

Assessment	Potential Nursing Diagnoses	Planning/Intervention	Evaluation/Expected Outcomes

Identify:
• Pain rating on a scale of 0 to 10 (0 = no pain, 10 = worst possible pain)
• Which methods of cutaneous stimulation were used previously and the results
• Which method the patient prefers to use now
• Which methods are available in the nurse's office and the patient's home
• Whether or not the patient is willing to try cold or ice if these have not been used before
• Whether or not the neck is too tender to apply stimulation directly to the neck
• Which stimulation sites were used previously and the results
	Pain, related to neck injury
	Anxiety related to pain and loss of income
	Activity intolerance related to pain
		Emphasize belief in patient's statements of severity of pain and limitations on activity.
		Explain that heat, cold, or ice probably will relieve the pain but only temporarily.
		Prevent further injury by advising the patient not to try to stretch or exercise the neck or do anything that increases pain until she has seen her physician and physical therapist.
		Explain that the underlying cause of the neck pain must be diagnosed and treated, emphasizing the following:
		  • The need for Ms. B. to be seen by her physician and physical therapist and to have her regular exercises reevaluated.
		  • That her work area will be evaluated for possible changes in the physical setup, and appropriate body mechanics will be reviewed when she returns to work.
		With the patient's consent, first apply a well-wrapped cold pack over the area of neck pain and another cold pack on the right arm if desired.
		Encourage the patient to allow the nurse to massage the right side of the neck with ice for about 10 min. If this relieves pain, suggest that patient find someone to do this for her (rather than strain her left arm trying to do it for herself).
		If ice or cold is effective explain to the patient how to make these at home (see Fig. 5-17 and pp. 146-147).
		If the site of pain on the right side of the neck is too tender to touch, apply a cold pack or ice massage to the left side of the neck, the right side of the head above the pain, the area surrounding the pain, and/or the right arm, explaining that stimulation of distant sites has been known to relieve pain, perhaps by distraction.
			Patient reports one or more of the following:
			• Decreased pain rating
			• Sensation is not as sharp and shooting, is more dull
			• Sensation of cutaneous stimulation, e.g., cold or menthol, distracts from pain
			• Confidence in ability to relieve pain both now and during rehabilitation
			• Optimism about returning to work soon and trying methods to prevent or relieve pain while at work
			Patient follows through with appointments with physician and physical therapist
			When she returns to work, she makes an appointment to see the nurse

Continued.

INDIVIDUALIZED NURSING CARE PLAN—cont'd.

Patient Who May Benefit from Cutaneous Stimulation—cont'd.

Assessment	Potential Nursing Diagnoses	Planning/Intervention	Evaluation/ Expected Outcomes
		Since arm and neck movement is limited by pain, suggest that for convenience at home alone the patient may alternate heat and cold packs placed on other sites found to be effective.	
		Explain to the patient how to probe for trigger points likely to be in the area of pain (see Fig. 5-9) and use pressure and/or massage with fingers or a tennis ball for pain relief (see p. 143).	
		Suggest how someone else could use a hand-held vibrator for about 25 min to the right side of the neck (pp. 144-145) if it is not too tender.	
		Explain that menthol-containing products may be used alone or in combination with cold packs.	
		Tell the patient how to avoid tissue damage associated with heat, cold, or ice massage.	
		Suggest that when she returns to work that a convenient method of pain relief while she is working might be TENS and that she should ask her physical therapist about this.	
		Suggest that the patient continue analgesics on a regular basis, e.g., q4h for acetaminophen and q6h for ibuprofen, until advised otherwise by her physician.	
		Plan follow-up with the patient, e.g., a phone call later that day and an appointment with the nurse on the day she returns to work.	

Gammon, BD, and Starr, I: Studies on the relief of pain by counterirritation, *J Clin Invest* **20**:13-20, Jan 1941. This report on several experiments continues to be cited as a basic reference in the literature on cutaneous stimulation. Selected findings are as follows. The *most effective intensity* of counterirritation was slightly less than that which produced discomfort. After the application of a counterirritant and after it was removed, there was often a period of sharp, but transient, increase in pain followed by pain relief. Relative *effectiveness of counterirritants* in descending order: cold (4° to 10° C), electrical stimulation (single shocks sufficient to cause muscle twitching), heat (40° C), tactile stimulation (rubbing with cotton or scratching with wooden edge), vibration, and air jet. However, sometimes heat or cold would relieve one pain and exaggerate another. In other cases both heat and cold were equally effective. By far the *greatest relief,* even for severe discomfort, was attained by interrupted counterirritation, consisting of a rhythm of approximately 5 seconds of application and 10 seconds without. When patients chose their own rhythms with heat and cold, the majority preferred alternating heat and cold or intermittent heat without cold. Intervals selected were generally about 40 seconds of heat and 30 seconds without it. The patients always preferred heat or cold to electrical or tactile counterirritation. The most effective *site of stimulation* for pain in the arm was over the pain, followed by a site 6 inches proximal to the painful area along the course of the nerve supplying it. Less but clearly detectable relief occurred with counterirritation distal to the pain, the back, or the contralateral arm.

Hansson, P, Ekblom, A, Thomsson, M, and Fjellner, B: Influence of naloxone on relief of acute oro-facial pain by transcutaneous electrical nerve stimulation (TENS) or vibration, *Pain*

24:323-329, 1986. Out of 28 patients with orofacial pain, 20 reported pain reduction during 100 Hz vibratory stimulation, low-frequency (2 Hz) TENS, or high-frequency (100 Hz) TENS. Application site was the skin overlying the painful area. This pain relief was *not* influenced by naloxone in 19 of the 20 patients. A review of research shows somewhat contradictory results regarding the naloxone reversibility of pain relief obtained with afferent stimulation, such as acupuncture and high frequency TENS. Relief of chronic pain from low-frequency TENS appears more likely to be reversed by naloxone, but not always. Thus pain relief from vibration or TENS is not necessarily mediated by opioid mechanisms.

Heng, MCY: Local necrosis and interstitial nephritis due to topical methyl salicylate and menthol, *Cutis* **39**:442-444, May 1987. A case report of a 62-year-old man illustrates the danger of using heat over the topical application of methyl salicylate and menthol. Used alone, these topical applications seldom cause significant problems; but combined with heat, skin necrosis and other complications may result. This particular patient suffered full-thickness skin and muscle necrosis as well as persistent interstitial nephritis following 15 to 20 minutes of heat over topical applications of Ben-Gay on several areas of his body, including both legs and arms.

Hillman, H, and Jarman, D: Freezing skin, *Nurs Times* **82**:40-41, May 1986. Immediately after a cube of ordinary ice was applied with slight pressure for 15 to 20 seconds to the upper arm of 10 subjects, sensations of touch and sharpness in the skin in that area were reduced. This use of ice was suggested as an inexpensive and safe way to decrease the discomfort of needle injections, e.g., IV or IM.

Hillman, SK, and Delforge, G: The use of physical agents in rehabilitation of athletic injuries. In Harvey, JS, ed: Rehabilitation of the injured athlete, *Clin Sports Med* **4**:431-438, July 1985. It is a common misconception that heat is invariably appropriate after 24 or 48 hours following an acute soft tissue injury. Application of cold, especially prior to therapeutic exercise, is recommended to reduce edema that commonly occurs when active exercise is used early in the recovery period, as is often done with athletes to avoid delay in return to competition.

Kunesch, E, Schmidt, R, Nordin, M, Wallin, U, and Hagbarth, K-E: Peripheral neural correlates of cutaneous anaesthesia induced by skin cooling in man, *Acta Physiol Scand* **129**:247-257, Feb 1987. Cooling of the skin by ice application for 3 to 5 minutes or by ethyl chloride spray for about 10 seconds resulted in "needle" or "sharpness" sensations being felt as blunt. Sensations for sharpness and pain did not fully return for 2 to 5 minutes.

Lehmann, JF, and de Lateur, BJ: Cryotherapy. In Lehmann, JF, ed: Therapeutic heat and cold, ed 3, pp 563-602, Baltimore, 1982, Williams & Wilkins. This is an extensive review of the therapeutic uses of local applications of cold, cryotherapy. Cold applications reduce *muscle spasm* secondary to underlying skeletal and joint pathology or nerve root irritation by breaking the cycle of secondary muscle spasm, ischemia, pain, and more muscle spasm. Arthritic joints are also treated with cold to reduce inflammation and pain. Cold produces an almost instantaneous drop in skin temperature with a slow reduction of muscle temperature, depending on thickness of subcutaneous fat. To reduce muscle temperature, cooling for a slender person should last longer than 10 minutes; for an obese person, longer than 30 minutes. When the muscle temperature does drop, it takes a long time to rewarm because the fat layer acts as an insulator. By contrast, a warmed muscle resumes normal temperature within a few minutes. Cold packs applied to the abdomen produce an increase in *peristalsis* in the stomach, small bowel, and colon.

Lehmann, JF, and de Lateur, BJ: Therapeutic heat. In Lehmann, JF, ed: Therapeutic heat and cold, ed 3, pp 404-562, Baltimore, 1982, Williams & Wilkins. This extensive review of the uses of heat includes the following information. The effect of heat on the contralateral extremity is referred to as *consensual reaction.* Heating the skin of one extremity increases the blood flow to that extremity and also the contralateral extremity but to a lesser degree. The degree of this reflex response is in proportion to the intensity of heat and the area of skin affected. When the skin of the abdominal wall is heated, e.g., with hot water bottles, within 5 to 10 minutes there is a reflex *reduction in blood flow to the mucous membranes of the stomach and intestines* along with relaxation of smooth muscle and a reduction in peristalsis and gastric acidity. *Contrast bathing,* a method of alternating heat and cold, results in increased blood flow and decreased joint stiffness. Initially the limb is immersed for 10 minutes in hot water (approximately 40° C, 104° F), followed by 1 minute in cold water (approximately 15° C, 59° F). Then 4 minutes in hot water and 1 minute in cold water is repeated for a total treatment time of 30 minutes.

Lundeberg, T, Nordemar, R, and Ottoson, D: Pain alleviation by vibratory stimulation, *Pain* **20**:25-44, 1984. In this study of 366 patients with acute or chronic musculoskeletal pain of various origins, 69% reported pain relief during vibratory stimulation at 100 Hz, most eventually reporting pain reduction of 50% or greater. The best site was the area of pain, the affected muscle or tendon, the antagonistic muscle, or a trigger point outside the painful area. Vibration applied with moderate pressure over a large area (i.e., a 200 cm cushioned applicator as opposed to 6 cm probe) produced the best pain relief. Maximal pain relief was experienced within about 10 to 20 minutes for most patients. After 45 minutes of vibration, many experienced pain relief for from 3 to 12 hours.

Mannheimer, JS, and Lampe, GN: Clinical transcutaneous electrical nerve stimulation, Philadelphia, 1984, FA Davis Co. This is a comprehensive text on the use of TENS for pain relief, both as adjunctive treatment while appropriate rehabilitation treatment occurs and as an analgesic while the body spontaneously heals, e.g., postoperatively. The book is heavily referenced and gives very specific guidelines regarding evaluation of numerous pain syndromes, electrode placement, stimulation modes, patient teaching, limitations of TENS, and available TENS units. This book is an invaluable guide to the appropriate use of TENS.

Melzack, R: Hyperstimulation analgesia. In Brena, SF, and Chapman, SL, eds: *Clin Anaesthesiol* **3**:81-92, Jan 1985. Hyperstimulation analgesia is identified as moderate to intense sensory input for a few seconds to 20 to 30 minutes, sometimes applied to a site distant to the site of pain, that may relieve pain for days. Pain relief may be due to neural inhibitory mechanisms followed by increased physical activity in the absence of pain that prevents the recurrence of memory traces of pain.

A review of research shows that stimulation of acupuncture

points or trigger points may effectively relieve pain. However, not only are the locations of trigger points very similar to acupuncture points, but these locations are not always discrete points—they may be a large area. That is, stimulation of exactly the precise point is sometimes the most effective, but other times stimulation over a large area is equally effective. As an example, ice massage of the back of the hand between the thumb and index finger (where the Hoku point is located) on the same side as pain decreases dental pain by 50% or more in most patients, but it may be equally effective to stimulate between the fourth and fifth fingers where no acupuncture point for the face is located. The entire hand or any point on it may be effective. As another example, research has shown that spinal cells excited by stimulation of the leg are inhibited by intense stimulation of the other leg or either hand.

The brainstem areas with mechanisms that exhibit a powerful descending inhibitory control appear to have a gross, complex somatotopic organization characterized by large receptive fields, making it possible for pain to be affected by stimulation at a distant site.

Melzack, R, and Bentley, KD: Relief of dental pain by ice massage of either hand or the contralateral arm, *Can Dent Assoc J* **49**:257-260, Apr 1983. An ice cube held in a gauze pad was used on 22 patients with dental pain to massage four sites for 7 minutes or until patient reported it was too painful to endure any longer. This was compared with a control procedure of tactile massage. Pain intensity was decreased by 40% to 50% after ice massage of the Hoku points (back of hand between thumb and index finger) ipsilateral and contralateral to the dental pain and ice massage of the contralateral arm (near the elbow) but not the ipsilateral arm. Pain relief was comparable to that obtained from TENS and acupuncture. This study and others suggest that intensity of stimulation is the significant factor rather than the precise site or mode of stimulation.

Melzack, R, Jeans, ME, Stratford, JG, and Monks, RC: Ice massage and transcutaneous electrical stimulation: comparison of treatment for low-back pain, *Pain* **9**:209-217, 1980. The results indicate that brief, intense cold from gentle massage with ice for lower back pain has analgesic effects comparable to those produced by transcutaneous electrical stimulation (TES). After being treated with TES and ice, 13 patients chose TES, 9 chose ice (even though some reported it was more painful than TES), and 5 asked for other therapy. Ice massage was performed for 7 minutes or less at each site with a 3-minute rest interval between stimulation until a total time of 30 minutes had elapsed. Treatment was stopped if the patient reported pain. Typically the sequence of sensations reported were cooling, burning, aching, and numbness. It was suggested that the analgesic effects of ice massage were a result of intense cold activating brainstem mechanisms that are known to exert descending inhibitory influences on pain signals.

Melzack, R, Stillwell, DM, and Fox, EJ: Trigger points and acupuncture points for pain: correlations and implications, *Pain* **3**:3-23, 1977. This study of trigger points and acupuncture points revealed a high degree of correspondence between them. Figures and tables clearly identify locations of numerous trigger points and acupuncture points.

Ramler, D, and Roberts, J: A comparison of cold and warm sitz baths for relief of postpartum perineal pain, *J Obstet Gynecol Neonatal Nurs* **15**:471-474, Nov-Dec 1986. In a study of 40 postpartum patients with episiotomies who took both cold (15.6° to 18.3° C) and warm (36.7° to 44.4° C) sitz baths, cold sitz baths were significantly more effective in relieving perineal pain. However, pain relief following the cold bath was of no longer duration than the warm bath. The latter differs from Droegemueller's (1980) findings of longer duration of pain relief following cold sitz baths, but he probably used colder water. Although 20 (50%) of the women in the study stated they preferred the cold to the warm bath, it is noteworthy that 119 women refused to participate in the study because they did not want to take a cold sitz bath. Of those 119, 58 stated they would not take a cold sitz bath no matter how severe their pain. This suggests that willingness to try a pain relief measure may be strongly influenced by beliefs or prior use.

Richardson, RR, Meyer, PR, and Raimondi, AJ: Transabdominal neurostimulation in acute spinal cord injuries, *Spine* **4**:47-51, 1979. Ileus is a common complication of acute spinal cord injuries. When abdominal TENS was used in 44 patients within 48 hours of spinal cord injury, none developed ileus, compared with ileus in 15% of 43 untreated control patients. Resolution of ileus in control patients treated with TENS occurred within 3 to 5 days. (Other studies discussing prevention and treatment of ileus include Hymes, Raab, Yonehiro, Nelson, and Printy, 1973; Hymes, Yonehiro, Raab, Nelson, and Printy, 1974; Perdikis, 1977; and Richardson and Cerullo, 1979.)

Shere, CL, Clelland, JA, O'Sullivan, P, Doleys, DM, and Canan, B: The effect of two sites of high frequency vibration on cutaneous pain threshold, *Pain* **25**:133-138, 1986. Cutaneous pain threshold was measured prior to, during, and following 5 minutes of vibration applied either proximal or distal to the site of pain. Significantly more temporary analgesia occurred when vibration was placed distally than when it was placed proximally, especially during vibration rather than before or after.

Talbot, JD, Duncan, GH, Bushnell, MC, and Boyer, M: Diffuse noxious inhibitory controls (DNICs): psychophysical evidence in man for intersegmental suppression of noxious heat perception by cold pressor pain, *Pain* **30**:221-232, 1987. Submerging the hand in painfully cold water (cold pressor pain) significantly, although not completely, reduced perception of painful heat stimuli applied to the face, and this effect continued briefly after the hand was removed from the cold water.

Travell, JG, and Simons, DG: Myofascial pain and dysfunction: the trigger point manual, Baltimore, 1983, Williams & Wilkins. This is the first of two planned volumes. It contains trigger points and related information for the upper half of the body. Numerous drawings clearly identify trigger points and pain patterns along with other details of the problem and its treatment.

Waylonis, GW: The physiologic effects of ice massage, *Arch Phys Med Rehabil* **48**:37-42, 1967. Ice massage to the thigh or calf for 5 to 10 minutes decreased skin temperature as much as 19.2° C, but not enough to present a danger of frostbite. Surface anesthesia occurred after 4.5 minutes and persisted for 30 minutes to 3 hours. Temperature reductions were smaller than those obtained with ice packs or ethyl chloride. No changes in blood pressure or pulse were observed. It was concluded that ice massage was safe even in inexperienced hands.

White, JR: Effects of a counterirritant on perceived pain and hand movement in patients with arthritis, *Phys Ther* 53:956-960, Sept 1973. In 30 patients with either rheumatoid arthritis or osteoarthritis, a placebo cream was applied to one hand and a counterirritant (10% menthol and 15% methyl salicylate, similar to Ben-Gay Greaseless/Stainless) to the other hand. Both significantly increased range of motion, but the counterirritant resulted in a significantly greater increase. Only the counterirritant reduced pain.

REFERENCES AND SELECTED READINGS

Aronoff, GM: Ice massage for pain, *Aches & Pains* 3:33-36, Feb 1982

Aronoff, GM: Massaging with ice, *RN* 48:84, June 1985

Arvidsson, I, and Eriksson, E: Postoperative TENS for pain relief after knee surgery: objective evaluation, *Orthopedics* 9:1346-1351, Oct 1986

Cailliet, R: Physical modalities and low back pain management. In Stanton-Hicks, M, and Boas, R, eds: Chronic low back pain, pp 171-176, New York, 1982, Raven Press

Cold may ease arthritis pain, *J Gerontol Nurs* 8:471, Aug 1982

Cooling more effective, *Aches & Pains* 3:37, Sept 1982

Crue, BL, Jr, and Hubrecht, G: Cutaneous vibrator—two models. In Crue, BL, Jr, ed: Pain: research and treatment, pp 293-296, New York, 1975, Academic Press

Crue, BL, Jr, Todd, EM, and Maline, DB: Postherpetic neuralgia—conservative treatment regimen. In Crue, BL, Jr, ed: Pain: research and treatment, pp 289-292, New York, 1975, Academic Press

Cyriax, JH: Clinical applications of massage. In Basmajian, JB, ed: Manipulation, traction and massage, ed 3, pp 270-288, Baltimore, 1985, Williams & Wilkins

Dalton, JA: Education for pain management: a pilot study, *Pat Educ Counsel* 9:155-165, 1987

Day, JA, Mason, RR, and Chesrown, SE: Effect of massage on serum level of β-endorphin and β-lipotropin in healthy adults, *Phys Ther* 67:926-930, June 1987

Diamond, S, and Freitag, FG: Cold as an adjunctive therapy for headache, *Postgrad Med* 79:305-309, Jan 1986

Dodi, G, Bogoni, F, Infantino, A, Pianon, P, et al: Hot or cold in anal pain? *Dis Colon Rectum* 29:248-251, Apr 1986

Droegemueller, W: Cold sitz baths for relief of postpartum perineal pain, *Clin Obstet Gynecol* 23:1039-1043, 1980

Fine, PG, Milano, R, and Hare, BD: The effects of myofascial trigger point injections are naloxone reversible, *Pain* 32:15-20, 1988

Green, BG: Menthol inhibits the perception of warmth, *Physiol Behav* 38:834-838, 1986

Halverson, GA: Sports-related injuries. In Kaplan, PE, ed: The practice of physical medicine, pp 490-525, Springfield, Ill, 1984, Charles C Thomas

Harvie, KW: A major advance in the control of postoperative knee pain, *Orthopedics* 2:26-27, 1979

Hendrixson, K: Alcohol on ice, *Nursing* 12:127, Nov 1982

Hofkosh, JM: Classical massage. In Basmajian, JB, ed: Manipulation, traction and massage, ed 3, pp 263-269, Baltimore, 1985, Williams & Wilkins

Howard-Ruben, J: Controlling pain from stomatitis, *Oncol Nurs Forum* 11:92, Jan-Feb 1984

Hymes, AC, Raab, ED, Yonehiro, EG, Nelson, GD, and Printy, AL: Electrical surface stimulation for control of acute postoperative pain and prevention of ileus, *Surg Forum* 24:447-448, 1973

Hymes, AC, Raab, ED, Yonehiro, EG, Nelson, GD, and Printy, AL: Acute pain control by electrostimulation: a preliminary report. In Bonica, JJ, ed: Advances in neurology, vol 4, pp 761-767, New York, 1974, Raven Press

Hymes, AC, Yonehiro, EG, Raab, DE, Nelson, GD, and Printy, AL: Electrical stimulation for the treatment and prevention of ileus and atelectasis, *Surg Forum* 25:222-224, 1974

Ice massage, *Nursing* 17:94, Aug 1987

Kamenetz, HL: Mechanical devices of massage. In Basmajian, JB, ed: Manipulation, traction and massage, ed 3, pp 289-308, Baltimore, 1985, Williams & Wilkins

Kirk, JA, and Kersley, GD: Heat and cold in the physical treatment of rheumatoid arthritis of the knee. A controlled clinical trial, *Ann Phys Med* 9:270-274, Aug 1968

Lehmann, JF, and de Lateur, BJ: Diathermy and superficial heat and cold therapy. In Kottke, FJ, Stillwell, CK, and Lehmann, JF, eds: Krusen's handbook of physical medicine and rehabilitation, pp 275-350, Philadelphia, 1982, WB Saunders Co

Lehmann, JF, and de Lateur, BJ: Ultrasound, shortwave, microwave, superficial heat and cold in the treatment of pain. In Wall, PD, and Melzack, R, eds: Textbook of pain, pp 717-724, New York, 1984, Churchill Livingstone

Levin, J: Fearless venipuncture, *Consultant* 27:122, Mar 1987

Licht, S: History of therapeutic heat and cold. In Lehmann, JF, ed: Therapeutic heat and cold, ed 3, Baltimore, 1982, Williams & Wilkins

Locsin, RG: Pinch-grasp technique, *Pain Res News Forum* 4:4-5, Mar-Apr 1985

Lublanezki, NC, and Cleary, RW: External analgesic products. In Handbook of nonprescription drugs, ed 8, pp 547-556, Washington, DC, 1986, American Pharmaceutical Association

Lundeberg, T: Long-term results of vibratory stimulation as a pain relieving measure for chronic pain, *Pain* 20:13-23, 1984

Lundeberg, T, Ottoson, D, Hakansson, S, and Meyerson, BA: Vibratory stimulation for the control of intractable chronic orofacial pain, *Adv Pain Res Ther* 5:555-561, 1983

Lundstrom, R, and Johansson, RS: Acute impairment of the sensitivity of skin mechanoreceptive units caused by vibration exposure of the hand, *Ergonomics* 29:687-698, 1986

Marshall, CM: The use of ice-cube massage for the relief of chronic pain following herpes ophthalmicus, *Physiotherapy* 57:374, Aug 1971

Mehus, AF: Cold comfort, *Nursing* 11:96, Oct 1981

Melzack, R, Guite, S, and Gonshor, A: Relief of dental pain by ice massage of the hand, *Can Med Assoc J* 122:189-191, 1980

Melzack, R, and Schechter, B: Itch and vibration, *Science* 147:1047-1048, Feb 26, 1965

Melzack, R, Stillwell, DM, and Fox, EF: Trigger points and acupuncture points for pain: correlations and implications, *Pain* 3:3-23, 1977

Mennell, JM: The therapeutic use of cold, *Am Osteopath J* 74:1146-1157, Aug 1975

Ordog, GJ: Transcutaneous electrical nerve stimulation versus oral analgesic: a randomized double-blind controlled study in acute traumatic pain, *Am J Emerg Med* 5:6-10, Jan 1987

Parsons, CM, and Goetzl, FR: Effect of induced pain on pain threshold, *Proc Soc Exp Biol Med* 60:327-328, 1945

Perdikis, P: Transcutaneous nerve stimulation in the treatment of protracted ileus, *South Afr J Surg* **15**:81-86, 1977

Pike, PMH: Transcutaneous electrical stimulation, *Anesthesia* **33**:165-171, 1978

Price, DD: Modulation of first and second pain by peripheral stimulation and by psychological set. In Bonica, JJ, and Albe-Fessard, D, eds: Advances in pain research and therapy, vol 1, pp 427-431, New York, 1976, Raven Press

Prudden, B: Pain erasure: the Bonnie Prudden way, New York, 1980, M Evans & Co

Richardson, RR, and Cerullo, LJ: Transabdominal neurostimulation in the treatment of neurogenic ileus, *Appl Neurophysiol* **42**:375-382, 1979

Roberts, DJ, Walls, CM, Carlile, JA, Wheaton, CG, and Aronoff, GM: Relief of chronic low back pain: heat versus cold. In Aronoff, GM, ed: Evaluation and treatment of chronic pain, pp 263-266, Baltimore, 1985, Urban & Schwarzenberg

Russell, WR: Discussion on the treatment of intractable pain, *Proc R Soc Med* **52**:983-991, Nov 1959

Russell, WR, Espir, MLE, and Morganstern, FS: Treatment of post-herpetic neuralgia, *Lancet* **1**:242-245, 1957

Schuster, GD, and Infante, MC: Pain relief after low back surgery: the efficacy of transcutaneous electrical nerve stimulation, *Pain* **8**:299-302, 1980

Snyder, M: Independent nursing interventions, New York, 1985, John Wiley & Sons

Solomon, RA, Viernstein, MC, and Long, DM: Reduction of postoperative pain and narcotic use by transcutaneous electrical stimulation, *Surgery* **87**:142-146, 1980

Stabile, ML, and Mallory, TH: The management of postoperative pain in total joint replacement, *Orthop Rev* **7**:121-123, 1978

Strodhoff, CC: Pathophysiology of rheumatoid arthritis, *Nurs Pract* **7**:32, June 1982

Swezey, RL: Low back pain in the elderly: practical management concerns, *Geriatrics* **43**:39-44, Feb 1988

Taub, HA, Beard, MC, Eisenberg, L, and McCormack, RK: Studies of acupuncture for operative dentistry, *J Am Dent Assoc* **95**:555-561, 1977

Veehoff, D: Put herpes pain on ice, *RN NV:*79, Oct 1985

Wachter-Shikora, HL: Does mechanostimulation control pain? *Am J Nurs* **82**:81, Jan 1982

Wagman, IH, and Price, DD: Responses of dorsal horn cells of *M. mulatta* to cutaneous and sural nerve A and C fiber stimuli, *J Neurophysiol* **32**:803-817, 1969

Wakim, KG: Physiologic effects of massage. In Basmajian, JB, ed: Manipulation, traction and massage, ed 3, pp 256-262, Baltimore, 1985, Williams & Wilkins

Wing, DM: A different approach to IM injections, *Am J Nurs* **76**:1239-1240, Aug 1976

Yeatman, GW, and Dang, VV: Cao gio (coin rubbing): Vietnamese attitudes toward health care, *JAMA* **244**:2748-2749, Dec 19, 1980

CHAPTER 6

Distraction

DEFINITION OF DISTRACTION

Distraction from pain may be defined as *focusing attention on stimuli other than the pain sensation.* At times, however, the focus may be on less bothersome qualities of the pain sensation such as pressure or warmth. Distraction is a kind of sensory shielding, i.e., the patient shields himself from the sensation of pain by increasing other sensory input, especially auditory, visual, and tactile-kinesthetic (hearing, seeing, touching, and moving). Attention to pain is sacrificed in favor of attention to other stimuli. The stimuli may be internal or external, e.g., the patient may hear music from a headset (external auditory stimuli) or he may hear himself singing mentally but silently (internal auditory stimuli).

In summary, the characteristics of distraction are:
- Attention is focused on stimuli other than the unpleasantness of pain.
- Pain is on the edge or periphery of awareness.
- When distracting stimuli cease, attention is again focused on pain.

KEY POINT: Usually distraction only makes pain more bearable and does not make the pain go away.

This section focuses on two types of distraction:
1. Strategies for brief episodes of pain, and
2. Maintaining a "normal" level of sensory input on a daily basis for ongoing or chronic pain.

BENEFITS AND LIMITS OF DISTRACTION

The possible *benefits* of being distracted from pain are:
1. Pain is more bearable; increase in pain tolerance; patient is not thinking about the pain.

2. Quality of pain sensation becomes more acceptable, e.g., feels less intense, less sharp, or more dull.
3. Improved mood from focus on pleasant things, e.g., less depressed while listening to music.
4. Gives the patient a sense of control over the painful experience.

TABLE 6-1 Assets and Liabilities of Distraction

Misconception:

The patient who can be distracted from pain does not have very severe pain, or the pain is not as severe as the patient would have us believe.

Correction:

Research and clinical observations show that distraction strategies are powerful techniques for making even severe pain more bearable for the patient.

Assets of Using Distraction:

↑ Pain tolerance
↑ Self-control
↓ Pain intensity
Renders quality of pain more acceptable, e.g., changes from sharp to dull.

Liabilities of Using Distraction:

Others doubt the existence or severity of pain because the patient does not look like he is in pain.
After the distraction is over:
↑ Awareness of pain
↑ Fatigue
↑ Irritability
Patient needs a pain relief measure that allows him to rest—usually asks for analgesic and health team reluctant to administer it since he did not look like he was in pain awhile ago.

IMMEDIATE HELP FOR DISTRACTION

Time involved: Reading time, 5 minutes; implementation time, 5 minutes.

Sample situation: A brief episode of pain, hopefully only a matter of a few minutes. The patient talks to you about this, saying he is afraid and he anticipates or is experiencing a lot of pain. The pain is sudden or unexpected and you have no special equipment, just yourself and a patient who wants help.

Possible solution: A structured distraction strategy.

Expected outcome: The patient says that the pain is more tolerable while he is using the distraction.

Don'ts

Do not expect or suggest that distraction will take away the pain.

Do not tell the patient he is just anxious or his pain is not as bad as he thinks.

Do not tell the patient everything will be all right.

Do not be afraid to laugh with the patient, *if* the patient begins to laugh as he tries to perform the distraction strategy. Laughter can be extremely effective.

Dos

Assure the patient you believe he hurts as much as he says he does.

If the patient is very frightened and if it is difficult to get his attention, start by asking the patient to look you in the eye. Then tell him your name and ask him to take a deep breath, hold it a moment, and then breathe out.

Tell him you will suggest and help him do a distraction method.

Tell him that you know distraction will not take away the pain but that you do know distraction can make pain a little more bearable.

Tell him you know that what you are about to suggest may sound silly or even disrespectful of his pain but that it may help.

Tell him you will do it with him so he will know you're serious and so he won't feel as self-conscious.

Explain that the two of you do not have much time to develop a plan so you will give him two ideas to choose from and make suggestions about.

Tell the patient you can help him do *either* of the following:
- Describe out loud each object he can see or use a magazine with pictures if one is available (see p. 179, patient/family teaching point regarding describing a series of pictures).

or
- Sing silently, whispering or mouthing out the words, a song such as "Jingle Bells" or "Happy Birthday" (see p. 177, patient/family teaching point regarding sing and tap rhythm). "Happy Birthday" can be sung over and over again to everyone he can think of including you and himself. Any song he knows is fine.

Ask the patient which he prefers.

If he chooses to describe objects in the room or a magazine, ask him to look at one picture or object at a time and ask him questions as often as necessary to help him keep talking.

If he chooses a song, ask him to look you in the eye and you will whisper or mouth out the words with him. Suggest he tap out the rhythm.

With either method, explain that when he hurts more he can talk or sing faster, slowing down when he hurts less.

Start the distraction *before the pain starts* if possible.

Explain to others present what you and the patient will be doing and why.

After the distraction and pain are over, or during the event, ask the patient if this helps him.

Regardless of the results, praise the patient for making the effort or being willing to listen to your ideas.

Some possible *limitations or disadvantages* of distraction from pain are:

1. Others may doubt the existence or severity of the patient's pain because he may not look or act like he is in pain while he is engaged in distraction. This may discourage the use of distraction.
2. Analgesics or other pain relief measures may still be needed during distraction because it does not usually make the pain go away.
3. When the distraction stops, the patient often experiences increased awareness of the pain, irritability, and fatigue.
4. Analgesics or other pain relief measures that allow the patient to rest may be required when the distraction ends.

KEY POINT: Watch for the misconception that the patient who can be distracted from pain does not have much pain.

The assets and liabilities of using distraction, along with the correction of a common misconception, are summarized in Table 6-1.

DISTRACTION STRATEGIES FOR BRIEF EPISODES OF PAIN

Appropriate/Inappropriate Situations/Patients

The distraction strategies described in the patient/family teaching points, pp. 176-179, are appropriate for episodes of pain lasting a matter of minutes up to 1 hour.

They are not appropriate for managing pain that lasts for hours, except under extreme circumstances where other methods of pain relief are not available. *Examples of brief episodes* of pain that might be made more bearable with a structured distraction strategy are:

- Lumbar puncture.
- Bone marrow aspiration.
- Tanking/debridement of burn or other wound.
- Suture removal.
- Dressing change.
- Removal of drainage tubes.
- Period of time between onset of pain and the onset of relief from an analgesic.
- Biopsy under local anesthetic.
- Unusually painful injections, e.g., IM hydroxyzine (Vistaril).
- Difficult venipuncture.
- Pain on movement, e.g., transfer from bed to chair.
- Uterine contractions during childbirth.

The *types of patients* who might be able to use and benefit from the distraction strategies are children or adults who:

- Understand the instructions.
- Possess the physical ability and energy to perform the activities.
- Are able to attend to, preferably concentrate on, the stimuli being offered.
- Are willing to try the technique, i.e., open-minded (initially the patient need not be convinced the technique will work).
- Desire some self-control over the painful experience.

Inappropriate patients/situations for structured distraction techniques may include:

- Patients who are hypersensitive to stimuli, e.g., patients with migraine or meningitis. Distraction may make them more uncomfortable.
- Long periods of moderate to severe pain. Structured distraction techniques require too much time and energy to be used repeatedly for long periods. Patient is also unable to engage in something else that may be a better contribution to his quality of life.

Patient/Family Teaching Points and Nursing Guidelines for Developing and Using Distraction for Brief Episodes of Pain

Both patients and nurses spontaneously devise effective distraction techniques for many unpleasant situations, including pain. Most people are accustomed to using distraction to some extent, e.g., watching TV to avoid thinking about or doing something unpleasant. To make distraction for brief episodes of pain more deliberate and structured, and hopefully more effective, both the nurse and the patient need to consider the following guidelines:

1. Individualize the content of the distraction technique. Assess whether or not the patient has used distraction

successfully for pain relief. If he has, try to utilize what he has done, perhaps improving upon it with the ideas that follow. Ask specifically if the patient (man or woman) has attended childbirth education classes. If so, the patient may already know distraction techniques such as rhythmic breathing patterns but may not realize these may work for any brief episode of pain. If the patient does not have a useful technique to suggest, assess his interests and use them to give him choices of distraction techniques.

2. Suggest distraction techniques consistent with the patient's energy level and ability to concentrate.

3. In developing the actual distraction strategy, use as many of the following as possible:
   - As pain increases in intensity, increase the complexity of the distraction, i.e., increase stimuli when pain increases. However, with very high intensities of pain, consider simple distractions since the patient may have limited energy and may not be able to concentrate well.
   - Try to provide stimuli through all the major sensory modalities, as illustrated in Figure 6-1, i.e.:
     Auditory: something to listen to, e.g., music.
     Visual: something to look at, e.g., picture, spot. (If the patient wishes to close his eyes, suggest a mental image or picture so that the patient will not begin to picture the pain or its cause.)
     Tactile: something to touch, rub, or hold.
     Kinesthetic: movement such as nodding or tapping.
   Avoid external or internal stimuli related to pain, e.g., looking at or mentally picturing the pain. Focus is away from pain.
   - Include and emphasize rhythm, e.g., use music and have patient keep time to music by tapping finger or foot. Keeping time to the music makes it necessary to pay attention to the music so less attention is paid to the pain; or alternatively, teach some type of rhythmic breathing and have the patient maintain the rhythm with silent counting or words or by nodding his head. (Characteristics of effective distraction strategies for brief episodes of pain are summarized in the box on p. 175.)

4. Perfect performance of the distraction is not necessary for success nor does it guarantee success. The patient can actually be distracted from pain by trying to learn a technique of distraction.

5. Identify the need for additional pain relief, i.e., an analgesic, during or after the distraction.

6. Plan to use distraction for a limited period of time, i.e., not for hours. Remember that most patients cannot use distraction for hours at a time as the only form of pain relief.

7. Whenever possible, practice the distraction technique with the patient prior to the time it is needed.

8. Use a preventive approach. Begin the distraction

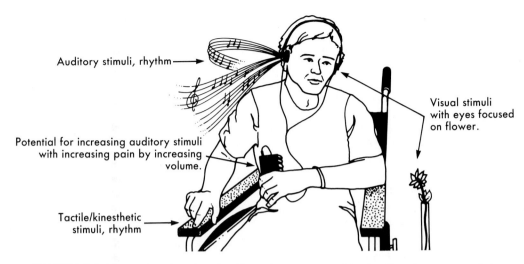

Auditory stimuli, rhythm ———→

Potential for increasing auditory stimuli
with increasing pain by increasing
volume.

Visual stimuli
with eyes focused
on flower.

Tactile/kinesthetic
stimuli, rhythm ———→

FIGURE 6-1 The patient is using the distraction strategy of "active listening to recorded music," p. 177. By listening to music through a headset, tapping out the rhythm, and focusing on the flower, the patient is making his pain more tolerable. Using the headset helps keep his attention focused on the music, helps him tune out other things in his environment, and prevents the music from disturbing others.

**Characteristics of Effective Distraction
Strategies for Brief Episodes of Pain**

1. Interesting to the patient.
2. Consistent with patient's energy level and ability to concentrate.
3. Rhythm is included and emphasized, e.g., keeping time to music.
4. Stimulates the major sensory modalities:
   • Hearing
   • Vision
   • Touch
   • Movement
5. Capable of providing a change in stimuli when the pain changes, e.g., ↑ stimuli for ↑ pain.

---

strategy before the pain begins or increases, or as soon as possible after the pain begins.

9. Inform others (health team, family) of what the patient will be doing, when, and why. This may help decrease the patient's self-consciousness about doing something different and avoid ridicule from those who do not understand the value of distraction. Explaining when the patient plans to begin the distraction, i.e., the importance of the preventive approach, may assure that the patient is warned prior to a painful procedure.
10. Consider giving the patient written instructions about how and when to use the distraction strategy.

Specific Distraction Strategies

Criteria for selection. The distraction strategies described on the following pages in the patient/family teaching points were selected with both the nurse's and patient's needs in mind. Most require little, if any, equipment; can be taught quickly and easily by the nurse; and have been shown to be effective on the basis of clinical experience or research. The directions for each strategy are stated in exactly the way the nurse might speak them to the patient, or the directions may be duplicated and a copy given to the patient. For the patient's benefit, most of the distraction strategies require very little physical exertion or intellectual ability and are low risk.

KEY POINT: Remember, **perfect performance of the distraction is not necessary for success.**

Problems and Possible Solutions

Getting the patient's attention. When the patient is very frightened about impending pain or is already experiencing severe pain, it may be difficult to distract him. All of his attention may be narrowly focused on the pain or his fears. To get his attention, try the following:

• Whisper in the person's ear.
• Use the person's first name.
• Ask a very simple question that focuses on you, e.g., How many fingers am I holding up? Or, what color is my blouse?
• Begin with a very simple distraction such as "Visual Concentration and Rhythmic Massage," previously described.
• Perform the distraction with the person and maintain eye contact.

Text continued on p. 180.

Patient/Family Teaching Point:
Distraction for Brief Pain with Visual Concentration and Rhythmic Massage

---

TO: _____ (patient's name)   DATE: _____

1. Keep your **eyes open and focus** steadily on one stationary spot or object. If you wish to close your eyes, decide upon a pleasant mental picture to keep in your mind's eye.
2. **Massage some part of your body** in a comfortable manner, perhaps slow, circular, rhythmic massage. You may wish to use a lotion or powder to keep contact smooth and comfortable.

   Additional points: This is very easy to do and may not be enough stimuli to distract effectively, yet it may be useful during periods of fatigue or difficulty concentrating.

From: _____ (nurse's name)   Phone: _____

■ May be duplicated for use in clinical practice. From McCaffery, M, and Beebe, A: PAIN: CLINICAL MANUAL FOR NURSING PRACTICE, St. Louis, 1989, The CV Mosby Company.

Patient/Family Teaching Point: Distraction for Brief Pain with Slow Rhythmic Breathing

---

TO: _____ (patient's name)   DATE: _____

1. Keep your **eyes open and focus** steadily on one stationary spot or object. If you wish to close your eyes, picture the air going in and out of your lungs.
2. To begin, **take a slow deep breath.**
3. Then **breathe slowly**, at whatever depth is comfortable for you. Breathe in slowly, breathe out slowly, at about 6 to 9 breaths per minute. Do not hold your breath and do not breathe too deeply, but do take a deep breath whenever you feel the need.
4. **Breathe in a slow rhythm.** Concentrate on your breathing, thinking of the air going in and out of your lungs. Establish your rhythm by counting or saying phrases silently to yourself. Example of counting: "In, 2, 3, out, 2, 3." Example of phrases: When you breathe in, say to yourself "Breathe in slowly." When you breathe out, say to yourself "Breathe out slowly."
5. **End with a slow, deep breath.**
6. If this is **not effective, try adding** one or more of the following: rhythmic massage of a body area; inhalation through nose and exhalation through lips; abdominal or chest breathing; raise and lower finger with inhalation and exhalation.

   Additional points: This technique does not require much physical or mental exertion and is fairly relaxing. It may be used for up to 10 or 15 minutes, or off and on for about an hour.

From: _____ (nurse's name)   Phone: _____

■ May be duplicated for use in clinical practice. From McCaffery, M, and Beebe, A: PAIN: CLINICAL MANUAL FOR NURSING PRACTICE, St. Louis, 1989, The CV Mosby Company.

Patient/Family Teaching Point: Distraction for Brief Pain with Sing and Tap Rhythm

TO: _____ (patient's name)   DATE: _____

1. Keep your **eyes open and focus** steadily on one stationary spot or object. If you wish to close your eyes, picture something about the song you will be singing.
2. **Select a song** that you know the words to (at least four or more lines), e.g., a hymn, nursery rhyme, popular song, or commercial jingle.
3. **Sing the song**. To avoid disturbing others or feeling self-conscious, most adults choose to sing silently. You may emphatically mouth the words silently or whisper the words.
4. **Mark time to the song**, e.g., tap out the rhythm with your finger or nod your head. This helps you concentrate on the song instead of your discomfort.
5. Begin singing slowly. **Sing faster if the pain increases**; sing slower when the pain decreases.
6. If this is **not effective enough, try adding or changing** one or more of the following: massage your body in rhythm to the song; try another song; ask someone to sing with you; or mark time to the song in more than one manner, e.g., nod your head at the same time you tap your finger.

   Additional points: This technique is easy to learn, but if you are already tired, you may find it physically exhausting if you do it for more than a few minutes. You may also feel self-conscious when you first do this, but you may find you don't mind as long as the technique helps you get through your discomfort.

From: _____ (nurse's name)   Phone: _____

■ May be duplicated for use in clinical practice. From McCaffery, M, and Beebe, A: PAIN: CLINICAL MANUAL FOR NURSING PRACTICE, St. Louis, 1989, The CV Mosby Company.

Patient/Family Teaching Point: Distraction for Brief Pain with Active Listening to Recorded Music

TO: _____ (patient's name)   DATE: _____

1. **Obtain** the following:
   - A cassette player or tape recorder. (Small, battery-operated ones are more convenient.)
   - Earphone or headset. (This is a more demanding stimulus than a speaker a few feet away, and it avoids disturbing others.)
   - Cassette of music you like. (Most people prefer fast, lively music, but some select relaxing music. Other options are comedy routines, sporting events, old radio shows, or stories.)
2. **Listen** to the music at a comfortable volume. **If the discomfort increases, try increasing the volume**; decrease the volume when the discomfort decreases.
3. **Mark time to the music**, e.g., tap out the rhythm with your finger or nod your head. This helps you concentrate on the music rather than your discomfort.
4. Keep your **eyes open and focus** steadily on one stationary spot or object. If you wish to close your eyes, picture something about the music.
5. If this is **not effective enough, try adding or changing** one or more of the following: massage your body in rhythm to the music; try other music; mark time to the music in more than one manner, e.g., tap your foot and finger at the same time.

   Additional points: Many patients have found this technique helpful. It tends to be very popular among patients, probably because the equipment is usually readily available and is a part of daily life—you see lots of people exercising and listening to a recording through a headset. Other advantages are that it is easy to learn and is not physically or mentally demanding. For these reasons, it may be used for up to an hour. If you are very tired, you may simply listen to the music and omit marking time or focusing on a spot.

From: _____ (nurse's name)   Phone: _____

■ May be duplicated for use in clinical practice. From McCaffery, M, and Beebe, A: PAIN: CLINICAL MANUAL FOR NURSING PRACTICE, St. Louis, 1989, The CV Mosby Company.

Patient/Family Teaching Point: Distraction for Brief Pain by Taking Laughter Seriously

===

TO: _____ (patient's name)   DATE: _____

Pain isn't funny, but you may have heard that Norman Cousins claimed that when he was sick he was able to get pain relief and sleep soundly after a bout of belly laughter. Some research has also supported this.

What's even more important is that this form of distraction seems to have a carry-over effect—pain relief continues after you stop laughing. With most types of distraction pain returns almost as soon as the distraction goes away. Here are some suggestions for using laughter.

1. Find something that makes you laugh frequently for up to 20 minutes. Consider the following:
   - Joke book.
   - Funny stories.
   - Audiotape of your favorite comedian.
   - Videotape of your favorite TV comedy show. If you know about a painful procedure far enough ahead of time or if you have painful episodes regularly (especially if you are at home and have a VCR) you may want to take advantage of Allen Funt's offer to let you borrow "Best of Candid Camera" videotapes. It's free! Write:

       Allen Funt's "Laughter Therapy"
       P.O. Box 827
       Monterey, CA 93942

2. Expose yourself to whatever is funniest to you prior to and/or during a painful event. But remember, **laughter is an especially useful technique to use prior to a painful procedure** that you cannot distract yourself from. For example, during some procedures you must participate by changing positions or taking deep breaths. Laughter is one of the few distractions that may help you immediately following its use. Other distractions seem to be helpful only while they are being used.

From: _____ (nurse's name)   Phone: _____

■ May be duplicated for use in clinical practice. From McCaffery, M, and Beebe, A: PAIN: CLINICAL MANUAL FOR NURSING PRACTICE, St. Louis, 1989, The CV Mosby Company.

Patient/Family Teaching Point: Distraction for Brief Pain by Describing a Series of Pictures

---

TO: _____ (patient's name)   DATE: _____

1. **Obtain pictures** that interest you.
   - Types of pictures. There are many possibilities, such as pictures from magazines; photographs of friends, family, or a vacation; merchandise catalogues; or books with pictures of a specific subject such as airplanes or the civil war. You may want pictures on the same subject or different subjects. Avoid any pictures that you find disturbing or that remind you of your discomfort.
   - Number of pictures. The number of pictures you need will depend on several factors, such as how long your discomfort will last, how much detail you describe, and how fast you talk.
2. You may need **assistance**. If you do not have much time or energy, you may consider asking a friend to obtain the pictures for you, e.g., cut out magazine pictures. You may also want someone to hold the pictures up for you to see as you describe them and help you with your descriptions by asking you for some of the details discussed below.
3. **Look at the pictures and describe them** in any manner that interests you. Usually it is best to continue looking at the pictures while you describe them (as opposed to looking at the picture briefly, hiding it, and then trying to remember the details of the picture). Ways of describing or talking about the pictures include the following—to help you keep your attention focused on the pictures, you may want a friend to have this list and ask you about these items:
   - Pretend you are in the picture. What would you do?
   - Count the number of items in the picture.
   - Name each item in the picture.
   - Name the colors.
   - What is happening in the picture? Make up a story about the picture.

      As soon as you are no longer interested in the picture, put it away and look at another picture. Proceed from one picture to another as rapidly as you wish. If the picture reminds you of something you would like to describe or discuss, try doing so. What the picture reminds you of may be more distracting than the actual picture.
4. If this is **not effective enough, try adding or changing** one or more of the following: massage an area of your body while you are describing the pictures; try different pictures or different questions; reverse the procedure and ask questions of the person who is assisting you; include at random some surprise pictures that may be difficult to describe but have novel value, e.g., simple cartoons or scantily clad figures; if the discomfort increases, try changing the pictures more rapidly; if you feel self-conscious talking aloud, try describing the pictures to yourself silently.

   Additional points: If you enjoy talking, you may find this technique useful in a number of situations. You may be able to use it for a few minutes during a very painful procedure, and use a variation of it for an hour or so with a visitor to help you with ongoing mild to moderate pain.

   This technique may be an ideal way to involve someone who has extra time and wants to help you with your pain. A friend or nurse may gather pictures in his/her spare time and give them to you prior to a painful event, or the person might be there to show you the pictures and ask questions.

From: _____ (nurse's name)   Phone: _____

Patient monitoring painful event. Some patients may feel a need to watch a painful procedure. This may give them a sense of control or reassurance that they are safe from or can prevent unnecessary harm to themselves. Naturally, while the patient is watching the painful event, he cannot be distracted from it. Try the following:

- Discuss the painful event with the patient prior to its occurrence. Ask if he wants more information or if he wants to be sure that the procedure is done in a particular manner.
- If the patient continues to monitor the procedure, respect his desire to do this, and suggest that he consider using the distraction before and/or after the painful procedure.
- Use another type of pain relief during the painful procedure, e.g., analgesic or application of cold near the site of pain.

Bedtime. Active involvement with distraction may very well prevent the patient from going to sleep. For distraction at bedtime, when sensory input needs to be reduced to allow the patient to go to sleep, try the following:

- Passive involvement with a distraction, e.g., simply listen to calming music or watch a calming TV program and perform no other activities along with this.
- Use another pain relief measure along with or instead of distraction, e.g., analgesic or back rub.

Emotional reactions. The specific content of the distraction may be unexpectedly upsetting to the patient. Fast music may make the patient feel more anxious. Certain pictures may remind the patient of a sad or irritating event. Obviously, these stimuli can simply be changed. However, not all emotional reactions, even sadness, are necessarily undesirable. For example, if a patient with pain knows he is terminally ill, using family photographs may precipitate part of the grieving process. The patient may actually benefit from this.

Ineffective technique. With each distraction strategy described, suggestions were given for making it more effective. If the patient is able to perform the technique reasonably well and if the suggested variations have failed to make the technique effective, try the following:

- If the patient says it is too simple, find a more complex technique.
- If the patient says it is too difficult to perform for very long, try a less complex technique.

INDIVIDUALIZED NURSING CARE PLAN

Patient with Brief Pain Who May Benefit from Distraction

Patient Description: An adult undergoing bone marrow aspiration (BMA).

Assessment	Potential Nursing Diagnoses	Planning/Intervention	Evaluation/ Expected Outcomes
Identify the following: • Knowledge of the type of pain usually felt during a BMA. • Types of distraction, if any, used previously and their effectiveness. • Mental ability to understand instructions and concentrate. • Level of physical energy. • Desire for some personal control over pain and behavior during BMA. • Special interests, e.g., music, family, shopping.	Pain related to BMA. Fear related to how pain will be managed. Knowledge deficit related to structured distraction techniques to use during BMA.	Describe benefits, limits, and types of distraction, see pp. 172-173, 176-179. Allow patient to choose the distraction he wishes to use and modify it to match his interests and abilities. Provide written instructions if needed. Practice technique with patient prior to BMA, if possible. Explain the importance of using the distraction before pain begins or increases. Inform person performing BMA and any assistants of the specific distraction the patient will use, stressing need to forewarn patient of pain so technique can be used preventively.	Patient reports pain during BMA is more bearable when distraction is used. Patient may report that distraction makes the pain sensation more acceptable, e.g., more dull than sharp, and perhaps less intense. Patient may feel a sense of pride in being able to handle part of the discomfort on his own. If future BMAs are anticipated, patient says he wishes to use distraction again and reports feeling less fearful of subsequent BMAs.

- If the distraction involves an activity the patient does not usually like anyway, such as the amount of talking that is involved with describing a series of pictures, switch to an entirely different distraction, such as listening to music.
- Use another method of pain relief, e.g., analgesic or relaxation.

MAINTAINING NORMAL SENSORY INPUT FOR ONGOING PAIN

A common problem for the patient with ongoing or chronic pain is frequent or almost constant exposure to a boring or monotonous environment. His level of sensory input may be less than usual simply because he is not engaged in his normal activities of daily living. Other patients may be exposed to excessive input that is largely meaningless to them, such as monitoring equipment in intensive care units.

In either case, the patient is deprived of sensory input that usually occupies his time and attention. This may result in the patient focusing more attention on his pain, making the pain seem more intense or less tolerable. Such environments may also contribute to anxiety or depression.

Appropriate/Inappropriate Situations/Patients

Examples of situations where there tends to be a lack of normal sensory input are:
- Isolation, protective or for infections.
- Decreased ability to be physically active, e.g., body traction, debilitating illness, arthritis, or artificial ventilation.
- Living alone with limited access to outside activities.
- Sedating medications (these decrease activity and interaction with others).
- Intensive care units, telemetry units.
- Hospitalized patient from a different culture and/or with language barrier.

Types of patients with pain who may benefit from plans to provide a more normal level of daily sensory input are adults and children who:
- Possess the physical energy and ability to engage in some activities similar to those in their previous daily lives.
- Are willing or motivated to make an effort to engage in more activities.
- Desire to regain some of their previous function or quality of life.
- Are aware of being adversely affected by the present environment, e.g., express feelings of loss, depression, frustration, or apprehension.
- Occasionally overextend themselves, i.e., "do too much," and precipitate more pain or retard their recovery.

Patients who may not be appropriate are:
- Those whose pain has produced an almost complete disability. The simple approaches recommended here may be insufficient. The patient may require a multidisciplinary approach in a structured program for several weeks along with systematic follow-up. This is discussed in greater detail in Chapter 9.
- Very withdrawn. Some patients feel very threatened by illness and the treatment inflicted upon them. They feel they have no control over the external environment, so they retreat to their internal environment. Such patients may first need to be given many choices about their care. Then they may be ready to participate more actively in creating a more normal day for themselves.

Nursing Care Guidelines and Patient/Family Teaching Points for Maintaining Normal Sensory Input

Here the focus is on simple and practical approaches to normalizing daily sensory input so that pain is more tolerable. This is done by avoiding an undue focus on pain and minimizing anxiety and depression. *Nursing care guidelines,* in addition to the patient/family teaching point for handling boring or strange days, p. 182, are:
1. Include some normal sensory input at regular intervals throughout the patient's waking day.
2. Identify the need for any pain relief methods that would allow the patient to engage in normal activities, e.g., aspirin and a cold pack prior to walking.
3. Identify the need for any special assistance needed for the activity, e.g., asking the patient's friend to bring in a videotaped movie or getting a prescription for physical therapy to provide range of motion and stretching of muscles daily for the inactive patient.
4. Realize the importance of providing input through all the major sensory modalities, e.g., music for auditory stimuli, physical exercise for tactile-kinesthetic stimuli, and selected TV viewing or magazines for visual stimuli.
5. Consider using the Daily Diary (p. 30) format for you and the patient to formulate a written daily schedule. The first and last columns may be helpful—each hour already written in with a space to write the major activity (see the example on p. 183).
6. Expect resistance from some patients. Some patients are self-motivated and will require little assistance. But many people need to have structure and well-stated expectations in order to perform. In a way, this is similar to the difference between a person who is self-directed and one who is not. To complicate the problem further, remember that for reasons not well understood, *boredom tends to lead to more boredom.* While the bored patient suffers the consequences of boredom such as disinterest, difficulty thinking, and less tolerance for pain, many are also surprisingly lack-

Text continued on p. 184.

===
Patient/Family Teaching Point: Handling Boring or Strange Days
===

TO: _____ (patient's name)   DATE: _____

Do you have this problem? Are most of your days boring or full of strange sights and sounds? Are you doing very little of what you did before this illness and pain? This may be causing you more trouble than you realize. Boring or strange days may make you more and more aware of your pain, and you may find it more difficult to tolerate. You may feel bored, tense, angry, frustrated, lonely, or sad. Getting back to a more normal daily life may help.

The *goal* is to plan your whole day, from getting up to going to bed, so that it includes specific activities that are somewhat like your more normal, healthy days. Try the following suggestions:

1. Think about the details of **what you used to do every day.** You might want to try making a list. What did you do almost every day? Which were most important? Most enjoyable? Little things like catching 10 minutes of morning news on the radio may be just as important as the big items such as working 8 hours. What were the special treats?

2. Which things could you still do with **just a little effort?** Examples that might apply to you: wear cologne, drink a second cup of coffee and read the morning newspaper, listen to the radio station you used to hear on the way to work, telephone a friend, get a copy of your favorite magazine, watch favorite TV programs, get a plant to water and feed.

3. Can you do some **small part of important, but currently impossible activities?** Examples that might apply to you: if you used to enjoy dressing carefully for the day, put on some personal and attractive clothing item or accessory each morning; if you enjoyed the conversation with peers at morning breaks or lunch, ask one of them to include you by telephone each day; if you enjoyed your work and if someone is taking over your work responsibilities, offer to assist (within your limits) by telephone each day, perhaps at a specified time; if you enjoyed a bedtime ritual with your child or anyone else, talk with the person by phone before retiring.

4. Be especially alert to the possibility of including something related to each of the following since they tend to have many benefits, such as the relaxing qualities of some types of music:
   - **Music** with headset (headset blocks out other sounds and avoids disturbing others with the music). Select music, note its effect on you, and make necessary changes in choices. Try listening to music about three times a day for 20 to 30 minutes. In some patients this makes pain more tolerable or reduces pain and the need for pain relievers.
   - **Physical exercise** at least once a day. At first this may be very limited, such as merely pointing toes and/or squeezing a ball with the hand. But some degree of physical activity tends to be a surprisingly important part of the daily plan.
   - **Conversation with a friend** at least once a day. Examples are telephone calls or arranging to stagger visitors from day to day.
   - Daily viewing of **specially selected videotapes or TV programs.** Avoid having the TV on most of the time. If you like them, **books or magazines** are a good substitute for TV.

5. Consider a **written schedule** of daily activities. You may want to ask a friend or your nurse to help with this.

6. Plan for periods of rest. Don't "overdo." **Pace yourself.**

7. **Vary your activities at regular intervals.** Anything can become boring after a while. If in doubt, try changing to a different activity at least every hour.

8. **Change your daily schedule.** Every day does not have to be the same. "Variety is the spice of life."

9. Consider a **special treat at the end of the day** as a reward for carrying through with your schedule.

10. It may be **difficult to get started** with your daily plans. But you may find that after you make the initial effort, it gets easier.

From: _____ (nurse's name)   Phone: _____

■ May be duplicated for use in clinical practice. From McCaffery, M, and Beebe, A: PAIN: CLINICAL MANUAL FOR NURSING PRACTICE, St. Louis, 1989, The CV Mosby Company.

Jazzing Up John's Day

DAILY DIARY

Name: __John__   Date: Tuesday __6-30-87__

Time	~~Pain rating scale~~	~~Medication type & amount taken~~	~~Other pain relief measures tried or anything that influences your pain~~	Major activity being done: lying sitting standing/walking
12 midnight	Sleep			
1				
2				
3				
4				
5				
6	↓			
7	Wake up to news report on radio.			
8 - 8:30	Listen to rock & roll on radio (during breakfast).			
9	Watch video tape of last night's late night TV—1 hr. ;			
10	apply aftershave cologne (during bath & dressing change).			
11:30	Expect call from work to talk to friends during their lunch.			
12 noon	TV if desired (during lunch).			
1-1:30	Listen to music via headset.			
2	Rest.			
3-3:30	Physical therapy—ROM & stretch per instructions.			
4-4:30	Read afternoon newspaper; coffee/beverage.			
5	Visitor from work.			
6-7	Watch evening news on TV during dinner.			
7	Talk with family at home on telephone.			
8-8:30	Listen to music via headset (20-30 min.).			
9	Special treat—can of beer with TV.			
10	Sleep.			
11	↓			

Comments: _____

_____

_____

ing in frustration. They become passive victims, even those who want to resume a more normal life-style. This circular process is illustrated below.

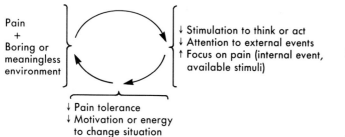

7. For patients who are able to read, consider duplicating the patient/family teaching point, p. 182, and giving it to the patient and family. The teaching points are stated in a manner suitable for the patient to have.
8. Inform other members of the health team of efforts to normalize the patient's day, explaining that this may increase his pain tolerance and possibly decrease the need for analgesics. However, warn the health team not to mistake more normal behavior for an absence of pain. When the patient engages in more activities, he may not look or act like he is in pain, but the pain is still there.

KEY POINT: Including regular periods of activity similar to the patient's usual routine when he is healthy is often surprisingly helpful in dealing with pain but also unexpectedly difficult to devise and carry out daily.

NURSING RESOURCES

Muralvision
(Scenic video tapes for patient viewing on TV, used in numerous hospitals to relieve boredom.)
Muralvision Studios
222 E 11th Ave
Eugene, OR 97401

INDIVIDUALIZED NURSING CARE PLAN

Patient Who May Benefit from Maintaining Normal Sensory Input

Patient Description: An adult male in isolation with antibiotic resistant infected lesions on both legs.

Assessment	Potential Nursing Diagnoses	Planning/Intervention	Evaluation/ Expected Outcomes
Identify the following: • Feelings of boredom, confusion, pain seems endless and tiring. • Amount of time focused on pain vs. amount focused on activity not related to illness. • Differences between activities now and those prior to illness. • Physical and mental ability to perform more activities. • Willingness to try —some activities similar to normal day —listening to music —visiting with family and friends —physical exercise • Special treats not now used. • Need for pain relief measures to facilitate more activity.	Pain related to infected, open lesions on legs. Diversional activity deficit related to isolation to prevent spread of infection and to inability to walk.	Patient along with nurse writes daily, hourly schedule of activities (see adaptation of "Daily Diary" format, p. 183) that includes daily: —music (× 2) —physical activity (× 1) —involvement with friends and family, visits or telephone (× 2-3) —different special treats at end of each day —rest periods. Nurse acknowledges/compliments patient at conclusion of each scheduled activity. Inform others that patient will be more active but that this does not mean pain has subsided. Provide analgesics or other pain relief as needed to facilitate patient's schedule of activity.	Patient states pain is less bothersome more of the time. Patient expresses positive feelings about the effects of activities, e.g., less bored, feels happier. Patient begins to initiate additional activities.

"Nurses for Laughter," an organization of nurses, can be reached through:
Debbie Leiber, R.N., M.N., Ph.D.
Oregon Health Sciences University
School of Nursing
3181 SW Sam Jackson Rd
Portland, OR 97201
(503) 279-7709

SELECTED ANNOTATED REFERENCES THAT CITE RESEARCH OR GIVE CLINICAL SUPPORT

Many of the noninvasive pain relief measures, such as distraction, have not yet been adequately researched. This sometimes makes it difficult to document or justify the use of these techniques. The following brief, annotated list provides some clinical or research support for use of distraction as discussed in this chapter:

Clum, GA, Luscomb, RL, and Scott, L: Relaxation training and cognitive redirection strategies in the treatment of acute pain, *Pain* 12:175-183, 1982. Cognitive redirection, consisting of focusing on pleasant images, during laboratory infliction of ischemic pain significantly reduced the perception of pain, whereas relaxation training did not.

Cogan, R, Cogan, D, Waltz, W, and McCue, M: Effects of laughter and relaxation on discomfort thresholds, *J Behav Med* 10:139-144, Apr 1987. Two experiments were conducted in a laboratory setting using human subjects to measure pressure-induced discomfort thresholds before and 10 minutes after listening to 20-minute long audio tapes. The first experiment compared effects of laughter-inducing, relaxation-inducing, dull-narrative, and no tape. Discomfort thresholds were higher for the laughter and relaxation tapes. The second experiment compared effects of laughter-inducing, interesting narrative, or uninteresting narrative audio tapes, completed multiplication tasks, or no intervention. This showed that only laughter significantly increased discomfort thresholds. In conclusion, it appears that laughter is more effective than other types of distraction and that the effects continue for at least 10 minutes after the laughter subsides.

Dalton, JA: Education for pain management: a pilot study, *Pat Educ Counsel* 9:155-165, 1987. An experimental study of cancer patients taught to use distraction, massage, and relaxation showed the greatest behavior change was in the use of distraction. The distraction technique taught was almost identical to "Active Listening to Recorded Music" on p. 177 of this chapter.

Eland, J: Personal communication, University of Iowa, Iowa City, Iowa, Feb 11, 1987. Use of patient-selected music via headset, similar to "Active Listening to Recorded Music" on p. 177 of this chapter, in 94 patients from pediatric, oncology, and burn units for brief, painful procedures such as bone marrow aspiration, was found helpful by all patients. Only one patient refused to try it.

Fritz, DJ: Noninvasive pain control methods used by cancer outpatients, *Oncol Nurs Forum* (suppl) p 108, 1988 (abstract). An itemized questionnaire about self-initiated, noninvasive pain control measures was administered to 53 oncology outpatients. Patients rated laughter as the most effective of these measures in relieving pain.

Schultz, DP: Sensory restriction: effects on behavior, New York, 1965, Academic Press. Presents findings of many studies regarding the effects of boredom on pain, e.g., boredom increases attention to pain, and studies that show the critical importance of physical exercise in reducing the effects of boredom.

Scott, DS, and Barber, TX: Cognitive control of pain: effects of multiple cognitive strategies, *Psychol Rec* 2:373-383, 1977. Very brief instructions, including examples of distractions, raised average pain tolerance 100% in a group of laboratory subjects. Pain intensity, however, did not change. They concluded it was much easier to change tolerance of pain than to change perception of pain.

REFERENCES AND SELECTED READINGS

Blitz, B, and Lowenthal, M: The role of sensory restriction in problems with chronic pain, *J Chronic Dis* 19:1119-1125, Nov-Dec 1966

Brody, R: Music medicine, *Omni* 6:24, 110, 1984

Chaves, JF, and Barber, TX: Cognitive strategies, experimenter modeling, and expectation in the attenuation of pain, *J Abnorm Psychol* 83:356-363, 1974

Cook, JD: Music as an intervention in the oncology setting, *Cancer Nurs* 9:23-28, Feb 1986

Cousins, N: Anatomy of an illness (as perceived by the patient), *N Engl J Med* 295:1458-1463, Dec 23, 1976

Davis-Rollans, C, and Cunningham, SG: Physiologic responses of coronary care patients to selected music, *Heart Lung* 16:370-378, July 1987

Dolan, MB: A drug you can't overuse, *RN* 48:47-48, Nov 1985

Glynn, NJ: The therapy of music, *J Gerontol Nurs* 12:6-10, Jan 1986

Hanswer, M, Larson, SC, and O'Connell, AS: Music therapy-assisted labor: effects on relaxation of expectant mothers, *Birth Psychol Bull* 4:2, 1983

Herman, EP: Music therapy in depression. In Podalsky, E, ed: Music therapy, New York, 1954, Philosophical Library

Herth, I: The therapeutic use of music, *Supervisor Nurse* 9:22-23, 1978

Isen, AM, Daubman, KA, and Nowicki, GP: Positive affect facilitates creative problem solving, *J Pers Soc Psychol* 52:1122-1131, 1987

Jacob, S: Bring on the music, *Am J Nurs* 86:1034, Sept 1986

Lavine, R, Buchsbaum, MS, and Poncy, M: Auditory analgesia: somatosensory evoked response and subjective pain rating, *Psychophysiology* 13:140-148, 1976

Locsin, R: The effect of music on the pain of selected postoperative patients *J Adv Nurs* 6:19-25, 1981

McCaffery, M: Nursing management of the patient with pain, ed 2, pp 89-116, Philadelphia, 1979, JB Lippincott

McCaffery, M: Relieving pain with noninvasive techniques, *Nursing* 10:55-57, Dec 1980

McClelland, DC: Music in the operating room, *ARON J 1979* 29:252-260, 1979

Melzack, R: Pain perception, *Percept Disord* 48:272-285, 1970

Melzack, R, Weisz, AZ, and Sprague, LT: Strategies for controlling pain: contributions of auditory stimulation and suggestion, *Exp Neurol* 8:239-247, 1963

OR patients tune in as they tune out, *RN*:12, Jan 1987

Osterlund, H: Humor: a serious approach to patient care, *Nursing* 13:46-47, 1983

Raber, WC: The caring role of the nurse in the application of humor therapy to the patient experiencing helplessness, *Clin Gerontol* 7:3-11, Fall 1987

Ruxton, JP, and Hester, M: Humor: assessment and interventions, *Clin Gerontol* 7:13-21, Fall 1987

Scott, DS, and Barber, TX: Cognitive control of pain: four seren-dipitous results, *Percept Mot Skills* 44:569-570, 1977

Snyder, M: Independent nursing interventions, New York, 1985, John Wiley & Sons

Wiener, CL: Pain assessment on an orthopedic ward, *Nurs Outlook* 23:508-516, Aug 1975

Ziporyn, T: Music therapy accompanies medical care, *JAMA* 252:986-987, 1984

CHAPTER 7

Relaxation

DEFINITION OF RELAXATION

Relaxation may be defined *as a state of relative freedom from both anxiety and skeletal muscle tension,* a quieting or calming of the mind and muscles. Subjectively, the person usually feels minimal or no anxiety or apprehension. Actually, the complete absence of anxiety is rare and not necessarily beneficial, since some level of arousal or anxiety is useful in alerting or motivating a person to take appropriate action.

In the strictest sense, relaxation should produce the relaxation response. Physiologically, the relaxation response is the opposite of the fight-or-flight response. It is characterized by a normal level of physiological functioning or a decrease in autonomic nervous system activity. However, many people use a relaxation technique and report feeling more relaxed and less distressed without necessarily demonstrating the traditional relaxation response, as summarized in the box below.

Relaxation Response

Physiological characteristics of the relaxation response are:
1. ↓ Oxygen consumption
2. ↓ Respiratory rate
3. ↓ Heart rate
4. ↓ Muscle tension
5. Normal blood pressure (↓ in patients with high blood pressure)
6. ↑ Alpha waves

Reference: Benson, H, Beary, JF, and Carol, MP: The relaxation response, *Psychiatry* 37:37-46, Feb 1974

Knowing *what relaxation is not* is important since many health team members, as well as patients, have naive attitudes about relaxation. Relaxation is *not* plopping down in front of the television set, sleeping, resting, sitting quietly, reading a book, working in the garden, or playing tennis. These activities may *promote* relaxation but should not be equated with it. During sleep, for example, dreams or subconscious thoughts can maintain or increase muscle tension. Further, even when the muscles are not being used, high levels of muscle tension may exist. In essence, people often think they are relaxed when in fact they are not. Most people must make a conscious attempt to relax, and many must learn the skill—it does not necessarily come naturally.

KEY POINT: It is common for people to think they are relaxed when they are not.

Techniques for accomplishing or learning relaxation comprise a wide variety of methods, including meditation, autogenic training, yoga, religion, and music. Some techniques are simple or utilize what the patient has already learned, while others constitute a training program of building skill in relaxation and incorporating this into daily life. Sometimes biofeedback in the form of skin temperature or muscle tension is used to help the person learn when he is relaxing, although there is little evidence that biofeedback is necessary or even helpful for learning relaxation (Roberts, 1987; Turner and Chapman, 1982).

Relaxation techniques are considered within the realm of professional nursing practice. The American Nurses Association, along with certain states such as California, specifically state that relaxation and suggestive therapies may be performed as an integral part of the individual registered nurse's area of nursing practice, assuming the nurse has appropriate education and experience.

IMMEDIATE HELP FOR RELAXATION

Time involved: Reading time, 5 minutes; implementation time, 5 to 7 minutes.

Sample situation: Patient is not only in pain but also in considerable distress about the pain. While you and/or others are trying to do something more to relieve his pain, you want to help him relax to relieve some of his distress about the pain.

Possible solution: He may be willing to try one of two or three methods of relaxation that you intend to suggest to him.

Expected outcome: Patient will feel his pain is acknowledged and someone cares. He will experience less distress with his pain.

Don'ts

1. Do not expect or suggest that relaxation will substitute for appropriate pain relief, e.g., adequate analgesic prescriptions.
2. Do not tell the patient "Just relax and it will be all right." Help him relax and assure him you are searching for appropriate pain relief methods.
3. Do not convey that the pain is largely due to anxiety.
4. Do not say that there is nothing else anyone can do.
5. Do not tell the patient he has to learn to live with this.
6. *Never* tell the patient his pain is not as bad as he thinks.
7. If relaxation helps, do not abandon the search for appropriate methods of pain relief.

Dos

1. Take a deep breath outside his room and relax a little yourself. Plan on 2 to 5 minutes with the patient.
2. When you enter the room, tell the patient you know he hurts.

3. Tell the patient you are still hoping (searching) for a better alternative, but that meanwhile relaxation may be helpful.

To convey points 2 and 3 above, you might say "I know that hurting this much often makes people feel frightened and anxious, and I know that the best way to relieve that anxiety is to relieve the pain. But since that isn't possible right now, maybe I can at least help you find a way to relieve some of the anxiety."

4. Tell the patient you have a few moments to help him learn a brief technique.

   If the patient is receptive to the idea of relaxation, try deep breath/tense, etc. (p. 199) or jaw relaxation (p. 200).

   If the patient is not receptive to the idea of relaxation, ask him to try to remember and concentrate on something peaceful that happened to him, suggesting recollection of being with a loved one, especially a child or parent. Or, if available, suggest relaxing music.
5. Tell the patient when you will try to return; give yourself leeway. It's better to return early than late.
6. When you return, ask the patient how the relaxation worked.
7. If the patient says the relaxation did not help, express your regrets, and tell him you admire his willingness to try the technique.
8. If the relaxation helped, praise his willingness to try it and encourage him to continue relaxation at least at intervals while you continue to try to find something to relieve his pain.

BENEFITS AND LIMITS OF RELAXATION

"Relax! Everything will be just fine!"

Questions	Answers
Can most people relax on command?	No, they need help.
Will relaxation really help with pain?	Not always, and when it does help, it may reduce distress, not pain.

KEY POINT: Relaxation may not relieve pain, but it has many other potential benefits for people with pain.

Relaxation techniques are incorporated in programs that have a multitude of purposes, such as stress reduction for those who have stressful lifestyles, an aid to weight reduction or abstinence from abused substances,

reduction of nausea and vomiting during chemotherapy, and treatment for hypertension. Here the focus is on using relaxation techniques to help people with pain.

The widely held belief that relaxation may be beneficial to patients with pain is illustrated by its use in almost every program for prepared childbirth, and for management of pain for patients with chronic nonmalignant pain. On the other hand, there is very little research to justify this widespread use. In fact, the exact benefits of relaxation for people with pain remain largely unknown. Thus relaxation should be used judiciously, not automatically.

For the person with pain, the *potential benefits* of using relaxation are related to the interaction between pain, muscle tension, and anxiety. The usual responses to pain, especially initially and when it cannot be avoided, are some anxiety-like feelings such as apprehension, fear, or panic, and some muscle tension such as restriction of movement, jaw-clenching, or splinting. The anxiety, pain, and muscle tension tend to intensify each other, and the situation proceeds from bad to worse. To help the patient with pain, relaxation attempts to interrupt this spiraling process with skeletal muscle relaxation. Quieting the body often quiets the mind.

KEY POINT: Muscle tension, anxiety, and pain may perpetuate each other and become a spiraling process.

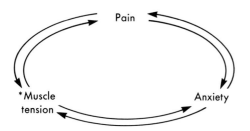

*Interrupting the cycle here with skeletal muscle relaxation may have many benefits, such as preventing the situation from worsening.

Relaxation, especially when it is used preventively, may produce one or more of the following *specific benefits* for the person with pain:

1. Aids sleep by helping the patient get to sleep faster, improving the quality of sleep by decreasing physical and mental tension, and helping the patient with frequent awakenings get back to sleep more quickly.
2. Strengthens the nurse-patient relationship through individualized attention. The manner in which the nurse offers to help the patient with relaxation can reassure the patient that the nurse is aware of his distress and wants to be of help.
3. Improves problem-solving and increases the likelihood that positive, adaptive ideas will reach consciousness. Helps prevent "catastrophizing."
4. Minimizes the detrimental effects of continued or repeated stress from pain or other sources. The patient may be able to learn to respond to stress with less autonomic nervous system activity and/or to recover more rapidly from a stress reaction, e.g., "fight or flight." (NOTE: Stress is a situation that makes it necessary for the person to readjust. However, stress is not necessarily negative, since happy as well as unhappy events may require an adjustment. In fact, people thrive on the right amount of stress. Stress becomes *distress* when there is a continual or intense need to readjust or adapt.)
5. Reduced skeletal muscle tension may reduce strain or pressure on pain-sensitive structures. This may relieve pain.
6. Increases confidence and a sense of self-control in coping with pain; better able to decide on appropriate action for handling the pain and avoid harmful or unproductive efforts.
7. Decreases fatigue, especially a technique done for 5 to 20 minutes. This may result in a more energized feeling than taking a nap for an hour.

8. Distracts from pain, since most relaxation techniques for pain include sufficient structure and activity to prevent thoughts from returning to pain. Certain types of relaxation imagery can give the patient a sense of freedom from being confined to bed or being hospitalized.
9. Increases the effectiveness of other pain relief measures. For example, even a quick and easy technique may increase the effectiveness of an analgesic. A relaxed person may be more susceptible to suggestions or intentions of pain relief.
10. Increases subjective reports of improved mood and decreased distress, e.g., pain is more tolerable and the patient increases involvement in various activities.
11. Decreases distress or fear during anticipation of pain, e.g., desensitizes the person to anxiety-producing aspects of a painful procedure.

Some *possible limitations or disadvantages* of relaxation for the person with pain are:

1. The suggestion to try relaxation techniques may be misinterpreted by the patient as meaning that the health team regards the pain as being of psychological origin or "not real pain."
2. The success of relaxation may be misinterpreted by the health team as meaning that the pain is mainly or exclusively caused by psychological problems.
3. Others may doubt the existence or severity of the patient's pain when he uses relaxation because he will not look like he is in pain. This may discourage the use of relaxation.
4. Relaxation is not a substitute for appropriate analgesics and other methods of pain relief.
5. It does not necessarily relieve pain and certainly is not a panacea for all pain-related ailments. There are exceptions, e.g., progressive relaxation has been shown to reduce pain of ulcerative colitis.
6. It is only an adjunctive treatment for pain—rarely will relaxation alone be sufficient to treat pain.
7. Once pain becomes severe, it is difficult to use relaxation even for the person who is well trained, e.g., relaxation may help prevent a migraine but may be useless once the migraine occurs.
8. Unwanted side effects are rare, but they may occur. This is most likely with the longer, meditative techniques. For example, the patient may experience anxiety or previously denied feelings of sadness or grief (see Table 7-1, p. 196).
9. Since not every relaxation technique works for everyone, with some patients it may take time to find or develop an effective technique for the individual.
10. Patient may find relaxation helpful without experiencing the traditional relaxation response (shown in the box on p. 188).
11. In some situations for some patients, relaxation may increase pain and distress.

12. Some elderly people do not seem to benefit as much or as quickly from relaxation training but do seem to benefit from more simple and brief techniques.

13. In spite of appropriate teaching and reassurance, some patients who are motivated to use relaxation will become more distressed. For example, failure to achieve profound relaxation or unrealistic expectations of the benefits of relaxation may result in frustration.

For an overview of practical guidelines for matching relaxation techniques to patients and situations, see the box below.

RELAXATION TECHNIQUES: ACTIVE PATIENT INVOLVEMENT

Some relaxation techniques require varying degrees of patient involvement, mentally and physically. Examples of those and specific instructions for teaching are on pp. 199 to 205. Following is an overview of patients and situations that may be appropriate or inappropriate opportunities to use these relaxation techniques.

Appropriate/Inappropriate Patients/Situations

The relaxation techniques described in this chapter may be appropriate for almost any person with pain. It is very difficult to say with any certainty that relaxation in general or any specific technique is or is not recommended for a certain person or a specific situation.

Examples of *patients who may be appropriate* candidates for using and benefiting from relaxation techniques requiring some active participation are children or adults who:

- Express a need or desire to use relaxation to cope with pain or have some control over the pain, or are open-minded enough to want to try.
- Understand the instructions.
- Are able to concentrate on the directions offered.
- Say they are anxious, tense, "up tight," or mildly depressed.
- Maintain a rigid posture or are unaware that they are tensing muscles, e.g., clenching fists or teeth.
- Have sleep disturbances or increased fatigue.
- Are adolescents or young to middle-aged adults with tension or migraine headaches.
- Have pain related to ulcerative colitis, temporomandibular joint (TMJ) problems, or surgery.
- Have ongoing muscle spasm.
- Have predictable pain periods.
- Have chronic pain, ongoing or recurrent, especially chronic nonmalignant pain.

Although research evidence of the effectiveness of relaxation for patients with pain is minimal, most pain specialists agree that relaxation is probably a significant part

---

Practical Guidelines for Matching Relaxation Techniques to Patients and Situations

1. Consider the *amount of time* the patient will experience pain vs. the time involved in teaching and using the technique. Usually:

Use the less time-consuming techniques for brief episodes of pain, e.g., jaw relaxation (p. 200) or slow rhythmic breathing (p. 201) for procedural or postoperative pain.

Be willing to invest more time for patients with chronic pain, e.g., peaceful past experiences (p. 201) or meditative relaxation (pp. 202 to 203) for cancer pain or recurrent headaches.

Beware of introducing time-consuming techniques to patients who are already under considerable stress, even if they have chronic pain, since this may add another stressor.

2. Consider how pain, fatigue, anxiety, and other factors influence the *patient's general ability to learn or engage in an activity.* Usually:

Use brief, simple techniques or massage during severe pain, lack of concentration, or along with other pain relief measures, e.g., deep breath/tense, exhale/relax, yawn (p. 199), when narcotic is given for renal colic.

Teach more time-consuming techniques when the patient is alert and comfortable, e.g., meditative relaxation (pp. 202 to 203) when severe back pain is in remission.

Even if the patient says relaxation is not helpful during pain or the anticipated pain will be too severe for him to use relaxation, suggest he use it before and after pain.

3. Note if the patient has *energy that needs to be dissipated,* e.g., restless, "up tight," or the "fight or flight" response (meaning that he has generated energy to fight or flee but has nowhere to go). Use a technique that releases energy, e.g., progressive relaxation (pp. 204 to 205).

4. For the *patient who misunderstands the purpose of relaxation,* use other terminology and suggest humor (p. 199), peaceful past experiences (p. 201), or passive recipient techniques such as a back rub (p. 206).

5. *Consider whether the focus is inward on the body or outward on peaceful scenes.* An inward focus can increase distress about changes in body image or feelings of failure about physical limitations. Be cautious about using an exclusively inward body focus for patients who are distressed about changes in body appearance or function, severely depressed, or have difficulty maintaining contact with reality.

of a successful pain management program for a person with chronic nonmalignant pain. When such a patient benefits from a tape-recorded 5- to 20-minute technique, they are usually so grateful and the technique is used so often (several times a day for months, even years) that the time required to discuss and record the technique often seems insignificant.

Patient Example

Mrs. N., 38 years old, requested her physician to refer her to someone who could help her learn relaxation. She had been diagnosed as having a form of cancer that was essentially always fatal, but she had responded to treatment and lived much longer than expected. Now she was in considerable pain and aware that her physician had lost hope in further progress. The physician referred the patient to a nurse and called the nurse to advise caution since the patient was prone to high achievement standards and might feel guilty if she could not relax well. The nurse and patient spent 3 hours discussing the possible benefits and limitations of relaxation, developing a personalized technique for this patient, and tape-recording it. Numerous relaxation techniques were described to her, and she was given complete control of what would be included in the tape. She chose a rhythmic breathing pattern, detailed description of a personally peaceful scene, and a psalm. She lived 2 more years. Until 2 days before her death she functioned well at her occupation of university professor. During those 2 years, as requested by the nurse, she regularly called to report her condition and problems. Never once did she indicate that she expected relaxation to be the answer to all her pain problems. Many other alternatives for pain relief were discussed and used. According to her reports and those of her husband, for those 2 years she listened to the tape at least twice a day, saying that it decreased stress and tension. Relaxation seemed to help her maintain her self-respect by enabling her to function in areas important to her.

While there are certainly situations where relaxation is inappropriate or unhelpful, quick and easy relaxation techniques are probably devoid of significant harm. Benefits probably exceed any undesirable side effects. However, use of those relaxation techniques that require the patient's time and effort should be carefully evaluated.

Examples of *patients who may be inappropriate* candidates for relaxation techniques, especially those that are *lengthy* (more than a few seconds) and *introspective or meditative* (focusing inward and excluding external stimuli) are children or adults who:
- State they do not want to try relaxation.
- Have a psychiatric history of hallucinations, loss of contact with reality, or delusion. Meditative or internally focused techniques may cause a loss of contact with reality and may be particularly troublesome, but such patients, if they are motivated, should be encouraged to try other brief or externally focused techniques, such as humor or jaw relaxation.

- Are significantly depressed. Time-consuming techniques, especially meditative or internally focused, may increase depression, rumination, or withdrawal.
- Are presently in extremely stressful situations and have no time or energy to devote to learning relaxation (practicing a relaxation technique may simply add another stressor).
- Have cardiac problems. Cardiac patients may be at increased risk for arrhythmias due to stimulation of the vagus nerve. Therefore if the technique involves muscle contraction, e.g., traditional active progressive relaxation, warn such a patient not to tightly tense muscles. If a hypotensive patient practices any type of relaxation regularly, monitor blood pressure.
- Some elderly people, since they do not seem to benefit as much or as quickly from relaxation training. However, they do seem to benefit from more simple and brief techniques, such as jaw relaxation.

Nursing Care Guidelines for Selecting, Developing, and Using Relaxation Techniques
Common Elements of Relaxation Techniques

This chapter provides only a small sample of the many available relaxation techniques. Numerous ones are offered on tape. Most relaxation techniques for patients with pain have certain elements in common (see below).

Common Elements of Effective Relaxation Techniques

Relaxation techniques often include one or more of the following:
- *Mental device* to reduce distracting thoughts, e.g., rhythmic breathing.
- *Passive attitude,* i.e., let it happen, it cannot be forced, worrying that it won't happen only creates more tension.
- *Quiet environment,* e.g., phone off hook, use headset to listen to tape.
- *Comfortable position,* e.g., lying down with support for neck and legs, not crossing extremities.
- *Behaviors already conditioned* to produce relaxation:
  Deep breath (big sigh following a stressful event is often paired with relaxing on exhalation)
  Yawn (paired with sleep)
  Abdominal breathing (paired with sleep)
  Peaceful images (patient reacts to pleasant, relaxing memories with same feelings experienced previously)
- *Repetition or practice* (using what the patient has already found helpful or selecting a technique and practicing it daily helps develop conditioning).
- *Patient controls* whether or not and when and where he performs the technique.

However, a technique may be effective without including all the items listed.

Specific Suggestions for Teaching Patients

The following suggestions for teaching patients about relaxation techniques are not necessarily indicated when a technique is used only once or a few times for quick, "on the spot" assistance with relaxation. However, the more time and effort required of the patient, the more important the following points become:

1. Emphasize that the reason for using relaxation is to reduce the distress caused by pain, not necessarily to reduce the pain. Be careful to avoid implying that the pain is caused by stress or psychological factors. Take care not to mislead the patient into thinking that the pain will go away if he relaxes.

2. Select terminology carefully. If the patient reacts negatively to or lacks understanding of the term "relaxation," select words from the patient's vocabulary. Examples of words that may be more acceptable or understandable to the patient are: comfort, hope, peace of mind, uplifting, renewal of faith or energy, time out, or collecting your thoughts.

3. Ask the patient if he has used any relaxation method in the past. If so, he may still be conditioned to it, so time and energy will be saved by using or building on that technique.

4. Be relaxed yourself when you talk with the patient about relaxation. Use a quick and easy technique, e.g., deep breath/tense, etc. (p. 199), before entering the patient's room.

5. Live, in person, assistance (your presence and voice) with relaxation is probably the most effective, but since it is time consuming, try to tape record instructions. This saves your time, and the patient may use the tape whenever he wishes rather than rely on your availability.

6. Demonstrate and practice the relaxation technique with the patient. Allow for a return demonstration if time permits.

7. Anticipate the need for the patient to use relaxation. Explain and teach relaxation prior to the patient being in pain or distress, e.g., preoperatively or prior to a course of chemotherapy.

8. Consider giving the patient and family copies of patient/family teaching points about preparing for and using relaxation techniques.

9. Offer to include and teach close friends and family members. They too may benefit from relaxation. In fact, sometimes the patient is under too much stress to learn relaxation but family or friends may be appropriate candidates.

10. If several patients in the hospital or clinic setting need to learn relaxation techniques, teach patients in groups.

11. Individualize the content of the relaxation technique by asking the patient to suggest changes. Whenever possible, let the patient select the technique after he has been exposed to several choices.

12. Inform others (health team, family) of what the patient will be doing, when, and why. This may decrease the patient's self-consciousness about doing something different, avoid ridicule from those who do not appreciate the value of relaxation, prevent others from discounting pain as simply anxiety, and minimize disruptions when the patient uses the technique. Others may also help by reminding the patient to use relaxation, but *caution them not to suggest relaxation as a substitute for other appropriate pain relief measures.*

13. Identify the need for additional pain relief before, during, or after the technique is used. Relaxation usually does not decrease pain, but it tends to enhance the effectiveness of other pain relief measures.

14. In selecting and recommending relaxation techniques, consider the specific situation as well as the characteristics of the specific patient. The techniques described in the chapter along with indications for use are summarized in the box on pp. 194 to 195, and practical guidelines for matching techniques to patients and situations are listed in the box on p. 191.

15. Give the patient a choice of closing his eyes or focusing on an object. Explain that this helps avoid disturbing sights. Do not insist that he close his eyes. Some patients fear loss of control or object to the degree of passivity inherent in closing their eyes.

16. If your time is limited, consider the following three-part time plan for time-consuming techniques that involve tape-recording a meditative or progressive relaxation script:

    Part 1. Plan 10 to 15 minutes for: discussion of the benefits of learning relaxation skills, general description of techniques you are able to provide, time for the patient to ask questions, and a specific description of the technique the patient chooses. Leave a copy of the script with the patient if he can read. Set a time with the patient for the next 15-minute visit, and ask the patient to provide a tape recorder with microphone and a blank cassette tape (unless these are already available). If possible, plan a way to tape record the relaxation technique with slow, non-lyric music in the background.

    Part 2. Plan about 15 minutes for: review of potential benefits and limitations of relaxation and time for patient to ask questions or make changes in the relaxation technique previously selected. Record the technique. Ask the patient about his reactions to the technique, when he intends to listen to it, and to let you know if he has any problems.

    Part 3. Contact the patient within 3 days and ask if he has used the technique. If not, determine why. If he has used the technique, ask him how he felt dur-

Characteristics of Specific Relaxation Techniques and Indications for Use

Deep Breath/Tense, Exhale/Relax, Yawn (p. 199)

This takes only a few seconds; is easily learned by patient; is appropriate to introduce when patient is already tense and in pain, e.g., during a procedure, or may be taught prior to brief painful procedures or preoperatively.

Humor (p. 199)

This takes very little of the nurse's time to suggest to patient; patient may spend as much time as he wishes using it. It may be appropriate for patients who are elderly; who resist or misunderstand the idea of relaxation; who are depressed or easily lose contact with reality; who have little time or energy for learning the skill of relaxation; or who are from a different culture (assuming a tape from his culture can be obtained). It may be used to relieve boredom of prolonged pain under confining circumstances; also appropriate for brief procedural pain.

Heartbeat Breathing (p. 200)

The nurse may have to teach the patient how to find and count the radial pulse, and some patients may have difficulty with this. If not, it takes very little of the nurse's or patient's time. Heartbeat breathing has an internal focus but is used only briefly. It may relieve a sudden, sharp increase in fear or anxiety and may be used without others noticing. It may be very helpful to patients who are aware of a sudden increase in heart rate during stress.

Jaw Relaxation (p. 200)

This takes very little time for the nurse to teach or for the patient to use. It is considered an abbreviated form of progressive relaxation. Its effectiveness may be due to relaxation of one area of the body leading to relaxation of the rest of the body. Useful for brief moderate to severe pain, e.g., postoperative pain, especially if taught in the absence of severe pain and tension. Effective with elderly patients.

Slow Rhythmic Breathing (p. 201)

This takes very little of the nurse's time to teach. It is very adaptable; patient can use for 30 to 60 seconds (a few breaths without others noticing) or for up to 20 minutes. It is also a useful technique for initial relaxation prior to engaging in more complex relaxation techniques.

Peaceful Past Experiences* (p. 201)

This may prove to be the best of all approaches to relaxation since it relies on what the patient has already found relaxing. It is usually an outward focus, i.e., not focused on the present body state. Recalling a peaceful experience is often a therapeutic process, and this approach may be most appropriate for patients with chronic pain, particularly those with terminal illness. Remembering certain past experiences may serve many purposes, e.g., releasing or letting go of treasured events or reinforcing the conviction that a valued event will occur again. However, the sharing of a valued past experience may require a trusting relationship between the nurse and patient. This may take a considerable amount of the nurse's time, but not always.

Give *priority* to this for terminally ill patients, and tape record it.

Meditative Relaxation Script (pp. 202-203)

This usually takes a minimum of three contacts with the patient. The first two take about 15 minutes each. The second usually involves tape recording the script. The third is a follow-up and may take only a minute unless problems occur. The script is highly effective in producing relaxation in English-speaking, middle-class Americans. It is permissive enough that the patient can individualize it on his own, and it combines an inward focus (breathing techniques and modified progressive relaxation) with an outward focus (peaceful place). Even when the patient says that certain options in the script are not helpful to him, it is seldom necessary to rerecord the tape, since the patient usually says he simply ignores what does not help him.

Give *priority* to this (or peaceful past experiences, or progressive relaxation) for patients with prolonged pain. It takes more time than you may have and it is not a miracle, but it often makes a significant difference.

Progressive Relaxation Script (pp. 204-205)

This also usually takes a minimum of three contacts with the patient for a total of 35 minutes or more. The first two contacts take about 15 minutes. The second usually involves tape recording the technique. The third is a follow-up and may take only a few minutes, unless problems have occurred.

Its potential advantages are that it involves physical activity that gives a sense of "doing something," e.g., muscle contraction, dissipates energy, is focused inward without the necessity of keeping the eyes closed, does not rely exclusively on mental activity, and easily gets the patient's attention by asking him to perform specific tasks.

Give this *priority* for patients with prolonged pain who exhibit signs of moderate to severe anxiety or "fight or flight," especially if they cannot engage in their customary physical exercise. They need to get rid of that muscular energy. Later they may benefit from a more meditative approach.

---

*Nurses attuned to this approach report they can engage a patient in conversation about a significantly relaxing event within moments of their first encounter with the patient, even in a stressful situation, e.g., emergency room. When I (McCaffery) ask the patient about peaceful or comforting memories, what is most striking to me is the intensity of the patient's description and the attention to details, especially the sensory aspects such as colors and tactile experiences. I find myself taking notes at top speed while the patient eagerly describes a scene or event. Terminally ill patients in general and any patients with prolonged pain seem to benefit enormously from talking about a significant past experience and then reliving it by listening to it on tape. Whether or not it produces relaxation is not clear to me. Its importance, however, is indisputable. Just ask someone this: Would you tell me where you were, who you were with, and what you were doing when you felt the greatest peace, joy, or comfort? The answers to these questions may enable the patient to use his own strengths and beliefs to increase his sense of identity and worth.

Continued.

Characteristics of Specific Relaxation Techniques and Indications for Use—cont'd.

Simple Touch, Massage, or Warmth (p. 206)

This may be done by the nurse or the patient's family or friends. It need not take much time and is indicated for patients who do not have time or energy to do for themselves whatever would produce relaxation. Loved ones who want to feel useful may benefit themselves and the patient by committing to body rubs of only 3 minutes, e.g., back, feet, hands. Help family and friends identify definite times for performing body rubs. This gives structure for the patient and the loved ones.

ing and after the technique. If there are problems, consult Table 7-1. Encourage the patient appropriately. Emphasize the positive and avoid any tension or urgency in relation to relaxation.

17. If the patient indicates that he does not want to try relaxation, never insist that the patient perform a technique against his will. This could result in severe side effects such as marked increase in depression or loss of contact with reality. Also, some patients endure pain with less distress by using muscle tension, i.e., relaxing may make the pain worse or less tolerable.

18. To evaluate the effectiveness of relaxation, simple measures include:

    a. Pulse rate before, during, and after relaxation. This is a type of biofeedback.

    b. Pain and distress scales before and after relaxation (see Figure 7-1; explain, draw, or show to patient).

    c. Gentle movement of body parts by nurse or others to determine any signs of tension before, during, and after relaxation. For example, carefully support the patient's arm or leg, and slowly flex or rotate the extremity. This too may provide the patient with biofeedback about the existence or absence of tension.

19. If pain is anticipated, e.g., a procedure, especially if the patient is fearful of it, suggest that the patient mentally rehearse the procedure while he is in a relaxed state, i.e., after he has used a relaxation technique. This may desensitize the patient to frightening aspects of the procedure.

20. Plan to provide regular reinforcement for the patient's use of relaxation. Patients using relaxation may be easily discouraged since relaxation is not consistently or dramatically effective, and it may use energy and time that are already in short supply. Indeed, for some patients, the benefits of relaxation do not warrant the time and effort required.

Serious or undesirable side effects from relaxation are not common but may occur in some patients. Relaxation lowers a person's defenses. Various unexpected, and sometimes unwanted, feelings or thoughts may emerge. This is more likely to occur with meditative techniques.

As a general guideline, if any problems are not quickly resolved, gently ask the patient to stop using that particu-

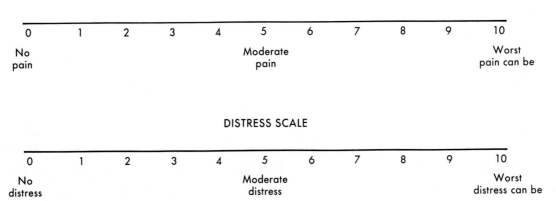

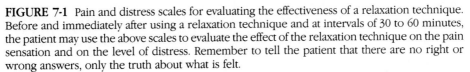

FIGURE 7-1 Pain and distress scales for evaluating the effectiveness of a relaxation technique. Before and immediately after using a relaxation technique and at intervals of 30 to 60 minutes, the patient may use the above scales to evaluate the effect of the relaxation technique on the pain sensation and on the level of distress. Remember to tell the patient that there are no right or wrong answers, only the truth about what is felt.

lar technique. To avoid feelings of failure, suggest the patient try a briefer technique with eyes open and/or a more structured or externally focused one. Certain problems may require referral or consultation. Table 7-1 lists problems most likely to occur with relaxation and suggests some possible solutions.

Patient/Family Teaching Points for General Use of Relaxation Techniques

For brief relaxation techniques, very little teaching or explanation may be required. However, for patients who are regularly using relaxation techniques that last 5 minutes or longer, the teaching points on p. 197 should be

TABLE 7-1 Relaxation: Possible Problems and Solutions

Problems	Possible Solutions
1. Falls asleep.	1. Set timer, or sit in straight-back chair. Ask about sleep patterns; especially inquire about sleep problems and medications. Patient may simply need to get more sleep.
2. Increased coughing or other respiratory problems.	2. May need to avoid deep breathing. Suggest breathing quietly, perhaps through pursed lips. To avoid changing the patient's normal breathing pattern, use a technique without a focus on breathing. Coughing is likely to be a problem with patients who smoke or have upper respiratory problems.
3. Prickly, tingling feelings, especially in the extremities.	3. Change positions; be sure extremities are not crossed.
4. Increased awareness of pain.	4. Add more distraction, such as activity, thoughts, or imagery to the technique. Avoid focusing on areas of pain. If this does not help, suggest shorter techniques.
5. Transient increase in heart rate, or increased awareness of heartbeat or breathing; eyelids flutter.	5. Assure patient this is normal. Encourage focus on other parts of relaxation technique or add external focus. Try heartbeat breathing at the beginning of the technique. If increased heart rate continues, gently suggest the patient discontinue the technique, report findings to physician, and see suggested solutions for item No. 10 below.
6. Feelings of suffocation.	6. Take a deep breath when desired. Adjust position to allow fuller expansion of lungs.
7. Restless legs (creeping or crawling sensation often of unknown cause, may result in the patient feeling the need to get up and walk around).	7. Mild cases may be relieved by keeping the legs cold; some patients report relief from heat. Otherwise, use brief relaxation techniques.
8. Increased focus on body functions and discomforts.	8. Change to a technique with an external focus, i.e., avoid a focus on the body; keep eyes open; try briefer technique.
9. Mild anxiety; fear of loss of control.	9. Reassure patient that he is in control and these feelings will probably subside. Consider shorter techniques or progressive relaxation with eyes open.
10. Hallucination, "out of body" feeling, loss of contact with reality, or general increase in depression or withdrawal.	10. Gently explain need to stop technique. To avoid feelings of failure, suggest short techniques with eyes open. Report finding to physician and obtain appropriate referral.
11. Sudden or increased crying, sadness, or extreme anxiety, such as perspiration, rapid respiration, and trembling.	11. Gently suggest discontinuing the technique. To avoid feelings of failure, suggest briefer techniques or progressive relaxation with eyes open. Ask patient if he wishes to deal with these feelings, and report finding to physician. If patient wants to deal with feelings, provide time for this or consider appropriate referral.
12. Patient uses technique frequently and this is associated with increased isolation and decreased function; patient may seem to "overdose" on relaxation.	12. Patient may desperately need other methods of pain relief that enable him to function at a higher level. Or, patient may try to use relaxation as an acceptable way to withdraw from others. Gently try to persuade patient to reduce use of that technique, and introduce briefer techniques. Present other methods of pain relief. Report findings to physician and ask for consult regarding mental health status. Evaluate patient frequently. May become an emergency, e.g., suicide threats.

NOTE: If the patient regularly uses relaxation techniques, periodically ask the patient how he feels during and after the technique. Be alert to:
- *Patient reluctance to report certain problems.* He may believe the problem is inevitable or unavoidable. Or, he may feel inadequate because he interprets a problem as his own failure.
- *The patient does not always consider the above to be problems,* e.g., items 10 and 12. They may be the patient's usual method of coping or they may be temporarily effective. Before suggesting solutions, note whether or not the patient considers it a problem. Of course, sometimes intervention is indicated even when the patient does not consider his reactions a problem, e.g., progressive withdrawal.

Patient/Family Teaching Point: Learning and Using Relaxation Techniques

TO: _____ (patient's name)   DATE: _____

1. Find a technique that works for you. Your nurse may be able to describe some alternatives. Also, you may wish to listen to some tape-recorded ones.
2. Stick with the same technique once you have selected one. You may combine several, but keep your relaxation exercise essentially the same each time. This helps you become conditioned to it, that is, you learn the skill faster and relax faster and better each time.
3. Be patient. It may take several practice sessions before you experience much benefit.
4. Practice at least once a day; twice a day is probably better. Relaxation is considered a skill that can be learned with repeated practice. Even if your pain subsides, continue to practice relaxation daily so you will remember how when you need to use it again.
5. When you are beginning to learn relaxation, practice when you feel fairly free of pain and tension. It's hard to learn anything when you're upset or in pain. Later, when you have learned the skill of relaxation, you will be able to use it more successfully during periods of distress or pain. However, try not to let things get that bad.
6. Use relaxation preventively, before pain and tension increase. Keep pain and distress under control.
7. During any given day, you may practice relaxation and then use it whenever needed to deal with pain and tension. If you find that your total time spent in relaxation is 1 hour or more, talk with your nurse. Other measures may be needed.
8. Do not expect success every time. Measure success by the fact that you tried. Your ability will vary. You cannot force relaxation to happen. You can only give it an opportunity. Everybody who practices anything, such as tennis or piano, knows that some days they perform well and some days they do not.
9. When you need to use something brief, select some small, helpful portion of the longer technique. Once you have learned a relaxation technique, note which parts are most helpful to you.
10. Check for tension at intervals throughout the day. For example, about every hour, quickly note your body from head to toe and use a brief technique to help decrease any tension you find.
11. Get ready to relax if you are using a relaxation technique lasting 5 minutes or longer. To obtain the maximal benefit from a relaxation technique, prepare for it in the following ways:
    - Get into a comfortable, well-supported position. Lying down or using a reclining chair may be best.
    - If you lie down, try elevating the legs and putting a small pillow under your neck as shown in the figure on the right. This gives you a head start on relaxing, since elevating the legs in this manner relieves a lot of tension in the muscles of the lower back and the neck.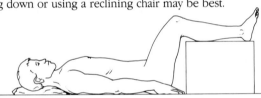
    - If you sit up, support your arms, e.g., place them in your lap, on a table in front of you, or on the chair's armrests. Do not dangle your arms.
    - Do not cross your legs or arms. They become heavy and may begin to cut off circulation, causing prickling sensations.
    - Try to create a quiet environment. Take the telephone off the hook, and consider placing a "Do not disturb" sign on your door. If there are noises that cannot be eliminated, listen to them before you begin your relaxation technique. This allows you to identify and, if necessary, respond to sounds so you may more easily ignore them later. Sometimes the steady noise of a fan, air conditioner, or "easy-listening" radio music will help override other distracting sounds. If your technique is taped, listen to it with a headset to minimize environmental noises.
    - Empty your bladder.
    - Loosen tight clothing, and take off any uncomfortable items, e.g., eye glasses.
    - Put down anything you are holding so you don't have to worry about dropping it as you relax.
    - If you are "cold natured," cover yourself.
    - If you wish to evaluate how well relaxation is working for you, try one of the following:
      Before and after relaxation, take your pulse rate. Sometimes you will notice a decrease in your heart rate after relaxation.
      Before and after relaxation, rate your pain and distress. Use a 0 to 10 scale for each. For distress, 0 equals no distress, and 10 equals worst distress can be. For pain, 0 equals no pain, and 10 equals worst pain can be. Sometimes you may note a decrease in both; other times, pain may remain the same, but your distress will decrease.
      Have someone gently move a body part, e.g., bend your arm for you, to test for any feelings of tension.
    Your nurse can show you pain and distress scales and help you learn to count your pulse.

From: _____ (nurse's name)   Phone: _____

■ May be duplicated for use in clinical practice. From McCaffery, M, and Beebe, A: PAIN: CLINICAL MANUAL FOR NURSING PRACTICE, St. Louis, 1989, The CV Mosby Company.

discussed with the patient and family. These suggestions are stated in the exact words that may be spoken to the patient, or the patient/family teaching point may be duplicated and given to the patient who can read.

Patient/Family Teaching Points for Specific Relaxation Techniques with Active Patient Involvement

The specific relaxation techniques covered in this section are presented in a sequence that roughly approximates the amount of time usually required for the nurse to teach the patient and for the patient to perform the technique or learn the skill. Naturally, the more experience and knowledge the nurse has about relaxation and the more time she can devote to individualizing the technique for the patient, the better the outcome is likely to be. However, a longer technique is not necessarily a more effective one for the individual patient. In reality the amount of time and energy available to both the nurse and patient may be a significant factor in determining which technique is chosen.

The presentation of the techniques begins with those that usually require the least amount of the nurse's or patient's time, progressing to those that are moderately time-consuming for the nurse or patient, and ending with those that are often referred to as training techniques (those that the patient will practice daily over a long period of time). At the end of the chapter a section on methods of touch and massage for relaxation is included for those patients who are not able or willing to be actively involved in achieving relaxation (p. 206).

The directions for each relaxation technique are stated in the exact words the nurse might say to the patient. If the patient can read, the appropriate patient/family teaching point(s) from pp. 199 to 205 may be duplicated and given to the patient and family.

Text continued on p. 206.

Patient/Family Teaching Point: Deep Breath/Tense, Exhale/Relax, Yawn for Quick Relaxation

---

TO: _____ (patient's name)   DATE: _____

1. Clench your fists; breathe in deeply and hold it a moment.
2. Breathe out slowly and go limp as a rag doll.
3. Start yawning.
    Additional points: Yawning becomes spontaneous. It is also contagious, so others may begin yawning and relaxing too.

From: _____ (nurse's name)   Phone: _____

■ May be duplicated for use in clinical practice. From McCaffery, M, and Beebe, A: PAIN: CLINICAL MANUAL FOR NURSING PRACTICE, St. Louis, 1989, The CV Mosby Company.

Patient/Family Teaching Point: Humor for Relaxation

TO: _____ (patient's name)   DATE: _____

Laugh when you hurt? Hurting is rarely funny, but people who hurt sometimes find that occasional humor is one of the most effective ways to deal with pain. Why not try some of the following?
1. Watch television programs that are really funny to you.
2. Listen to recordings by comedians that you find hysterical.
3. Read books that make you laugh.

Something funny can certainly be distracting, but its value seems to go beyond a momentary redirection of thoughts. Humor may produce relaxation.

For example, when you laugh, it is almost impossible to maintain muscle contraction. A simple example of this is when two or more people attempt to lift a heavy object in unison. One of them may be in charge of coordinating the efforts. That person counts or gives some cue to signal everyone to lift at the same time. But if they laugh, they fail. The result is familiar: the lifters become limp, drop the object, and sometimes actually fall to the floor. Laughter causes skeletal muscle relaxation; the skeletal muscles become too limp to hold or lift an object.

When Norman Cousins reported on his painful illness, he noted that 10 minutes of belly laughter resulted in 2 hours of sound sleep. Many have speculated about the reason. Could laughing have relaxed him?*

From: _____ (nurse's name)   Phone: _____

*For more information on use of humor, see patient/family teaching point on "Taking Laughter Seriously," p. 178.

■ May be duplicated for use in clinical practice. From McCaffery, M, and Beebe, A: PAIN: CLINICAL MANUAL FOR NURSING PRACTICE, St. Louis, 1989, The CV Mosby Company.

Patient/Family Teaching Point: Heartbeat Breathing for Relaxation

---

TO: _____ (patient's name)   DATE: _____

Before you do this, if you are unsure about how to find and count your pulse rate (usually radial pulse at the wrist), ask your nurse to help you.

1. Take a deep, comfortable breath.
2. Close your eyes or focus on your hands.
3. Count your radial pulse (at the wrist) for two beats.
4. Inhale while you count the next two beats.
5. Exhale while you count the next three beats.
6. Inhale and exhale in this manner several times.

Additional points: You can do this quickly if you are suddenly anxious or fearful. You can do this without drawing attention to yourself. The pulse (heart) rate usually slows noticeably.

From: _____ (nurse's name)   Phone: _____

■ May be duplicated for use in clinical practice. From McCaffery, M, and Beebe, A: PAIN: CLINICAL MANUAL FOR NURSING PRACTICE, St. Louis, 1989, The CV Mosby Company.

Patient/Family Teaching Point: Jaw Relaxation

TO: _____ (patient's name)   DATE: _____

1. Let your lower jaw drop slightly, as though you were starting a small yawn.
2. Keep your tongue quiet and resting in the bottom of your mouth.
3. Let your lips get soft.
4. Breathe slowly, evenly, and rhythmically: inhale, exhale, rest.
5. Allow yourself to stop forming words with your lips and stop thinking words.

Additional points: This technique may reduce both pain and distress, especially postoperatively.

From: _____ (nurse's name)   Phone: _____

■ May be duplicated for use in clinical practice. From McCaffery, M, and Beebe, A: PAIN: CLINICAL MANUAL FOR NURSING PRACTICE, St. Louis, 1989, The CV Mosby Company.

Patient/Family Teaching Point: Slow Rhythmic Breathing for Relaxation

---

TO: _____ (patient's name)   DATE: _____

1. Breathe in slowly and deeply.
2. As you breathe out slowly, feel yourself beginning to relax; feel the tension leaving your body.
3. Now breathe in and out slowly and regularly, at whatever rate is comfortable for you. You may wish to try abdominal breathing.
4. To help you focus on your breathing and breathe slowly and rhythmically:
   Breathe in as you say silently to yourself, "in, two, three."
   Breathe out as you say silently to yourself, "out, two, three."
   or
   Each time you breathe out, say silently to yourself a word such as peace or relax.
5. You may imagine that you are doing this in a place you have found very calming and relaxing for you, such as lying in the sun at the beach.
6. Do steps 1 through 4 only once or repeat steps 3 and 4 for up to 20 minutes.
7. End with a slow deep breath. As you breathe out you may say to yourself "I feel alert and relaxed."
   Additional points: If you intend to do this for more than a few seconds, try to get in a comfortable position in a quiet environment, and close your eyes (or focus on an object). If you are not sure you know how to do abdominal breathing, ask your nurse for help. This technique has the advantage of being very adaptable in that it may be used for only a few seconds or for up to 20 minutes. For example, you may do this regularly for 10 minutes twice a day and then use it for one or two complete breaths any time you need it throughout the day or when you awaken in the middle of the night.

From: _____ (nurse's name)   Phone: _____

■ May be duplicated for use in clinical practice. From McCaffery, M, and Beebe, A: PAIN: CLINICAL MANUAL FOR NURSING PRACTICE, St. Louis, 1989, The CV Mosby Company.

Patient/Family Teaching Point: Peaceful Past Experiences

TO: _____ (patient's name)   DATE: _____

Something may have happened to you a while ago that can be of use to you now. Something may have brought you deep joy or peace. You may be able to draw on that past experience to bring you peace or comfort now. Think about these questions.

Can you remember any situation, even when you were a child, when you felt calm, peaceful, secure, hopeful, comfortable?

Have you ever laid back, kicked off your shoes, and daydreamed about something peaceful? What were you thinking of?

Do you get a dreamy feeling when you listen to music? Do you have any favorite music?

Do you have any favorite poetry that you find uplifting or reassuring?

Are you now or have you ever been religiously active? Do you have favorite readings, hymns, or prayers? Even if you haven't heard or thought of them for many years, childhood religious experiences may still be very soothing.

Very likely some of the things you think of in answer to these questions can be tape recorded for you, such as your favorite music or a prayer read by your clergyman. Then you can listen to the tape whenever you wish. Or, if your memory is strong, you may simply close your eyes and recall the events or words.

From: _____ (nurse's name)   Phone: _____

■ May be duplicated for use in clinical practice. From McCaffery, M, and Beebe, A: PAIN: CLINICAL MANUAL FOR NURSING PRACTICE, St. Louis, 1989, The CV Mosby Company.

Patient/Family Teaching Point: Meditative Relaxation Script

TO: _____ (patient's name)   DATE: _____

This script takes approximately 6 minutes and contains four parts:
1. Ways of using breathing to relax.
2. Passive progressive relaxation, i.e., thinking of body parts relaxing as you breathe out.
3. Remembering a place where you felt peaceful and calm.
4. Method for ending the relaxation experience.

This technique should be tape-recorded. You may choose your nurse or someone else to record this. Listening to the tape with a headset helps reduce distracting noises from the environment.

The script is usually most effective if it is read slowly in a quiet, monotone voice with frequent, brief pauses. There is a pause at the end of each sentence, a bit longer pause between paragraphs, and pauses within the script are also suggested by "...". Change the script in any way you wish. At the end, some changes are suggested for specific portions of the script; they are indicated within the script by one or more asterisks (*). Consider including background music, something you like that is "easy-listening" without lyrics (without words).

You may use this relaxation technique in any comfortable, well-supported position, sitting or lying down. To get the most out of relaxation, prepare yourself and the environment. Your nurse can give you a list of suggestions.

Following are the exact words that may be used in the script:

(*Name of patient*), this is (*name of person speaking*). I believe you have chosen to listen to this because you want to give yourself a chance to experience and benefit from relaxation. Together we will do what we can at this moment. We cannot make it happen, but each time we will try to find a way to help you allow it to happen, if it will. We cannot make it happen, but together we will try to create an opportunity for you to experience relaxation.

Please close your eyes now.... Breathe in slowly and deeply. As you breathe out slowly, perhaps you can feel yourself beginning to relax.... Now you may breathe in your usual way, just slowly and regularly—whatever is comfortable for you. You may find that breathing from your abdomen helps you relax a bit more.... Each time you breathe out, perhaps you can allow yourself to feel you are relaxing more and more.

*You may be able to begin to identify your own special feelings of relaxation. Perhaps you feel heavy, or maybe you feel light, weightless, as if you're floating.... You may feel limp, warm, or you may feel the tension draining from your body. Perhaps you can let these relaxed feelings spread throughout your body.

**You may wish to try certain ways of breathing to help you relax more. You may wish to think about your breathing, feel the air enter your nose and lungs,... feel the air leave your lungs and nose, and feel the tension leaving your body as you breathe out.

Or, you may wish to select a word such as peace or calm... and say the word silently to yourself each time you breathe out.

Or, you may find you relax more if you imagine that you breathe in through your fingertips, up your arms and shoulders. Then breathe out down your trunk, abdomen, legs, and leisurely out your toes.

I will pause now for a few moments while you use whichever method of breathing seems to help you relax more and more. (Length of pause to be determined by patient, or arbitrarily set at 20 seconds minimum.)

***Now you may wish to relax separate parts of your body. If so, you may begin by thinking of your feet, ankles, and calves. The next time you breathe out, feel these areas relax.

You may think of your legs. The next time you breathe out, you may feel the tension draining down your legs and out the tips of your toes.

You may think of your abdomen, pelvis, and lower back. As you breathe out, feel these areas relax.

You may think of your arms and hands. The next time you breathe out, you may feel the tension draining down your arms and out the tips of your fingers.

You may think of your shoulders and neck. Feel these areas relax as you breathe out.

You may think of your face, forehead, mouth, and scalp. Feel these tiny muscles relax the next time you breathe out....

****Now if you wish you may remember a place where you felt very peaceful, calm, secure.... Perhaps you can allow yourself to go there in your imagination. You may look around. Notice what there is to see, the objects, the colors.... Notice the sounds... the smells... the temperature of the air.... Perhaps you can find a comfortable place to sit or lie down in this peaceful environment and continue to relax more and more....

■ May be duplicated for use in clinical practice. From McCaffery, M, and Beebe, A: PAIN: CLINICAL MANUAL FOR NURSING PRACTICE, St. Louis, 1989, The CV Mosby Company.

Continued.

Patient/Family Teaching Point: Meditative Relaxation Script—cont'd.

*****When you are ready, there is a method you may use to end this relaxation experience for yourself. You may listen to this and remember it, but you do not have to use it until you are ready. . . . When you are ready, you may count slowly and silently to yourself from one to three. At the count of one, move your lower body slightly. At the count of two, move your upper body slightly. At the count of three, breathe in deeply, hold it a moment, and open your eyes. As you breathe out, say silently to yourself, "I feel relaxed and refreshed." (End of script.)

Other ideas or suggestions for the script (the asterisks below correspond with those in the script):
*If you can identify your own feelings of relaxation prior to taping, the alternatives can be omitted and your own feelings can be repeated, added, or elaborated upon.

**If you can identify the most effective method of breathing for yourself prior to taping, the alternatives can be omitted and your preference for relaxing breathing can be repeated, added, or elaborated upon.

***You may wish to reverse or change the sequence of body parts. You may also want to omit certain body parts if you find that focusing on them causes discomfort. Some people find it helpful to omit the body parts that hurt, while others find it helpful to increase a focus on and effort to relax the areas that hurt. Or, you may wish to spend more time focusing on particular body parts that do not hurt.

****If possible, tell your nurse or person recording the tape details about the peaceful place you have chosen. This may help you imagine it more vividly and recapture the peace you felt then. Focus on the specific sensations that were most important to you, e.g., some people remember more of what they saw; others, what they heard.

*****The ending may be omitted or ignored if you want to use this to go to sleep. But, if you intend to function after using the relaxation technique, give yourself time to go through the transition from relaxed to active. If you have experienced a true relaxation response, you need time to journey from that particular level of awareness to the level of being aware of external expectations and requirements.

Additional points: Once you have gained skill in using this technique to produce relaxation, you may find that when your time is limited you can benefit from using one small part of it, e.g., briefly imagining your peaceful place. This can be a practical way of integrating relaxation into your daily life. To prevent tension from building up, at intervals throughout the day you might take a slow, deep breath, close your eyes for a few seconds and imagine your peaceful place.

From: _____ (nurse's name)   Phone: _____

■ May be duplicated for use in clinical practice. From McCaffery, M, and Beebe, A: PAIN: CLINICAL MANUAL FOR NURSING PRACTICE, St. Louis, 1989, The CV Mosby Company.

Patient/Family Teaching Point: Progressive Relaxation Script

TO: _____ (patient's name)   DATE: _____

This technique consists of:

1. Tense (or contract) and then relax specific muscle groups.
2. Usually tense/relax is done twice with each muscle group.
3. In the following script, 14 muscle groups are used, but many different groups may be used.

You may perform this technique from memory or by referring to the written directions. However, most people prefer to have it tape-recorded. Listening to the tape with a headset helps decrease distracting noises in the environment. You may choose your nurse or someone else to record this.

Before this is recorded, follow the directions for at least one or two sets of tense/relax. Have your recorder note approximately how many seconds you prefer to contract your muscles and how many seconds you prefer to remain relaxed between muscle contractions.

You may do this relaxation technique in any comfortable, well-supported position, sitting or lying down. To get the most out of relaxation, prepare yourself and the environment. Your nurse can give you a list of suggestions.

Changing the script. The script may be changed in several ways. In the script, each muscle group is noted with a bullet (•). Go over each of these. If you do not understand the directions for the muscle contraction, ask for an explanation or change the directions. If you want a longer technique (up to 20 minutes), divide the muscle groups into smaller groups; if you want a shorter technique, combine some muscle groups into one group or perform each muscle contraction only once with each muscle group. Determine if any muscle groups should be omitted. Some muscle contractions may increase your pain. If you are prone to leg cramps, you may wish to omit all muscle contractions involving the legs and feet. Also, the sequence may be changed, e.g., you may begin at the toes and progress to the upper body.

Following are the exact words, designed for tape-recording, that may be used in the script:

(*Name of patient*), this is (*name of person speaking*). I believe you have chosen to listen to this because you want to give yourself a chance to experience and benefit from relaxation. Together we will do what we can at this moment. We cannot make it happen. Sometimes you will feel relaxed, sometimes you won't. All we can do is go through the technique and give it a chance to work.

You may close your eyes now or find something to focus on. Breathe in deeply, hold it a moment, and breathe out slowly. Now you may breathe in your usual way, just slowly and regularly.

• Clench your right fist and hold it.
  Feel the tension. Now let it relax. Feel the difference. Notice the feelings of relaxation.
  Now, with less tension, clench your right fist again and hold it.
  Feel this level of tension. Now let it relax. Notice the feelings of relaxation in your hand.
• Clench your left fist and hold it.
  Feel the tension. Now let it relax. Feel the difference. Notice the feelings of relaxation.
  Now, with less tension, clench your left fist again and hold it.
  Feel this level of tension. Now let it relax. Notice the feelings of relaxation in your hand.
• Press your upper right arm toward your ribs and press the elbow back. Hold it.
  Feel the tension. Now let it relax. Feel the difference. Notice the feelings of relaxation.
  Now, with less tension, once again press your upper right arm toward your ribs and press the elbow back. Hold it.
  Feel this level of tension. Now let it relax. Notice the feelings of relaxation in your arm.
• Press your upper left arm toward your ribs and press the elbow back. Hold it.
  Feel the tension. Now let it relax. Feel the difference. Notice the feelings of relaxation.
  Now, with less tension, once again press your upper left arm toward your ribs and press the elbow back. Hold it.
  Feel this level of tension. Now let it relax. Notice the feelings of relaxation in your arm.
• Wrinkle your forehead and hold it.
  Feel the tension. Now let it relax. Feel the difference. Notice the feelings of relaxation.
  Now, with less tension, once again wrinkle your forehead and hold it.
  Feel this level of tension. Now let it relax. Notice the feelings of relaxation in your forehead.

■ May be duplicated for use in clinical practice. From McCaffery, M, and Beebe, A: PAIN: CLINICAL MANUAL FOR NURSING PRACTICE, St. Louis, 1989, The CV Mosby Company.

Continued.

===
Patient/Family Teaching Point: Progressive Relaxation Script—cont'd.
===

- Wrinkle your nose and shut your eyes tightly. Hold it.
  Feel the tension. Now let it relax. Feel the difference. Notice the feelings of relaxation.
  Now, with less tension, again wrinkle your nose and shut your eyes. Hold it.
  Feel this level of tension. Now let it relax. Notice the feelings of relaxation in your nose and eyes.
- Clench your teeth, pull back the corners of your mouth, and press your tongue against the roof of your mouth. Hold it.
  Feel the tension. Now let it relax. Feel the difference. Notice the feelings of relaxation.
  Now, with less tension, again clench your teeth, pull back the corners of your mouth and press your tongue against the
    roof or your mouth. Hold it.
  Feel this level of tension. Now let it relax. Notice the feelings of relaxation in your mouth and jaw.
- Press your head backwards and hold it.
  Feel the tension. Now let it relax. Feel the difference. Notice the feelings of relaxation.
  Now, with less tension, again press your head backwards and hold it.
  Feel this level of tension. Now let it relax. Notice the feelings of relaxation in your neck.
- Bring both shoulders upward toward your ears and hold it.
  Feel the tension. Now let it relax. Feel the difference. Notice the feelings of relaxation.
  Now, with less tension, bring both shoulders upward toward your ears and hold it.
  Feel this level of tension. Now let it relax. Notice the feelings of relaxation in your shoulders.
- Make your stomach hard, pull it inward, and hold it.
  Feel the tension. Now let it relax. Feel the difference. Notice the feelings of relaxation.
  Now, with less tension, again make your stomach hard, pull it inward, and hold it.
  Feel this level of tension. Now let it relax. Notice the feelings of relaxation in your stomach.
- Press your right leg backwards and hold it.
  Feel the tension. Now let it relax. Feel the difference. Notice the feelings of relaxation.
  Now, with less tension, again press your right leg backwards and hold it.
  Feel this level of tension. Now let it relax. Notice the feelings of relaxation in your leg.
- Press your left leg backwards and hold it.
  Feel the tension. Now let it relax. Feel the difference. Notice the feelings of relaxation.
  Now, with less tension, again press your left leg backwards and hold it.
  Feel this level of tension. Now let it relax. Notice the feelings of relaxation in your leg.
- Point your right toes, stretch, and hold it.
  Feel the tension. Now let it relax. Feel the difference. Notice the feelings of relaxation.
  Now, with less tension, again point your right toes, stretch, and hold it.
  Feel this level of tension. Now let it relax. Notice the feelings of relaxation in your leg and foot.
- Point your left toes, stretch, and hold it.
  Feel the tension. Now let it relax. Feel the difference. Notice the feelings of relaxation.
  Now, with less tension, again point your left toes, stretch, and hold it.
  Feel this level of tension. Now let it relax. Notice the feelings of relaxation in your leg and foot. (End of script.)

    Additional points: Once you have gained skill in using this technique to produce relaxation, you may find that when your time is limited you can benefit from using one small part of it, e.g., briefly clenching and relaxing your fists. This can be a practical way of integrating relaxation into your daily life. To prevent tension from building up, at intervals throughout the day you might clench your fists, note the tension, and then relax, noting the feelings of relaxation. Relaxation of one part of the body may spread throughout the body.

From: _____ (nurse's name)   Phone: _____

RELAXATION TECHNIQUES: THE PATIENT AS PASSIVE RECIPIENT

The relaxation techniques previously discussed require the patient's active participation to some extent, and for the most part, are techniques the patient can learn to do for himself. However, some patients are simply unable to participate actively in achieving relaxation and need to have something done for them to help them relax.

Appropriate/Inappropriate Patients/Situations

Examples of *appropriate patients* are those who are:
- Debilitated or acutely ill, i.e., limited physical or emotional energy.
- Babies and young children; elderly.
- Confused or agitated.
- In acute or sudden distress or pain.
- Extremely fatigued or sedated, e.g., immediate postoperative period.

- Those with families or friends who would like to do something to help the patient and who can learn to perform these relaxation techniques for the patient.
  Examples of *inappropriate patients* are those who:
- Are uncomfortable with physical touch.
- Dislike feelings of passivity or dependence.

Nursing Care Guidelines and Patient/Family Teaching Points for Specific Techniques

The patient/family teaching point for simple touch, massage, or warmth (below) includes information for all caregivers and may be duplicated and given to the patient, family members, or friends.

For additional information about massage and for a teaching guide that can be duplicated and given to the patient/family, see Chapter 5, Cutaneous Stimulation, p. 141 on superficial massage, including "Patient/Family Teaching Point: Massage of Body, Hands, or Feet," p. 142.

Patient/Family Teaching Point: Simple Touch, Massage, or Warmth for Relaxation

---

TO: _____ (patient's or massager's name)   DATE: _____

Touch and massage are age-old methods of helping others relax. Some examples are:
1. Brief touch or massage, e.g., handholding or briefly touching or rubbing a person's shoulder. These are so common and quickly done that we sometimes forget they are methods of helping someone relax.
2. Warm foot soak in a basin of warm water, or wrap the feet in a warm, wet towel.
3. Massage (3 to 10 minutes) may consist of whole body or be restricted to back, feet, or hands. If the patient is modest or cannot move or turn easily in bed, consider massage of the hands or feet.
   Use a warm lubricant, e.g., a small bowl of hand lotion may be warmed in the microwave oven, or a bottle of lotion may be warmed by placing it in a sink of hot water for about 10 minutes.
   Massage for relaxation is usually done with smooth, long, slow strokes. (Rapid strokes, circular movements, and squeezing of tissues tends to stimulate circulation and increase arousal.) However, try several degrees of pressure along with different types of massage, e.g., kneading, stroking, and circling. Determine which is preferred.
   Especially for the elderly person, a back rub that effectively produces relaxation may consist of no more than 3 minutes of slow, rhythmic stroking (about 60 strokes/minute) on both sides of the spinous process from the crown of the head to the lower back. Continuous hand contact is maintained by starting one hand down the back as the other hand stops at the lower back and is raised.
   Set aside a regular time for the massage. This gives the patient something to look forward to and depend on.

From: _____ (nurse's name)   Phone: _____

■ May be duplicated for use in clinical practice. From McCaffery, M, and Beebe, A: PAIN: CLINICAL MANUAL FOR NURSING PRACTICE, St. Louis, 1989, The CV Mosby Company.

INDIVIDUALIZED NURSING CARE PLAN

Patient Who May Benefit from a Brief Relaxation Technique

Patient Description: Ms. P., age 47, is admitted for a cholecystectomy the following day. Preoperative teaching and postoperative follow-up include the following.

Assessment	Potential Nursing Diagnoses	Planning/Intervention	Evaluation/ Expected Outcomes
Identify: • Ability to understand and follow directions. • Previous use of relaxation. • Desire or willingness to try a brief relaxation technique following surgery. • Possibility of including family or friends in relaxation teaching.	Pain, related to impending surgery. Fear related to outcome of surgery and pain. Sleep pattern disturbance before and after surgery related to hospital environment and to the pain and stress of surgery.	Describe one or two brief relaxation techniques and let the patient choose Teach the relaxation technique by including the following: • Detailed explanation (consider patient/family teaching tools). • Provide demonstration and period for patient to practice (include family or friends if possible). • Encourage practice again before surgery. • Review technique with patient as soon as feasible following surgery. Emphasize that learning a simple relaxation technique may have the following benefits: • Aid sleep periods and decrease fatigue during day. • Reduce distress of hospitalization, surgery, and discomfort. • Reduce strain on the incisional area, thereby reducing some pain. • Enhance the effectiveness of pain relief measures such as analgesics. • Facilitate a return to comfort following an uncomfortable activity such as deep breathing or turning. Teach the patient to try to remember to use relaxation at the following times: • Before, after, and if possible during painful activities. • Before pain occurs or increases. • Along with, not instead of, pain relief measures, such as analgesics. Inform health team members about patient's use of relaxation and the need to forewarn patient of pain so relaxation can be used preventively.	Patient reports one or more of the following occur when she uses relaxation: • Less discomfort during a painful activity. • More rapid return to comfort following a painful activity. • Less distress following a painful activity. • More rapid onset of analgesia following medication. • Greater pain relief from analgesics. • Improved ability to return to sleep when awakened during the night. • Decrease in fatigue during the day. • Ability to decrease incisional pain. Patient appears to feel pride and a sense of control in relation to using relaxation.

INDIVIDUALIZED NURSING CARE PLAN

Patient Who May Benefit from Regular Daily Use of a Relaxation Technique

Patient Description: Mr. C., age 34 years, is recuperating at home following a work-related back injury 6 weeks ago. He has ongoing pain from muscle injury and spasm. He comes to the clinic for physical therapy three times a week, in addition to performing daily exercises at home, sees the physician once or twice a week for trigger point injections, and meets with the clinic nurse once a week to review his progress and coordinate his care. Medications include muscle relaxants and nonnarcotic analgesics.

Assessment	Potential Nursing Diagnoses	Planning/Intervention	Evaluation/ Expected Outcomes
Identify: • Level of pain and distress. Consider teaching patient to use pain and distress scales (Figure 7-1). • Use of medications and their effectiveness. • Sleep disturbance. • Fatigue or excessive undirected physical energy. • History of psychiatric disorders and current level of depression. • Ability to understand and follow directions. • Time available to patient for use of relaxation. • Desire for personal control of distress, pain, fatigue. • Previous use of relaxation. • Desire or willingness to try relaxation. • Possibility of including family or friends in relaxation training.	Pain, potential chronic, related to back injury. Anxiety, moderate, related to pain and lack of control over ability to progress and return to work. Sleep pattern disturbance related to pain and distress.	Emphasize belief in patient's pain and in the primary cause being related to work injury. Describe benefits, limits, and types of relaxation available. Unless contraindicated, encourage use of techniques lasting 3 minutes or longer. Allow patient to choose technique. Teach relaxation technique by including the following: • Give more detailed description of technique. • Ask if patient wants any changes. • Provide demonstration and/or period of patient practice. • Provide relevant patient/family teaching points and/or tape recording. • List of ways to prepare to get the maximal benefit from the use of relaxation, e.g., positioning. • Emphasize learning skill by practicing the same technique daily during periods of minimal pain and stress. • Include family member or close friend during instructions. If patient desires objective evidence or record of achieving relaxation, suggest use of pain and distress scales or pulse rate before and after using technique. If available, someone can test extremities for tension during or after use of technique. Emphasize use of relaxation preventively and as an addition to, not as a substitute for, other appropriate treatment. Suggest use of relaxation before and after distressing or painful activities, and at bedtime and if awakened during night. Plan a time within the next 3 days to check with patient regarding his response during and after use of relaxation. Plan regular follow-up to determine if any problems occur and to provide reinforcement, including assurance that immediate and dramatic effects are not expected.	Patient reports one or more of the following: • Less distress from daily discomfort and from pain related to physical therapy exercises, perhaps indicated as a lower number on the distress scale. • Less sleep disturbance. • Less fatigue. • Generally improved mood. • Better pain relief from nonnarcotics and muscle relaxants when he uses relaxation at the time he takes the medications. • Sense of control over his progress. If patient reports problems with relaxation and suggested solutions are not effective, gently explain that the technique should be discontinued and obtain appropriate consultation or referral.

RESOURCES FOR PATIENTS

BMA Audio Cassettes (Guilford Publications). This series includes tapes with instruction and information about relaxation as well as tapes of various relaxation techniques. Address: 200 Park Ave S, New York, NY 10003; toll free 1-800-221-3966 or in New York 212-647-1900. Many other companies have similar offerings.

CompCare Publishers sells several tapes on relaxation and visualization as well as videos for stress control. Address: Comprehensive Care Corporation, 2415 Annapolis Lane, Minneapolis, MN 55441; toll free 1-800-328-3330 or in Minnesota call collect 612-559-4800; call between 8:30 AM and 5:00 PM central time, Mon-Fri.

Plain Talk About the Art of Relaxation. Two pages, defines relaxation, explains some causes of stress, and suggests ways to relax. Single copy free from the Public Inquiries Branch, National Institute of Mental Health, Parklawn Bldg Room 15C-05, 5600 Fishers Lane, Rockville, MD 20857; 301-443-4513.

Psychology Today Tapes. This series includes tapes with instruction and information about relaxation as well as tapes of various relaxation techniques. Address: Dept. 728, Box 059073, Brooklyn, NY 11205-9061; toll free 1-800-345-8112. Many other companies have similar offerings.

"Relax Your Self." This 40-minute audiotape consists of two relaxation exercises with music in the background. Address: Self Health Cassettes, 16661 Ventura Blvd, Suite 822, Encino, CA 91426-1914 (about $11.00).

"The Relaxation Tape." This was developed by S. Sampson to help patients with headaches learn to relax. To order, send $9.00 to: National Headache Foundation, 5252 N Western Ave, Chicago, IL 60625.

SELECTED ANNOTATED REFERENCES THAT CITE RESEARCH OR GIVE CLINICAL SUPPORT

Many of the noninvasive pain relief measures, such as relaxation, have not yet been adequately researched. This sometimes makes it difficult to document or justify the use of these techniques. The following brief, annotated list provides some clinical or research support for use of relaxation as discussed in this chapter.

American Nurses' Association. For statements on generic and specialty nursing practice, including use of relaxation and suggestive therapies, write: ANA, 2420 Pershing Rd, Kansas City, MO 64108.

Bruya, MA, and Stevertsen, B: Evaluating the effects of music on electroencephalogram patterns of normal subjects, *J Neurosurg Nurs* 16:96-100, Apr 1984. Electroencephalogram (EEG) responses of 47 adult volunteers were compared while they listened to music by Chopin and by the new age composer Steven Halpern. Brain wave activity did not support the claim that Halpern's music puts subjects into a state of relaxed, alert consciousness. The study raised many questions and no conclusions were possible. However, some subjects said that they found Halpern's music disturbing and irritating.

Ceccio, CM: Postoperative pain relief through relaxation in elderly patients with fractured hips, *Orthopaed Nurs* 3:11-19, May-June 1984. Patients aged 56 to 89 years were taught jaw relaxation prior to surgical repair of fractures and compared to a control group that was not taught relaxation. Pain and distress scores after the painful activity of turning during which the experimental subjects used jaw relaxation showed significantly lower pain and distress compared to the control group. Overall intake of analgesics was also lower. Other studies (e.g., Flaherty and Fitzpatrick, 1978) have also demonstrated that relaxation taught preoperatively could reduce pain and analgesic intake postoperatively.

Cleeland, CS: Nonpharmacological management of cancer pain, *J Pain Sympt Manag* 2:S23-S28, Spring 1987. This overview emphasizes that relaxation is never a substitute for other appropriate therapies such as analgesics for the patient with cancer; it is most clearly indicated for patients without significant prior psychiatric history. Successful use of relaxation should never be misunderstood as indicative of the pain being psychogenic.

Clum, GA, Luscomb, RL, and Scott, L: Relaxation training and cognitive redirection strategies in the treatment of acute pain, *Pain* 12:175-183, 1982. A laboratory study using ischemic pain showed that relaxation training appears to reduce distress attendant upon experiencing pain, but does not reduce pain perception during the actual infliction of pain.

Graffam, S, and Johnson, A: A comparison of two relaxation strategies for the relief of pain and its distress, *J Pain Sympt Manag* 2:229-231, Fall 1987. This study compared the effectiveness of taped transcripts of guided imagery and progressive muscle relaxation in 30 oncology patients. The patients' pain and distress ratings before and after listening to each tape showed that both strategies were equally effective in reducing pain and distress. However, most patients preferred the progressive muscle relaxation technique, some saying it was difficult for them to clear their minds to visualize the peaceful scene described in the guided imagery tape. Although the authors did not mention this, it seems possible from the patients' comments that the progressive muscle relaxation may have served as a distractor from pain. Thus distraction, either instead of or in addition to relaxation, may have produced pain relief.

Horowitz, BF, Fitzpatrick, JJ, and Flaherty, GG: Relaxation techniques for pain relief after open heart surgery, *Dimens Crit Care Nurs* 3:364-371, Nov-Dec 1984. This study compared the effects of jaw relaxation with generalized passive relaxation in patients following open heart surgery. Generalized passive relaxation was more effective than jaw relaxation, significantly reducing distress postambulation. There was no apparent effect on pain sensation in either group. Both techniques apparently were effective to some extent, e.g., both reduced systolic blood pressure on postambulation.

Kulich, RJ, and Warfield, CA: Relaxation in the management of pain, *Hosp Pract* 20:117-121, Dec 15, 1985. This excellent overview of benefits of relaxation training for chronic nonmalignant pain emphasizes relaxation, not as pain relief but as adjunctive treatment and only as partial rather than perfect control. It gives specific ideas about teaching relaxation, including contraindications and problems.

Lapp, JE: Music vs. biofeedback for migraine headache, unpublished paper, Calif. State Univ., Fresno, Calif., 1986. Patients with migraine who were taught relaxation and imagery skills and listened to self-selected, non-lyric, "easy-listening" music reported significantly fewer and less intense migraine head-aches 1 year later than did those who used biofeedback in-stead of music. This difference was probably due to the fact that the music group practiced significantly more, stating that music heard randomly throughout the day served as a stim-ulus to practice.

Mast, D, Meyer, J, and Urbanski, A: Relaxation techniques: a self-learning module for nurses: Unit III, *Cancer Nurs* 10:279-285, 1987. This article includes specific instructions for teaching the patient deep breathing, passive muscle relaxation, and relaxing imagery. An example of a relaxation log is included.

Mogan, J, Wells, N, and Robertson, E: Effects of preoperative teaching on postoperative pain: a replication and expansion, *Int J Nurs Stud* 22:267-280, 1985. Preoperatively one group of patients was taught a relaxation technique consisting of rhyth-mic breathing, pleasant imagery, and generalized muscle re-laxation. Equal time was spent with a control group. Follow-ing elective abdominal surgery, the group taught relaxation reported less distress caused by the pain, but the pain sensa-tion itself did not seem to be affected.

Peveler, RC, and Johnston, DW: Subjective and cognitive effects of relaxation, *Behav Res Ther* 24:413-419, 1986. This study shows that passive muscular relaxation with pleasant mental imagery and meditation was as effective as simple information when both were conducted by a therapist, but in solo practice relaxation was much more effective. Based on this study and a review of the literature, the suggestion is made that regular practice of relaxation can make adaptive thoughts more ac-cessible, i.e., if relaxation improves mood, there may be greater likelihood that positive, helpful thoughts will emerge. It is noted that the beneficial effects of relaxation persist well beyond the period of practice of the technique.

Turner, JA, and Chapman, CR: Psychological interventions for chronic pain: a critical review. I. Relaxation training and bio-feedback, *Pain* 12:1-21, 1982. Based on this extensive review of the literature up to 1981, the authors conclude that the efficacy of relaxation techniques has only been shown for headache and to some extent for temporomandibular joint pain. They also find that evidence to date indicates that biofeedback is not more effective than relaxation training for headaches. They suggest that relaxation could be a valuable therapeutic tool for patients with chronic nonmalignant pain if it is taught as a coping skill to assist in learning better ways of responding to life stresses that trigger or exacerbate pain. A later review (Turner and Romano, 1984) arrived at the same conclusions. An even more recent review (Roberts, 1987) again concluded that biofeedback has not been shown to be essential or to be superior to other treatments for chronic pain and may even exacerbate pain in some patients.

REFERENCES AND SELECTED READINGS

Bailey, LM: Music therapy in pain management, *J Pain Sympt Manag* 1:25-28, Winter 1986

Barsevick, A, and Llewellyn, J: A comparison of the anxiety-reducing potential of two techniques of bathing, *Nurs Res* 31:22, 1982

Bayuk, L: Relaxation techniques: an adjunct therapy for cancer patients, *Semin Oncol Nurs* 1:147-150, 1985

Benson, H: The relaxation response, New York, 1975, William Morrow

Benson, H: Beyond the relaxation response, New York, 1984, Times Books

Blanchard, EB, Andrasik, F, Evans, DD, and Hillhouse, J: Biofeed-back and relaxation treatments for headache in the elderly: a caution and a challenge, *Biofeedback Self-Regul* 10:69-73, Mar 1985

Bresler, DE: Free yourself from pain, New York, 1979, Simon and Schuster

Brown, BB: Stress and the art of biofeedback, 1978, New York, Bantam Books

Cogan, R, Cogan, D, Waltz, W, and McCue, M: Effects of laughter and relaxation on discomfort thresholds, *J Behav Med* 10:139-144, 1987

Copp, LA: The spectrum of suffering, *Am J Nurs* 74:491-495, Mar 1974

Davis-Rollans, C, and Cunningham, S: Physiologic responses of coronary care patients to selected music, *Heart Lung* 16:370, July 1987

DiMotto, JW: Relaxation, *Am J Nurs* 84:754-758, June 1984

Donovan, MI: Relaxation with guided imagery. In Donovan, MI, ed: Cancer care: a guide for patient education, pp 242-256, New York, 1981, Appleton-Century-Crofts

Donovan, MI: Relaxation with guided imagery: a useful tech-nique, *Cancer Nurs* 3:27-32, Feb 1980

Dossey, B: A wonderful prerequisite, *Nursing* 14:42-45, Jan 1984

Fakouri, C, and Jones, P: Relaxation Rx: slow stroke back rub, *J Gerontol Nurs* 13:32-35, Feb 1987

Flaherty, GD, and Fitzpatrick, JJ: Relaxation technique to increase comfort level of postoperative patients: a preliminary study, *Nurs Res* 27:352-355, 1978

Freedberg, PD, Hoffman, LA, Light, WC, and Kreps, MK: Effects of progressive muscle relaxation on the objective symptoms and subjective responses associated with asthma, *Heart Lung* 16:24-30, Jan 1987

Graffam, S: Report of survey of untoward reactions to relaxation strategies, *Pain Res Nurs Forum* 3:3, Mar-Apr 1983

Hanswer, M, Larson, SC, and O'Connell, AS: Music therapy-assisted labor: effects on relaxation of expectant mothers, *Birth Psychol Bull* 4:2, 1983

Heide, FJ, and Borkovec, TD: Relaxation-induced anxiety: mech-anisms and theoretical implications, *Behav Res Ther* 22:1-12, 1984

Herman, JA: The effect of progressive relaxation on valsalva response in healthy adults, *Res Nurs Health* 10:171-176, 1987

Kaempfer, SH: Relaxation training reconsidered, *Oncol Nurs Forum* 9:15-18, Spring 1982

Kutz, I, Caudill, M, and Benson, H: The role of relaxation in behavioral therapies for chronic pain, *Int Anaesth Clin* 21:193-200, Winter 1983

Lapp, J: Music hath charms to soothe a throbbing head, *Psychol Today* 21:14, Feb 1987 (as reported by P Chance)

Larson, B, Daleflod, B, Hakansson, L, and Melin, L: Therapist-assisted versus self-help relaxation treatment of chronic head-aches in adolescents: a school-based intervention, *J Child Psychol Psychiatry* 28:127-136, Jan 1987

Levin, RF, Malloy, GB, and Hyman, RB: Nursing management of postoperative pain: use of relaxation techniques with female cholecystectomy patients, *J Adv Nurs* 12:463-472, July 1987

Longworth, JCD: Psychophysiological effects of slow stroke back massage in normotensive females, *Adv Nurs Sci* 4:44-61, July 1982

Lyles, JN, Burish, TG, Krozely, MG, and Oldham, RK: Efficacy of relaxation training and guided imagery in reducing the aversiveness of cancer chemotherapy, *J Consult Clin Psychol* 50:509-524, Aug 1982

Mast, D, Meyer, J, and Urbanski, A: Relaxation techniques: a self-learning module for nurses: Unit I, *Cancer Nurs* 10:141-147, 1987

Mast, D, Meyer, J, and Urbanski, A: Relaxation techniques: a self-learning module for nurses: Unit II, *Cancer Nurs* 10:217-225, 1987

McCaffery, M: Nursing management of the patient with pain, pp 137-155, Philadelphia, 1979, JB Lippincott

McCaffery, M: Relieving pain with noninvasive techniques, *Nursing* 10:55-57, Dec 1980

Miller, KM: Deep breathing: a pain management technique, *AORN J* 45:484-488, Feb 1987

Newman, RI, Seres, JL, Yospe, LP, and Garlington, B: Multidisciplinary treatment of chronic pain: long-term follow-up of low-back pain patients, *Pain* 4:283-292, 1978

Registered Nurses as Providers of Relaxation and Suggestive Therapies: A position statement, San Francisco, Mar 1982, California Nurses Association

Restless Legs Syndrome, *Harvard Medical School Health Letter* 12:2-3, Aug 1987

Roberts, AH: Literature update: biofeedback and chronic pain, *J Pain Sympt Manag* 2:169-171, Summer 1987

Shaw, L, and Ehrlich, A: Relaxation training as a treatment for chronic pain caused by ulcerative colitis, *Pain* 29:287-293, 1987

Snyder, M: Progressive relaxation as a nursing intervention: an analysis, *Adv Nurs Sci* 6:47-58, Apr 1984

Snyder, M: Independent nursing interventions, New York, 1985, John Wiley & Sons

Stuckey, SJ, Jacobs, A, and Goldfarb, J: EMG biofeedback training, relaxation training, and placebo for the relief of chronic back pain, *Percept Mot Skills* 63:1023-1036, 1986

Swinford, P: Relaxation and positive imagery for the surgical patient: a research study, *Periop Nurs Q* 3:9-16, Sept 1987

Trygstad, L: Simple new way to help anxious patients, *RN* 43: 28-32, Dec 1980

Turner, JA, and Romano, JM: Evaluating psychologic interventions for chronic pain: issues and recent developments, *Adv Pain Res Ther* 7:257-296, 1984

Wortz, E: A yawn a day, *Psychol Today* 21:8, May 1987

CHAPTER 8

Imagery

DEFINITION OF IMAGERY FOR PAIN RELIEF

Imagine not having pain. In a way, that is what imagery for pain relief is—the use of one's *imagination* to control pain. This involves mental images or internal representations. Imagining is a form of thinking that most people use rather regularly. It is commonly referred to as "trying to picture" something, visualizing, daydreaming, or fantasizing.

Imagery techniques for physical healing date back hundreds of years. Recently, imagery has been used in the treatment of medical conditions such as cancer, hypertension, acne, alcoholism, arthritis, and in the management of symptoms such as depression, anxiety, and nausea and vomiting, as well as pain related to cancer, backache, and headache.

The use of imagery for pain relief does not imply that the pain is imagined. *No pain is truly imaginary. All pain is real.* This chapter does not discuss using imagination to deal with imaginary pain. It does focus on how imagery may be of help to certain patients with acute or chronic pain, whether or not physical causes are known.

KEY POINT: Caution! Are people saying any of the following about your patient's pain? "It's just his imagination." "It's all in his head." "It's psychogenic." "He just thinks he hurts; it isn't that bad." If so, this *is not* the chapter you need to read. Look up pp. 11 to 12 on misconceptions in Chapter 2 on assessment.

The use of imagery in relation to pain control is suggested elsewhere in this book in Chapter 6 on distraction (e.g., imagining dancing to music while listening to it) and Chapter 7 on relaxation (e.g., imagining a peaceful place). Obviously, imagery may be used for a number of purposes. Common uses of imagery in relation to pain are summarized in the box on the right.

Many structured pain relief imagery techniques are preceded by a relaxation technique or involve a relaxing image. These imagery techniques may result in relaxation and distraction in addition to decreased pain. In other words, there may be considerable overlap between imagery techniques for pain relief, distraction from pain, and relaxation.

Imagery for the purpose of pain relief may be *defined* as using one's imagination to develop sensory images that decrease the intensity of pain or that become a pleasant, more acceptable, or nonpainful substitute for pain, e.g., numbness or coolness. In other words, imagery may act as an analgesic or anesthetic. Images may vary from brief, such as those used in ordinary conversation, to lengthy, such as those developed systematically for the individual. The latter is often referred to as *therapeutic guided imagery.* The purpose is to use it for pain relief. The patient deliberately or purposefully imagines something about pain that will provide pain relief, rendering this activity *therapeutic,* or helpful. The nurse may assist the patient in

---

Common Uses of Imagery or Imagination in Relation to Pain

1. Imagery may be used for *distraction* from pain, resulting in increased tolerance for pain (see Chapter 6 for examples).
2. Imagery may be used to produce *relaxation*, resulting in decreased distress associated with pain (see Chapter 7 for examples).
3. Imagery may be used to produce an *image of pain relief,* resulting in a decrease in the perceived intensity of pain (see examples in this chapter).

IMMEDIATE HELP FOR IMAGERY

Time involved: Reading time, 5 minutes; implementation time, 10 minutes.

Sample situation: Patient is in pain and probably will continue to be for about 30 to 45 minutes while you and/or others are trying to do something more to relieve his pain, e.g., obtain appropriate analgesic orders.

Possible solution: Patient may be willing to try a simple type of imagery or use his own spiritual beliefs.

Expected outcome: Patient will feel his pain is acknowledged and someone cares. He finds the sensation of pain is relieved by becoming less intense or by changing to a more acceptable sensation. Or, he merely finds the pain more tolerable because this distracts him momentarily. He may note that he feels less anxious.

Don'ts

1. Do not expect or suggest that imagery will substitute for appropriate pain relief, e.g., adequate analgesic orders.
2. Do not attempt to present imagery for pain relief if you feel unsure or uncomfortable about it. *Or,* admit these feelings before you proceed, and explain why you think it's worth a try.
3. Do not say there is nothing else anyone can do.
4. Do not tell the patient that he must learn to cope with pain on his own. (He may learn to do this, but not in 10 minutes.)
5. Never tell the patient his pain is not as bad as he thinks.

Dos

1. Take a deep breath outside his room and relax a little yourself. Plan on spending up to 10 minutes with the patient. You are about to discuss something the patient may find strange; you need to be relaxed and confident.
2. When you enter the room tell the patient you know he hurts. Be certain that you have assured the patient that you consider his pain real, not imaginary, and that you believe it is just as intense as he says.
3. Tell the patient you are still hoping (searching) for a better alternative, but that meanwhile you would like to *offer* him the opportunity to try a technique that may ease his pain for just a little while.
4. Explain that you are going to describe a method of using concentration and imagination to help with pain for a brief time. Tell the patient that this may sound strange and he may not want to try it. If so, that is per-

fectly all right, but you want to offer it just in case it turns out to be something he wants to try and finds helpful.
5. Ask the patient if he daydreams or has a good imagination, or if prayer or any kind of faith helps him with pain or illness.

   If he gives a negative reply, tell him he may be better at it than he thinks. Ask him if he remembers a bedroom from his childhood (progress to any bedroom he remembers). Ask him how many windows it had and how many doors. If he can answer with confidence, point out that this is a result of memories that are mental pictures of some sort and not a result of storing numerical information. It is one example of how people who do not even have vivid mental pictures still use their imagination, e.g., images from the past. If he cannot answer these questions, admit that you might be wrong about the appropriateness of this method for him. Ask him if he wants you to continue. If so, try either of the following.

   If he gives a positive reply to daydreaming or a good imagination, use simple symptom substitution (p. 219), stressing that you are hoping that this will at least reduce unpleasant aspects of the pain for a short time. If the patient cannot concentrate well, try providing another sensation, e.g., cold, to focus on.

   If he gives a positive reply to some type of faith, use the ball of healing energy (p. 225), suggesting that he substitute his personal faith for the healing energy and that this may reduce his pain.
6. Tell the patient you will return to find out if he decided to try this and if it helped. Tell the patient when you will return, but give yourself leeway. It's better to return early than late.
7. When you return, ask the patient what he decided about the imagery.

   If the patient says he did not try the imagery, tell him you appreciate his considering it.

   If it did not work, tell him you admire his willingness to try the technique, reassuring him that it does not always work.

   If it did help, tell him you do not expect him to rely on it as his only source of pain relief.
8. In all cases, continue to explore and explain other plans for pain relief.

doing this by *guiding* him through the use or development of an imagery technique.

BENEFITS AND LIMITS OF PAIN RELIEF IMAGERY

The use of imagery for pain relief is based in part upon *two interrelated beliefs:*
1. Images may affect the functioning of the body in ways

over which we ordinarily have little or no control. Mental images or representations may be a key to partial control over body functions that we do not usually consciously control by rational thoughts.
2. The body may react to images (or memories of an event) in a manner very similar to its functioning or response during the actual event. For example, even when a person remains physically inactive, imagining jumping can increase heart and respiratory rates or

imagining bending the arm can result in minimal but measurable muscular activity. However, simply imagining *watching* rather than performing these activities may produce little if any effects. Likewise, trying to increase heart rate simply by desiring it to happen has little or no effect (Jacobsen, 1930; Jones and Johnson, 1980; Mast, 1986).

When conflict exists between imagination and the will, it has been said that imagination always wins. A simple example experienced by many people is the fear of speaking in front of a large audience. Perhaps this has happened to you. As you wait to give your speech you may find that your hands and knees are trembling and your heart is pounding. You may very much want to stop the trembling and pounding, but your will is not as strong as the threat or danger you imagine in relation to public speaking. Your imagination has won over your attempt to will your body to act in a different manner.

The potential benefits of imagery are perhaps best appreciated by seeing imagery in the context of a total situation. Imagery occurs naturally in relation to many everyday events as well as health care situations. Imagery may be conceptualized as *occurring within a sequence of events*:

1. An object or event is sensed, e.g., seen, felt, or heard. Example: The patient feels back pain.
2. An emotional response to the event or objects occurs. Example: The patient is afraid the back pain will not be relieved and will interfere with his plans to go to work.
3. Plans or images such as a mental rehearsal are evoked, sometimes only for a split second. Example: The patient thinks about taking an analgesic that never works very well, imagines himself at home alone instead of going to work, and wonders how he will pay his rent that month.
4. The body responds, i.e., a physiological response occurs, such as increased heart rate and increased muscle tension. Example: The patient feels his back muscles tighten and his heart pound.

KEY POINT: Possible Effect of Imagery

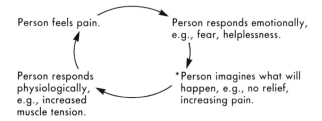

*Imagery may interrupt the process here to change the image of what will happen thereby changing the physiological response. A positive image may result in a helpful physiological response.

The power of imagery is considered by some to be primarily the image's physiological effect on the body.

For this reason, some view imagery as a potential self-healing technique. With regard to pain control, imagery may decrease pain by altering the physical cause of pain.

However, imagery may be beneficial without affecting the physiological aspects of pain, i.e., the cause of pain or the physiological response to it. Imagery may be used to render a painful sensation more acceptable, e.g., changing burning pain to a warm sensation. Imagery may also be beneficial without either altering the pain sensation or reducing the intensity of pain. Like relaxation, imagery may at times simply reduce the distress associated with pain.

Admittedly, the scientific basis of imagery is elusive, and health professionals are obliged to be cautious about what cannot be explained or understood. However, the professional literature refers to imagery as a useful technique that is within the realm of nursing practice. Not every nurse will feel comfortable helping patients with imagery, but every nurse can encourage and respect the use of it. Total dismissal of imagery is close-minded thinking and inhibits careful exploration of its potential. Let it not be said that we would rather see a patient suffer according to the rules than recover in an unorthodox manner.

The following discussion of the specific, potential benefits and limitations or disadvantages for patients who use imagery to relieve pain are especially relevant to more involved imagery techniques. Subtle, conversational images may have some of the same benefits or limitations, but this use of imagery is initiated by the nurse, is brief, and should occur naturally. Hence, as long as these are positive images, there is little danger in using them, and the benefit may range from being great for a susceptible patient to being negligible for others.

Potential benefits of pain relief imagery for the person with pain may include one or more of the following:

1. Forms and strengthens a close, trusting nurse-patient relationship.
2. Assists expression of feelings about pain and associated problems.
3. Encourages exploration and understanding of personal beliefs about illness and may alter erroneous or harmful ideas about pain.
4. Increases confidence in and ability to control or heal the painful experience. Imagery techniques tend to capitalize on the patient's strengths such as his creativity and ability to concentrate. When imagery is successful, the patient may feel very proud of himself.
5. Increases the effectiveness of other pain relief measures. For example, imagining increased warmth at an injection site may increase circulation to the area, cause faster absorption of an analgesic, and result in quicker onset of pain relief.
6. Decreases intensity of pain or changes the pain sensation into one that is more acceptable.

7. Dramatic and long-lasting pain relief from imagery has occurred in some patients. However, effectiveness remains highly unpredictable.

The *possible limitations or disadvantages* of pain-relieving imagery techniques are:

1. The suggestion to try an imagery technique may be misinterpreted by the patient as meaning that the health team regards the pain as being imaginary or "not real."
2. The successful use of imagery for pain relief may be misinterpreted by the health team as meaning that the pain is primarily imaginary or caused by psychological problems. Or, they may conclude the pain is not severe or significant if it can be controlled with a nontraditional method.
3. Successful use of imagery is rarely a substitute for other appropriate pain relief measures. In the majority of cases, imagery is only an adjunctive treatment for pain.
4. Some patients and health team members inaccurately regard imagery as unscientific and may scoff at the nurse or patient who uses it. The possibility that imagery may effectively relieve pain may be contrary to their belief systems.
5. Unwanted side effects may occur, especially with the longer, meditative imagery techniques (see Table 8-2, p. 218). Some side effects may be similar to those that may occur with relaxation (see Table 7-1, p. 196). Other side effects may be a result of the specific image, e.g., imagining cold may decrease the blood supply to an ischemic area and contribute to increased pain.
6. Imagery does not work for every patient with pain, even when the patient believes in its effectiveness and is highly motivated to use it.
7. It may take time to find or develop an effective technique for the individual.
8. Occasionally, the actual use or development of imagery is not only time-consuming for the nurse but also an emotionally exhausting experience.
9. Imagery that focuses on the pain sensation may increase pain or distress.
10. Unsuccessful use of imagery for pain relief may lead to feelings of failure in the patient.

IMAGERY TECHNIQUES FOR PAIN RELIEF

Numerous imagery techniques for pain relief have been developed and used successfully. However, in keeping with the purposes of this book, this chapter includes only selected examples that appear to be reasonably effective with appropriately chosen patients, are minimally time-consuming, low risk, and do not require knowledge or skills beyond those expected of the professional nurse with basic education.

Overview of Types of Imagery and Indications for Their Use

Four basic types of imagery are discussed here, summarized along with their indications for use in Table 8-1.

1. *Subtle,* or conversational. These may be contained in the nurse's routine statements and questions to the patient, e.g., during patient teaching or discharge planning. The nurse may already automatically or consciously use images to increase the likelihood of the patient understanding or remembering certain ideas. Common examples are explaining that antibiotics "fight" infection and a well-balanced diet helps "resist" infection.

2. *Simple, brief symptom substitution.* For example, for a short period of time the patient may be able to imagine his pain as being a sensation that is more acceptable, e.g., pressure rather than aching. This technique may be suggested and developed during a brief conversation with the patient.

3. *Standardized imagery techniques.* Certain techniques are brief and stated permissively enough to be used safely, quickly, and also effectively. The images are vague enough that the patient can individualize them in his own imagination.

4. *Systematically individualized imagery techniques.* These are developed in specific detail by the individual patient with guidance from the nurse. For example, the patient may develop an elaborate image of the antibiotic being many soldiers that successfully kill invading bacteria.

Appropriate/Inappropriate Patients/Situations

For subtle, conversational images and for some of the simple symptom substitution or release techniques, there

TABLE 8-1 Imagery Techniques and Indications for Their Use to Relieve Pain

Techniques	Possible Uses
1. Subtle, conversational.	1. Routine explanations of how pain relief measures work or how and when recovery takes place.
2. Simple, brief symptom substitution.	2. Brief, painful experiences or procedures.
3. Standardized imagery techniques.	3. Brief or prolonged pain in a patient who wants to use imagery, but the nurse lacks time for or experience in development of individualized imagery techniques.
4. Systematically individualized imagery techniques.	4. Brief or prolonged pain in a patient who wants to use imagery, and the nurse has time for and experience in (or a willingness to attempt) development of imagery.

are few restrictions or dangers. These may be used or suggested by the nurse in a casual manner that ensures that the patient will simply reject the idea if it is inappropriate. The more involved the development and use of imagery becomes, the more important are the following guidelines for selecting appropriate patients and situations and avoiding patients who are inappropriate.

Examples of *patients who may be appropriate* candidates for use of the more involved imagery techniques for pain relief include a child or adult who:

- Requests imagery or desires nontraditional approaches to health care (in addition to traditional methods).
- Has repeated contacts with the nurse over a long period, e.g., patients in long-term care facilities or home care.
- Understands the instructions.
- Is able to concentrate on the image.
- Has acute or chronic pain, especially a patient at the beginning of potentially long-term pain problems.
- Has artistic abilities, e.g., draws or paints pictures, writes stories, or is an actor/actress.
- Uses imagery in conversation, reads a lot, or admits to or talks about daydreaming or intense concentration during an activity.
- Is a verbal child, especially between the ages 8 to 11 years.
- Has strong religious beliefs.
- Has used nontraditional health care, e.g., studied Transcendental Meditation, is familiar with Simonton's imagery for cancer therapy, or takes yoga classes.

KEY POINT: Imagery techniques for pain relief may be helpful to patients who have pain of clearly defined physical origin.

The nurse whose educational background is limited to basic preparation or who has not specialized in mental health, counseling, or psychotherapy should probably avoid using meditative, lengthy, or intense imagery with certain patients, mainly because of possible adverse effects of imagery. (However, health professionals who are specially trained in counseling or psychotherapy may be able to work with the following patients in the use of imagery.) *Patients who may be inappropriate for the more involved or lengthy imagery techniques* are children or adults who:

- State they do not want to try imagery.
- Have severe emotional problems.
- Have a history of psychiatric illness.
- Report hallucinations for whatever reason, e.g., psychosis, drug reaction, or sensory restriction of ICU.
- Have no time or energy to devote to using lengthy imagery. Patients may use imagery for pain relief successfully for a while but finally become exhausted and unable to continue to use it.
- Cannot concentrate.

- Are or recently have been exposed to the unfortunate experience of health team members discounting their pain or failing to provide appropriate and effective pain relief. An exception may be made if the nurse is absolutely positive that she has communicated to the patient that she believes what the patient says about his pain and wants to help him find relief in spite of what others say or do.

Sometimes the nurse's inappropriate attempt to get a patient to use imagery is related to well-meant but misguided enthusiasm. Be alert to your own motivation to have the patient try imagery for pain relief. Occasionally, the nurse's successful use of imagery for her own pain or with other patients will result in an overly optimistic view that imagery can be effective for almost anyone if he or she will only try it. The nurse should carefully monitor her own motivation or purpose in suggesting imagery for pain relief to a patient. The following quotes from Steven Levine (1982) serve as helpful guidelines:

This offering [imagery for pain relief] should not be accompanied by even the subtlest suggestion that if those in pain use these techniques they will be "doing the right thing," that if they accept your advice they are good and that if they don't they are weak. (p. 126.)

As I offered this alternative, I watched closely for any quality in myself that wished her to be in any state other than the way she was, any desire that might in some subtle way motivate me to be "selling" her something that I imagined was best for her. (p. 127.)

KEY POINT: Imagery techniques for pain relief are merely *offered* to the patient as one way of dealing with pain. Never force or even strongly suggest imagery to a patient.

Nursing Care Guidelines for Developing and Using Imagery Techniques

To use or develop any type of pain relief imagery, ranging from brief conversational to lengthy individualized techniques, the following are useful *general guidelines:*

1. If you feel uncomfortable or unsure about imagery techniques, avoid trying to help a patient with pain relief imagery. If you think the patient is an appropriate candidate for imagery, try to find someone else to assist him. If this is not possible and if the patient has asked you for help with pain relief imagery, admit your feelings but encourage him to try on his own.
2. Always acknowledge the reality of and your belief in what the patient says about his pain. Before you introduce imagery techniques for pain relief, try to be sure that the patient knows you believe that most or all of the cause of his pain is physical, and you believe what he says about the nature of his pain sensation.
3. If the patient himself discounts his pain in any way, e.g., suggests that maybe he is imagining his pain or

he must be crazy to hurt when others can find no reason, tell the patient that you seriously doubt that he is crazy or is imagining the pain.

4. Listen for and incorporate the patient's spontaneous use of images. Use the positive, helpful images, but try to rephrase negative, unhelpful images. For example, the patient may comment that it feels like the muscles in his back are in knots. If you later give him a muscle relaxant, suggest that this will help untie those knots in his back muscles. Pain relief and/or recovery may be impeded if the patient maintains an image of his pain or an image that causes pain.

5. Images need not be anatomically or physiologically correct to be useful. For example, the patient may imagine that his incisional pain is a red, hot, hard square that becomes a pale pink, cool, soft circle as it begins to hurt less. On the other hand, the next guideline is also important.

6. Consider the potential effect of an image if it is taken literally. Images may affect the functioning of the body. For example, avoid using anything the patient is allergic to, e.g., picturing himself in a field of wheat if he is allergic to wheat. Consider the effect of the image on circulation, e.g., warmth may increase peripheral circulation, whereas coolness may decrease it. Therefore if a sensation of cold is suggested in the imagery, consider whether or not applications of cold would be contraindicated for that particular patient. Another example of the need for caution might be the patient who has a cardiac condition that requires complete bed rest and reduced oxygen needs. His heart and respiratory rate may increase if he uses an image that involves imagining he is running as fast as he can to escape pain.

7. Consider using the patient's religious or spiritual beliefs or practices, if any. Many religious writings and practices involve imagery that can be helpful in relieving pain, e.g., "God's healing hand" and scripture such as the 23rd Psalm.

8. Consider using the patient's artistic ability and interest, if any, e.g., drawing or painting pictures. For example, musicians or painters may more easily relate to or create auditory or visual images, respectively. Perhaps a connoisseur of fine wines would relate best to the taste or smell of pain.

9. Use the individual patient's preferences, if any, for sensory descriptors. The person may use several sensory modalities when he describes pain, but one modality may be predominant or specific words may be used repeatedly. For example, the patient may describe his pain using mainly visual descriptions such as the color, size, and shape of pain. "Screaming" pain is an example of an auditory description. "Bitter" pain is related to the gustatory (taste) and olfactory (smell) senses. "Writhing," "fast," and "crawling" are kines-

thetic (movement) descriptions; "rough," "burning," and "hard" are tactile (touch) descriptions.

10. Stress to the patient the importance of his developing his own images and that they may be vague or clear. When standardized images or systematically individualized images are used, examples of what others have done may be helpful, but avoid giving the patient specific images of his own pain sensation or methods of pain relief. However, to help the patient develop his own images, offer to answer any questions he has about his pain and methods of relief.

11. Try to focus more attention on soothing and positive descriptions of pain than on the word pain or on disturbing aspects of the pain. For example, rather than limiting your remarks to saying that pain in the legs is getting smaller and smaller, it may be more effective to focus more on the leg becoming more comfortable and relaxed with accompanying soft, smooth, healing sensations.

12. If the patient has difficulty imagining a method of relieving his pain, use imagery involving the desired result or state. Images may be either or both of the following:
    a. *Process image,* a method of achieving the desired result, e.g., imagining how the pain is relieved. This usually involves focusing on the pain and the pain relief measure. Not all patients can imagine this. Further, a focus on pain may increase pain.
    b. *Final state image,* a representation of the desired state, e.g., the body without pain. The dying patient may remember his body without pain or imagine the effective result of a pain relief measure. A recovering patient may imagine his body at a future time, relieved of pain by some pain relief measure, or healed and without pain. The patient need not focus on the pain nor have any idea of how the process of healing or pain relief will take place.

13. Use permissive directions and suggestions when you discuss or guide imagery. Simply offer the image rather than force it upon the patient. Use words and phrases such as "Perhaps...," "If you wish you may...," or "You might like to...."

14. If the patient seems easily frustrated or overly anxious to succeed, suggest that he sneak up on the image instead of trying to imagine it immediately. For example, a relaxation technique prior to the image may help him calm down and concentrate better. Or, if he has chosen to achieve warmth by imagining himself sunbathing at the beach, suggest he begin by imagining getting ready to go to the beach. Another method is to work with an image over time. The patient may imagine his pain as a red-hot poker and want to try to relieve it by imagining a stream of cool water flowing over it. The patient might practice this

TABLE 8-2 Imagery for Pain Relief: Possible Problems and Solutions

Problems	Possible Solutions
1. Reports problems with working out the logic of the specific imagery, e.g., unable to figure out how to move healing energy in or out of a certain area.	1. The patient may observe some rules of logic when he uses his imagination. Offer to listen and try to help him solve the problem. If this fails to help, remind him that anything is possible in one's imagination. If the patient continues to dwell on the problem, gently explain that this is not achieving the desired goal of pain relief and suggest that he try another imagery technique or stop using imagery.
2. Increased pain.	2. Most likely to occur if a process image is used because of a focus on pain. Try changing the image of how pain is relieved. If this fails, suggest switching to a final state image, i.e., focus on a pain-free image from the past or future, not on the pain sensation and how it will be relieved.
3. Increased distress, e.g., anxiety, depression, withdrawal.	3. Suggest that he try an entirely different image, explaining that sometimes a person chooses what he thinks is a pleasant or desirable image but it may contain unidentifiable sources of conflict or emotional disturbance.
4. Feels drowsy, sluggish, or tired afterwards.	4. Patient may simply be fatigued and need more sleep or rest. Or, try shortening length of imagery technique. Add a technique that slowly ends the imagery with suggestions of being rested and alert, e.g., count slowly from 1 to 5 while feeling more alert and beginning slight body movements, starting at the feet and progressing up to the head.
5. Fear that imagery will be so effective that it will eliminate pain as a useful warning signal, i.e., fear that bodily harm will occur without his awareness.	5. Be sure imagery is not being forced on this patient. If patient does want to use imagery, explain that imagery can be restricted to a specific area or pain, that he may retain some of the pain if he wishes, and that numbness rarely results and can be deliberately avoided.
6. Very difficult to arouse following imagery.	6. This is rare if imagery is used with the patient's full consent and the patient has been fully informed of the content of the imagery technique, especially if he has participated in developing the imagery. This is most likely to occur when imagery is guided by someone. Patient usually will spontaneously become aroused within a short time, e.g., may go to sleep and awaken refreshed. To arouse sooner, try asking the patient, "Why don't you want to be fully awake?" Then deal with the answer. If he says he is sleepy, suggest that he awaken now and plan to sleep later, giving a specific and appropriate time. When he is alert again, gently explain that drowsiness could be bothersome and that it is best if you do not conduct his imagery again. He may be able to conduct imagery on his own without extreme drowsiness, or drowsiness may be an indication of a severe, underlying mental or emotional disturbance.

NOTE: If any of the above problems are not easily resolved, gently explain to the patient the need to stop using imagery and consider a consultation from a professional hypnotherapist.

two or three times a day for days, starting with a small trickle of warm water that gradually becomes a cooler and larger stream.

15. Provide additional pain relief if needed, e.g., an analgesic in addition to imagery.

16. When imagery effectively relieves pain, be sure the patient is also assessed and treated appropriately for the underlying cause of the pain.

17. Inform others (health team, family) of what the patient is doing, when, and why. This may decrease the patient's self-consciousness about doing something different, avoid ridicule from those who do not appreciate the potential value of imagery, and minimize disruptions when the patient uses the technique. Others may also help by reminding the patient to use imagery for pain relief, especially preventively. But, *caution others not to suggest imagery as a substitute for appropriate pain relief measures.*

18. Be alert to problems that may result from the use of pain relief imagery and their possible solutions, summarized in Table 8-2 (see also problems related to relaxation, Table 7-1, p. 196).

Subtle, Conversational Imagery

Subtle imagery may be contained in the nurse's usual statements and questions to the patient. This need not take any additional time if images are already a natural part of the nurse's thinking and conversation. Many nurses already automatically use images in their routine discussions with patients, e.g., patient teaching or discharge planning. Teachers who are regarded as exceptionally good usually include imagery as one of their many teaching methods.

To develop your ability to use images more naturally in conversation with patients for the purpose of assisting with pain relief, *specific guidelines* are:

1. Identify a specific pain relief measure and try to explain how it relieves pain by using words that paint a mental picture or create sounds or tactile-kinesthetic feelings.

    Example: When you administer an analgesic you might say, "Now it's as if the medication is slowly floating through your body to find your pain and make it smaller and smaller, leaving feelings of comfort and healing."

2. Use words and phrases that tend to convey relaxing, pain relieving images.

    Examples:

    - Floating
    - Smaller
    - Softer
    - Melting
    - Dissolving
    - Smooth
    - Lighter
    - Quieting

    - Releasing
    - Slowly leaving
    - Healing
    - Cool or warm
    - Letting go
    - Soothing
    - Less and less
    - Loosening

    Notice when you use these words naturally. Practice using them more often in relation to pain relief.

3. Notice when a patient is given an image of what causes his pain, and try to make sure he is also given an image of how the pain will subside or be relieved.

    Example: The physician may explain how he will make an incision in a certain place and remove or repair something internally. The nurse may then add one or more of the following:

    - Afterwards a soft comfortable dressing will be in place.
    - A well-wrapped, lightweight cold pack may be placed over the area to make it feel soothingly cool.
    - Medication (narcotic) will help the brain feel fewer nerve impulses from the area.
    - Another medication (nonnarcotic) will go to the area to help soothe any swelling or irritation.
    - As you rest and take in nutrients the area will begin repairing and healing itself.
    - Within a week (or whatever period of time is reasonable) you will feel healed and healthy again.

4. Use only those images or descriptors that feel natural to you. You need to be at ease and comfortable with what you describe to the patient.

Simple, Brief Symptom Substitution

Helping a patient develop an image that substitutes pain with a more acceptable sensation, or perhaps a pleasant sensation, for a brief period of pain need not take much of the nurse's time. *Specific guidelines* are:

1. When pain is known to the patient because it is present or an impending painful procedure has been experienced before, the nurse's conversation with the patient may include the following:

    - Ask the patient, "How would you describe this pain?"
    - Note any words that seem more acceptable or less

uncomfortable than the actual sensation, such as stinging versus knifelike. Suggest "Perhaps it would help if you try focusing on just that feeling and try to ignore the total discomfort for a little while." Or the nurse could say "You might try pretending for a little while that this is what is happening instead of the actual discomfort."

Patient Example

Ms. C. had tonsilitis. Mouth care, drinking fluids, and eating were especially painful events. Upon questioning, Ms. C. described the pain as stinging, aching, like a rock in her throat, and pressure. The nurse suggested "Maybe you could try pretending that for some strange reason a rock is pressing into your throat—maybe you have to lie on it for a while. Swallowing just might hurt less if you imagine this silly, inconvenient rock being there." Ms. C. laughed, said she would try it, and reported that she was able to drink more fluids when she imagined the rock.

2. When pain is anticipated but not previously experienced by the patient, the nurse may describe what the sensation usually feels like to other patients, being careful to use descriptive words that are not necessarily unpleasant or very bothersome sensations.

    Examples of what the nurse might say:

    - If burning pain is typical, suggest to the patient "This procedure may hurt less (or be less troublesome) if you concentrate on or try to imagine it as being simply warm instead of burning. Maybe you can imagine the sun shining on you and warming the area."
    - If a procedure involves cleansing with an antiseptic, suggest to the patient "When you feel the cool sensation of the area being cleaned, you may want to try to focus on that coolness and try to ignore some of the other more uncomfortable and bothersome sensations."

3. For any type of brief pain, known or unknown to the patient, the nurse may try to help the patient substitute a sensation by actually providing a separate sensation for the patient to focus on. The nurse may say "I can give you a cube of ice to hold in your hand and you can try for a while to concentrate on the extreme cold rather than the discomfort in the rest of your body. You may even try to imagine the numbness in your hand transferring to numbness in the areas that hurt."

KEY POINT: Suggestions for symptom substitution are probably best used for brief pain (a matter of minutes, not hours) and should merely be offered to the patient as possible alternatives.

The remainder of the pain relief images are more time-consuming. The specific images and some overall considerations are explained in the patient/family teach-

---

Patient/Family Teaching Point: Using Imagery for Pain Relief

TO: _____ (patient's name)   DATE: _____

Definition of imagery for pain relief: deliberate use of your imagination to help you reduce your pain.

Your pain is certainly real, but you may be able to use your imagination in some way that helps relieve the pain. If you decide to try this, consider the following:

1. Find a technique that you like, one that makes sense to you. You may want to develop your own. The trick, of course, and it is admittedly a big trick, is to find the image that will relieve your particular pain.

2. Use your own image or representation of your pain and what relieves it. Although some imagery techniques suggest certain images for pain relief, these images are fairly vague because it is important for you to substitute your own personal images. Also, some techniques simply refer to areas of discomfort without much description. Again, use your own personal image of your pain.

3. If you feel you do not know enough about the cause of your pain or how it might be relieved, ask your nurse or doctor for information.

4. You need not use "medically correct" images. For example, some people have achieved pain relief by imagining their pain as a sound that gets quieter, a shape that becomes smaller, or a vicious animal that becomes friendly or eventually disappears.

5. Include your religious, spiritual, or "good luck" charms or rituals. For example, you may want to recite a passage of scripture, hold a rosary or rabbit's foot, or visualize a white light surrounding your body.

6. You may imagine how your pain is relieved and/or imagine the final result of being comfortable. If you prefer, you need not focus on your pain or imagine how it is relieved—just that it is relieved and you are comfortable. You may remember how you felt before the pain occurred or imagine how you will feel when you are recovered.

7. If you wish you may practice your imagery technique or develop it over time. You may practice it in the absence of pain. Especially at first, some people like to practice imagery so they feel more familiar with it when they need it. You may decide on an image that relieves a little bit of pain each day rather than one that relieves all of the pain at once, especially if your pain is prolonged and severe.

8. If you decide to use more than one image or technique, use only one at a time. Most people concentrate more intensely and get a better effect this way. Trying to concentrate on two different images may dilute the effect of both.

9. Consider using a relaxation technique first, right before you begin the imagery. The imagery for pain relief may work better if you are relaxed and ready to concentrate.

10. Get comfortable. Get into a position with good support, e.g., lying down or sitting in a reclining chair. Loosen clothing or take off anything uncomfortable, e.g., your shoes. Empty your bladder before you begin.

11. Try to prevent interruptions. If your technique is tape-recorded, using a headset will help eliminate some of the noises around you. Taking the phone off the hook and posting a "Do not disturb" sign may help.

12. You may keep your eyes closed or open during the imagery technique. You may concentrate better with your eyes closed.

13. If you cannot concentrate, try counting each breath you take, saying each number silently to yourself before or after you breathe in or out. If this doesn't work, try again later. Perhaps you are too tired and need to rest. Or, you may be in too much pain and need another type of pain relief now.

14. If you are using an imagery technique that lasts several minutes or more than a few seconds, remember that you do not always have to use the entire technique. You may select part of the image and focus on it only momentarily, perhaps as you stare into space. When the total imagery technique is used and effectively relieves pain, sometimes this effect can be maintained by frequently but briefly recalling a portion of the technique. Also, brief recall of the image may be helpful when you are unable to concentrate on using a lengthy imagery technique.

15. The amount of time spent using an imagery technique for pain relief probably should not be more than 20 minutes at a time, and total time spent each day should not exceed 1 hour. If you are spending more time than this, discuss it with your nurse. You may need additional pain relief measures.

16. Expect the effect of imagery to vary. It may not work every time you use it, or it may work better some times than others. Measure success by the fact that you gave it a try.

17. Use other methods of pain relief, too. Rarely is imagery all that is needed for acceptable pain relief.

18. Use your imagery technique preventively, if possible. If you can predict when pain will return, use imagery before pain returns to try to prevent it from returning. At the very least, use imagery before pain increases to an intense level.

■ May be duplicated for use in clinical practice. From McCaffery, M, and Beebe, A: PAIN: CLINICAL MANUAL FOR NURSING PRACTICE, St. Louis, 1989, The CV Mosby Company.

Continued.

Patient/Family Teaching Point: Using Imagery for Pain Relief—cont'd.

---

19. Be selective about the people you talk to about your use of imagery. Not everyone is open-minded about its possible value. Find out how others feel about imagery before you tell them what you do. If you want to close your eyes and prevent interruptions while you use imagery, you may simply tell others that you would like a few moments to rest your eyes. In preparation for a painful procedure, you could explain that you will be trying to concentrate on something else while the procedure is performed.
20. If you have any concerns about imagery or if you experience any unwanted side effects from using it, let your nurse know at once.

From: _____ (nurse's name)   Phone: _____

■ May be duplicated for use in clinical practice. From McCaffery, M, and Beebe, A: PAIN: CLINICAL MANUAL FOR NURSING PRACTICE, St. Louis, 1989, The CV Mosby Company.

---

ing points on pp. 220 to 227. They are suitable for copying and giving to the patient. It may be appropriate to offer to tape-record these lengthier images for the patient. If so and if your time is limited, you may wish to consider the three-part time plan, as suggested on pp. 193 and 195, Chapter 7, item No. 16, for taping relaxation techniques.

Patient/Family Teaching Points for General Use of Imagery for Pain Relief

This chapter includes two types of imagery for pain relief that require at least a moderate amount of patient involvement: (1) standardized imagery and (2) systematic, individualized imagery. These techniques may be used in a concentrated manner for several minutes or more. The patient is asked to consider the content, approve or disapprove of what is included, and perhaps suggest specific content. The patient may also devote time to practicing the imagery or may use it fairly often.

For the above types of imagery, the patient/family teaching point titled "Using Imagery for Pain Relief" may be used (pp. 220 to 221). If the patient can read, it may be duplicated and given to the patient.

Comparison of Hypnosis and Imagery

Some patients will ask about possible similarities between imagery and hypnosis, either because of unfounded fears of hypnosis or because of a desire to try hypnosis. In either case, the nurse needs to provide accurate, reassuring information. The patient/family teaching point on p. 222 may be discussed, copied, and given to the patient who has questions about the relationships between hypnosis and imagery.

Patient/Family Teaching Points for Specific Images for Pain Relief

The specific imagery techniques for pain relief covered in this section are presented in a sequence that roughly approximates the amount of time usually required for the nurse to teach the patient and for the patient to perform or learn the technique. The least time-consuming techniques are presented first.

The more experience and knowledge the nurse has about imagery and the more time she can devote to individualizing the technique for the patient, probably the better the outcome. However, some of the standardized techniques are permissive and vague enough that the patient may interpret or individualize them as he listens. Further, although research evidence is lacking, clinical experience has demonstrated that the standardized techniques selected for this chapter have a reasonable success rate.

The directions for each imagery technique are stated in the patient/family teaching points in the exact words the nurse might say to the patient and family. Following are five image techniques. Four are standardized images for pain relief: (1) emptying the sandbag, p. 223, (2) breathing out pain, p. 224, (3) ball of healing energy, p. 225, and (4) opening around pain, p. 226 (Levine, 1982). The fifth technique is comprised of questions and suggestions for helping a patient create highly individualized imagery for pain and its relief, pp. 226 to 227. If the patient can read, the directions for any of these techniques may be duplicated and given to the patient.

If you talk to guide the patient through the technique or if you tape-record it for the patient, speak slowly and

Text continued on p. 229.

Patient/Family Teaching Point: Hypnosis and Imagery

TO: _____ (patient's name)   DATE: _____

    When you use imagery to relieve pain, you are usually alert, concentrating intensely, and imagining various sensations. Is this the same as hypnosis?

    Truthfully, it is somewhat difficult to distinguish between hypnosis and imagery since they overlap in some areas. The following may be helpful:

- Hypnosis is a broad concept and has been used for numerous purposes. Therapy with hypnosis (hypnotherapy) involves the use of many techniques, one of which is imagery.
- There is no single, accepted definition of hypnosis. However, it is generally believed that all hypnosis is self-hypnosis (sometimes directed by another person, e.g., psychologist) and that hypnotic thinking is a state of alertness and intense concentration, very similar to normal, everyday thinking. Concentration is not only intense but also narrowly focused with diminished peripheral awareness. Hypnosis is not loss of consciousness nor is it mind-control initiated by someone else. The following example takes some of the mystery out of hypnosis.

    Example: Have you ever driven along a familiar road and suddenly realized you could not remember the past 10 minutes and were not sure if you had passed your turn-off? That's hypnotic thinking accompanied by amnesia for about 10 minutes. You were concentrating intently on something other than driving, and although you were fully alert you were not consciously aware of what was going on around you and you could not remember what you had driven past.

- Hypnosis is recognized by the American Medical Association as a legitimate treatment method. It is not quackery. Also, its use does not indicate that pain is regarded as imaginary or "all in the mind." One of the oldest uses of hypnosis is for surgical procedures. Very few people can use hypnosis to replace anesthesia during surgery, but when they can it does not mean the pain of surgery is not real!
- Hypnosis often begins with a hypnotic induction technique. Certain relaxation techniques may be used for hypnotic induction. When imagery techniques are preceded by a relaxation technique, imagery then becomes quite similar to traditional self-hypnosis, but it is an alert state over which you may maintain complete control. (The results of some studies suggest that hypnosis need not be preceded by any hypnotic induction technique, e.g., suggestions of imagery given without hypnotic induction have effectively relieved pain.)
- Use of an imagery technique ordinarily requires your active participation. You decide whether or not to use a technique; you use your own imagination (you help create your own image); and you must be able to concentrate on the imagery.

From: _____ (nurse's name)   Phone: _____

■ May be duplicated for use in clinical practice. From McCaffery, M, and Beebe, A: PAIN: CLINICAL MANUAL FOR NURSING PRACTICE, St. Louis, 1989, The CV Mosby Company.

Patient/Family Teaching Point: Emptying the Sandbag

TO: _____ (patient's name)   DATE: _____

1. This imagery technique is usually used to relieve pain in one area at a time. If you have pain in several areas of your body, decide which area of discomfort you want to relieve first.
2. Get into a well-supported, comfortable position. You may want to use a reclining chair or lie down.
3. Close your eyes, unless you feel better with them open. Most people can concentrate and imagine better with their eyes closed.
4. A brief relaxation technique at the beginning may be helpful, especially if you feel tense or find it hard to concentrate. Use whatever relaxes you, e.g., music. Or, ask your nurse about a brief technique such as slow, rhythmic breathing.
5. Breathe in slowly, deeply; breathe out slowly. Then continue to breathe slowly and evenly in whatever way is comfortable. This may be all that is needed to help you feel reasonably calm and comfortable.
6. Concentrate on your body being an empty sack or bag.
7. Gradually, at your own pace, focus on or imagine filling the bag slowly with sand. Feel your body get heavier and heavier as this happens. You may begin anywhere. For example, you may imagine filling your body from your toes up to your head. You may want to think of each area of your body as it fills with sand and gets heavier.
8. Continue filling the sandbag, your body, until it is completely full of sand; until the skin or covering has no more room, and until the bag, or your body, feels very heavy.
9. If a second person is available, indicate to them when you are ready to have help with this part. When the sandbag is completely full, you might raise your hand as a signal that you are ready for the following assistance: place one hand on top of the area of pain and the other hand underneath. If this is impossible or uncomfortable, place the hands near the pain. The use of someone's hands is merely to help you focus on where the pain is. Another person is not essential. If a second person is not available, simply think about or focus on where the pain is.
10. Imagine making a small slit in the sandbag, usually in the back.
11. Imagine the sand slowly trickling out.
12. Begin to imagine the pain also trickling out slowly with the sand.
13. Continue thinking about, imagining, or visualizing the sand and pain slowly trickling out until the sandbag empties completely, is flat, depleted, and weightless.
14. Repeat the above steps 6 through 13 for each area of pain.

Additional points: This technique can be done from memory. But, you may concentrate better if you tape-record the above steps or ask someone to read them to you each time you want to use the technique. Beginning with step #2, each step may be read in a slow monotone voice with pauses between each step. You may want to omit #4 or add a brief relaxation technique. Except for #4, each step may be read almost exactly as it is written.

You may wish to develop your own image of your pain, e.g., color, size, weight, temperature, sound, texture (e.g., feeling sharp or jagged around the edges), and smell of the pain. You may then imagine these sensory images changing or leaving the body as the sandbag empties.

From: _____ (nurse's name)   Phone: _____

Patient/Family Teaching Point: Breathing Out Pain

TO: _____ (patient's name)   DATE: _____

NOTE: In this script for pain relief imagery, a blank is left (i.e., _____) for you to fill in your own area(s) of discomfort. Before using this script, decide what words you will use for the blanks.

Script: You may close your eyes, if you wish, and take a slow, deep breath. You may feel yourself relax as you breathe out. Continue breathing comfortably and slowly, at whatever depth is natural for you, feeling your body relax each time you breathe out.

If you wish, the next time you breathe in you may imagine that your breath goes to your _____, bringing

nutrients, comfort, and calm. As you breathe out, you imagine that the air goes out through your _____, taking with it the discomfort, leaving behind relaxed, healthy, comfortable tissues.

Each time you breathe in you may picture the air flowing through to your _____, bringing health and

comfort. As you breathe out, the air once again flows out through your _____, leaving calm, relaxation, health, and comfort behind.

I will pause now and you may continue to breathe slowly and imagine more and more comfort with each breath that

flows through your _____.

When you are ready, you may end this image by counting silently to yourself from one to three. At the count of three inhale, open your eyes, and say to yourself that you feel alert and relaxed.

I will wait now until you are ready to end this for yourself. Take your time. Enjoy the experience.

Additional points: If you already have a mental image of your pain, you may try to work with your image by breathing through it, gradually changing it to a more comfortable image. For example, if you see your pain as red and hard you may try to use your breaths to change the image to soft and white, or whatever you think of as a comfortable image.

Another variation is to imagine that there is a hole in your body near the painful area. During exhalation, you may imagine the pain going out of your body through the hole.

From: _____ (nurse's name)   Phone: _____

■ May be duplicated for use in clinical practice. From McCaffery, M, and Beebe, A: PAIN: CLINICAL MANUAL FOR NURSING PRACTICE, St. Louis, 1989, The CV Mosby Company.

Patient/Family Teaching Point: Ball of Healing Energy

TO: _____ (patient's name)   DATE: _____

NOTE: This script for pain relief imagery uses the phrase "area that hurts," but you may substitute the name of your area of discomfort, e.g., "lower back."

Script: Now, if you wish, you may close your eyes. Take a slow, deep breath. You may feel yourself relax as you breathe out. Continue to breathe comfortably and slowly, at whatever depth is natural for you. Perhaps you can feel yourself relax each time you breathe out.

Now if you wish, you may begin to imagine a ball of white light, or healing energy, forming on your chest or in your lungs. This ball of white light or healing energy need not be terribly clear or vivid. Anything you want to imagine is suitable. It may be dim or abstract or very clear. Anything may be effective as long as you understand it as being positive, helpful, or healing.

When you are ready you may circulate this ball of white light and healing energy to the area that hurts. The next time you breathe in you may use that air to send the ball of healing energy to the area that hurts. When you breathe out you may use that air to send the ball away from your body, letting it take with it the hurt and tension, leaving behind feelings of comfort and healthy tissue.

You may, if you wish, continue to circulate the ball of healing energy with every breath you take. The ball of healing energy enters your body again, purified, and as you breathe in you may send the ball of healing energy to the area that hurts. As you breathe out you may send the ball of healing energy away from your body, letting it leave behind comfort and health.

Each time the ball of healing energy leaves your body it may take away twice as much of the hurt and leave behind twice as much comfort and health. The ball may get larger and larger as it does this.

I will pause now to allow you time to circulate the ball of healing energy or white light. When you are ready to end this, you may signal to me by raising your hand.... Take your time....

Now that you are ready to end this technique, count silently to yourself from one to three. At the count of three inhale deeply, open your eyes, and as you breathe out, say to yourself "I feel relaxed and alert."

Additional points: Healing energy is an ancient concept, and visualizing the sun or a white light is considered by many to be a powerful image for healing and pain relief. However, you may wish to substitute something else for this ball of energy. For example, you may prefer to use "God's healing power." You may wish to begin or end with scripture you find comforting, e.g., the 23rd Psalm or I Corinthians 10:13: "There hath no temptation taken you but such as is common to men: but God *is* faithful, who will not suffer you to be tempted above that ye are able; but will with the temptation also make a way to escape, that ye may be able to bear *it.*"

Or, you may want to decrease or change certain specific qualities of the pain sensation. If you have burning pain, you may want to substitute something cool or cold, e.g., cold water, for the ball of energy.

Another variation is to have the ball of energy take away specific items, such as swelling, toxins, tension, or bacteria.

Obviously, you need not have someone read this script to you. You may be able to do it well from memory.

From: _____ (nurse's name)   Phone: _____

■ May be duplicated for use in clinical practice. From McCaffery, M, and Beebe, A: PAIN: CLINICAL MANUAL FOR NURSING PRACTICE, St. Louis, 1989, The CV Mosby Company.

Opening Around Pain*

Sit or lie down in a position you find comfortable. Allow yourself to settle into this position so that the whole body feels fully present where it sits or lies.

Bring your attention to the area of sensation that has been uncomfortable.

Let your attention come wholly to that area. Let the awareness be present, moment to moment, to receive the sensations generated there.

Allow the discomfort to be felt.

Moment to moment new sensations seem to arise.

Does the flesh cramp against the pain? Feel how the body tends to grasp it in a fist, tries to close it off.

Begin to allow the body to open all around that sensation.

Feel the tension and resistance that comes to wall off the sensation.

Don't push away the pain. Just let it be there. Feel how the body tries to isolate it. Tries to close it off. Picture that fist. Feel how the body is clenched in resistance.

Feel how the body holds each new sensation.

Begin gradually to open that closedness around sensation. The least resistance can be so painful. Open. Soften. All around the sensation. Allow the fist, moment to moment, to open. To give space to the sensation.

Let go of the pain. Why hold on a moment longer?

Like grasping a burning ember, the flesh of the closed fist is seared in its holding. Open. Soften all around the sensation. Let the fist of resistance begin to loosen. To open.

The palm of that fist softening. The fingers beginning to loosen their grip. Opening. All around the sensation.

The fist loosening. Gradually opening. Moment to moment, letting go of the pain. Release the fear that surrounds it.

Notice any fear that has accumulated around the pain. Allow the fear to melt. Let tension dissolve, so that the sensations can softly radiate out as they will. Don't try to capture the pain. Let it float free. No longer held in the grasp of resistance. Softening. Opening all around the sensation.

The fist opening. The fingers, one by one, loosening their grip.

The sensation no longer encapsulated in resistance. Opening.

Let the pain soften. Let the pain be. Let go of the resistance that tries to smother the experience. Allow each sensation to come fully into consciousness. No holding. No pushing away. The pain beginning to float free in the body.

All grasping relinquished. Just awareness and sensation meeting moment to moment. Received gently by the softening flesh.

The fist opened into a soft, spacious palm. The fingers loose. The fist dissolved back into the soft, open flesh. No tension. No holding.

Let the body be soft and open. Let the sensation float free. Easy. Gently.

Softening, opening all around the pain.

Just sensation. Floating free in the soft, open body.

*Reprinted by permission from the publisher. From Levine, S: Who dies? An investigation of conscious living and conscious dying, pp. 134-135, Garden City, NY, 1982, Anchor Books. Permission to duplicate more than one copy may be obtained by writing: Doubleday, 666 Fifth Avenue, New York, NY 10103.

Patient/Family Teaching Point: Individualized Imagery Technique for Pain Relief

TO: _____ (patient's name)   DATE: _____

If you have the time and interest, you may create your own personalized image of what your pain is like and how it can be relieved. Following are some questions, suggestions, and examples that may help you create your own imagery technique.

1. The parts of an imagery technique may include any or all of the following, presented in the sequence in which they are often used:
   - Getting into a comfortable position.
   - Closing your eyes.
   - Beginning with a relaxation technique (if you don't know one, ask your nurse).
   - Imagining or focusing on the pain sensation.
   - Imagining or focusing on what will relieve the pain.
   - Imagining yourself as you were before you had pain or at a future date when you are free of the pain.
   - Using a technique to end the imagery, unless you wish to go to sleep at the end.

■ May be duplicated for use in clinical practice. From McCaffery, M, and Beebe, A: PAIN: CLINICAL MANUAL FOR NURSING PRACTICE, St. Louis, 1989, The CV Mosby Company.

Continued.

Patient/Family Teaching Point: Individualized Imagery Technique for Pain Relief—cont'd.

2. Suggestions for various types of images are given in items 4, 5, and 6 below. (When you read over these suggestions, you may want to pause with your eyes closed from time to time to consider the ideas more carefully.) After considering the possible types of images, you will eventually need to decide which of the following you want to do:
   - Focus on your pain and develop an image for pain relief. (Use No. 4 and No. 5 below; you may want to consider some points in No. 6.) Imagining pain or what relieves it may increase pain or otherwise be difficult. If so, you may choose the following instead.
   or
   - Focus on developing an image of yourself without pain. That is, you decide not to focus on your pain and a specific method of relieving it. Instead, you decide to focus on yourself as free of pain, either as you were before you had pain or as you expect to be at some future date. (Omit No. 4 and No. 5 below; use No. 6.)
3. Regardless of the type of imagery you decide to use, remember that imagery tends to be more effective if you:
   - Whenever possible, use your memories of what you have actually experienced.
   - Work with only one image at a time, i.e., do not include two or more very different images in your technique.
4. To develop your own image of your pain, consider the questions below. Skip those that don't make sense to you. You may use none, one, or several of these ideas:
   - How do you picture your pain? Is it an object? an animal? a vague presence?
   - Does it remind you of something else (e.g., running water, outer space, prison)?
   - What would you have to do to someone else to make them feel the same pain you are feeling?
   - What is the pain doing?
   - What color is it?
   - What are the edges of the pain like?
   - Does it have weight?
   - Does it have a sound? Can you hear it?
   - Does it have a temperature? Cool? Hot?
   - Can you smell or taste the pain?
   - Can you draw a picture of you and your pain?
5. Now that you have a picture of your pain, try to imagine a way it can be decreased, eliminated, or changed to a more acceptable sensation. To develop your own image of pain relief, consider the questions below. Again, use only what makes sense to you.
   - How would your picture of your pain change to make the pain better? Would it change colors? Become lighter in weight? Sound quieter? Soften around the edges? Feel cooler or warmer? Become a tamer animal? Be released or freed? Become smaller?
   - Is there a particular way you can imagine this change taking place so that the pain is better? For example, if your pain is large and hot, can it be cooled by running water and slowly become smaller as it is washed away?
   - Is this image of pain relief something you can imagine taking place all at once, or will it happen over a period of time? Sometimes imagery develops slowly over days or weeks, e.g., each day the running water feels cooler and takes away more of the pain.
6. To develop a picture of yourself without pain, consider the following suggestions, using only what you find helpful:
   - Try to remember yourself at a specific point in time before you had pain, a time when you were especially happy, comfortable, or relaxed. Where were you? What were you doing? How were you dressed?
   - Or, imagine yourself in the future when you will be healthy, comfortable, and doing something you enjoy. Again, imagine the details of this, e.g., how you are dressed, where you are, what you are doing.
   - Try constructing this picture of yourself by beginning at your feet or head; mentally draw, paint, or picture one body part at a time.
7. To end your imagery technique, you may simply count slowly and silently to yourself, e.g., from one to three. When you count one, move your lower body slightly; when you count two, move your upper body slightly; when you count three, breathe in deeply, open your eyes and as you breathe out say to yourself that you feel relaxed and comfortable.

From: _____ (nurse's name)   Phone: _____

INDIVIDUALIZED NURSING CARE PLAN

Patient Who May Benefit from a Pain Relief Imagery Technique

Patient Description: Ms. M., 23 years old, is 8 months pregnant with her first child. Over the last 6 weeks she has experienced increasing low back pain of mild to moderate intensity with the most discomfort in the evening and at bedtime. Daily physical exercises plus a cold pack for 30 minutes several times a day have reduced her pain during the day, but she has requested additional assistance with pain relief due to difficulty sleeping at night. She wants to avoid medications because of their potential harm to her unborn child.

Assessment	Potential Nursing Diagnoses	Planning/Intervention	Evaluation/Expected Outcomes
Identify: • Interests/abilities in art, nontraditional health care, religion. • Ability to understand directions and concentrate. • Mental picture or image of pain. • Use of sensory descriptors of pain and nonpainful terms. • History of emotional or psychiatric disorders.	Pain, related to strain on back muscles. Sleep pattern disturbance related to low back pain. Knowledge deficit related to nonpharmacological methods of pain relief.	Emphasize belief in patient's statements about pain and in the cause of pain being related to muscle strain. Describe the benefits, limits, and types of imagery techniques available. Help patient choose imagery technique, explaining difference between final state and process images. Help the patient develop own pain relief imagery by using the Patient/Family Teaching Point: Individualized Imagery Technique for Pain Relief (pp. 226 to 227) and including the following: • Use permissive directions and suggestions. • Offer to answer any questions patient may have about imagery or the cause and relief of pain. • Emphasize need for patient to develop own image, using memories of actual experiences if possible, and focusing on one image rather than several. • Explain that images need not be "medically correct" or vivid. • Incorporate patient's spontaneous use of positive images or nonpainful descriptions of pain or its relief, as well as any spiritual aspects desired by patient. • Consider potential effect of images if taken literally. • Suggest use of a brief relaxation technique prior to imagery. • Offer to provide written instructions and/or tape recording of technique. Encourage patient to use imagery early before pain becomes severe. Suggest patient select one brief part of the imagery technique to focus on if she awakens during night or is bothered by pain while busy during day. Suggest simultaneous use of other pain relief measures, e.g., positioning, cold pack. Plan a time during the next 3 days to check with patient regarding effects of imagery, and ask if any problems occurred. Plan regular follow-up to assess continuing effects of imagery and any changes in pain.	Patient reports one or more of the following: • Decreased intensity of pain. • Pain sensation becomes a different and more tolerable sensation. • Improved sleep, e.g., gets to sleep quicker, able to fall asleep readily if awakened, feels more rested in the mornings. • Pride or increased confidence in ability to handle discomfort. If patient reports problems with imagery and suggested solutions are not effective, gently explain that the technique does not always work no matter how hard one tries and that it should be discontinued while other pain relief measures are explored. Obtain appropriate consultation, if needed.

quietly in a monotone, pausing at regular intervals. Usually there is a pause at the end of each sentence, between paragraphs, and wherever you see "..." within a script.

If you are teaching a standardized pain relief image to a group of patients, use the phrase "area of discomfort" instead of the specific body part that hurts—unless they all have pain in the same area.

Patient Example

Mr. L., age 78, and an artist for most of his adult life, was terminally ill with cancer that had metastasized to many areas of his body. Pain in his left shoulder was the most severe and the least responsive to analgesics. He did not want to increase any of his medications because of accompanying sedation and confusion that occurred in spite of various medication changes. He lived with his wife, Mrs. L. His daughter, Ms. S., was visiting and was familiar with yoga. She discussed relaxation and imagery techniques with her father, and they decided to try "emptying the sandbag." Mr. L. lay in bed while Ms. S. talked him through this technique and Mrs. L. put her hands on the painful left shoulder when it was time to make a "slit in the sandbag." Mr. L. was asleep at the conclusion and slept for 2 hours. He later said that the technique not only completely relieved his pain but also allowed him a more restful sleep than usual. He said the pain gradually returned after he awakened. The three of them, Mr. and Mrs. L. and their daughter, used this technique several times a day for the remaining 4 days of Mr. L.'s life.

RESOURCES FOR PATIENTS

Bresler, D: Learning to control pain. This audiotape focuses on how to use guided imagery to control chronic pain. Available as tape #20098 from Psychology Today Tape Program, Dept PTC 77, Box No 059073, Brooklyn, NY 11205-9061.

Bresler, D: Mind-controlled analgesia: imagery in the treatment of chronic pain. A lecture tape on imagery, available for about $10.00 from Insight Publishing, PO Box 2070, Mill Valley, CA 94942; phone 415-388-8825.

Bresler, DE: Free yourself from pain, New York, 1979, Simon and Schuster. This is written for the layman. Chapter 10, pp 347-396, discusses how to use guided imagery for pain relief. The book is out of print but may be available in libraries.

Levine, S: Audiotapes of his guided meditations for pain control are available from the Hanuman Tape Library, Box 61498, Santa Cruz, CA 95061.

SELECTED ANNOTATED REFERENCES

Many of the noninvasive pain relief measures, such as imagery, have not yet been adequately researched. This sometimes makes it difficult to document or justify the use of these techniques. The following brief, annotated list provides some clinical or research support for the use of imagery for pain relief, as discussed in this chapter.

Barber, TX, Chauncey, HH, and Winer, RA: Effect of hypnotic and nonhypnotic suggestions on parotid gland response to gustatory stimuli, *Psychosom Med* 26:374-380, 1964. This study suggests that an image may exert more control over physiologic response than does the actual stimulus. When subjects were told to imagine that water applied to their tongues was sour, measures of saliva showed a significant increase. When subjects were asked to imagine that citric acid applied to their tongues was tasteless, measures of salivation showed a decrease as compared to salivation during baseline treatment with citric acid.

Burish, TG, and Lyles, JN: Effects of relaxation training in reducing adverse reactions to cancer chemotherapy, *J Behav Med* 4:65-78, 1981. This study suggests that relaxing imagery can decrease distress without changing the physiological response. Experimental subjects who engaged in therapist-guided relaxation and imagery showed significantly lower systolic blood pressure and reported significantly lower anger, anxiety, and nausea before and after chemotherapy than the control subjects. However, there was no difference in the frequency of vomiting in the two groups.

Harano, K, Ogawa, K, and Naruse, G: A study of plethysmography and skin temperature during active concentration and autogenic exercise. In Luthe, W, ed: Autogenic training, pp 55-58, New York, 1965, Grune & Stratton. This study suggests the superiority of imagination over will or desire. Each subject was asked to focus on the idea of his arms being warm and repeat to himself "My arms are warm." This thinking and imagining resulted in the sensation of warmth, an increase in surface temperature, and an increase in blood volume in the arm. However, these changes did not occur when the subject tried to raise the temperature without thinking or imagining that the arm was warm.

REFERENCES AND SELECTED READINGS

Achterberg, J, and Lawlis, F: Imagery and health intervention, *Topics Clin Nurs* 3:55-60, Jan 1982

*Barber, J, and Gitelson, J: Cancer pain: psychological management using hypnosis, *CA-Cancer J Clinic* 30:130-136, May-June 1980

Barber, TX, Spanos, NP, and Chaves, JF: Hypnosis, imagination, and human potentialities, New York, 1974, Pergamon Press

Bresler, DE: Free yourself from pain, pp 347-396, New York, 1979, Simon and Schuster

Crowther, JH: Stress management training and relaxation imagery in the treatment of essential hypertension, *J Behav Med* 6:169-187, 1983

Donovan, MI: Relaxation with guided imagery: a useful technique, *Cancer Nurs* 3:27-32, 1980

Greene, RJ, and Reyher, J: Pain tolerance in hypnotic analgesic and imagination states, *J Abnorm Psychol* 79:29-38, Feb 1972

Grinder, J, and Bandler, R: The structure of magic, II, pp 6-12, Palo Alto, Calif, 1976, Science & Behavior

*Free reprints available through American Cancer Society. Professional Education Publication (Spiegel, 85-50M-No. 3344-PE; Barbar and Gitelson, 80-50M-No. 3385-PE).

Horan, JJ, Layne, FC, and Pursell, CH: Preliminary self-regulation of chronic pain, *Am J Clin Hypn* 20:106-113, 1977

Jacobsen, DE: Electrical measurements of neuromuscular states during mental activities. II. Imagination and recollection of various muscle acts, *Am J Physiol* 94:22-34, 1930

Jones, GE, and Johnson, HJ: Heart rate and somatic concomitants of mental imagery, *Psychophysiology* 17:185-191, 1980

Kroger, WS, and Fezler, WD: Hypnosis and behavior modification: imagery conditioning, Philadelphia, 1976, JB Lippincott

Lankton, S: Practical magic: a translation of neurolinguistic programming into clinical psychotherapy, pp 18-19, Cupertino, Calif, 1980, Meta Publications

Levine, S: Who dies? An investigation of conscious living and conscious dying, Garden City, NY, 1982, Anchor Books

Lyles, JN, Burish, TG, Krozely, MG, and Oldham, RK: Efficacy of relaxation training and guided imagery in reducing the aversiveness of cancer chemotherapy, *J Consult Clin Psychol* 50:509-524, Aug 1982

Mast, DE: Effects of imagery. *Image J Nurs Scholarship* 18:118-120, Fall 1986

McCaffery, M: Nursing management of the patient with pain, pp 156-183, Philadelphia, 1979, JB Lippincott

Pearson, BD: Pain control: an experiment with imagery, *Geriatric Nurs* 8:28-30, Jan-Feb 1987

Peterson, GH: Birthing normally: a personal growth approach to childbirth, pp 57-73, Berkeley, Calif, 1981, Mindbody Press

Raft, D, Smith, R, and Warren, N: Selection of imagery in the relief of chronic and acute clinical pain, *J Psychosom Res* 30:481-488, 1986

Sachs, LB: Feuerstein, M, and Vitale, JH: Hypnotic self-regulation of chronic pain, *Ann J Clin Hypn* 20:106-113, Oct 1977

Samuels, M, and Samuels, N: Seeing with the mind's eye: the history, techniques and uses of visualization, New York and Berkeley, Calif, 1975, Random House and The Bookworks

Schwartz, GE, Fair, PL, Salt, P, Mandel, MR, and Klerman, GL: Facial muscle patterning to affective imagery in depressed and nondepressed subjects, *Science* 192:489-491, 1976

Scott, DS, and Barber, TX: Cognitive control of pain: effects of multiple cognitive strategies, *Psychol Record* 2:373-383, 1977

Sheikh, AA: Imagery: current theory, research and application, Somerset, NJ, 1983, John Wiley & Sons, Inc

Simonton, OC, Simonton, SM, and Creighton, JL: Getting well again, New York, 1978, Bantam Books

Sodergren, KM: Guided imagery. In Snyder, M: Independent nursing interventions, pp 103-124, New York, 1985, John Wiley & Sons

*Spiegel, D: The use of hypnosis in controlling cancer pain, *CA-Cancer J Clinic* 35:221-231, July-Aug 1986

Swerdlow, B: A rapid hypnotic technique in a case of atypical facial neuralgia, *Headache* 24:104-109, Mar 1984

White, KD: Salivation: the significance of imagery in its voluntary control, *Psychophysiology* 13:196-203, 1978

CHAPTER 9

Chronic Nonmalignant Pain

Special Considerations

The saddest story in all of pain management may well be about chronic nonmalignant pain. There is more chronic nonmalignant pain than any other kind of pain. The person who has it has suffered a long time, sometimes years. The health professionals providing care for the patient have most likely felt helpless as they failed in their repeated efforts to help the patient.

Perhaps no aspect of pain control is as humbling for both sufferer and caregiver as chronic nonmalignant pain, sometimes referred to as chronic benign pain. However, it is far from being benign; it may be devastating, not only for the person with the pain but for his family, friends, and caregivers. Chronic nonmalignant pain is capable of driving a destructive pathway through the lives of all it touches, at some point bringing each one to his knees. Chronic nonmalignant pain, by definition, is prolonged because it has not responded to whatever treatment has been tried. It exacts a high price from the sufferer, his family, and caregivers. To society in general in the United States it literally represents a yearly cost well in excess of $100 billion (Sternbach, 1986).

KEY POINT: By definition, chronic nonmalignant pain continues in spite of efforts to relieve it. This pain is not benign—it is destructive.

DEFINITION OF CHRONIC NONMALIGNANT PAIN

A truly satisfactory or generally agreed upon definition of chronic nonmalignant pain simply does not exist. In fact, some professionals do not use the phrase, preferring other terminology, such as chronic benign pain or chronic intractable benign pain syndrome. It encom-

passes diverse types of pain that may occur in virtually any area of the body and vary in intensity from mild to excruciating. The cause may or may not be known. The characteristics of the pain may fit a well-known pattern, or the patient may be told that his type of pain makes no sense.

A review of the literature shows that there is strong disagreement among health professionals in almost every area of managing chronic nonmalignant pain. This is not surprising since this type of pain covers such an enormous variety of conditions and people. What to call it, what it encompasses, and how to treat it remain areas of controversy. To try to settle these differences or even offer a comprehensive definition of chronic nonmalignant pain would be truly presumptuous. Thus, for this chapter, we have merely chosen from among the currently used terms, defined how the terminology is used in this chapter, and identified the general conditions it covers.

Our decision to use the terminology chronic *nonmalignant* pain rather than chronic *benign* pain is because the word benign is potentially misleading. Benign suggests a mild condition, which is rarely true of any chronic pain, regardless of its intensity. In oncology, malignant refers to conditions that are potentially life-threatening. Thus we have chosen nonmalignant because this chapter focuses on types of pain that result from causes that are not life-threatening.

Working Definition

For the purposes of this chapter the *working definition* of chronic nonmalignant pain is: *pain that has lasted 6 months or longer, is ongoing on a daily basis, is due to non–life-threatening causes, has not responded to currently available treatment methods, and may continue*

IMMEDIATE HELP FOR CRISIS WITH CHRONIC NONMALIGNANT PAIN

Time involved: Reading time, 7 minutes; implementation time, 20 minutes (longer if telephoning the physician is required or if the team conference with the physician is included).

Sample situation: From the 7:00 AM nursing report it is obvious that a crisis is occurring in the relationship between the nurses and a patient who has chronic nonmalignant pain and has been admitted to the hospital for an exacerbation of this pain. This is the fifth hospitalization for this patient in the last 18 months. The patient does not describe his pain as any worse or different from what it was yesterday when he was admitted, but the staff's relationships with the patient have steadily deteriorated—the patient and staff seem to be "at war." The nurses say the patient is "demanding," "uncooperative," "addicted," a "clock-watcher," "never satisfied," and sometimes verbally abusive to the nurses. The nurses say there is no known cause for his pain but they believe he does hurt. However, the nurses say he makes his pain worse by getting upset, and sometimes if they only go in his room and talk to him about baseball, he seems very happy. Right now, the patient is alternating between refusing to talk to the staff and yelling that he wants his pain medication changed, that it doesn't work, and that he wants to see his physician. The physician was informed of this by telephone about 6:00 AM and would not change his prescription for analgesics. The physician will be making rounds in early afternoon.

Possible solution: There is no immediate, truly satisfactory solution, but there may be a temporary answer that will pave the way to a better long-range plan. Use whatever analgesics are currently available, and find a nonpharmacological method of pain relief. Defuse the situation—get the staff and patient to talk to each other, and plan a patient-staff conference involving the physician to determine goals of this hospitalization. Focus on the most positive aspects of the patient and staff. This situation encompasses long-standing misconceptions and misunderstandings on the part of both staff and patient.

Expected outcome: The immediate result, hopefully, is somewhat better pain relief within about an hour and a specific plan for determining the goals of this hospitalization. Overall, the desired outcome is that the patient feels that the staff believes that he hurts; the staff knows that chronic pain is frustrating to the patient; and all staff members acknowledge that at this time there does not appear to be any way to cure the cause of the pain, but that a plan for managing the pain is needed.

Don'ts

1. Do not "take sides" by agreeing with the staff or with the patient that the other is unreasonable.
2. Do not avoid the patient.
3. Do not expect to provide immediate, satisfactory pain relief.

Dos

1. State the problem as clearly as possible to both staff and patient, i.e., the patient is in pain and the nurses do not know what more to do for the patient. It is frustrating to the patient to ask for help and not get it; it is frustrating to the staff to use what they can and still not relieve the pain.
2. Give whatever analgesics are prescribed as often as allowed. Set up a schedule, e.g., q4h.
3. Regarding the patient's behavior, tell the patient:
   You understand he hurts and is very frustrated by this.
   Exactly when he can expect his next analgesic and you are not allowed legally to give him more.
   If he wants more analgesic, he and you must discuss this with his physician that afternoon during rounds. If narcotic injections have been prescribed, suggest the regular use of an oral nonnarcotic and a strong oral narcotic (see pp. 106-107 on how to change from IM to PO analgesics for moderate to severe pain).
   He sounds angry and, if he is, you want him to tell you why and also, if he wishes, you will help him tell the nurses or physician what has upset him. (This is a lesson in assertiveness—the patient has a right to be angry, and he needs to learn how to tell others when he is angry and why without using abusive language.)
4. See if there is an order for heat or cold for pain relief (see pp. 131 and 145-152). If not, try to obtain one (or use massage instead, p. 141) and do the following:
   Ask the patient which he prefers, heat or cold, explaining that this will relieve some of the pain for right now. Encourage use of cold, if possible, since it works faster and relieves more pain than heat or massage.
   Stay with him until it begins to relieve pain.
   Say that you have heard he does a good job of getting his mind off pain for a while by talking about baseball and suggest that he tell you about a recent game while the cold (or heat, massage) begins to work. Of course, he may prefer to be silent and relax, especially if massage is done.
5. Regarding the nurses' attitudes and observations, discuss with them and include in the nursing care plan where appropriate:
   Arguing with the patient creates an adversarial rather than therapeutic or helpful relationship.
   You personally will not argue with the patient about his pain because no one can prove or disprove the existence of pain.
   They are correct when they say that the patient makes his pain worse when he gets upset, but explain that being anxious and depressed does not cause pain—it just makes pain more difficult to handle.
   We cannot make the pain go away right now, but we can stop contributing to the patient's anxiety and depression and help him gain control simply by ceasing to argue with him about his pain.
   Taking narcotics for pain relief is not the same as addiction.
   Clock-watching is usually a result of inadequate pain relief, particularly from a short-acting analgesic.
   The patient's anger is understandable if he came to the hospital expecting pain relief and it is not provided.

Continued.

IMMEDIATE HELP FOR CRISIS WITH CHRONIC NONMALIGNANT PAIN—cont'd.

Dos—cont'd.

They have identified some of the patient's strengths, i.e., he maintains an interest in outside events, e.g., baseball, is able to be distracted from his pain by baseball, and is using a lot of energy to try to keep the pain from being overwhelming. Remind them that distraction is a powerful method of dealing with

pain but does not make the pain go away, and distraction should be encouraged.

6. Talk with the patient, nurses, and physician to set a time, within the next 24 hours, for a patient-staff team conference to identify the specific goals of this hospitalization and how they will be accomplished.

---

for the remainder of the patient's life. To some extent the patient must live with this pain, but hopefully certain strategies or approaches will effectively manage or control the pain. To the extent possible the patient himself is enabled to control his own pain. (Basic differences between acute and chronic pain along with a review of types or causes of chronic pain and general recommended approaches are presented in Chapter 2, pp. 19-20.)

Examples of chronic nonmalignant pain, somewhat overlapping and of various origins, that may or may not be under control or managed are:

Low back pain
Headaches
Rheumatoid arthritis
Osteoarthritis
Neck pain such as whiplash
Causalgia
Neuralgia
Phantom limb pain
Peripheral neuropathy
Postherpetic neuralgia
Trigeminal neuralgia
Fibrositis or diffuse myofascial pain
Vascular diseases of the limbs such as Raynaud's disease
Crohn's disease
Irritable bowel syndrome
Chronic pancreatitis
Ankylosing spondylitis
Burning mouth syndrome
Reflex sympathetic dystrophy

The above examples make it clear that chronic nonmalignant pain may very well have an identifiable physical or organic cause. Some of these may even be cured with proper diagnosis and treatment, e.g., sympathetic nerve blockade for classic causalgia. The intensity may be just as severe as any other type of pain. What distinguishes this pain from other types of pain is that it is ongoing because a cure for it is unknown and that the cause has more or less stabilized, i.e., no additional injury or healing is occurring.

Many of the suggestions in this chapter for controlling chronic nonmalignant pain are covered elsewhere in this

book and certainly are appropriate for other types of pain as well. To say that the suggestions are inappropriate for other types of pain is inaccurate. Rather, it is important to realize that there is lack of agreement about approaches to chronic nonmalignant pain, that different approaches are recommended for different types of pain, and for the individual patient the type of pain may not clearly fit one category. In general, more conservative approaches aimed at self-management are usually indicated when it is obvious that the patient has a normal life expectancy but will also have continuous pain that is not life-threatening and is due to causes that have stabilized.

Perhaps more important than a definition of chronic nonmalignant pain is a reminder to the reader that this chapter is written in keeping with our philosophy of believing what the patient says about his pain, or at the very least giving him the benefit of the doubt, and working with the patient in the context of full disclosure, always being honest with the patient and conveying as much information as the patient can receive.

The health team sometimes fails to appreciate what the person with chronic nonmalignant pain experiences. Following are examples of both a physician's and a patient's views of chronic nonmalignant pain.

A Health Team Member's View of Chronic Nonmalignant Pain

It was in the middle 1970s, and a neurosurgeon and nurse were discussing their concerns about the difficulties of relieving prolonged pain. The physician's patients had chronic nonmalignant pain; the nurse's patients had cancer pain and many were terminally ill. Both told stories of patients who continued to hurt despite their efforts. The physician said "I give them analgesics and they say the pills don't work but they want more anyway. I tell them not to take the pills if they don't help. Lots of them still go to work so you know they aren't hurting all that much. I tell them they're doing OK and don't need any more pills. Then there are those I know are hurting badly—discs protruding, muscles in spasm. But how many laminectomies can you do? And I don't want to keep giving them narcotics and make addicts out of them. So I tell them for their own good that they just have to learn to live with this." The physician concluded the conversation by saying to the nurse "At least your patients usually die." As uncaring as it may sound, this statement probably reflects the physician's genuine distress over seeing the same patients month after month without being able to help them. In truth, he wants to end the patient's pain, not the patient's life.

In the 15 years following this conversation much has been learned about the treatment of chronic nonmalignant pain. For example, back pain without neurological complications is now seldom treated surgically. Professional attitudes toward patients with chronic nonmalignant pain have also begun to change.

However, through the years some of the remarks heard about patients with chronic nonmalignant pain seemed angry and derogatory. Many were no doubt borne out of the frustration of seeing so many efforts fail and not knowing what else to do. Following are examples of some of the statements that have appeared in the literature and have been heard in clinical settings about people who suffer chronic nonmalignant pain:
Uses his pain
Addicted
Enjoys his drugs
Drug-dependent
Wants only drugs for pain relief
Uncooperative
Noncompliant
Plays pain games
Malingering
Exaggerates his pain
Hypochondriac
Controls others with his pain
Psychological overlay
Psychogenic pain
Imagines his pain
Not willing to learn to live with his pain
Low pain tolerance (a somewhat sophisticated way of
    suggesting that the patient is a sissy)
Doesn't want to get better
Wants to keep his pain
Secondary gains
Makes a career out of pain
Has a bachelor's or master's degree in pain
A professional pain patient
A pain-prone person
Wishes to occupy the sick role
Unmotivated
Dependent on the health care system
A "crock"

The above remarks suggest a lack of respect or a degree of dislike for the patient with chronic nonmalignant pain, whether or not they are intended to do so. The attitudes potentially conveyed by such phrases serve no useful purpose in the relationship with the patient. As the

years have gone by, it is increasingly recognized that collaborating with, working with, the person with chronic nonmalignant pain has the potential for far superior results than does being in an adversarial position and waging a war with the patient. There is still at tendency, however, to discount patient's descriptions of pain when it is chronic as opposed to acute. There seems to be an assumption that the emotional problems found in chronic pain patients confound the quality of information they give about pain (Tearnan and Dar, 1986).

A Composite of the Patient's View of Chronic Nonmalignant Pain

The previously mentioned conversation between the physician and nurse reflects the health team's view of patients who are probably similar to the patient in the following example whose remarks present the patient's view. A woman with chronic nonmalignant pain said "I've lived with this pain every day for over 5 years. I've had doctors tell me I couldn't be hurting this much, that I was addicted, that I should be strong enough to learn to live with this, and all sorts of things. I take these pain relievers but they don't really help. Oh, they do help a little though, and I'm afraid the doctor will stop prescribing them so I only take them when I really need them. I've tried to keep going to work and take care of my family, but no one believes I hurt any more. I know people at work think I'm lazy when I go home early once in a while. They just don't know I barely made it there in the first place. My husband says it's just my nerves, and maybe it is. Sometimes I think I must be crazy. How could I hurt this much? I try to ignore it and just do all the things I used to do, but then I end up hurting so much I'm knocked out for a day or so. I'm so irritable and tired all the time. I feel so ashamed when I can't do what I used to do. Inadequate, like a bad person. I feel guilty. You know, I think about those hospice patients with pain and sometimes I envy them. At least they know they'll die soon. And because they're dying, lots of doctors will give them all the pain relievers they need."

How can you help this patient feel worthwhile again? You can't take away the pain right now, maybe never, but you can begin to help her by treating her with respect and believing her.

PURPOSE AND LIMITATIONS OF THIS CHAPTER

By definition, in this chapter we are dealing with pain that has not responded to our best efforts to eliminate it. Therefore approaches suggested in this chapter are not expected to put an end to chronic nonmalignant pain. Rather, the hope is to suggest ways the health team can assist the patient to learn to manage the pain.

The patient, family, friends, and health professionals no doubt wish they could get rid of the pain—

find a cause and cure it. However, pain has now become a chronic condition that requires daily management, very much like other chronic illnesses such as diabetes or hypertension. The goals of patient care now become two-fold: (1) decreasing the pain intensity to the extent possible, but not expecting that it will disappear, and (2) helping the patient obtain an optimal quality of life and level of function.

To accomplish these goals, the purposes of this chapter are:

- To improve the quality of interaction between the nurse and the person with chronic nonmalignant pain by addressing the common misconceptions that hamper this and suggesting some approaches to collaborating with, or working with, the patient.
- To present guidelines for establishing realistic goals and identifying appropriate nursing interventions for helping the patient with chronic nonmalignant pain in various settings under limited circumstances (i.e., not within a structured rehabilitation program), including helping the patient learn self-management techniques for dealing with chronic nonmalignant pain.
- To identify professional and self-help resources the nurse may suggest for the patient with chronic nonmalignant pain, including pointers on selecting a pain management program.

This chapter will not, however, include the nurse's role in structured inpatient or outpatient pain management programs designed to rehabilitate the person with chronic nonmalignant pain, nor will guidelines for establishing a pain management program be discussed. References at the end of the chapter will enable the nurse to pursue these interests.

MISCONCEPTIONS ABOUT CHRONIC NONMALIGNANT PAIN

Nurses often admit that caring for a patient with chronic pain is frustrating. Typically the patient with chronic nonmalignant pain returns again and again to the health care setting, whether it is the physician's office, the emergency room, or an orthopedic inpatient unit. Such a patient may be called a "repeater." The patient's diagnosis, or cause of pain, may not be clear, such as is often true with low back pain. The patient's report of pain, such as a migraine headache, may not be objectively verifiable by a physical examination or by X-ray; and although the patient may report severe pain, the patient is not always acting like he is in pain since he has been in pain for so long. However, the patient is often depressed and there may also be signs of anxiety. Nevertheless, the patient may be smiling when he asks for his narcotic analgesic. He may also know the names and doses of his analgesics and related medications along with how often he needs them, watching the clock and reminding the nurse well in advance of when they are due.

Nurses may say they feel like they have lost control in such situations, failing to realize they never had control in the first place. Only the patient knows when and how much he hurts. Therefore the patient is in control, i.e., the final authority about his pain. Further, in any chronic illness, optimal results depend on the patient himself learning how to control his illness. In fact, in programs for chronic pain management, an attitude of self-control and control over pain is fostered. If a patient with diabetes or chronic hypertension knows all about his medications and when he should take them, this is viewed as desirable. When the patient with chronic pain has the same information and has learned to use it to manage his pain, ironically this tends to upset the health team.

One study of 268 registered nurses' responses to descriptions of patients with various types of pain showed that many nurses have a negative stereotype of the patient with chronic pain. They tend to believe that pain is less intense in patients with chronic vs. acute pain, especially if there are no signs of pathology. Nurses are particularly likely to have negative attitudes about patients with chronic low back pain as compared with their attitudes toward patients with headache or joint pain. There is also a tendency for nurses to believe that pain relief measures are less effective when the patient is depressed, failing to appreciate that pain may cause the depression (Taylor, Skelton, and Butcher, 1984).

Patients seem to be aware that expressions of depression may be viewed negatively. They may defend themselves against the possibility of their pain being psychologically interpreted by making a great effort to represent themselves as cheerful and nondepressed. Thus the patient is in a no-win situation. If he acts like his pain is emotionally disturbing, he may be diagnosed as having a "mental problem," and his pain may be labeled as largely psychogenic. If he does not appear depressed, the intensity of his pain may not be believed.

KEY POINT: The health team's reaction to a patient with chronic nonmalignant pain may present an impossible dilemma for the patient. If the patient expresses his depression, the health team may believe the pain is psychogenic or is largely an emotional problem. If the patient tries to hide the depression by being cheerful, the health team may not believe that pain is a significant problem.

Misconceptions that hamper assessment and treatment of patients with pain are especially difficult to correct when the patient has chronic nonmalignant pain. (Many of the reasons for failing to believe the patient when he says he has pain of any sort have already been reviewed in Chapter 2, pp. 6-17.) This time we are faced not only with the fact that pain is subjective and cannot be proven or disproven, but also that it is not going away. It continues or returns. Further, we are also often dealing with the chronic or repeated administration of narcotics, drugs about which we have many exaggerated fears (see reasons for undertreatment with narcotics, pp. 67-74).

For all catastrophic events there seems to be the final question of "Why me?" How do we explain this? Uncertainty is very difficult. A bad reason may be better than no reason at all. When pain is chronic, has no clear cause, and is not life-threatening, the question of blame arises, probably because we would rather have a reason than believe that our lives might be determined by an arbitrary and uncontrolled force. Thus with chronic nonmalignant pain sometimes the patient blames himself and feels inadequate and depressed. Then, unfortunately, as if having the prolonged pain were not enough, the health team also tends to blame the patient or fails to believe him. Following are some of the misconceptions that surround these and other issues about chronic nonmalignant pain.

KEY POINT: Health team members have many misconceptions about the cause and treatment of chronic nonmalignant pain. Some emotional or personality characteristic of the patient is often mistakenly blamed for the cause of chronic nonmalignant pain.

Misconception: The patient with chronic pain lasting for years becomes less sensitive to pain and better able to tolerate it.

Correction: Research shows that, unfortunately, as pain continues through the years, the patient's own internal narcotics, endorphins, decrease and the patient perceives even greater pain from the same stimuli. Further, most patients with chronic pain become more frightened and feel they have less control over pain as time goes by, perhaps mainly because they begin to learn how severe unrelieved pain can be. In their repeated encounters with health professionals they also may learn that their pain may not be believed, and they may not receive assistance with pain relief (see annotated reference: Kosten and Kleber, 1987).

Misconception: Pain, especially chronic pain, for which there is no known organic cause, is a symptom of psychological disturbance, e.g., psychogenic pain.

Correction: Psychogenic pain is often inaccurately diagnosed simply because a physical cause cannot be found or because the patient does not respond to treatment. It is presumptuous to believe that diagnostic testing is always thorough or precise enough to identify all physical causes of pain. The health team's inability to identify a physical cause for the pain does not justify diagnosing the pain as psychogenic (see annotated references: Fischer, 1984; Hendler, 1984).

Misconception: A patient who is very expressive about pain, i.e., "exaggerates" his pain, and/or has a greater decrease in function than can be explained by the physical cause is consciously trying to manipulate others or obtain secondary gains.

Correction: Patients with symptomatology incongruent with the physical cause for pain are very likely to have poor, or ineffective, coping styles and are also likely to be considerably distressed by the pain. The patient's lack of adaptive coping styles may predate the onset of pain. The patient may never have been able to cope with any stressful life events very well. His attempts to cope, such as withdrawing or being passive, may have prolonged the problems and created others. Thus when the patient who is already barely coping with life events also experiences pain, he is poorly equipped to handle it and may very well be overwhelmed by it.

The patient's intense reaction to pain often causes the staff to discount the pain and believe that the patient has emotional problems, forgetting that many of these patients do have significant, identifiable organic damage. When the patient senses the staff's disbelief, the patient simply increases his behavioral reaction in an effort to get the staff to believe him. This becomes a vicious cycle that is disruptive for both patient and staff. Just because the patient's response to pain seems out of proportion to the degree of physical cause does not mean the patient hurts any less.

Many patients with chronic nonmalignant pain who have repeated crises with pain, manifested by frequent emergency room visits or hospital admissions, may have an underlying psychiatric illness or simply ineffective coping styles. Realizing this may enable the health team to be less frustrated and judgmental about them. Such patients may be handling their pain to the best of their ability, and it may be unrealistic to expect more without intensive therapeutic intervention.

No pain is imaginary, and outright fabrication of chronic pain is considered rare. Further, some pain specialists believe that certain causes of pain, e.g., myofascial syndrome and sympathetic dystrophy, are commonly overlooked (see annotated references: Crook and Tunks, 1985; Fischer, 1984; Hendler, 1984; Leavitt and Sweet, 1986; Reesor and Craig, 1988).

Misconception: If the patient is depressed, especially if there is no known physical cause for the pain, then depression is causing his pain. The pain would subside if the depression could be effectively treated.

Correction: It is *normal* to be depressed because of chronic pain. Chronic pain causes depression. Further, an additional variety of types of depression may accompany chronic pain. Some types of depression are present prior to the onset of pain but are not likely to be the cause of pain. A preexisting depression does, however, make it more difficult for the patient to handle chronic pain. For a patient experiencing a localized sensation of pain to be told that he is simply depressed is infuriating to the patient. Depression of any sort is a form of suffering (see annotated references: Ahles, Yunus, and Masi, 1987; Bouckoms, Litman, and Baer, 1985; Hendler, 1984; Krishnan, et al, 1985, Parts I and II; Pilowsky, Crettenden, and Townley, 1985).

Thus the vast majority of people with chronic pain will

TABLE 9-1 Features of Chronic Nonmalignant Pain and Depression

Depression without Pain	Responses to Chronic Nonmalignant Pain
The first five symptoms are not only features of depression but also common responses to chronic pain in the absence of or independent of depression.	
1. Weight loss or gain.	1. Usually weight gain, often partly due to decreased physical activity; or overeating out of boredom and inability to be involved with other desirable activities.
2. Insomnia or hypersomnia.	2. Same. Insomnia due to unrelieved pain; or hypersomnia due to medication, or due to extreme fatigue from severe or prolonged unrelieved pain or from exerting extra energy required to perform certain activities.
3. Decreased involvement in social, sexual, and work activities.	3. Same, but not usually due to lack of interest; usually due to decreased physical ability or increased pain from activity.
4. Fatigue and loss of energy.	4. Same. May be related to increased energy required to adapt to pain, e.g., change life style to keep pain under control; or due to general body deconditioning from inactivity; or due to sedating medications, e.g., narcotic/sedative.
5. Difficulty concentrating.	5. Same. Due to unrelieved pain or sedating medications, e.g., narcotic/sedative.
These last two are not only features of depression of any type but are also features of depression caused by chronic pain.	
6. Feelings of worthlessness.	6. Same. Due to loss of ability to function as did in past; due to degrading actions of others, e.g., not believing reports of pain, suggesting patient should be able to handle pain better, avoiding patient.
7. Suicidal ideas or attempts.	7. Same. Due to belief that lack of control over present pain and/or inability to function will continue, or due to self-blame for situation.

be depressed. They may suffer from a form of depression that would exist in the absence of pain but are also likely to experience some depression from the chronic pain. To make it even more complicated, the symptoms of chronic pain are somewhat like those of depression in general. That is, even if the person with chronic pain were not depressed, the person would still exhibit some of the same symptoms as depression, e.g., decreased involvement in activities, sleep disturbances, and difficulty concentrating. When the symptoms of chronic pain are compared with those of depression, the similarities between the two make it easy to see how they can become confused and how the patient can be mistakenly identified as being only depressed. Table 9-1 illustrates how features common to most types of depression may also be a result of chronic pain alone, while others are likely to be a result of the depression caused by chronic pain.

Misconception: If the patient's pain occurs or increases soon after a traumatic life event, e.g., divorce or death in the family, this stress is probably what precipitated the occurrence or exacerbation of pain.

Correction: Studies fail to show that increases in tension or anxiety are predictive of an exacerbation of pain in patients with low back pain (see annotated reference: Feuerstein, Carter, and Papciak, 1987). Furthermore, this is retrospective speculation. Most people have experienced some disturbing event within the last 6 months and not all have developed chronic pain. To say that an upsetting event is the cause of chronic pain is probably neither true nor very helpful. On the other hand, it is also true that if a person is having difficulty coping with an upsetting event, and this person additionally experiences pain,

the person will be at a disadvantage for dealing with the pain.

Misconception: Patients who are awaiting litigation after an injury or who receive worker's compensation are very likely to exaggerate their pain for financial gain, or may be malingerers. This is sometimes referred to as "compensation neurosis."

Correction: Numerous studies have failed to support this view. For example, Melzack, Katz, and Jeans (1985) found that patients who receive compensation do not report higher levels of pain than patients who do not receive compensation. These authors say "Compensation is not a *cause* of pain. . . . This does not mean that malingerers or neurotics do not exist. It suggests instead that they may be relatively rare and unfortunate patients have been misdiagnosed, mistreated and allowed to suffer under the shroud of unfair labels instead of receiving appropriate therapy" (p. 111). (See annotated references: Dworkin, et al, 1985; Leavitt and Sweet, 1986; Peck, Fordyce, and Black, 1978; Reesor and Craig, 1988.)

Litigation, of course, is not limited to worker's compensation. Other types of litigation that the patient with chronic nonmalignant pain may be involved with are divorce or insurance payments following an automobile accident. Again, there is no basis for suspecting that the patient is exaggerating his pain.

Misconception: Narcotics are totally inappropriate for all patients with chronic nonmalignant pain.

Correction: There is little evidence to support this view. However, this belief has been held for many years, and even in very recent years this opinion has been strongly stated by some pain specialists. The majority of books written for the layman with chronic nonmalignant pain are biased against the use of narcotics, and many articles in professional journals express this bias. For years most pain management programs have considered detoxification from narcotics and sedatives as one of their major rehabilitation goals. However, patients referred to pain clinics are not typical of people in the general population who suffer chronic pain and are not referred to these clinics.

Further, several studies have shown that prolonged narcotic therapy for selected patients with chronic nonmalignant pain can be a safe and humane alternative to surgery or no treatment. Most researchers suggest that prolonged narcotic therapy for chronic nonmalignant pain be considered only after other reasonable attempts to control pain have been unsuccessful and only in patients without a history of drug abuse (see annotated references: Crook and Tunks, 1985; Halpern and Robinson, 1985-86; Portenoy and Foley, 1986). On the other hand, one study showed that patients with alcohol use disorder, compared with those who had no history of this, were *not* more likely to be prescription medication users (Holzman and Gulliver, 1986).

Misconception: People with chronic pain who have been taking narcotics for months or years are very much like street drug users or addicts.

Correction: Street drug users or narcotic addicts are not taking narcotics to relieve physical pain, nor do they claim to need or want narcotics for pain relief unless they are trying to obtain narcotics illicitly via the health care system, e.g., emergency rooms. Prolonged use of narcotics for pain relief may not be appropriate for all patients, but it is not addiction since narcotics are legally and medically sanctioned for use as analgesics. Further, unlike narcotic addicts, patients who take very high doses of narcotic for weeks or months, even years in some cases, will almost always stop using narcotics when the pain stops (refer to pp. 67-72 regarding differences and incidence of addiction, physical dependence, and tolerance to analgesia; see annotated reference: Halpern and Robinson, 1985-86).

Although the term "drug abuse" may appear in a patient's record, the fact that a person has used narcotics for pain relief for a long time does not necessarily mean he is abusing them. If the long-term use of narcotics is inappropriate, then the term *misuse* is applicable. A patient may misuse narcotics for pain relief for years because they are misprescribed by a physician (misprescribed in the sense that for some patients another method of pain relief might be a better choice).

Patient Example

Ms. N., 42 years old, sustained a neck injury in an automobile accident that was diagnosed 10 months later as a disc protrusion at cervical vertebra 5 and 6. Due to complicated circumstances, a cervical laminectomy was not performed until 2 months later. For approximately 1 year, from the time of the accident until the time of surgery, this patient was cared for at home by nurses and family members. During that entire year she received meperidine IM, usually 200 mg every 2 hours. This, of course, was a very poor choice of drug and route if the goal was to relieve severe pain with a narcotic (see pp. 83-85). This situation illustrates misprescribing and what usually happens with drug intake in a patient who is not an addict. When this patient was admitted to the hospital, most nurses referred to her as being addicted because they believed that anyone who stayed at home and "shot up Demerol" for a year automatically became addicted. If this were true, one would expect the patient to continue to request narcotic injections after surgery relieved her pain. However, postoperatively this patient requested meperidine injections for 3 days, oral codeine plus nonnarcotic for an additional 2 days, and nonnarcotic analgesics thereafter. She was totally off analgesics within 20 days after surgery. A patient who indeed "looked like an addict" was not—she stopped taking the narcotic and all other analgesics when the pain was relieved.

Misconception: When patients with chronic nonmalignant pain are "noncompliant," it is probably because they do not want to give up their pain.

Correction: When patients with chronic nonmalignant pain do not follow the recommendations of the health team and this results in a continuation of significant problems, such as lack of improvement in physical function or an exacerbation of pain, it may well be that the health team's recommendations are inappropriate for the patient. Noncompliance has a negative connotation, and often patients who are noncompliant are considered "difficult." Such patients tend to take more time to treat, both per visit and over time, and to have more complications and multiple treatments. Health team members are understandably frustrated when the patient fails to follow recommendations that they feel would benefit the patient. However, noncompliance is widespread in all chronic diseases, e.g., asthma and diabetes, and should be expected to occur with chronic nonmalignant pain as well.

It may help to reconsider the situation in terms of two features: (1) the implications of the term "compliance," and (2) reasons that the health team's recommendations may not be appropriate for the individual.

First, "compliance" implies an undemocratic and authoritarian relationship between a knowledgeable health care provider and an informed patient who is the passive recipient of directions. It is not likely that the use of the term compliance will be discontinued, but hopefully a different attitude can be fostered. To help patients who have any chronic condition, a more collaborative relationship is desirable. The patient must be an active member of the relationship, plan his care with the health care professional, and be given respect for his opinions and goals. Hence, a more acceptable term for this relationship might be therapeutic alliance, and compliance might be replaced with the term adherence.

Second, why might the patient fail to follow recommendations? The recommendations may be too complicated for the patient. He may not remember all the recommendations, some may be unrealistic for him, he may be overwhelmed from being asked to accomplish too many things, or some recommendations may have increased his pain or related problems and now need to be modified. The patient may also feel that control has been taken away from him, and he may fail to follow recommendations as a means of reasserting his right to control his own life.

Asking the following questions may be helpful: Were the recommendations written down for the patient and discussed with him, encouraging him to ask questions and suggest revisions? Did the patient agree to each item, as well as consider the total time and effort required by all the recommendations? What happened when the patient attempted to follow the recommendations?

NURSING CARE GUIDELINES FOR HELPING THE PERSON WITH CHRONIC NONMALIGNANT PAIN IN THE GENERAL CLINICAL SETTING

In general clinical settings, e.g., on an inpatient orthopedic unit, outside of a structured rehabilitation program for chronic nonmalignant pain, taking care of the patient with chronic nonmalignant pain is often frustrating to nurses. Such patients are commonly referred to as difficult. However, following the guidelines below may prevent difficulties. If the patient is already angry, complaining, dissatisfied, ordering nurses around, perhaps shouting, it is still not too late to use these guidelines. The suggestions may not result in instant success, but consistent persistence usually succeeds.

Meanwhile, remember that the patient's initial reaction to you is probably based on countless unsatisfying and perhaps adversarial encounters with caregivers. Most patients who have pain for very long have been told some of the following: "It can't hurt that much." "It's all in your head." "You're just using your pain." "You're going to get addicted." "You'll just have to learn to live with this." So the patient is likely to be upset at the outset.

A Guide to Setting Realistic Goals

A less than ideal solution for the patient with chronic nonmalignant pain is often necessary when the patient is cared for in clinical settings other than those specifically designed for pain management, e.g., a pain clinic. Setting realistic goals for helping the patient in these varied settings is far from simple. However, it is essential that the goals be attainable and important for both patient and nurse. Otherwise, more harm than good may be done.

Pursuing unattainable goals or expecting the patient to do something he does not value becomes a negative and frustrating experience for all concerned.

Three practical considerations are: (1) the patient's stage of acceptance of his condition, (2) the patient's ability to follow through independently with recommendations, and (3) time and available resources.

Patient's Stage of Acceptance

The health team may recognize that the patient's pain is not life-threatening and is likely to persist, possibly for the remainder of the patient's otherwise normal life. However, the patient may not have accepted this fact. Understandably, the patient may still prefer to find a cure for the pain. It may be years before the patient accepts that a cure probably is not realistic and that he needs to make plans to handle pain on an ongoing, usually daily basis. This acceptance cannot be forced on the patient. It is similar to a form of grief that must be endured and worked through gradually.

At least four stages of dealing with chronic nonmalignant pain have been described (Hendler, 1984):

1. During the first few weeks or months of having pain, the patient may hope it will go away or begin seeking a cure for it.
2. During the following months, as the pain persists, the patient may wonder if he has been misdiagnosed or if he has received inappropriate or harmful treatment for the pain. Bodily concerns tend to increase. This patient is still cure oriented vs. accepting that the pain will persist.
3. As years go by the increasing realization that the pain is permanent may trigger increasing anger, resentment, and depression. This patient may vacillate between looking for a cure and looking for daily pain management techniques.
4. At some point, usually several years after the onset of pain, the patient may partially or sometimes completely accept that the pain will persist for the rest of his life. At this point the patient is much more likely to consider permanent alterations in his life-style and to accept or seek strategies to help him deal with the pain on a daily basis. Depression may decrease but is likely to continue to some extent. Compared with other chronic health problems such as decreasing eyesight, diabetes, or limb amputation, the patient with chronic nonmalignant pain is probably more likely to encounter unsympathetic attitudes in family, friends, and caregivers, e.g., disbelieving the existence or severity of the pain. Such attitudes increase the patient's distress and reinforce feelings of inadequacy.

Obviously, patients who are less oriented to seeking a cure will tend to be more accepting of self-management techniques, such as relaxation and pacing. Patients more oriented to finding a cure may be more accepting of physical therapy, medications, and other more tangible and health-team directed approaches to pain management.

As long as the patient believes a cure is possible or believes that control of the pain is dependent upon medical or surgical interventions, the patient is unlikely to be very committed to self-directed strategies for pain control. They may be offered, but the patient's rejection of them is understandable, since to him they seem inappropriate.

Patient's Ability to Handle Recommendations Independently

Regardless of the patient's state of acceptance of chronic pain, he may wish to pursue certain recommendations for pain control that he simply is not able to do. Physical limitations such as living in an isolated area with no public transportation or living in a dangerous neighborhood may prohibit engaging in activities outside the home. Regular supervision of exercises by a physical therapist is hampered if the patient lives several hundred miles away from one. Physical problems such as diminished eyesight or a memory deficit may render even the simplest medication regimen difficult or unsafe.

Further, the patient's coping style of active and independent vs. passive and dependent will influence the skill with which he is able to implement certain recommendations. No matter how good the patient's intentions may be, if he has very little experience in taking active control of his daily life, his efforts may not be very successful, e.g., keeping an accurate or complete daily diary or remembering to make or keep appointments.

Time and Available Resources

In spite of what the patient is willing and able to do to control his pain, the nurse simply may not have the time to help the patient with all or even most of the possibilities. The nurse in the emergency room who sees a patient return every week for "shots" for his low back pain probably knows that this is not the best approach to helping the patient. But how much time does she have to do more than this?

Further, resources such as a psychologist, a physician specializing in pain, certain medications, or a pain clinic may not be available or affordable. Thus referral to other resources is not always a reasonable option.

Trying to identify goals that are not only a priority for the individual but also realistic is no small matter. The specific nursing care guidelines summarized on p. 242 pinpoint some frequently relevant and important approaches, and they are listed in somewhat of a hierarchy from the most commonly and easily done to the more complex activities. Although they are admittedly not comprehensive, it often is not even possible to follow all of them. Thus realistic goals may sometimes seem not only less than ideal but also less than the acceptable minimum.

KEY POINT: To set goals that are important, realistic, and attainable requires acknowledgment of limitations in the nurse, patient, and surrounding circumstances.

At the very least, the goal is to work as effectively as possible with whatever is presented in the immediate situation. This usually includes the attitude expressed toward the patient, basic assessment of any changes in the patient's condition, and appropriate use of whatever analgesics are prescribed. This involves the first eight nursing care guidelines listed on p. 242.

For example, the emergency room nurse, mentioned above, who sees the patient with low back pain return weekly for a narcotic injection can find time to follow most of the first eight nursing care guidelines on p. 242, i.e., she can believe the patient, refrain from referring to him as an addict, not try to fool him with a placebo, ask him about any changes in his pain, discuss the cause of the low back pain, recognize that an acute exacerbation may require narcotics, avoid suggesting that the patient simply stop taking all medications, and advise the patient to take whatever the physician has prescribed on a regular basis to help prevent back pain from escalating to the point of needing to return to the emergency room.

When the nurse is able to see the patient with chronic pain over a period of days, the goal is broadened to addressing the patient's methods of handling pain on a daily basis in addition to the problems in the immediate situation. Even when the patient is seen only briefly, if it is repeatedly but without the stress of an emergency, broader goals are also appropriate. Examples of such situations are recurrent hospitalizations, weekly home visits by a nurse, or regular patient visits to the office of the industrial nurse or a physician. Repeated or prolonged contacts allow time for gradual assessment and introduction of alternative methods of dealing with chronic pain. Several or all of the nursing care guidelines numbered 8 through 22 on p. 242 may be indicated.

Specific Nursing Care Guidelines

The nursing care guidelines below are one of the few places in this book where the word "never" is used repeatedly. This is probably because there are more misconceptions about the treatment of chronic nonmalignant pain than other types of pain. Nursing care guidelines for helping the patient with chronic nonmalignant pain (or, at the very least not making the situation worse) are discussed in the text and summarized in the box on p. 242.

1. Never argue with the patient about whether or not the patient feels the pain he says he has. Whatever the patient says about his pain, or whatever indications he gives about his pain, are treated with respect. Even if the health team doubts some or all of what the patient is saying, the patient is given the benefit of the doubt. To do otherwise is to call the patient a liar and to begin a battle

Specific Nursing Care Guidelines
for Helping the Person with Chronic Nonmalignant Pain: Summary

1. Never argue with the patient about whether or not the patient feels the pain he says he has.

2. Never refer to the patient as a narcotic addict.

3. Never use a placebo to try to determine if the patient has "real" pain, has a physical cause for pain, or is lying about his pain.

4. Be especially alert to any changes in the patient's condition as well as any advances in treating the patient's pain.

5. Recognize and treat acute pain or exacerbations of chronic pain differently than ongoing chronic nonmalignant pain.

6. Be sure the patient receives what he feels is an adequate explanation from the appropriate person of why he has pain.

7. Avoid sudden withdrawal of narcotic and sedative medications, but when medication reduction is indicated, give priority to reduction of sedatives rather than narcotics.

8. When analgesics are required, give them orally, if at all possible, at high enough doses to provide satisfactory pain relief, and often enough on a regular schedule ATC to prevent the return of pain.

9. Review analgesics being used for relief of chronic (vs. acute) pain, usually with the goals of avoiding narcotics, encouraging nonnarcotic analgesia, and suggesting trials of appropriate classes of drugs recently found to have analgesic properties for specific conditions, e.g., anticonvulsants and antidepressants for neuropathic pain.

10. When it is obviously very likely that the patient will return for treatment of chronic pain, e.g., to the orthopedic unit, try to develop a summary of the present treatment and a plan for the return visit.

11. Decreasing the severity of a chronic sleep disturbance is a priority, and the appropriateness of antidepressants and/or relaxation techniques should be evaluated.

12. Offer pain relief alternatives likely to be most consistent with the patient's coping style, e.g., active vs. passive methods of coping with pain.

13. Help the patient learn and plan to use coping strategies, especially relaxation, that avoid catastrophizing.

14. Help the patient develop his own daily commitment to specific activities, e.g., physical and/or social, especially a return to employment of any type, if appropriate.

15. Help those living with the patient, especially the spouse, to work with the patient to establish expectations and limitations regarding the activities of the patient and others in relation to the patient's pain.

16. Review with the patient his support systems, and suggest additional ones, if appropriate.

17. Consider obtaining the assistance of a physical therapist to help the patient identify physical exercises that are appropriate, especially a reasonable quota for the patient.

18. Review with the patient any types of help he has sought outside traditional medical practice, providing appropriate encouragement or suggesting precautions.

19. All recommendations to the patient regarding management of his chronic pain need to be specific and detailed, in writing with a copy for the patient and health team, and incorporated with any other recommendations so that a picture of the total plan is readily available.

20. Evaluate the effectiveness of each specific recommendation made to the patient for pain management, with regular follow-up and possibly written, daily diaries kept by the patient.

21. Assess the need for requesting a consultation to identify and treat depression, anxiety, or posttraumatic stress disorder.

22. Assess suicidal risk.

---

with the patient over a matter that can never be proven or disproven.

As early as the 1970s this approach was recognized as important and addressed by pain specialists. For example, at one multidisciplinary pain center during that time, about 15 health team members met for their weekly discussion of the patients admitted to the inpatient unit. While a particular patient was being reviewed, a physician began to shake his head slowly from side to side. Finally a colleague asked him to share the meaning of his reaction. The physician said he found it difficult to believe that this patient had any pain, certainly not as much as the patient said he had. The colleague responded in a routine, matter-of-fact fashion, saying that the physician was entitled to his personal opinion, but that professionally it was their responsibility to respond to the patient's report of pain.

2. Never refer to the patient as a narcotic addict. Pain relief is a legal, medical reason for the use of narcotics. When a patient is taking narcotics for pain, no matter how long or how much narcotic, he is not an addict. Even if the patient has developed tolerance to analgesia and requires more narcotic to relieve his pain, or even if the patient develops withdrawal syndrome when narcotics are abruptly stopped, he is not an addict (see Chapter 4, pp. 67-72 for definitions and distinctions between these terms). Sometimes the words tolerance, withdrawal, and addiction are used interchangeably, but by current definitions they are separate entities.

Not only is it inaccurate to refer to the patient who takes narcotics for chronic nonmalignant pain as an addict, it is degrading to the patient. Considerable stigma is attached to the term. In our society, to be an addict is to be a "bad" person.

3. Never use a placebo to try to determine if the pa-

tient has "real" pain, has a physical cause for pain, or is lying about his pain. Pain relief from a placebo proves nothing. It merely confirms the pharmacological fact that 33% of the time or more, placebos will provide adequate pain relief for patients with obvious physical causes for pain of moderate to severe intensity (see Chapter 2, p. 16).

4. Be especially alert to any changes in the patient's condition as well as any advances in treating the patient's pain. Note the need for additional diagnostic testing. Significant changes in the patient's condition may go unnoticed because it is altogether too easy to become accustomed to chronic reports of pain. Thus a diagnosis may be missed. It is always possible that the patient will develop additional pain problems requiring different treatment, e.g., a malignancy or myocardial infarction.

Further, the condition underlying pain may change or may be eventually diagnosed and treated as advances are made in pain management. Progress is being made in many areas of pain control. It is possible that some new treatment will be indicated for the patient's pain. For example, in recent years adjuvant analgesics (pp. 113 and 116-123) have been found effective with some types of pain, such as anticonvulsants for phantom limb pain.

5. Recognize and treat acute pain or exacerbations of chronic pain differently than ongoing chronic nonmalignant pain. To treat acute pain differently than chronic nonmalignant pain requires careful assessment to distinguish between the two. Unfortunately, it is common for some types of acute pain to be mistaken for chronic nonmalignant pain. When acute pain is prolonged, e.g., lasting weeks or months, is recurrent, e.g., weekly or monthly episodes for a few days, or is an exacerbation of chronic nonmalignant pain, these situations may be misunderstood as chronic nonmalignant pain. Examples of acute pain that may be erroneously treated as chronic nonmalignant pain are sickle cell crisis, burn pain that lasts for weeks or months, weeks or months of pain related to multiple orthopedic injuries following an accident (e.g., unhealed fractures, infected wounds), exacerbation of neck pain from excessive strain, or postoperative pain from a laminectomy performed on a patient with chronic low back pain. Analgesics and limited activity may be indicated temporarily for acute pain, but with ongoing chronic nonmalignant pain the goal is usually to increase activity. Fear of causing addiction or allowing the patient to become accustomed to the relief of stronger analgesics, especially narcotics, often results in inadequate treatment of acute pain, e.g., postoperative pain. However, intravenous morphine is entirely appropriate for sickle cell crisis, postoperative pain, or burn tanking and debridement. High doses of oral narcotics on a regular basis are appropriate while complicated orthopedic injuries heal or during an exacerbation of musculoskeletal pain. At the same time, techniques often recommended for chronic nonmalignant pain may be used, such as relaxa-

tion and pacing, e.g., taking a break before pain increases (see p. 247). On the other hand, for daily chronic nonmalignant pain, intravenous morphine is obviously not the answer.

The difference between acute and chronic pain must be clear to both patient and health team. Just because pain is prolonged and not life-threatening is not justification for treating it as chronic nonmalignant pain as defined in this chapter. For pain to be classified and treated as chronic nonmalignant pain, it must have also failed to respond to current treatment, further medical and surgical interventions to cure the cause of the pain should not be indicated, and pain must be expected to continue indefinitely. This is not the case with the above examples. Either the pain will subside as healing takes place, e.g., orthopedic injuries, or the pain is a time-limited episode, e.g., exacerbations of chronic nonmalignant pain, postoperative pain, or sickle cell crisis.

6. Be sure the patient receives what he feels is an adequate explanation from the appropriate person of why he has pain. Ask the patient what he has been told about the cause of his pain and whether or not this makes sense to him. If not, identify if there is anyone in particular, such as the physician, whom the patient would like to have explain the reason for his pain. The nurse also needs to be prepared to explain to the patient why he hurts. An explanation from the nurse may suffice or be very helpful in addition to explanations from others. The explanation need not be detailed or time consuming.

Every attempt needs to be made to provide an explanation acceptable to the patient. This increases the patient's satisfaction with his care and tends to reduce the patient's requests for diagnostic tests, the extent to which he uses health care services, and changes from one agency or physician to another (Deyo and Diehl, 1986).

Patient Example

Ms. A., 39 years old, is seen by her physician in his office for her first evaluation and treatment of "whiplash," or cervical neck syndrome, resulting from being rear-ended in an automobile accident 36 hours previously. In addition to specific information about medications and physical therapy, the nurse reinforces the physician's explanation to the patient about the cause of pain by saying "From our assessment and from what you have said about the accident and your pain, it's clear that the pain is mostly a result of injury to your neck and shoulder muscles and not an injury to your spinal cord or any major nerves. It's typical not to feel pain immediately after a muscle injury. Remember when you did some strenuous yard work last year and had that backache the next day? When muscles are strained they tend to hurt worse a day or so later. Your muscles react to being injured by contracting and that causes more pain. That's why we have suggested physical therapy to help you learn how to keep your muscles as stretched out as possible. Later there will be strengthening exercises to prevent further injury from muscle weakness that develops while you rest the muscles and allow them to heal. You'll also get some information on how to use aspirin and cold packs to help relieve the pain. Pain often causes tension and guarding that increases the muscle spasm and pain. So we try to break the cycle of pain and muscle tension in several ways, such as the stretching, cold packs, and regular use of aspirin."

7. Avoid sudden withdrawal of narcotic and sedative medications, but when medication reduction is indicated, give priority to reduction of sedatives rather than narcotics. Some patients have tried the "grand stand" approach of suddenly stopping all narcotic/sedative drugs. The results are often devastating to the patient. Not only does the patient face sudden return of pain, anxiety, and other emotional disturbances but he also experiences very uncomfortable withdrawal, described as "super-flu" with narcotic withdrawal, and characterized by irritability, motor tremor, and other sometimes more severe symptoms with tranquilizer/sedative withdrawal.

Suggest a gradual reduction of narcotics and sedatives for patients who wish to discontinue their use and have been on them for 3 weeks or longer. Gradual reduction over periods ranging from as short as 1 week for narcotics and as long as 8 weeks for benzodiazepines helps prevent significant withdrawal symptoms and gives the patient time to find alternate methods of dealing with pain and emotional or sleep disturbances. With benzodiazepines and barbiturates, it is best to err on the side of slow detoxification by giving larger doses for longer than may be necessary in order to avoid severe, and sometimes life-threatening, withdrawal (Busto et al, 1986).

When contacts with the patient are limited, it is probably wise to decrease only one drug at a time by small amounts over a long period. Try to eliminate the drug that causes the most detrimental effects on functioning, especially a drug that causes sedation. Usually the most offensive drug is a tranquilizer or sedative, such as benzodiazepine or barbiturate.

Because of exaggerated fears about addiction to narcotics, narcotics are usually mistakenly thought to be the most important drug to eliminate. Narcotics do not necessarily cause much sedation after the patient has taken them for a long time. Tolerance to sedation tends to occur rapidly and to a greater extent than tolerance to analgesia. Research shows that certain patients with chronic nonmalignant pain have been successfully maintained on narcotics for long periods and that use of narcotics enabled patients to return to work when other approaches failed (Portenoy and Foley, 1986; Tennant et al, 1988).

8. When analgesics are required, give them orally, if at all possible, at high enough doses to provide satisfactory pain relief, and often enough on a regular schedule ATC to prevent the return of pain. Analgesics should never be withheld until the pain becomes severe. During an exacerbation of chronic pain, the IV route may be used initially to relieve severe pain quickly, but then the patient should be changed to oral analgesics as soon as possible, probably both narcotic and nonnarcotic (see Chapter 4, p. 88, regarding how to use oral analgesics for severe pain).

KEY POINT: Either use narcotics well or use them not at all. If narcotics are prescribed, the frequency and dose must be adequate to relieve the pain.

9. Review analgesics being used for relief of chronic (vs. acute) pain, usually with the goals of avoiding narcotics, encouraging nonnarcotic analgesia, and suggesting trials of appropriate classes of drugs recently found to have analgesic properties for specific conditions, e.g., anticonvulsants and antidepressants for neuropathic pain. Narcotic analgesics are not strictly prohibited in the treatment of chronic nonmalignant pain, but because of side effects, such as sedation, constipation, and possible increased doses over time due to tolerance to analgesia, narcotics are avoided unless other treatment measures fail. Then narcotics may be considered appropriate if they enable the patient to maintain or improve his quality of life or level of function.

Muscle relaxants are another class of drug that is used with caution. The effectiveness of muscle relaxants when they are taken orally is somewhat questionable. If they do produce muscle relaxation, this is often accompanied by some sedation. Thus they are usually used on a time-limited basis, sometimes for an acute injury or exacerbation or in conjunction with active physical therapy until the patient is able to do exercises that keep the muscles from contracting (see pp. 119-120).

Since nonnarcotic analgesics such as acetaminophen or naproxen rarely interfere with daily function, their regular use may be indicated when analgesics are needed for a patient with chronic nonmalignant pain. The most effective nonnarcotic with the fewest side effects for the individual is given at the highest appropriate dose and on a regular ATC basis (see pp. 54-61).

Recently certain types of neuropathic pain have been successfully treated with drugs other than the usual analgesics. Dull, aching neuropathic pain may respond to antidepressants (see pp. 118-119). Lancinating or shooting neuropathic pain may be relieved by anticonvulsants (see p. 119).

Careful selection and adjustment of medications for pain relief may result in good pain control without the use of narcotics.

10. When it is obviously very likely that the patient will return for treatment of chronic pain, e.g., to the orthopedic unit, try to develop a summary of the present treatment and a plan for the return visit. It is especially important to identify which pain relief measures have been effective and which have not, hopefully enabling the staff to avoid repeating any approaches that were not effective.

The goal of the following is to use the information available from this hospitalization to facilitate arriving at the best possible plan for pain relief for the next hospitalization. This may also be used to develop a plan for outpatient treatment. Further, by involving the patient and showing respect for his opinion, other desirable outcomes of this interaction may be that an adversarial relationship is avoided or minimized and the patient feels less angry, anxious, or helpless when he is readmitted. Within the constraints of time, try the following:

• About 24 hours before discharge, make a list of all pain relief measures used during this hospitalization, e.g., all analgesics, sedatives, muscle relaxants, and other pain related medications administered during this hospitalization, any noninvasive pain relief measures used, and physical therapy (involve the physical therapist, if possible, or at least obtain specific information about what was done and what exercises are recommended now).

• Review this list with the patient and ask him if he has any additions.

• Ask the patient to give his estimate of how helpful each item was. Use information from flow sheets (e.g., p. 27), if available.

• Based upon the patient's answers, identify with the patient what would seem to be a logical plan of treatment when he returns. Findings may suggest a revision of the previous plan. For example, if the patient had both narcotics and nonnarcotics ordered but they were never given together, the future plan may be to try this combination.

• Provide the patient with a written copy of the plan, and keep a copy on the unit.

• Integrate this plan with medications, exercises, and any other approaches for pain control following discharge. The patient/family teaching point "Planning for the Future: Review of Pain Relief Measures," p. 246, may be copied and used for this purpose. This form may be completed by both patient and nurse. One copy is given to the patient and another is kept in the patient's record by the agency or facility treating the patient.

11. Decreasing the severity of a chronic sleep disturbance is a priority, and the appropriateness of antidepressants and relaxation techniques should be evaluated. Sleep disturbances are common in chronic nonmalignant pain, and their continuation may have an increasingly detrimental effect on the patient's efforts to manage his pain. A poor night's sleep contributes to depression, muscle soreness, difficulty thinking, and decreased motivation. Avoid sedative/hypnotic medication to which the patient may become tolerant, especially benzodiazepines and barbiturates. Tricyclic antidepressants (p. 121) at subtherapeutic doses are often excellent bedtime sedatives. Also offer to help the patient learn relaxation techniques (pp. 197 and 199-205) that may help him get to sleep faster and get back to sleep if he awakens during the night.

12. Offer pain relief alternatives likely to be most consistent with the patient's coping style, e.g., active vs. passive methods of coping with pain. When the pain is brief, or acute, passive coping styles, e.g., depending on others for help, are generally more effective than active coping, and probably should be encouraged. The patient may very well recover from acute illness more rapidly if he decreases physical and emotional demands and allows others to care for him for a brief time.

However, as pain becomes chronic, maintaining quality of life and a high level of function is usually better accomplished with active coping styles, e.g., learning self-management techniques, than passive ones. In an acute care setting or when structured time with the patient is limited, it is difficult to change the patient's coping style. However, knowing the type of coping the patient uses helps determine which pain relief measures might be most successfully offered to the patient.

Patients with passive coping styles tend to avoid physical activity and to depend on others to tell them what to do about pain control. Their coping style may consist mainly of taking medication for pain relief, accepting or requesting help from others, talking about their pain, and resting frequently. These patients might most readily accept not only medication regulation, but also use of heat, cold, and perhaps TENS, listening to music for distraction, relaxation if it is made easily available, a backrub, or group support such as maintaining contact with their church or being visited by a member of their church or a person from a local chapter of American Chronic Pain Association.

Patients who have active coping styles may use medication and other approaches used in the more passive coping style but they also tend to try to ignore the pain, stay busy, and engage in physical activities. These patients might most readily accept experimenting with various types of pain relief, including cutaneous stimulation (Chapter 5), distraction (Chapter 6), relaxation (Chapter 7), and imagery (Chapter 8), consulting with the physical therapist to determine appropriate daily exercise, or contacting a self-help organization such as American Chronic Pain Association (see p. 257). Usually active coping styles should be encouraged, but caution the patient to pace himself (see "Patient/Family Teaching Point: Pace Yourself," p. 247).

13. Help the patient learn and plan to use coping strategies, especially relaxation, that avoid catastrophizing. Catastrophizing is a form of thinking that focuses on the negative characteristics of a situation and escalates to feeling helpless to control pain and believing that the worst may happen. This prevents the patient from making realistic choices about how to keep pain under control.

A variety of coping strategies may also help the patient regain control, including taking time out such as going into a room alone for 5 minutes, silently repeating hopeful statements such as "I can handle this. I know what to

Text continued on p. 249.

Patient/Family Teaching Point: Planning for the Future—Review of Pain Relief Measures

TO: _____ (patient's name)   DATE: _____

Purpose: To use the information available from a recent episode of pain to plan the best possible pain relief for any future occurrence of similar pain. This is accomplished by identifying the effect of pain relief measures used for a recent episode of pain.

Nature of pain: _____

From (date) _____ to _____
Medications used in relation to problem of pain (e.g., narcotic and nonnarcotic analgesics, tranquilizers, antidepressants, sleeping pills, muscle relaxants):

Medication name, dose, frequency: Helpful? Other comments:

Nonpharmacological (non-drug) pain relief measures (e.g., relaxation, distraction, TENS, exercise):

Method, frequency: Helpful? Other comments:

Summary of what did help: Summary of what did not help:

Plans for pain relief if situation occurs again (e.g., at home, or if readmit to hospital, return to emergency room):

Plans for pain relief at home or in immediate future, if applicable:

From: _____ (nurse's name)   Phone: _____

■ May be duplicated for use in clinical practice. From McCaffery, M, and Beebe, A: PAIN: CLINICAL MANUAL FOR NURSING PRACTICE, St. Louis, 1989, The CV Mosby Company.

Patient/Family Teaching Point: Pace Yourself

TO: _____ (patient's name)   DATE: _____

What is pacing? It's doing things throughout the day for periods of time that do not make your pain worse. Many people with chronic pain push or force themselves for a day or so, and then end up with much worse pain and are unable to do much for several days. Pacing is the opposite of this. The purpose of pacing is to make it possible for you to be active every day. Pacing and the big push are compared below.

Pacing

Take a break before you need it.

Benefits:

1. Pain stays manageable.

2. Able to maintain a certain level of activity day after day. No need to take time off.

3. Every day you are able to accomplish something you want or need to do.

Big Push

Force yourself.

Results:

1. Pain increases significantly. Medication intake increases. Irritability increases.

2. Must take time off to recover. Recovery may be slow and depressing.

3. You accomplish your goal but while you are recovering you can't do much at all.

By trial and error you can find out what you can do and for how long without your pain increasing or returning. For example, you may find that you can work at a certain activity for 30-minute periods, taking off 5 minutes every half hour. Setting a timer helps you remember. At the end of the day you may discover that you have worked productively for a total of 5 hours without increasing your pain. However, if you had pushed yourself to work 3 hours straight without a break, you might have increased pain and gotten less done.

From: _____ (nurse's name)   Phone: _____

■ May be duplicated for use in clinical practice. From McCaffery, M, and Beebe, A: PAIN: CLINICAL MANUAL FOR NURSING PRACTICE, St. Louis, 1989, The CV Mosby Company.

Patient/Family Teaching Point: Overall Daily Plan

TO: _____ (patient's name)   DATE: _____

   As a general rule, keep your pain under control by using your approaches to coping with pain before you really need them. Figure out a daily schedule that includes each of the following to some extent in some way. Keep your pain under control. Don't wait until your pain is severe before you use something like relaxation, rest periods, or medication.

1. **Pacing.** Plan to rest before your pain increases and before you get tired.
2. **Exercises.** At least once a day, perform exercises that are appropriate for you. You may need to be advised by a physical therapist. The main purposes of the exercises are:
   - Stretch muscles to reduce soreness and muscle spasm
   - Strengthen muscles
   - General physical fitness (this helps avoid further injury)
   - Increased ability to perform other activities
3. **Relaxation.** Allow yourself to relax completely for at least 10 minutes once a day. You may use a relaxation tape, prayer, listening to music, or anything else that brings you peace of mind and contentment. Pain is stressful and frustrating, so you need to give yourself a real break from stress by truly relaxing. Just sitting down watching TV is not really profound relaxation. You may want to ask your nurse about relaxation techniques. Relaxation is a way to recharge yourself. Afterwards you'll feel more energetic and able to think clearly.
4. **Medications** for pain should be taken regularly by the clock, or at least before pain begins or increases.
5. **Things to do every day.** Do something every day that involves these three things:
   - Work (for wages, volunteer work, or study). Be sure you feel capable.
   - Family or close friend. Be sure you hug somebody.
   - Fun. Be sure you laugh.

From: _____ (nurse's name)   Phone: _____

■ May be duplicated for use in clinical practice. From McCaffery, M, and Beebe, A: PAIN: CLINICAL MANUAL FOR NURSING PRACTICE, St. Louis, 1989, The CV Mosby Company.

---

do," using imagery (Chapter 8), or performing a distraction strategy (see Chapter 6). Help the patient anticipate problems and decide on a course of action in advance. Try writing down the specific problem in one column and the possible solutions in the adjacent column. This is an exercise in problem-solving, and it gives the patient something tangible to turn to when he is distressed and unable to think clearly.

Relaxation techniques seem particularly helpful to people with chronic pain of any type (see Chapter 7). Explain to the patient that using a relaxation technique, such as a tape, prayer, or music, is a way of slowing down and calming down so that it is easier to think of ways to cope with the pain instead of becoming more upset and overwhelmed by the pain. Relaxation may also relieve some types of chronic nonmalignant pain, e.g., low back pain (Stucky, Jacobs, and Goldfarb, 1986).

14. Help the patient develop his own daily commitment to specific activities, e.g., physical and/or social, especially a return to employment of any type, if appropriate. Physical or mental activity is important for all patients who must cope with pain daily, but it seems especially important for the depressed patient (consider using "Patient/Family Teaching Point: Overall Daily Plan," p. 248, as a guide). Return to employment is not always appropriate. The patient may be far too disabled to return to his former employment, and reeducation for a new job may not be feasible. For the very disabled patient, guidelines for simply maintaining the normal sensory environment may be appropriate (pp. 181-184). Or, the patient may have been retired from work for some years and have no desire to return. A female patient may never have worked outside the home.

However, if at all possible, for the patient who was employed prior to the onset of pain, a return to some level of employment is helpful in many ways, ranging from earning money to increasing feelings of worthiness. Even volunteer work without financial compensation may have many advantages such as providing one type of support system for the patient, distracting the patient from pain, and increasing feelings of being capable and adequate because of making some sort of contribution to others.

15. Help those living with the patient, especially the spouse, to work with the patient to establish expectations and limitations regarding the activities of the patient and others in relation to the patient's pain. Any person living with the patient may experience uncertainty and helplessness, even physical problems, due to activities or changes necessitated by the patient's pain. Such persons may benefit from identifying the extent to which they can realistically control the pain and daily living activities. It may be helpful to emphasize the following:

• The patient is in charge of controlling his own pain.
• Pain should not become the family's dictator.
• What can the patient commit himself to doing regard-

less of what his pain is like? A list of specific activities is helpful. Others close to the patient need to know what they can depend on. This also helps the patient feel responsible and adequate.

• What can family members do to help the patient but not place a burden on them?
• Are there things the patient does not want the family to do for him? For example, the patient may feel embarrassed or "babied" by certain types of help.
• Which activities or plans include the patient but should be carried out even if the patient is unable to participate?
• Are there certain times when the patient should avoid talking about his pain?
• Should the patient consider using resources outside the family to meet some of his needs, e.g., someone else to talk to about his pain, engaging in recreational or social activities without the family? If the patient has sources of satisfaction outside the family, the family need not feel totally responsible for the patient's well-being and the patient need not feel completely dependent on the family.

16. Review with the patient his support systems, and suggest additional ones, if appropriate. Support systems include groups or individuals to whom the patient may turn for assistance with managing his pain. Family members or those living with the patient are a common support system. However, the entire burden of support should not fall on the family or spouse alone. Family members need to be able to set limits on what they can do for the patient.

Other support systems that the patient can contact on a regular basis include friends not living in the home, members of the health team such as a psychologist or nurse, members of various groups to which the patient belongs such as church groups, people who regularly engage in the activities with the patient such as volunteer projects or card games, and coworkers if the patient is employed.

The need for a contact person 24 hours a day is especially important for the patient with severe pain and depression. It is likely to be a difficult need to meet. For reasons mentioned above, this person should not be someone living with the patient. The contact person might be a health professional such as a nurse in home care or an outpatient clinic, someone in a crisis center, a friend outside the home, or a member of a local organization of patients with chronic pain.

The contact person and all members of the patient's support systems need to realize that attempting to rescue the patient from his pain is not the answer and that a permanent "happy ending" is not likely. It is very difficult to be the person the patient contacts when he needs help with unrelieved pain. By definition, there is no instant or magic remedy. The helping person must know that the pain is likely to continue.

The most important help that others can offer the patient is to believe what the patient says, not argue with the patient, and validate with the patient that it is indeed difficult to try to cope with ongoing pain. The most reassuring assistance is usually an emphasis on the patient's attempts to handle the pain and an acceptance of the fact that attempts will not always be successful. Continued attempts must be encouraged. The patient can benefit from knowing that his reactions to this devastating situation are understandable, that someone believes the pain is exactly what he says, and that someone likes him enough to continue a relationship.

17. Consider obtaining the assistance of a physical therapist to help the patient identify physical exercises that are appropriate, especially a reasonable quota for the patient. Patients with chronic pain tend to become inactive and physically deconditioned. Many have an exaggerated fear that exercise will increase the pain. Thus the patient may benefit in several ways from closely supervised physical activity.

The patient needs to know exactly what exercises to do, how many repetitions, for how long, and how often. It is very important to help the patient avoid doing exercises to the point of causing pain. Hence the emphasis is on doing exercises to quota, not pushing until there is pain. The patient's quota is set at a level that hopefully will not precipitate pain.

The exercises should be written down for the patient. Encourage the patient to keep a written record of his performance and any problems he has. The daily diary (p. 30) or a modification of it may be used for this purpose. A written record helps the patient feel a sense of achievement and enables the physical therapist to make appropriate changes.

18. Review with the patient any types of help he has sought outside traditional medical practice, providing appropriate encouragement or suggesting precautions. It is not unusual for patients with chronic pain to seek nonmedical health care such as naturapathy, various so-called health foods, acupuncture, faith healing, and especially chiropractic if the patient has musculoskeletal problems. In fact, patients with pain are probably the largest group of patients utilizing these services. These nonmedical modalities are not necessarily harmful and may prove somewhat helpful if they are appropriately supervised by the nurse or physician. Stress to the patient the importance of using these approaches in addition to rather than instead of traditional health care.

Chiropractic is scorned by many health professionals but it is the largest licensed "unorthodox" health profession in the United States, and its services are covered by most health insurance. Exactly what chiropractors do other than spinal manipulation is extremely varied. However, they provide a drugless treatment option, and they have a high success or satisfaction rate, apparently due in

large part to the chiropractor-patient interaction. Basically the patient's needs are met for validation and explanation of his pain, physical treatment, and a treatment plan. Used in combination with appropriate physical therapy and medical supervision, it can be enormously beneficial.

19. All recommendations to the patient regarding management of his chronic pain need to be specific and detailed, in writing with a copy for the patient and health team, and incorporated with any other recommendations so that a picture of the total plan is readily available. To put all of this in writing is admittedly time consuming and may not seem very practical in an acute care setting. However, with any chronic health problem, the patient is likely to receive numerous instructions from various health team members. It is difficult for the patient to remember these, and health team members are not always aware of what other recommendations have been made. It is also likely that some instructions may be incompatible or contradictory. Thus in the long run, it undoubtedly saves time for the patient and health team if all attempts to help the patient are organized into one plan.

It is also helpful if one person, e.g., the primary care nurse, is designated as being responsible for coordinating the total plan. Then both patient and health team members know whom to contact when conflict or confusion occurs. To begin such a plan, it may be necessary to spend an hour or more obtaining information from the patient, verifying this with other health team members, and putting it in written form. When simple problems or crises occur, this information facilitates evaluating the circumstances and deciding on a course of action, saving time and making the situation go much smoother for everyone.

20. Evaluate the effectiveness of each specific recommendation made to the patient for pain management, with regular follow-up and possibly written daily diaries kept by the patient. Too often the assumption is made that a recommendation is safe, effective, and useful unless the patient reports a problem. However, the patient may encounter problems following through with a recommendation and decide to discontinue it without realizing that a simple modification might enable him to benefit from it. Or, the patient may continue with something in spite of problems and cause a worsening of his condition. In either case, considerable time may be lost before the health professional is contacted and able to rectify the situation.

Whether the recommendation involves medication, relaxation, physical therapy or some other approach, make specific plans for follow-up. This may involve making another appointment to see the patient or asking the patient to telephone in a few days to report the results.

If a period of days or weeks goes by, the patient is likely

to have difficulty remembering exactly what happened in relation to his pain. Also, memory may be adversely affected by many factors, such as pain, medications, and a desire to forget or deny how severe the pain has been. When the patient is unable to give a specific or complete history of his pain and its management, a daily diary is probably indicated (see p. 30).

21. Assess the need for requesting a consultation to identify and treat depression, anxiety, or posttraumatic stress disorder. Anxiety and depression often accompany pain, especially prolonged pain, and may respond to various types of treatment. For example, if depression predates the onset of pain, psychotropic medication may be indicated. There is growing recognition that pain incurred as a result of unexpected trauma, e.g., an accident, may lead to posttraumatic stress disorder. This may have a paralyzing effect on the patient but may respond well to therapy that gradually desensitizes the patient to fearful aspects.

However, suggesting a psychological or psychiatric evaluation may well be misunderstood by health team members and the patient. Try to approach this by clarifying that depression and anxiety rarely cause pain, but pain often causes depression and anxiety that make the pain more difficult to handle. Reassure the patient that after even a few weeks of pain, it would be abnormal if he felt no depression or anxiety. It may be more acceptable to the patient and less misleading to others to refer to the *frustration,* rather than the depression, of dealing with pain.

22. Assess suicidal risk. Many people with chronic nonmalignant pain become depressed, and it is not unusual for them to express suicidal thoughts. The risk of suicide is high in some patients, particularly those with prolonged, uncontrolled, severe pain. Remember, too, that the angry patient may also be suicidal. When a patient expresses hostility toward us for our failure to help him, it is altogether too easy to withdraw and become self-protective, forgetting momentarily how devastated the patient may be.

Identify whether or not the patient has a suicide plan and has the ability to carry it out. Document your findings, inform the physician, and obtain an appropriate referral.

PATIENT/FAMILY TEACHING POINTS

Once as much of the pain as possible has been relieved, the major goal in assisting the patient with chronic nonmalignant pain is to maintain as good a quality of life as possible on a daily basis. Many approaches discussed elsewhere in the book may be helpful. But no matter what strategies are used by the patient, it is almost always necessary to focus on how to incorporate these into the patient's daily living. Two recurring themes in helping patients accomplish this are pacing and looking at the total day. The patient/family teaching tools on pp. 247-248 address these issues. They may be duplicated and given to the patient/family.

REFERRAL TO A PAIN MANAGEMENT PROGRAM

Pain management programs are extremely varied. Presently there is no comprehensive listing of all such programs nor is there a group or agency empowered to license or accredit all pain programs. Therefore determining the need for a pain program and then selecting the appropriate one is a complicated matter. General information about pain programs can be obtained from the American Pain Society (p. 5) and CARF (p. 257), from whom pain programs may voluntarily request certification.

Types of Pain Management Programs

One way of distinguishing between the various pain management programs is to ask the following four questions.

1. What types of pain are treated? Some pain programs treat only certain types of pain or are open to only certain types of patients. A program may offer assistance only to patients with cancer, headache, neck and spine problems, or arthritis.

2. How are services offered? Some pain programs offer services on an individual level, possibly with some group involvement, e.g., group therapy. Others have a rather structured program in which the patient is treated in a group of patients and receives some individual attention.

Programs may be on an inpatient or outpatient basis. Pain *clinic* usually refers to outpatient facilities only; pain *center,* to both inpatient and outpatient. Many outpatient programs and most inpatient (hospital based) programs are structured for groups of patients. Structured programs tend to involve specific blocks of time, e.g., 2 to 6 weeks, during which the patient, and usually his family, is intensively involved in the program.

3. Which services are offered? Some programs offer only a few treatment approaches, while others offer a wide variety of treatment strategies.

The *restricted* ones are sometimes referred to as modality oriented and may offer mainly biofeedback for relaxation or stress reduction, TENS, acupuncture, or nerve blocks.

The more *comprehensive* programs are also referred to as multidisciplinary or interdisciplinary and should offer most of the following, either on a regular and continuing basis or through affiliation or consultation arrangements:

• Thorough assessment to determine the need for further medical or surgical intervention. If additional treatment

Text continued on p. 256.

Important Information About a Pain Management Program

Name of pain program: _____ Telephone: _____

Address: _____

General information:
Name of person giving initial information about the program (e.g., the person on the telephone):

_____ Date _____

Director of program: _____

Other staff members met or talked with: _____

Specific questions:
1. What types of pain problems are treated? (Describe the pain problem and ask if it is treated here; if not, do they have a recommendation?)

2. How are services offered? (e.g., individual appointments, in groups, inpatient, outpatient, structured, specific period of time such as a 2-week program)

3. Which services are offered? For convenience, the following may be used as a checklist (probably not all will be included, and some may not be desired):
   - _____ Thorough initial assessment to determine need for further medical or surgical approaches.
   - _____ Team of health professionals, i.e., more than one person (e.g., physician, physical therapist, nurses).
   - _____ Medication adjustments, detoxification. (If so, which drugs? _____)
   - _____ Physical therapy. (How often? _____ Hours per day _____ Pool? _____ Written exercise program? _____)
   - _____ TENS (transcutaneous electrical nerve stimulation).
   - _____ Acupressure.
   - _____ Acupuncture.
   - _____ Relaxation. (Biofeedback? _____)
   - _____ Individual psychotherapy or counseling.
   - _____ Family group therapy or counseling. (When? _____)
   - _____ Assertiveness training.
   - _____ Recreational therapy. (Types: _____)
   - _____ Occupational therapy. (Types: _____)
   - _____ Vocational counseling. (Training? _____)
   - _____ Self-hypnosis.
   - _____ Imagery.
   - _____ Nutritional counseling. (Weight loss required? _____)
   - _____ Expressive therapies (e.g., art, dance, music).
   - _____ Follow-up after completion of program. (By whom? _____ How often? _____ Alumni group? _____)
   - _____ Mechanisms for working with those involved or affected by participation in the program (e.g., present physician, employer, worker's compensation case worker).
   Other:

Continued.

Important Information About a Pain Management Program—cont'd.

4. What are the goals or benefits for the patient who completes the program? (e.g., Are the goals the same for every patient? Are the goals established by the program or by the individual patient? Is detoxification required?)

5. Exactly what is expected of persons who participate in the program? (e.g., participation in certain activities or all activities, hospitalization, weekly appointments, no smoking, special diet)

6. Exactly what is expected of the patient's family? (e.g., accompany patient on the initial visit, weekly therapy)

7. What are other sources of information about the program?
   _____ Brochures, videotapes.
   _____ Names and telephone numbers of "graduates" of the program who may be contacted:

   _____ Journals or magazines with articles about the program or articles written by health team members who staff the program:

8. How long has the program been in operation? Especially if the program is new, ask what other programs the director and staff have been associated with.

9. By what agencies has the pain program been certified or accredited? (e.g., CARF—Commission on Accreditation of Rehabilitation Facilities)

10. How much does the program cost? Are there incidental expenses? Does insurance or Medicare pay for any of this? If so, is there anyone connected with the program who can help investigate third-party payment?

11. What is the earliest date open for an initial appointment? If this is a structured group program, what is the earliest date the person could expect to be admitted?

Comments and impressions:

■ May be duplicated for use in clinical practice. From McCaffery, M, and Beebe, A: PAIN: CLINICAL MANUAL FOR NURSING PRACTICE, St. Louis, 1989, The CV Mosby Company.

INDIVIDUALIZED NURSING CARE PLAN

Patient with Chronic Nonmalignant Pain

Patient Description: Ms. G., 35 years old, has had neck and shoulder pain often accompanied by headaches for 5 years, initially caused by lifting heavy objects at work and later precipitated by simple, daily tasks involving use of the arms. She is divorced and has three children living with her, ages 7, 9, and 12 years. None of her family live near her but she mentions several friends and she attends church one or more times each week. She is presently employed as a salesperson in a department store, but she misses an average of 4 days a month due to pain. She cries easily and says that she is unable to do all that is expected of her and that her frequent absences from work occur when she does too much. Her history includes regular emergency room visits (about twice a month) for narcotic injections, numerous medical consultations including neurology, completion 3 years ago of a structured inpatient pain management program in another city, a variety of analgesic prescriptions, and several physical therapy referrals that included an unsuccessful trial of TENS. Now she has been referred to an outpatient orthopedic facility for ongoing care. Her present prescriptions include Tylenol #3 (codeine 30 mg and acetaminophen 300 mg) for pain and diazepam (Valium) 10 mg for nervousness and sleep. She reports taking diazepam once during the day, usually in the morning, and two at night (30 mg/day) and Tylenol #3 only on days when she really hurts, approximately five a day at times.

Assessment	Potential Nursing Diagnoses	Planning/Intervention	Evaluation/ Expected Outcomes
Identify: • Satisfaction with explanations given for cause of pain. • Location and intensity of present pain, using a scale of 0-10 (0 = no pain, 10 = worst pain). • Increases or changes in pain. • What has and has not been effective in relieving pain, using a modification of the form "Planning for the Future," p. 246). • Degree of sleep disturbance. • Coping style. • Regular daily activities in relation to pain and methods of pain relief, especially analgesic consumption, requesting the patient to complete the daily diary (p. 30) for 2 weeks. • Support systems. • Use of nontraditional medical care. • All current recommendations from others regarding pain management, e.g., exercises suggested by physical therapy.	Pain, chronic, related to myofascial problems in the neck and shoulders. Ineffective individual coping related to mostly dependent and passive approaches to pain control. Knowledge deficit related to methods of formulating a comprehensive plan for daily management of chronic pain.	(The following would be attempted over a period of several months in approximately the sequence listed.) Express belief in what she says about her pain and respect for the frustration of dealing with daily pain. Obtain a prescription for the strongest nonnarcotic she can take without side effects, and instruct her in regular daily dosing (use Patient/Family Teaching Point for NSAIDS, p. 65) to relieve ongoing pain and prevent increased pain. Use whichever method of cutaneous stimulation has been most effective in the past, encouraging regular use for ongoing pain as well as use as soon as pain begins to increase. Encourage cold if it has not been tried. For episodes of increased pain, suggest the following: • Take Tylenol #3 as soon as pain begins to increase rather than waiting until pain is severe, and take it every 4 hours until pain begins to subside. • Continue regular doses of nonnarcotic. • Use cutaneous stimulation. • Contact nurse (yourself) by phone (use of nurse as support system). • Ask a friend to take care of her children for a while (use of friends as support system). Further increase her support systems by encouraging her involvement with church activities and suggesting she talk with her clergyman about calling him when her pain becomes distressing.	Returns for each clinic appointment with partially completed daily diaries. Expresses increased confidence in managing pain by using prayer, relying on friends, calling the nurse, and planning her total day. After a few days on regular doses of nonnarcotic, reports decrease in daily pain level from 5 to 3 on a scale of 0 to 10. Decrease in days absent from work. Reports improved sleep from antidepressant. Gradual decrease in daily dose of diazepam. When pain increases, calls nurse or clergyman, takes Tylenol #3 on a regular basis, asks a friend to help with responsibilities, and does not go to the emergency room.

Continued.

INDIVIDUALIZED NURSING CARE PLAN—cont'd.

Patient with Chronic Nonmalignant Pain—cont'd.

Assessment	Potential Nursing Diagnoses	Planning/Intervention	Evaluation/ Expected Outcomes
• Need for a consult to treat depression, anxiety, or post-traumatic stress disorder. • Suicidal risk.		Help prevent catastrophizing by incorporating her frequent use of prayer as a relaxation strategy, encouraging her to pray regularly for about 5 minutes at least two or three times a day, especially at bedtime and when she becomes agitated or fearful of increasing pain. Introduce pacing by encouraging her to give priority to safe care of her children and going to work, spending less energy on housekeeping chores and delegating some to her children (use form "Pace Yourself," p. 247). For sleep disturbance, suggest use of an antidepressant and a gradual decrease in diazepam. Avoid sudden withdrawal of diazepam. Suggest decreasing the total daily dose by 2½ mg every 3 weeks. Provide a written copy of all recommendations for pain management made by all health team members. Review this to establish feasibility of accomplishing all of it. Formulate a reasonable daily plan, incorporating recommendations of health team plus instructions on form "Overall Daily Plan," p. 248. Evaluate all recommendations using the "Daily Diary," or telephone calls if necessary, and establish regular clinic appointments, perhaps every 3 weeks.	

for the cause of chronic nonmalignant pain is indicated, the patient may be referred elsewhere.

(NOTE: Usually patients with chronic nonmalignant pain are not admitted to any type of structured pain program until it is clear that the pain will persist but no additional medical or surgical intervention is indicated.)

- Team of health professionals who specialize in pain management, including physician, psychiatrist, psychologist, nurses, and others who are involved in specific treatment approaches listed below, e.g., physical therapists and specialty consultations.
- Physical therapy, e.g., stretching, strengthening, pool.
- TENS.
- Medication counseling or adjustment, possibly detoxification from narcotics/sedatives and use of newer adjuvant analgesics, e.g., antidepressants.
- Relaxation, possibly with biofeedback.
- Individual psychotherapy or counseling.
- Family group therapy and counseling.
- Assertiveness training.
- Recreational therapy.
- Occupational therapy.
- Vocational counseling, training.
- Social services.
- Self-hypnosis, imagery.
- Nutritional counseling.
- Expressive therapies, e.g., dance, music, art.
- Regular follow-up after completion of the program, e.g., visits to the physical therapist, program director, or psychologist, perhaps participation in alumni activities.
- Mechanisms for working with present physician, employer, or others (especially family) relevant to involvement in and progress after the program.

4. What are the goals of the pain management program? Sometimes the outcomes are explicitly stated by the program. Other programs may request that the patient set specific goals. Still others may use a combination of these approaches. For the patient with chronic nonmalignant pain, *examples* of outcomes, hopefully long-term, that may be expected as a result of participating in a pain management program are (not all are expected in every program or of every patient):

- Ability to keep pain intensity at a bearable level (elimination of pain is not expected), e.g., through pacing, use of TENS.
- Overall increased independence in activities of daily living.
- Decreased depression or increased sense of well-being.
- Increased daily physical activity, e.g., endurance, strength.
- Increased involvement with family/social activities.
- Decreased use of health care system, e.g., fewer visits to physicians, no further diagnostic testing or surgical procedures.

- Decreased intake of or elimination of narcotic/sedative medications.
- Return to work.

Selection of a Pain Management Program

Factors to consider in selecting a pain management program are numerous. Obtain as much information about the program as possible before an actual appointment or commitment is made. Ideally the patient and his family would collect information about two or more programs (for comparison purposes) in the following ways:

- Write or telephone for written information, including cost and insurance coverage (some programs are very expensive), types of patients served, types of services offered, and goals patients may accomplish as a result of participating in the program.
- Attend any public lectures or orientation sessions provided by the program.
- Visit the facility to ask questions and meet the staff, especially the director.
- Ask for names of "graduates" of the program who are willing to discuss their experiences and for citations of any lay or professional articles concerning the program or published by staff working with the program.
- Find out what types of certification or accreditation the program has, how long the program has existed, and how long most of the staff has been involved with the program.

Obviously, not all patients are capable of this effort. Some patients are not assertive or self-directed enough to pursue information; others have become almost completely disabled by the pain and are confined to bed. The more disabled the patient is by the pain the more likely he is to need a structured, comprehensive pain management program, but the less likely he is to be able to identify one that suits his particular needs. With any patient suffering chronic nonmalignant pain, it is quite possible that the patient will not know exactly what he needs or what possibilities exist for assistance.

Thus the patient often needs the guidance of the health team and family in selecting an appropriate program. Cost, convenience of location, disruption of normal life, and other factors must be weighed against the potential benefits of the particular program. Further, it is imperative that the patient understand as fully as possible what is expected of him in the program and what the goals of the program are before he commits to the program. The form "Important Information About a Pain Management Program," pp. 252-253, may be duplicated and used as a guide by the patient, family, or nurse for finding out about pain management programs.

A specialized program in pain management is not necessary for every person with chronic nonmalignant pain. However, when pain becomes the central feature of a person's life, some type of special help is indicated. Effective treatment and management may be offered by a concerned and knowledgeable health care professional. Often the primary care physician is able to do this in conjunction with appropriate consultations and referrals. Under the guidance of such a physician, use of a less comprehensive pain program may be very helpful.

Whatever is selected, the patient should always be cautioned not to expect a miracle or a magic answer. Remind the patient that his chronic pain has existed for a very long time and that it may well take a long time to arrive at a satisfactory approach to managing it.

RESOURCES FOR PATIENTS/NURSES

American Chronic Pain Association. This is a self-help organization for people with chronic pain. It is open to all persons with chronic pain, and each group is led by a person with chronic pain. Chapters are being formed in different parts of the country. They provide individual and group support along with information such as a manual to help people with chronic pain and guidelines for what to look for in a pain clinic. Write: 257 Old Haymaker Rd, Monroeville, PA 15146-1711; phone: 412-856-9676.

Ankylosing Spondylitis Association. This volunteer organization provides support and information; regional chapters are being formed. Membership (about $15/year) includes their newsletter. Write: 511 N La Cienega, Suite 216, Los Angeles, CA 90048; phone: 231-652-0609.

Arthritis Foundation. Provides a variety of information. Write: 1314 Spring St NW, Atlanta, GA 30309; phone: 404-872-1700.

Barja, RH, and Sherman, RA: What to expect when you lose a limb. A 55-page booklet available for $1.75 by writing: US Government Superintendent of Documents Office, Washington, DC 20402.

CARF (Commission on Accreditation of Rehabilitation Facilities). They provide various types of information, including a list of facilities that have chronic pain management programs and a booklet titled "Program Evaluation in Chronic Pain Management Programs." Write: 2500 N Pantano Rd, Tucson, AZ 85715; phone: 602-886-8575.

Catalano, EM: The chronic pain control workbook: a step-by-step guide for coping with and overcoming your pain, 1987 (207 pages, paperback $12.50; hardcover, $22.50). This is written for the person with chronic pain and is a fairly comprehensive guide to understanding and coping with pain. Special sections cover specific types of pain such as headaches, irritable bowel syndrome, and temporomandibular joint disorders. The publisher also offers many other workbooks and tapes for the layman on problems of daily living such as stress and grief and specific approaches such as assertiveness that may be helpful for any person with chronic pain. Write: New Harbinger Publications, 5674 Shattuck Ave, Oakland, CA 94609; phone: 415-652-0215, or toll free 1-800-621-0851, ext 287 (credit card orders accepted).

Chronic Pain Letter. This bimonthly publication is an information source for people with chronic pain. To subscribe (about $20/year for laymen; $35/year for professionals), write: Box 1303 Old Chelsea Station, New York, NY 10011.

National Chronic Pain Outreach Assn, Inc. This is a nonprofit organization that serves as a clearinghouse for information on chronic pain for the layman and professional. Information resources include quarterly newsletter, cassette tapes, and many publications. Membership: $25 a year for patients, $50 a year for professionals. Write: 4922 Hampden Lane, Bethesda, MD 20814; phone: 301-652-4948.

National Directory of Pain Treatment Centers. In April 1988, The Oryx Press reported that they were in the process of compiling information for a comprehensive directory of chronic pain treatment centers throughout the United States and Canada. The purpose of the directory is to enable those that need specific types of pain treatment to find it and to help physicians and clinicians find the treatment centers which are appropriate for their patients. For information write: The Oryx Press, Suite 103, 2214 N Central at Encanto, Phoenix, AZ 85004; phone: 602-254-6156.

National Headache Foundation (formerly National Migraine Foundation). Membership (about $15/year) includes a quarterly newsletter with articles on current research findings and treatment techniques. Write: 5252 N Western Ave, Chicago, IL 60625. For a free copy of "52 Proven Stress Reducers" send a self-addressed, stamped envelope.

Nuprin Pain Report. This is data from the first national (USA) pain survey, conducted in August and September of 1985. It provides a comprehensive view of the nature and impact of acute, chronic, and recurrent pains in the adult population. It shows that pain problems have an enormous social and economic impact, justifying efforts to increase research and education of health professionals. For a free copy, write: The Nuprin Pain Report, PO Box 14093, Baltimore, MD 21203.

Pain Program Registry. This registry collects and compiles data submitted voluntarily by pain programs. The purpose of the registry is to facilitate effective communications and national delivery of clinical services. "The 1988 Pain Program Registry" appears in the Nov/Dec 1988 issue of *Pain Management*. For further information write: Pain Program Registry, Pain Management, Greenville General Hospital, 100 Mallard St, Greenville, SC 29601.

Pain Resources, Ltd. This company publishes several booklets written by Barbara J. Headley, M.S., P.T., Cbt., for people with chronic nonmalignant pain and their families. For information, write: Pain Resources, Ltd., 1940 S Greeley St, #202, Stillwater, MN 55082. Phone: 612-430-3892.

PMS (premenstrual syndrome) Access. This organization offers a number of resources, including symptom charts, diets, and education for professionals. Write: Madison Pharmacy Associates, Inc, 1603 Monroe St, Madison, WI 53711.

Plain Talk About Handling Stress, DHHS No (ADM) 85-502; Plain Talk About the Art of Relaxation, DHHS No (ADM) 85-632. For a free copy of these 2-page publications, write: Public Inquiries Branch, National Institute of Mental Health, Parklawn Bldg, Room 15C-05, 5600 Fishers Lane, Rockville, MD 20857.

RSDS (reflex sympathetic dystrophy syndrome) Association. This organization is open to laymen and professionals and offers support and information. Regional chapters are being formed. Write: PO Box 821, Haddonfield, NJ 08033.

SELECTED ANNOTATED REFERENCES THAT CITE RESEARCH OR GIVE CLINICAL SUPPORT

Since so much controversy exists about what chronic nonmalignant pain includes and how it should be treated, the content of this chapter reflects, to the extent possible, the conclusions of research studies rather than the sometimes divergent opinions expressed in the literature. Following are the references most pertinent to the approaches suggested in this chapter.

Ahles, TA, Yunus, MB, and Masi, AT: Is chronic pain a variant of depressive disease? The case of primary fibromyalgia syndrome, *Pain* 29:105-111, 1987. The responses of 45 patients with primary fibromyalgia (PFS), 29 with rheumatoid arthritis (RA), and 31 people with no pain showed no differences between the PFS and RA groups regarding depression, although the PFS group has no known organic pathology, unlike the RA group. The data do not support the hypothesis that chronic pain in the absence of a known organic problem is a variant of depressive disease.

Bouckoms, AJ, Litman, RE, and Baer, L: Denial in the depressive and pain-prone disorders of chronic pain, *Clin J Pain* 1: 165-169, 1985. In this study of 63 patients admitted to an inpatient center for treatment of chronic nonmalignant pain, depressive symptoms were present in 60%, but major depression in only 24%, a lower percentage than previously thought. Evidence strongly suggested developmental deficit in the childhood of 37% of these patients, but findings failed to support the diagnosis of pain-prone disorder as a masked depressive equivalent.

Busto, U, Sellers, EM, Naranjo, CA, Cappell, H, et al: Withdrawal reaction after long-term use of benzodiazepines, *N Engl J Med* 315:854-859, Oct 2, 1986. The 40 patients included in this study met the following criteria: 18 to 79 years of age; daily use of a benzodiazepine for at least 3 months, with a cumulative benzodiazepine exposure above 2700 mg of diazepam (or the equivalent); and either reported problems attributed to the use of a benzodiazepine or an inability to stop taking the drug because of symptoms that occurred during attempts at discontinuation. In a double-blind, placebo-controlled trial, patients were switched to placebo or to diazepam in a dose approximately equivalent to their usual dose and then tapered during an 8-week period. Patients who received placebo had more symptoms, assessed their symptoms as more severe, and stopped taking the study drug at a higher rate than those receiving the tapering doses of diazepam. Seven in the placebo group not only used additional doses of their prestudy benzodiazepine but also refused to continue in the study. Withdrawal symptoms gradually disappeared over a 4-week period in both the placebo and the diazepam groups. The withdrawal syndrome observed was not severe but was easily detectable and disturbing to patients. Symptoms consisted of twitching, tinnitus, paresthesias, vision disturbances, and depersonalization. The authors noted that although this group had no seizures, disorientation, or psychotic reactions, these symptoms have been observed after withdrawal from higher doses of benzodiazepines.

Crook, J, and Tunks, E: Defining the "chronic pain syndrome": an epidemiological method, *Clin J Pain* 1:159-163, 1985. This study suggests that people suffering persistent pain attending chronic pain clinics are not typical of people in the general population who suffer persistent pain but who are not referred to such clinics. Pain clinic patients are likely to be deficient in coping skills, have greater adaptive problems with work and social roles, and suffer greater emotional distress. The authors suggest that because the pain of pain clinic patients is more often related to work injuries and there is a greater probability of litigation or compensation, the adversarial relationships may be a significant factor.

Crue, BL, Jr: Multidisciplinary pain treatment programs: current status, *Clin J Pain* 1:31-38, 1985. In this review article the author addresses the practical problem of defining and classifying pain, suggesting that an acceptable pragmatic definition of pain is simply anything the patient says it is and that all pain is real (exclusive of the malingerer who consciously fakes pain). He explains the differences between the centralist and peripheralist concepts of chronic pain and the implications of this controversy. In brief, the peripheralist believes that chronic pain results from peripheral input; the centralist believes that the initial peripheral input no longer exists but has become some type of central "memory of pain" that now produces chronic pain. Both the peripheralist and centralist mechanisms of pain may exist and may occur together. He traces the evolution of pain treatment facilities and suggests what should be included in a comprehensive pain center.

Deyo, RA, and Diehl, AK: Patient satisfaction with medical care for low-back pain, *Spine* 11:28-30, Jan-Feb 1986. In a questionnaire survey of 140 patients seen in a walk-in clinic for mechanical low back pain (70% of less than 2 weeks duration), the most frequently cited source of dissatisfaction was failure to receive an adequate explanation of the problem. In comparison with patients who felt they received an adequate explanation, those who did not thought more diagnostic tests were needed, were less satisfied with their physicians, and were less likely to want to see the same physician again. Explanation of symptoms has a high priority among these patients, and the data suggest that giving this explanation does not take additional physician time and might reduce future utilization of the health care system. Patients not given an explanation seem inclined to see more physicians and request more testing.

Dworkin, RH, et al: Unraveling the effects of compensation, litigation, and employment in treatment response in chronic pain, *Pain* 23:49-59, 1985. The relationships among compensation, litigation, employment, and short- and long-term treatment response in a series of 454 chronic pain patients was examined. Only employment at the time of the initial evaluation significantly predicted long-term outcome, whereas compensation and litigation did not. A review of the literature confirmed that there are very few differences between patients who do and do not receive compensation and between patients who do and do not have litigation pending with respect to organic basis for pain and psychological distress. Litigation also does not influence pain behavior. Further, there is little support for the view that patients typically resume employment when litigation is settled (Mendelson, 1982). The authors suggested that attention be directed away from concern about "compensation neurosis" and directed toward returning the patient to appropriate employment as soon as possible. The article ends with a quote made in another article over 20 years ago, suggesting that returning injured workmen to a job within the limitations imposed by their pain might maintain morale and allow sufficient time for the problem to subside (White, 1966).

Feuerstein, M, Carter, RL, and Papciak, AS: A prospective analysis of stress and fatigue in recurrent low back pain, *Pain* **31**: 333-344, 1987. This study compared 33 ambulatory chronic low back pain patients with an asymptomatic control group. Both groups recorded mood states for 14 consecutive days. No mood state was predictive of pain onset, but fatigue was associated with pain 24 hours following onset. Overall the patients had a higher level of anxiety than the control group, but the results do not support the notion that negative mood states initiate or exacerbate pain.

Fischer, AA: Diagnosis and management of chronic pain in physical medicine and rehabilitation. In Ruskin, AP, ed: Current therapy in physiatry, pp 123-149, Philadelphia, 1984, WB Saunders Co. The author makes an interesting point about diagnosing the cause of pain. A diagnosis of "chest pain" is recognized as inadequate and requires identification of cause. No physician would seriously consider treating a patient with a diagnosis of chest pain without identifying the cause, e.g., lung infection, coronary occlusion. However, a large number of patients have a diagnosis of "low back pain" without identification of the cause. He notes that the origin of pain is crucial for treatment. Then he states an interesting opinion. On the basis of his personal experience of treating patients with pain for 10 years, he concludes that 80% of patients with chronic pain suffer from undiagnosed or improperly treated myofascial pain syndromes, which require triggerpoint injections and appropriate physical therapy.

Halpern, LM, and Robinson, J: Prescribing practices for pain in drug dependence: a lesson in ignorance, *Adv Alcohol Subst Abuse* **5**:135-161, Fall 1985/Winter 1986. Patients with the type of chronic nonmalignant pain syndrome usually referred to pain management programs often rely on opiates and sedative medications for long periods of time, sometimes at high doses. These medications are generally believed to contribute to the chronic pain problem, especially increased dysfunction. Most pain programs consider detoxification from sedatives and opiates a mandatory part of successful rehabilitation. In addition, the same negative biases directed toward street drug users seems to be expressed toward chronic pain patients who have been taking narcotics for months or years. However, a literature review reveals an amazing lack of research to support the widely held belief that medications contribute to dysfunction in patients with chronic pain.

Regarding prolonged use of narcotics, a review of the literature shows no serious medical complications resulting from months or years of daily narcotic use (exclusive of accidental overdose). The fear that prolonged use of narcotics will result in tolerance to analgesia, necessitating increasing doses, may be unfounded; if pathology remains stable, so may the narcotic dose. Detoxifying chronic pain patients from narcotics is usually done in 1 to 2 weeks with minimal, if any, symptoms of withdrawal. Compared to narcotic street addicts, detoxification is brief and successful, apparently with no indication of compulsive drug-seeking behavior later. Patients with chronic pain accompanied by prolonged use of narcotics are probably physiologically dependent but not psychologically dependent, i.e., not addicted. Clearly the prolonged use of narcotic/ sedative drugs in some patients will produce cognitive impairment, and detoxification will result in increased function, but no evidence exists that suggests this will be true for all or even the majority of patients.

The relationship between functional ability and analgesic intake is simply unknown. Narcotics can impair function but so can chronic pain. Therefore it is important to continue to ask if narcotic therapy can improve function in some patients with chronic nonmalignant pain.

Hendler, N: Depression caused by chronic pain, *J Clin Psychiatry* **45**:30-38, Mar 1984. The author believes that the psychogenic pain diagnosis is made far too freely, arising from the mistaken belief that chronic pain without organic disease is largely imaginary. He also notes that chronic pain almost always leads to depression and that this is normal. Four stages of pain are reviewed, from acute through the patient's acceptance of chronic pain. He notes that patients who exaggerate their pain are showing that they are devastated by their problem, not that they are imagining or faking pain. He feels outright fabrication of chronic pain is rare and that a patient's report about pain should not be challenged. He believes that the following are commonly missed causes of chronic pain: myofascial syndrome (or fibromyositis), sympathetic dystrophy, facet syndrome, and temporomandibular joint syndrome. He says there is evidence that sleep disorder contributes to myofascial syndrome.

Holzman, AD, and Gulliver, S: The relationship of a history of alcohol use disorder to treatment completion in chronic pain management, *Clin J Pain* **2**:115-118, 1986. An assessment of 104 patients referred to a pain management program did *not* show that patients with a history of alcohol use disorder were more likely to be current prescription medication users. However, these patients were less likely to complete the treatment program.

Kosten, TR, and Kleber, HD: Control of nociception by endogenous opioids, *Mediguide Pain* **3**:1-5, 1987. This recent review of the literature suggests that individual endorphin response to each pain exposure is substantially less for later exposures than it was for early exposures. Patients with ongoing chronic pain reportedly have decreased endorphin in the cerebrospinal fluid.

Krishnan, KRR, et al: Chronic pain and depression. I. Classification of depression in chronic low back pain patients, *Pain* **22**:279-287, 1985. An association between chronic pain and depression has been recognized for a long time. This study of 71 patients with chronic low back pain revealed 31 with major depression and 8 with minor depression. In most patients the depression developed after the onset of pain; however, 10 patients had major depression preceding the onset of pain. The data suggest that there is more than one type of depression involved with chronic pain.

Krishnan, KRR, et al: Chronic pain and depression. II. Symptoms of anxiety in chronic low back pain patients and their relationship to subtypes of depression, *Pain* **22**:289-294, 1985. This study of the same 71 patients with chronic low back pain (above) showed that anxious mood and other symptoms of anxiety are common, especially in patients with depression.

Leavitt, F, and Sweet, JJ: Characteristics and frequency of malingering among patients with low back pain, *Pain* **25**:357-364, 1986. A survey mailed to orthopedic surgeons and neurosurgeons in six geographic regions of the United States resulted in 105 responses. The purpose was to determine if a consensus of opinion underlies clinical judgment concerning malingering in the low back pain patient. (The purpose was not to identify the actual existence of malingering.) The majority of surgeons (60%) agreed that malingering was relatively infrequent, occurring in 5% or less of patients who present with low back pain. Data suggested that high estimators of malingering (20% or more of patients) place more importance on the patient receiving compensation or having seen an attorney. (Note that numerous studies in this annotated reference section do not support a high incidence of malingering related to compensation or litigation.) The symptoms defined as most important in determining malingering were related to exaggeration, such as overreaction during the examination or disablement disproportionate to objective findings, or incongruity, such as pain complaints not following organic patterns and weakness to manual testing not seen in other activities. These opinions, of course, need validation.

Linton, SJ: Behavioral remediation of chronic pain: a status report, *Pain* 24:125-141, 1986. A review of publications, especially those from 1982 and later, concerning the outcome of behavioral treatment of chronic nonmalignant pain showed that relaxation training was a particularly valuable tool in decreasing reported pain intensity. However, data did not support the need to use biofeedback with relaxation.

Melzack, R, Katz, J, and Jeans, ME: The role of compensation in chronic pain: analysis using a new method of scoring the McGill pain questionnaire, *Pain* 23:101-112, 1985. A study of 145 patients with chronic low back or musculoskeletal pain revealed that, contrary to popular opinion, compensation and noncompensation patients had virtually identical pain scores and pain descriptor patterns. In fact, the patients receiving compensation had significantly fewer visits to health professionals. Apparently receiving compensation decreases anxiety. Results for the two groups were also similar on the MMPI pain triad of depression, hysteria, and hypochondriasis.

Nathan, RG, et al: Alternative treatments for withdrawing the long-term benzodiazepine user: a pilot study, *Int J Addict* 21:195-211, 1986. A review of studies from 1976 to 1983 concerning benzodiazepine dependence and withdrawal reveals inconclusive results. However, it appears that at least some patients will become physically dependent on benzodiazepines, but withdrawal reactions usually are not life-threatening. A few other studies have reported occasional severe symptoms, e.g., seizures (Levy, 1984). Withdrawal of benzodiazepines probably should be gradual. Relaxation techniques and other forms of stress reduction may be helpful during withdrawal.

Peck, CJ, Fordyce, WE, and Black, RG: The effect of the pendency of claims for compensation upon behavior indicative of pain, *Washington Law Review* 53:251-278, 1978. From files in the state of Washington, the medical treatment of a group of 105 recently closed cases involving third-party tort claims was compared with a control group of 103 cases with similar injuries who received workmen's compensation awards but did not have third-party claims. Further, a group of claimants who were represented by lawyers in presenting their claims were compared with a group of claimants who lacked representation by a lawyer. Given the popularity of the belief that lawyers and litigation aggravate pain, it was surprising to find that for almost all types of behavior selected for analysis there was no significantly greater occurrence of pain behavior (e.g., days lost from work) in the group having third-party claims than in the group having only claims for workmen's compensation. In fact, contrary to expectation, the control group saw significantly more different physicians than did the persons with third-party claims. Narcotic use was greater in the control group during the first month but dropped off sharply for both groups by the sixth month. In the comparison of the lawyer and no-lawyer groups, the lawyer group saw a significantly greater number of physician specialists, but there was not a significant difference in the total number of physician contacts between the two groups. The lawyer group also used significantly more physical therapists, suggesting the fallacy of the belief that lawyers resist attempts to cure their clients. Further, the percentage of the lawyer group having no prescriptions for drugs was higher than the percentage of the no-lawyer group, suggesting that lawyers may even have an analgesic rather than aggravating effect upon pain. The authors suggest that physicians who have observed psychogenic or operantly conditioned pain in certain patients who have claims pending may have erroneously concluded that this was a significant factor in producing pain behavior.

Philips, HC: The effects of persistent pain: the chronic headache sufferer, *Pain* 21:163-176, 1985. In a survey of 360 patients with chronic headache, including migraine and tension, sleep disturbance was common, but depression was not found to be elevated.

Pilowsky, I, Crettenden, I, and Townley, M: Sleep disturbance in pain clinic patients, *Pain* 23:27-33, 1985. In a study of 100 outpatients with chronic pain, only 10 reported good sleep, while 70 reported poor sleep. Patients with poor sleep had significantly more affective disturbance, especially depression, than patients reporting good sleep, and also greater pain and physical disability. Sleep disturbance may provide an index to the severity of symptoms. Possibly treatment that is aimed specifically at alleviating sleep disturbances will in turn reduce emotional and physical symptoms.

Portenoy, RK, and Foley, K: Chronic use of opioid analgesics in non-malignant pain: report of 38 cases, *Pain* 25:171-186, 1986. Although the use of narcotic analgesics for relief of chronic nonmalignant pain is currently viewed with disfavor, this study shows that prolonged narcotic therapy can be a safe and more humane alternative to the options of surgery or no treatment if there is no history of drug abuse. Out of 38 patients maintained on narcotics (for 4 or more years in 19 patients), management became a problem in only 2 patients, both with a history of prior drug abuse. Patients occasionally required escalation of dose for exacerbation of pain, but doses usually returned to a stable baseline afterward. Acceptable or fully adequate relief of pain occurred in 24 patients; inadequate relief in 14. No patient underwent a surgical procedure while receiving narcotics, but there were few gains in employment or social function. Patients were on a variety of narcotics, e.g., oxycodone, propoxyphene, codeine, and for 23 patients the total daily dose was less than the equivalent of 20 mg morphine IM.

The authors suggest that opioid maintenance therapy be instituted only after other reasonable attempts at pain control have failed, have been documented in the patient's record, and pain continues to be a major impediment to improved function; that a single physician with committed involvement oversee the therapy, seeing the patient monthly and determining the monthly medication requirement; and that the patient gives fully informed consent, perhaps in writing, including discussion of the risks of using alcohol and other drugs along with opioids.

The authors review three other studies that reported similar success with prolonged use of opioids for chronic nonmalignant pain. Taub (1982) treated 313 such patients with narcotics for up to 6 years with problems in only 13 patients, all of whom had prior histories of substance abuse. Tennant and Uelman (1983) treated 22 patients who failed to benefit from pain clinics with the result that all reduced medical visits and two-thirds returned to work. France, Urban, and Keefe (1984) treated 16 patients with narcotics as a part of a comprehensive pain management program, resulting in improved function.

Reesor, KA, and Craig, KD: Medically incongruent chronic back pain: physical limitations, suffering, and ineffective coping, *Pain* 32:35-45, 1988. Forty chronic low back pain (CLBP) patients with pain and symptomatology incongruent with physical findings were compared with 40 CLBP patients without incongruent findings. Incongruent pain patients engaged in less effective coping styles, such as catastrophizing, feeling less control, and perceiving the pain as more disturbing and debilitating, than the other CLBP patients. Those with incongruent pain also had more restricted physical functioning. Pending litigation and compensation was not associated with incongruent pain, and there was no difference between the two groups regarding medication intake. The authors suggest that clinicians are more likely to *conclude incorrectly* that patients with incongruent pain symptomatology have minimal organic basis for pain and that they are malingering. This in turn may prompt the patient to display more exaggerated pain expression to convince the clinician of the reality of the pain. These results suggest, however, these patients most likely have problems with their coping styles and their confidence in their ability to cope with the pain.

Rowat, KM, and Knafl, KA: Living with chronic pain: the spouse's perspective, *Pain* 23:259-271, 1985. In this study of 40 spouses of patients with chronic nonmalignant pain, 83% of spouses reported experiencing some form of health disturbance attributed directly to the pain. The most frequently named source of difficulty for 40% of spouses was the sense of helplessness over how to help with their mate's pain. Uncertainty concerning management of the pain and daily family life were central to the spouses' distress. Enabling spouses to recognize what control they have over the pain and their daily lives seems an important feature of working with families where an adult has chronic nonmalignant pain.

Roy, R, and Thomas, MR: Elderly persons with and without pain: a comparative study, *Clin J Pain* 3:102-106, 1987. This study of 205 elderly subjects who were members of an organization devoted to providing social and recreational programs for the elderly revealed that nearly 70% reported a pain problem, but disability due to pain was virtually unknown. Firm conclusions are not possible but it appears that the lack of disability due to pain was related to an attitude of acceptance of limitations accompanying aging, a zest for living, well-planned days, and continued social integration with the community at large.

Sternbach, RA: Survey of pain in the United States: the Nuprin pain report, *Clin J Pain* 2:49-53, 1986. In the United States in August and September 1985, a nationwide telephone survey was made of 1254 persons aged 18 and older, representing a cross section of the adult population. An additional group of 165 "executive types" was included. The purpose of the survey was to provide data on several aspects of pain, such as the prevalence and severity of different kinds of pain and the impact of pain on work. The results showed that the most common complaint was headache (73%), followed by backache (56%), muscle pains (53%), joint pains (51%), and stomach pains (46%). Menstrual related pains were reported by 40% of women. Interestingly, the younger adults were more likely to report pains of every type than older persons, with the exception of joint pains. For all pains and all adults more than 4 billion workdays were lost in the past year, about 23 days per person. For full-time employees, days lost from work were only about 5 days per person. Yet approximately $55 billion in productivity was lost in the preceding year as a result of pain in full-time employees. If one adds disability incomes and other costs of chronic pain, the economic cost is staggering, not to mention the toll this takes on the quality of life.

Stucky, SJ, Jacobs, A, and Goldfarb, J: EMG biofeedback training, relaxation training, and placebo for the relief of chronic back pain, *Percept Mot Skills* 63:1023-1036, Dec 1986. Twenty-four patients with low back pain were randomly assigned to three groups: (1) EMG biofeedback, (2) relaxation training (varied, individualized techniques), and (3) placebo condition. Relaxation training was significantly superior to the other groups in several of its effects on chronic low back pain, including a decrease in pain during function tests. Practicing at home in between training sessions also produced better overall results than no practice. Interestingly, relaxation or the feeling of calmness is not necessarily directly related to the actual state of tension in the painful area.

Swanson, DW, Maruta, T, and Wolff, VA: Ancient pain, *Pain* 25:383-387, 1986. Of approximately 1000 patients evaluated for an inpatient pain program, 45 (about 4%) had pain for 25 years or more, called ancient pain. This group was compared with a group of subjects with a mean duration of pain of 6.6 years. Compared with those with pain of shorter duration, those with ancient pain used more analgesics and sedatives, with more women than men misusing drugs; had a higher incidence of face and head pain; had more frequent diagnoses of depression; and had a greater elevation of nearly all clinical MMPI scales. The importance of continuing careful medical evaluation was illustrated in one case-study of a 60-year-old man with a 40-year history of back pain who obtained limited benefit from the pain rehabilitation program. He returned 1.5 years later with no change in his complaints of pain but with a fever. Evaluation revealed renal cell carcinoma. This was treated, but the patient died of the malignancy about 1.5 years later.

Tennant, FS, Robinson, D, Sagherian, A, and Seecof, R: Chronic opioid treatment of intractable, nonmalignant pain, *Pain Manag* 18-26, Jan-Feb 1988. This is a report on a pilot program that accepted referral of 52 patients who had severe, nonmalignant pain, who were already dependent upon the daily administration of opioids for pain relief, and who had unsuccessfully attempted all other acceptable pain treatments. These patients were evaluated and treated between 1979 and 1986. Almost all patients had a history of numerous emergency room visits or repeated hospitalizations. The usual reason for referral was inadequate pain relief. Four techniques were used to control pain: raising the daily dose of the patient's usual opioid; changing to a longer-acting opioid, usually methadone or oxycodone (some patients, however, got better pain relief from a short-acting opioid); combining low doses of methadone, 10 to 40 mg per day, with a short-acting opioid such as codeine; or supplementing the patient's usual dose with morphine or hydromorphone suppositories. Interestingly, in a few patients who complained of inadequate pain relief on large doses of opioid, plasma concentrations were low, indicating inadequate absorption from the gastrointestinal tract. They obtained relief by taking another opioid. After systematic changes in opioid dosage were done using the four techniques described above, 46 of the 52 patients achieved adequate pain control according to the patient's self-report. Further, there was a marked reduction in hospitalizations and emergency room visits. The authors conclude that chronic administration of opioid is a relatively safe and effective treatment and should be made available as a last resort to this population of patients.

REFERENCES AND SELECTED READINGS

Ahern, DK, Adams, AE, and Follick, MJ: Emotional and marital disturbance in spouses of chronic low back pain patients, *Clin J Pain* 1:69-74, 1985

Anderson, EF, Hegstrum, JA, and Charboneau, GJ: Multidisciplinary management of patients with chronic low back pain, *Clin J Pain* 1:85-90, 1985

Aronoff, GM: Pain centers: a revolution in health care, New York, 1988, Raven Press

Auld, AW, Maki-Jokela, A, and Murdoch, DM: Intraspinal narcotic analgesia in the treatment of chronic pain, *Spine* 10:777-781, 1985

Brena, SF, and Chapman, SL, eds: Chronic pain: management principles, *Clin Anaesthesiol* 3:1-236. Philadelphia, WB Saunders, Jan 1985

Brena, SF, and Chapman, SL, eds: Management of patients with chronic pain, New York, 1983, SP Medical & Scientific Publications

Brown, GK, and Nicassio, PM: Development of a questionnaire for the assessment of active and passive coping strategies in chronic pain patients, *Pain* 31:53-64, 1987

Corey, DT, Etlin, D, and Miller, PC: A home-based pain management and rehabilitation program: an evaluation, *Pain* 29:219-229, 1987

Coulehan, JL: Adjustment, the hands and healing, *Cult Med Psychiatry* 9:353-382, Dec 1985

Crue, BL, Jr, ed: Chronic pain: further observations from City of Hope National Medical Center, New York, 1979, SP Medical & Scientific Books

Duckro, PN, Margolis, RB, Tait, RC, and Korytnyk, N: Long-term follow-up of chronic pain patients: a preliminary study, *Int J Psychiatry Med* 15:283-292, 1985-86

Dworkin, RH, Richlin, DM, Handlin, DS, and Brand, L: Predicting treatment response in depressed and non-depressed chronic pain patients, *Pain* 24:343-353, 1986

Edwards, PW, Zeichner, A, Kuczmierczyk, AR, and Boczkowski, J: Familial pain models: the relationship between family history of pain and current pain experience, *Pain* 21:379-384, 1985

Feinmann, C: Pain relief by antidepressants: possible modes of action, *Pain* 23:1-8, 1985

France, RD: Chronic pain and depression, *J Pain Sympt Manag* 2:234-235, Fall 1987

France, RD, Urban, BJ, and Keefe, FJ: Long-term use of narcotic analgesics in chronic pain, *Soc Sci Med* 19:1379-1382, 1984

Guck, TP, Skultety, FM, Meilman, PW, and Dowd, ET: Multidisciplinary pain center follow-up study: evaluation with a no-treatment control group, *Pain* 21:295-306, 1985

Haley, WE, Turner, JA, and Romano, JM: Depression in chronic pain patients: relation to pain, activity, and sex differences, *Pain* 23:337-343, 1985

Holzman, AD, and Turk, DC, eds: Pain management: a handbook of psychological treatment approaches, New York, 1986, Pergamon Press

Jensen, J: Life events in neurological patients with headache and low back pain (in relation to diagnosis and persistence of pain), *Pain* 32:47-53, 1988

Karen, H: Rehabilitation research review, rehabilitation of persons with chronic low back pain, Washington, DC, 1986, ATA Institute

Kotarba, JA: Chronic pain: its social dimensions, Beverly Hills, Calif, 1983, Sage Publications

Levy, AB: Delirium and seizures due to abrupt alprazolam withdrawal: case report, *Clin Psychiatry* 45:38-39, Jan 1984

Low back pain: what about chiropractors? *Harvard Med School Health Letter* 13:1-4, Jan 1988

Mendelson, G: Chronic pain and compensation: a review, *J Pain Sympt Manag* 1:135-144, Summer 1986

Mendelson, G: Not "cured by a verdict": effect of legal settlement on compensation claimants, *Med J Aust* 2:132-134, 1982

Merskey, H: Classification of chronic pain: descriptions of chronic pain syndromes and definitions of pain terms, *Pain* (suppl 3):S1-S225, 1986

Merskey, H, et al: Psychological normality and abnormality in persistent headache patients, *Pain* 23:35-47, 1985

Miro, J, Garcia-Monco, C, Leno, C, and Berciano, J: Pelvic pain: an undescribed paroxysmal manifestation of multiple sclerosis, *Pain* 32:73-75, 1988

Muse, M: Nonadversarial pain management, *Clin J Pain* 3:61, 1987

Muse, M: Stress-related, posttraumatic chronic pain syndrome: behavioral treatment approach, *Pain* 25:389-394, 1986

Muse, M: Stress-related, posttraumatic chronic pain syndrome: criteria for diagnosis, preliminary report on prevalence, *Pain* 23:295-300, 1985

Parris, WCV, Jamison, RN, and Vasterling, JJ: Follow-up study of a multidisciplinary pain center, *J Pain Sympt Manag* 2:145-151, Summer 1987

Perlman, SL: Modern techniques of pain management, *West J Med* 148:54-61, Jan 1988

Portenoy, RK: Postherpetic neuralgia: a workable treatment plan, *Geriatrics* 41:34-48, Nov 1986

Russel, ML: Behavioral counseling in medicine: strategies for modifying at risk behavior, London, 1986, Oxford University Press

Sammons, EE: Drug use and misuse in chronic pain patients, *Clin Anaesthesiol* 3:169-181, Jan 1985

Stanton-Hicks, M, and Boas, RA, eds: Chronic low back pain, New York, 1982, Raven Press

Stimmel, GL, and Escobar, JI: Antidepressants in chronic pain: a review of efficacy, *Psychopharmacol Bull* 22:865-869, 1986

Swerdlow, M: Anticonvulsant drugs and chronic pain, *Clin Neuropharmacol* 7:51-82, 1984

Taub, A: Opioid analgesics in the treatment of chronic intractable pain of non-neoplastic origin. In Kitahata, LM, and Collins, D, eds: Narcotic analgesics in anesthesiology, pp 199-208, Baltimore, 1982, Williams and Wilkins

Taylor, AG, Skelton, JA, and Butcher, J: Duration of pain condition and physical pathology as determinants of nurses' assessments of patients in pain, *Nurs Res* 33:4-8, Jan-Feb 1984

Tearnan, BH, and Dar, R: Physician ratings of pain descriptors: potential diagnostic utility, *Pain* 26:45-61, 1986

Tennant, FS, and Uelman, GF: Narcotic maintenance for chronic pain: medical and legal guidelines, *Postgrad Med* 73:81-94, 1983

Turk, DC, Rudy, TE, and Stieg, RL: Chronic pain and depression. I. "Facts," *Pain Manag* 1:17-25, Nov-Dec 1987

Turk, DC, and Stieg, RL: Chronic pain: the necessity of interdisciplinary communication, *Clin J Pain* 3:163-167, 1987

Turner, JA, and Clancy, S: Strategies for coping with chronic low back pain: relationship to pain and disability, *Pain* 24:355-364, 1986

Urban, BJ, et al: Long-term use of narcotic/antidepressant medication in the management of phantom limb pain, *Pain* 24:191-196, 1986

Wall, PD, and Melzack, R, eds: Textbook of pain, New York, 1984, Churchill Livingstone

Ward, NG: Tricyclic antidepressants for chronic low-back pain: mechanisms of action and predictors of response, *Spine* 11:661-665, Sept 1986

Ward, N, et al: Antidepressants in concomitant chronic back pain and depression: doxepin and desipramine compared, *J Clin Psychiatry* 45:54-57, Mar 1984

Whipple, B, and Komisaruk, BR: Elevation of pain threshold by vaginal stimulation in women, *Pain* 21:357-367, 1985

White, AWM: Low back pain in men receiving workmen's compensation, *Can Med Assoc J* 95:50-56, 1966

Pain in Children

Special Considerations

The younger the child, the more defenseless he is against pain. Yet it seems that the younger the child is, the less adequately is pain controlled. Problems of under-treatment of pain that adults encounter are even more extensive with children. For example, the first operating hospice for care of terminally ill patients in the United States was established in 1974 (such hospices were established much earlier in some countries such as England), but a survey conducted by Children's Hospice International in 1984 revealed that less than 10% of 1400 hospice programs provided services to children (Martin, 1985). Incredibly some health professionals still debate issues such as whether or not the young child (especially the newborn) hurts at all, and if he does, whether or not it matters.

Certainly not all children in pain receive inadequate relief. However, inadequate or inconsistent pain relief for children appears to be widespread.

The causes of inadequate pain relief in the young may more likely be due to lack of knowledge than to lack of concern. Fortunately, in the last few years interest in pain control in children has increased significantly. A search of the literature published between January 1970 and August 1975 produced a total of only 1380 articles on pain, and a meager 33 dealt with pain in children (Eland and Anderson, 1977). A quick glance at the reference section of this chapter shows we have come a long way since then. Further, by the late 1980s two books devoted entirely to

pain in children were published: *Pain in Children and Adolescents* by McGrath and Unruh (1987) and *Childhood Pain* by Ross and Ross (1988).

However, we are still far from a satisfactory approach to assessing and relieving pain in children. In an early study of pain in children one school-age child completed the sentence "Pain is . . ." like this: "When you scream for help and nobody comes" (Schultz, 1971, p. 672). To this child we may now say that we are coming, too slowly perhaps, but we are on our way.

This chapter provides basic information and practical approaches to assessing and relieving pain in children. Specifically, the *purposes of this chapter* are:
- To apply previously discussed methods of assessment and pain relief to children from birth through adolescence.
- To add selected age-related considerations (see Table 10-1 for age-related terminology).
- To encourage the reader to explore beyond this chapter to obtain additional knowledge and to develop greater skills in caring for children with pain.

Thus throughout this chapter the reader will be referred to previous chapters and will also be introduced to new material. The level of material presented assumes that the reader has basic knowledge about growth and development of children and about the care of children during health and illness.

However, this chapter is neither a complete nor a thorough guide to pain in children. Not only is pediatrics itself a specialty area but also there are many subspecialties within pediatrics. The *limitations of this chapter* are:
- Specialties within pediatrics are addressed only briefly and some not at all. Separate discussions of the various specialty areas such as those related to age groups (e.g.,

■ The authors would like to thank Joann M. Eland, PhD, RN, Associate Professor of Nursing, The University of Iowa, Iowa City, Iowa, and Donna L. Wong, MN, RN, PNP, Nurse Counselor in Private Practice, Tulsa, Okla, for their review of this chapter and for their many helpful comments and suggestions.

TABLE 10-1 Guide to Definitions of Age Groups*

Age Group Terminology	Approximate Age
Premature neonate or preterm infant	Gestational age equal to or less than 37 weeks
Neonate (full term) or newborn	Gestational age approximately 38 weeks
	Postnatal age less than 1 month
Infant	1 to 12 months
Toddler	1 to 3 years
Preschooler	3 to 5 or 6 years
School age	6 to 10 or 12 years
Adolescent	12 or 13 to 18 years

*Terminology for the different age groups in the very young is not yet standardized and is probably one of the reasons for inconsistent research findings regarding assessment and relief of pain in the very young.

neonatology), and those related to specific diagnostic entities (e.g., colic, cancer, headache, or abdominal pain), are beyond the scope of this chapter.

• This chapter is an introduction to some of the many possible ways of helping children with pain and their parents. Due to space limitations, many methods of assessment and relief that are included in this chapter are not discussed in detail.

References at the end of the chapter will guide the reader in pursuit of additional information and more depth in various specialty areas. Further, considerable research is in progress, and the reader is reminded to refer to the current professional literature for the most recent advances in the care of children with pain.

MISCONCEPTIONS

Pain in children tends to be doubted more often and to a greater degree than pain is doubted in adults. Children with pain are not only subjected to the many misconceptions that exist about pain in the adult patient but also encounter misconceptions specific to their young age. Pain in preverbal children seems especially likely to be questioned. But even when the child is verbally fluent, adults unfortunately tend to behave as if children are less credible or less accurate when they report pain.

An article published in 1968 (Swafford and Allan) illustrates the confusion that seems to have existed for some years about pain in children. These inconsistent statements appeared within the same article: "As long as the onset of remembrance of pain is unknown, the neonatal infant has the same right to analgesia and anesthesia as older patients" (p. 132). Yet the authors also state "Pediatric patients seldom need medication for relief of pain after general surgery" (p. 133) and "Infants and children below the age of 10 years rarely require narcotics" (p. 135).

In an attempt to clarify confusion about pain and its treatment in children, some of the more common misconceptions are presented below. Each misconception is accompanied by information that corrects it.

Misconception: Young children, particularly neonates, do not feel pain.

Correction: There is more evidence to support the belief that neonates, including premature infants, feel pain than there is evidence that they do not. In any debate of this point, the burden of proof now rests with those who believe the neonate or young child feels no pain. Further, there is some evidence that younger children are more sensitive to pain than older children.

Although it is simply not yet known whether children experience more, less, or the same pain as adults, it is far from a proven fact that pain in infants and children is absent or even less than that of adults. Many years ago it was thought that the infant did not feel pain because of an immature nervous system in which the nerves were not completely myelinated. However, it is now known that myelination progresses rapidly after birth and in any case is not necessary for pain transmission.

Several recent studies clearly document that newborns and infants respond with dramatic physiological and observable behavioral changes to stimuli that adults would feel as painful, such as heel lance, immunization, and circumcision and other surgical procedures.* Pain during circumcision without anesthesia is so well established and widely recognized that circumcision has become a model for analysis of pain and stress responses in the newborn. Further, a recent article in *The New England Journal of Medicine* (Anand and Hickey, 1987) listed 201 references pertaining to pain in the human neonate. There is little doubt that neonates and infants feel pain, or, more specifically, react to noxious stimuli with distress indicative of pain.

Several preliminary studies of children's reports of pain have suggested that there is increased pain with decreased age, i.e., given comparable stimuli, younger children may perceive a greater intensity of pain than older children (e.g., Fowler-Kerry and Lander, 1987; Haslam, 1969; Katz et al, 1982). Further, in a study of analgesic requirements of terminally ill children, those age 1 to 4 years required higher doses of PO narcotics than those 5 to 14 years old (Burne and Hunt, 1987). Infants and toddlers also seem to require higher doses of IV fentanyl for procedural pain than do older children (Billmire, Neale, and Gregory, 1985; Maunuksela, Rajantie, and Silmes, 1986).

Whenever pain in infants and young children is questioned by the health team, the above articles may be cited along with the following examples of *statements made by*

*Bell and Ellis, 1987; Craig, McMahon, Morison, and Zaskow, 1984; Dale, 1986; Franck, 1986; Izard, Hembree, Dougherty, and Coss, 1983; Owens and Todt, 1984; Stang et al, 1988; Williamson and Williamson, 1983.

professional organizations regarding pain and its control in the child:

- In a joint statement from the American Academy of Pediatrics, the chairmen of the Committee on Fetus and Newborn, Committee on Drugs, Section on Anesthesiology, and Section on Surgery state, "There is an increasing body of evidence that neonates, including those born preterm, demonstrate physiologic responses to surgical procedures that are similar to those demonstrated by adults and that these responses can be lessened by anesthetic agents. . . . (We) believe that local or systemic pharmacologic agents now available permit relatively safe administration of anesthesia or analgesia to neonates undergoing surgical procedures and that such administration is indicated according to the usual guidelines for administration of anesthesia to high-risk, potentially unstable patients . . . the decision to withhold such medication should be based on the same medical criteria used for older patients" (Poland, Roberts, Gutierrez-Mazorra, and Fonkalsrud, 1987, p. 446).
- In a joint statement, presidents of both the International Pain Foundation and the International Association for the Study of Pain state, "We are appalled by the needless pain that plagues the people of the world. . . . We are appalled, too, by the fact that pain is most poorly managed in those most defenseless against it—the young and the elderly. Children often receive little or no treatment, even for extremely severe pain, because of the myth that they are less sensitive to pain than adults and more easily addicted to pain medication" (Liebeskind and Melzack, 1987, p. 66).
- In the publication of the proceedings of the 8th World Congress of Anaesthesiologists, Steward (1984) states, "The extent of pain perception of the preterm infant is unknown, but it is generally accepted that pain can be felt, and therefore, that anesthesia is indicated during surgical procedures" (p. 189).

Misconception: If a child can communicate well verbally, his denial of pain should be regarded as true.

Correction: Certain fears will cause children to conceal the fact that they have pain. Also, children with prolonged or gradually increasing pain may not be able to identify that pain is what they are experiencing.

Children may deliberately and effectively disguise or deny their pain, since admitting to pain may result in various frightening possibilities. Many children are extremely fearful of injections. If the child learns that a report of pain results in "the needle," he may decide he would rather endure the ongoing pain than be subjected to this method of providing pain relief. Also, many children do not comprehend the logic underlying the administration of a painful injection in the buttocks to obtain relief in the abdomen 30 minutes later. Further, the child may believe if he says he has no pain, he can go home from the hospital sooner or avoid some painful procedure.

Sometimes the issue is not denial of pain but rather an inability to recognize pain, particularly chronic pain. As time goes on, the child seems to lose his basis of comparison and forgets what it was like not to have pain. Even short-term pain that has a gradual onset may be difficult for the child to identify. Pain that suddenly occurs or increases usually evokes an immediate response from even the neonate, but when pain sneaks up, the child's awareness and response may be minimal or less dramatic. Awareness of the underlying pathology, e.g., what a tumor may be compressing, and trial doses of analgesic accompanied by careful observations of the effect are important ways to uncover this type of pain. (See discussion of denial of pain and refusal of analgesics in Chapter 2, pp. 17-19.)

Patient Example

A 13-year-old with far advanced Ewing's sarcoma repeatedly denied pain. However, he was silent and withdrawn and his pathology strongly suggested that pain was present. Therefore trial doses of analgesics were administered regularly, and 36 hours later the child's behavior had changed into that of an outgoing teenager. When he was questioned about why he had not admitted that he hurt, he replied, "I think I had been hurting for so long that I forgot what it was like not to hurt" (Eland, 1985b, p. 109).

Misconception: If the child neither reports pain nor requests pain relief, he is not in pain.

Correction: Children do not necessarily know that they must report pain or ask for pain relief. Once they have done so, they may not understand the need to persist.

Obviously, the neonate or older child who cannot verbalize well will not be able to request or demand pain relief. Neonates and preverbal children simply have no choice about whether or not they must tolerate pain since they are unable to defend themselves.

Due to a lack of experience with pain, older children may not know the alternatives to suffering pain nor the socially expected methods of obtaining pain relief. Like some adults, they may not even know it is necessary to report the fact that they feel pain, assuming that the health professionals caring for them are aware of this and are in control of it (Stevens, 1987). Apparently, it is not unusual for the parents of a child with pain to fail to request an analgesic for the child because they think the nurse is aware of what is needed and can be given (Eland, 1988a).

Patient Example

One of the authors had a teenage daughter who had an emergency appendectomy while this chapter was being written. Afterward, during a discussion of the experience, this 17-year-old remarked, "I just lay there afraid of more pain." She was asked, "Why? Didn't you know you could tell the nurse you hurt and ask for medication to relieve it?" She replied, "I didn't know I had to tell the nurse. I thought the nurses were taking care of me. I think most teenagers would just lie there like me and think the nurses know they hurt and are doing whatever they can to stop it. I thought the nurses had done all they could do." When her mother asked her what she thought should be included in this chapter, she answered, "Tell the nurses we're younger than adults and more scared so we need more attention." (Reported with the patient's permission.)

Misconception: If the child sleeps, plays, or can be otherwise distracted from pain, he does not have much pain.

Correction: Children are especially talented in the effective use of distraction and physical activity to handle pain, and children may also sleep or pretend to do so as a method of handling pain. The child, like the adult, need not act like he is in pain to be in pain (see pp. 12-14). Further, the coping mechanisms of distraction, physical activity, and sleep cannot be used indefinitely.

Children are perhaps even better able than adults to use distraction to make pain more bearable. Children also seem to make greater use of physical activity to cope with pain. Adults in pain tend to "take to the bed" but, especially for young children, physical activity is often an effective coping strategy. A toddler usually becomes more, not less, active when he is in pain. This, coupled with the belief that if he gets out of his room and keeps moving he may avoid painful procedures, results in a big incentive for early ambulation in this age group.

Playing may provide both distraction and physical activity as well as give the child a sense of control. Many children in pain play until they almost drop from exhaustion. Escape to the playroom is especially likely since it serves the dual purpose of removing him from his room and providing the opportunity for play.

On the other hand, children may sleep or pretend to do so to withdraw from pain or procedures. The child may fake sleep, hoping to avoid or delay a painful procedure, e.g., burn debridement. Or, a child may close his eyes to block out a distressing environment, e.g., monitors and tubes. Even the baby may use sleep as a coping strategy. In response to postoperative pain following circumcision, healthy newborns may sleep quietly without eye movement rather than fuss and cry, as do older infants. When they are aroused, some are irritable. Others are lethargic and difficult to arouse (Marshall et al, 1980). These behaviors may persist for up to 24 hours. Thus many of the child's effective coping strategies preclude expressions of pain. If the child is pretending to be asleep or playing and laughing to distract himself from pain, he cannot at the same time show expressions of pain such as crying.

Misconception: Children are able to tolerate pain better than adults.

Correction: The above misconception is the culmina-

tion of several previously discussed misconceptions, e.g., that children often do not act like they are in pain since they may play, engage in physical activity, or sleep, and may not report pain or ask for pain relief.

Actually, to some extent children may be able to use certain coping strategies, such as distraction and physical activity, better than adults. Thus at times the child may be better able to tolerate pain than the adult, but the adult's overall ability to cope with pain is considerably greater than the child's. The adult with pain usually has more control over his situation, including more knowledge about pain relief measures such as medications or cold packs, more outside sources of help such as friends to telephone, and more ability to persist in obtaining pain relief such as asking the physician to increase a dose or requesting a consultation.

The child's apparent tolerance for pain may also depend upon which painful experience is being observed, e.g., how distressing that type of pain is for the child and which coping strategies the child is permitted to use. During a venipuncture, the adult may simply talk and seem to ignore it, but a child may protest or scream. On the other hand, following a herniorrhaphy, an adult may walk bent over for a week, but a child may be playing actively within a few hours. One study showed that children who were not afraid did not always demonstrate behavioral distress even though they reported pain (McGrath, de Veber, and Hearn, 1985).

Further, as the duration of pain increases, some children, like adults, seem to have less tolerance for pain, e.g., they may scream with greater forcefulness (Katz, Kellerman, and Siegel, 1980; Savedra, 1976). It is difficult to know if this is because perception of pain increases or because the child feels more distress.

However, most children probably tolerate pain simply because they cannot or do not pursue pain relief as well as adults. As discussed above, older children, may assume that "the nurse is taking care of me and knows when I hurt and what I need."

Misconception: The potential side effects of narcotics make them too dangerous to use to relieve pain in children.

Correction: If the pharmacokinetics are understood and the child is properly observed, narcotics may be used safely in children, even in newborns, premature infants, and children being weaned from a ventilator (e.g., Bell and Ellis, 1987; Lynn, Opheim, and Tyler, 1984; Lynn and Slattery, 1987).

All drugs have potential dangers. But in spite of the danger of anaphylactic shock from allergy to antibiotics, children continue to receive them when they are indicated. The potential for dangerous side effects from narcotics does not preclude their use, since the most dangerous side effects, such as respiratory depression, can be easily monitored. Further, should respiratory depression or any other life-threatening side effects occur from narcotics, the effects are almost always easily and quickly reversed by the antidote naloxone.

Misconception: Narcotics should be avoided or used sparingly in teenagers because they are at high risk for developing narcotic addiction. Indicators of abuse or addiction in teenagers are when they enjoy themselves after narcotic injections, prefer the "needle" to the pill, or ask for narcotics before they are due.

Correction: The risk of narcotic addiction in adults being treated with adequate doses of narcotic for pain relief is considerably less than 1%, and there is no reason to suspect it is any greater with children. When a person's pain is relieved, it is natural and even desirable for them to enjoy being free of pain. A preference for injections instead of oral narcotics is most likely related to the fact that a dose of narcotic given IM provides 2 to 6 times more pain relief than the same dose given orally. Requesting narcotics frequently is usually a sign of inadequate pain relief; a short duration of action should be expected in children since they tend to metabolize narcotics rapidly (Kaiko, 1980). All of the above misconceptions about addiction are discussed in greater detail in Chapter 4.

Further, research on children fails to support fears that addiction will result from use of narcotics to treat severe pain. In one study of 38 children and adolescents with sickle cell crisis, 76 episodes were treated with continuous IV narcotic infusion, and no addictive behavior was observed in any of the children (Cole, Sprinkle, Smith, and Buchanan, 1986). Similarly, in three adolescents using IV PCA for sickle cell crisis pain, no evidence of abuse was noted (Schechter, Berrien, and Katz, 1988).

On the other hand, physical dependence (withdrawal) may occur after a course of narcotics. Parents and children as well as health team members need to understand that this is not the same thing as addiction.

The increase in substance abuse during the 1980s, especially among adolescents and young adults, has resulted in increased concern about narcotic addiction in this age group when their pain is relieved with narcotics. Not only does this probably contribute to undertreatment of pain in children on a daily basis in many clinical areas, but also it prevents research efforts. Deeply entrenched beliefs about the addiction proneness of adolescents with sickle cell disease resulted in the medical staff of one hospital withdrawing previously granted approval to perform research on the use of IV PCA (patient controlled analgesia) in these adolescents. The researchers state, "In light of the complete absence of studies demonstrating an increased risk of addiction in adolescents with sickle cell disease, the rejection of our study before it was begun suggests the degree to which assumptions and stereotypes can define clinical practice and hamper investigation" (Schechter, Berrien, and Katz, 1988, p. 112).

Misconception: Pain is not life-threatening and has no lasting effect on infants and young children, and they will not remember it anyway.

Correction: Pain may have adverse and even life-threatening consequences in the neonate. The onset of memory is unknown, and absence of conscious memory of an event is not evidence that it has no physical or psychological effect on the person.

While some argue that the neonate cannot feel pain, others fear that pain in neonates may be life-threatening, especially if the baby responds with crying and decreased oxygenation, which may in turn cause intraventricular hemorrhage, a major cause of death among premature infants (Beaver, 1987). Heel lance is considered a relatively benign procedure, yet research has shown that it causes increased heart rate and blood pressure and decreased transcutaneous oxygenation in premature infants (Beaver, 1987). Neonates with various physical causes for pain have been noted to be agitated, cyanotic, bradycardic, hypoxic, and hypercarbic (Bell and Ellis, 1987). In newborns, circumcision without a local anesthetic results in a greater adrenocortical stress response than circumcision preceded by lidocaine injection (Stang et al, 1988). Obviously, pain is far from safe.

Regarding the onset of memory of pain, a study of behavioral responses of infants in an immunization clinic strongly suggests that by 9 months of age some infants cry in anticipation of an immunization based on having had an immunization 6 weeks earlier (Levy, 1951, 1960). One mother of a newborn who was subjected to numerous heel sticks in the first few days after birth reported that once the infant was home and the sticks were discontinued, the infant continued for 2 weeks to grimace and to withdraw his feet whenever his feet were touched.

Very little data exists about the later effects of past experience with pain, but one study of adults revealed that those who had more pain during childhood had greater sensitivity to pain and less tolerance for pain as adults (Collins, 1965). A study of children showed that those who had endured extensive periods of pain were developmentally retarded or regressed (Quinton and Rutter, 1976).

COMMUNICATING WITH THE CHILD AND HIS PARENTS

One of the ways that assessment and relief of pain in the child differs from the adult is that additional communication skills are necessary. Involvement of the parents or family is usually more essential in the care of the child than the adult. Further, communication with the child requires an appreciation of the cognitive abilities and concerns of the various age groups along with the usefulness of play as a communication tool.

Talking with the Parents

When the patient is an infant or child, the rights to which a patient is entitled are essentially transferred to the parents. As guardians of those rights, the parents need information that will enable them to make decisions about the care of their child. Further, the child's family can be a great asset in the assessment and relief of the child's pain.

Family members other than the parents may also be important and helpful resources. The child's grandparents or brothers and sisters may offer valuable information and assistance. And of course, the parents are not always the major caretakers. For convenience, however, the major caretakers are usually referred to in this chapter as parents.

Talking with the parents provides not only an opportunity to obtain helpful information about assessing and relieving the child's pain and to show respect for the parents' knowledge about the child but also an avenue for increasing the parents' sensitivity to their child's pain and increasing their ability to be involved in providing pain relief. Regarding assessment and relief of a child's pain, important topics to discuss with the child's parents are:

- Their priorities in the current situation. The parents may have more immediate concerns than pain and may not be able to focus on identification and relief of pain until other matters have been settled. Try to sit down with them in a quiet place to discuss this, and offer to talk and to answer questions then and later. Decreasing the parents' fears usually also decreases the child's apprehension. Even the very young child tends to assimilate his parents' attitudes about painful or distressing events.
- Clarification of what is meant by the word pain. Many adults associate the word *pain* with discomfort that is excruciating and intolerable. Identify the words the parents use to refer to pain, e.g., *uncomfortable* or *hurting,* and try to use these terms in the discussion. Also, ask them what words the child uses for pain.
- The child's previous experiences with pain. A history of the child's pain experiences may be very helpful, including types of pain, how the child reacts to pain, and what the parents do for the child (Hester and Barcus, 1986). Talking with the parents about the child's past pain experiences and reactions to them may help improve their ability to detect pain in their child. In particular, it may help to review the differences in the child's behavior when pain is sudden and when it is ongoing.
- Their assessment of the child's current pain. The parents have the potential for understanding their child better than anyone else by virtue of having spent more time with the child under a variety of circumstances. They possess a wealth of information about the child. Remember, however, that the parents may be at a disadvantage in some situations. The parents may never have seen the child in as much pain before, or they may be upset about the illness or surrounding circumstances. Parents may have emotional reactions of helplessness, fear, or guilt that may prevent them from admitting to

themselves that the child has pain, e.g., guilt over allowing an accident to happen. Or, they may need to feel in control of the child's behavior or need to feel that the child is being brave.

- The need to inform the health team whenever they think the child is hurting. Remind the parents, as well as the child, that the health team does not necessarily know when the child is hurting.
- How the "Flow Sheet" (see p. 27) may be used to identify the safety and effectiveness of pain relief methods. Ask for the parents' help in devising a flow sheet specific to their child. For example, even when the child is preverbal, the nurse and parent may use the flow sheet together to titrate analgesics. A continuous IV infusion of morphine was successfully titrated for several days in a 10-month-old child with prolonged cancer pain simply by the mother and nurse making independent pain ratings based on observation of various behaviors, such as sleep and crying (Dothage, Arndt, and Miser, 1986). Examples of how the "Flow Sheet" may be modified for a young child are shown in Figure 10-1.
- How they feel about staying with the child while he is in pain, especially during painful procedures. Explain that no matter how old they are, children often want their parents with them when they are hurt and scared. Preschool children in particular fear abandonment. Help the parents recognize the value of their presence when the child is in pain. This is difficult for many parents. To help the parents feel more comfortable, offer to answer questions about the child's condition and care. The more frightening the circumstances, the more important the parents' presence may be. Therefore during an emergency room visit, allow the parents to sit near the child and touch him. Prior to surgery, let parents stay during induction of anesthesia. Allow and encourage parents to visit the intensive care unit. When the parents and other family members must be absent, encourage them to bring toys or pictures from home. If possible, have the family make tape recordings for their child, e.g., conversation over dinner or bedtime stories.
- What they usually do to relieve the child's pain or to comfort the child. Ask them what is the most effective and what they would like to try now. Also, ask parents if they know how far in advance the child wants to be informed about painful events. Children between 5 and 12 years of age have greatly different preferences for the timing of information about pain (Ross and Ross, 1984).
- Their interest in learning new ways to comfort the child and relieve his pain, e.g., noninvasive techniques for pain relief such as helping the child distract himself with a favorite story or blowing bubbles.

KEY POINT: For the benefit of both the child of any age and his parents, allow the parents to be with, touch, and hold the child to the extent possible without causing undue distress for either.

Age: 6 mo.

FLOW SHEET—PAIN

Patient ___Jim_____   Date _4/13_

~~*Pain rating scale used~~ Behaviors indicating pain: cry, whimper, restlessness, frowning
or angry looking face, inability to sleep, parent unable to elicit smile.
Purpose: ~~To~~ evaluate the safety and effectiveness of the analgesic(s).

Analgesic(s) prescribed: _acetaminophen 80mg PO q4h; MS IV 0.2 mg/hr._

Time	Possible ~~Pain rating~~ behaviors	Analgesic	R	P	BP	Level of arousal	Possible ~~Other†~~ comfort behaviors	Plan & comments

Age: 6 years

FLOW SHEET—PAIN

Patient ___Joy_____   Date _5/29_

Pain rating scale used _Faces (0=no pain, 5=worst pain)_
Other common pain behavior is crying easily and wanting to be held.
Purpose: To evaluate the safety and effectiveness of the analgesic(s).

Analgesic(s) prescribed: _codeine 30 mg + acetaminophen 300 mg_

Time	# of Face Pain rating	Analgesic	R	P	BP	Level of arousal	Other† Pain behaviors	Plan & comments

FIGURE 10-1 Examples of how the flow sheet from p. 27 can be adapted for infants and young children. *See Figure 10-2 on p. 279 for illustration of the "faces" rating scale.

Parent interview. The topics discussed above may be formulated as statements and questions to use in ongoing discussions with parents about assessing and relieving pain in their child, presented in an interview format on pp. 272-273. A copy of this form along with a copy of the Flow Sheet on p. 27 may provide an efficient and fairly complete approach to obtaining information. As mentioned previously, it may also be a useful format for teaching the parents about assessment and relief of pain in their child and involving them in this process.

Thus the *purposes* of the "Parent Interview Regarding Child's Pain/Hurt" are:

1. To obtain information from the parent(s) regarding assessment and relief of a child's pain, especially if the child is reluctant or has minimal or no ability to communicate the information himself.
2. To increase the parent(s)'s ability to assess and relieve pain in the child.
3. To involve the parent(s) in providing comfort and relief for the child.

Ideally, the interview is conducted with the nurse and both parents present. Of course, a formal interview with a written record of the responses is not always possible or desirable. It is probably most important for those children with prolonged or frequent hospitalizations or illnesses. The questions may be discussed with the parent without actually using the written tool, or the tool may be used as a guide to discussions without making a written record of the parents' responses.

Further, the interview is an ongoing process, and certainly need not be completed at one sitting. Not all the questions need to be asked of all parents. Simply begin with the questions that seem most relevant. When time is limited, give priority to identification of verbal and nonverbal behaviors that indicate pain so that a meaningful flow sheet can be implemented to evaluate pain relief measures. In some instances the parents might wish to keep a copy of the interview and make their own notations on it to share with the nurse later.

Talking with the Child

Even when a child has no verbal ability, such as the infant, talking to the child may convey at least an attitude of caring. Remember, too, that the child's ability to understand what is said is almost always greater than his ability to communicate verbally. Nonverbal communication, such as some form of play or physical contact, may be an important aspect of interacting with any age child.

General guidelines for communicating with infants and older children (adapted and expanded from Whaley and Wong, 1989) are:

- Allow the child time to feel comfortable with the nurse.
- Avoid sudden or rapid advances.
- Talk to the parent initially if the child is shy.
- Try talking through objects such as dolls or puppets before directly questioning a young child.

- Give the older child an opportunity to talk without parents or friends being present.
- Assume a position that allows for eye contact but do not force eye contact or maintain it for long periods.
- Speak in a quiet, unhurried voice.
- Use simple words and sentences, but avoid upsetting terms such as "shot" instead of injection or "deaden" instead of numb.
- Offer physical contact. Once an infant or toddler makes eye contact and shows no fear, hand him a toy and gradually increase physical contact with him, eventually holding him. A similar approach may be used with the older child, beginning with handing him a toy or touching his arm or shoulder, eventually offering physical comfort such as an arm around the shoulder or holding his hand.
- *Be honest,* especially about the possibility of pain occurring.
- Give the child an opportunity to express his concerns and ask questions. Ask open-ended questions, wait for answers, and do not interrupt. Avoid "putting words in his mouth."
- Use actual equipment or pictures in explanations. Demonstrate on self or doll, or use figure drawings (e.g., p. 21 or p. 281). Be sensitive to the older child's desire not to be treated childishly.

Specific guidelines for discussing assessment and relief of pain with the child are:

- Talk with the child about previous hospitalizations and painful experiences. Note the exact words the child uses for pain. Children may not know the names of body parts or the meaning of the word *pain*. Pain is actually a difficult concept that includes numerous different sensations as varied as pricking from a needle, deep aching visceral pain, headache, and indigestion.
- Regardless of age, remind any child who has verbal ability, even the adolescent, to tell the health team when he has pain. Explain that nurses and doctors cannot always tell when he has pain and that we need his help.
- Establish the child's understanding of time. For example, can he tell time using a clock or watch? Use this information to help the child understand when pain will occur and how long it will last and how long before analgesics take effect. A timer may be set to illustrate the passage of time before the analgesic relieves pain or the length of time it takes to perform a certain procedure. Ask the child if he has any preferences about when he would like to be told about an impending painful event, e.g., the day before or an hour before.
- Give the child choices in relation to pain, whenever possible. For example, allow the child to choose which hip will receive an injection. Offer two or more methods of handling pain, e.g., holding your hand, looking at a pop-up book, breathing slowly and deeply. Adolescents are particularly resistant to rigid rules and tend to respond well to mature reasoning and explanations.

Text continued on p. 274.

Parent Interview Regarding Child's Pain/Hurt

Child: _____ Parent/caregiver: _____ Date: _____

I. Total Current Situation

What are your major concerns (unrelated to pain), if any, about the current situation/hospitalization in general, e.g., finances, care of other children, cause or seriousness of illnesses?

What are your child's major concerns (unrelated to pain), if any, about the current situation/hospitalization in general, e.g., being separated from parent, sleeping in a different bed or room, missing a birthday party, school work?

II. Child's Previous Experiences with Pain/Hurt

What types of pain has your child had before? Include descriptions of cause, duration, severity, frequency, and other important aspects.

What words, if any, does your child use for pain or hurt?

How does your child usually act when he is *suddenly* hurt, e.g., falls down?

How does your child usually act when he has been *hurting for a long time,* e.g., with a sore throat or earache?

III. Assessment of the Child's Current Pain

Since no one but the child knows if he hurts, the health team needs your help in finding out when your child is hurting and whether or not efforts to relieve the pain are working.

What behaviors indicate that your child is or is not in pain right now? For example, can you get your child to smile at you?

A written record, called a "Flow Sheet" can be very helpful. What do you suggest be recorded on the flow sheet? List of behaviors that probably indicate pain:

List of behaviors that probably indicate comfort:

■ May be duplicated for use in clinical practice. From McCaffery, M, and Beebe, A: PAIN: CLINICAL MANUAL FOR NURSING PRACTICE, St. Louis, 1989, The CV Mosby Company.

Continued.

Parent Interview Regarding Child's Pain/Hurt—cont'd.

IV. Comforting the child and/or Relieving the Pain

When your child hurts, what do you usually do to comfort your child or relieve the pain? Which work best? Which could you do now?

When your child hurts, what does the child do for himself that seems to help? How can we help the child help himself?

Considering the pain your child has now or will have, what are your concerns about being with your child while he is hurting or is having a painful procedure?

What would you like to learn about how you can soothe or distract your child during pain?

If painful procedures are performed, do you wish to be with your child? If this varies, during which procedures do you wish to be present and which ones would you rather avoid?

Do you have any ideas about how far in advance your child would like to be informed about a painful procedure?

Other Comments

Is there anything special we should know about your child and pain? Is there anything disturbing to the child that we should *not* do?

- State directions firmly and positively along with the exact time an event will occur, especially something painful. Toddlers, preschoolers, and even older children are likely to try to postpone a painful procedure, but after appropriate choices have been given, it is important to proceed. Give one direction at a time and wait until the child has responded; e.g., instruct the child to lie down, then wait until he has done so before directing him to turn on his side. Praise the child for doing what is requested, e.g., "that's right," "very good."
- Perform painful procedures outside the child's room, whenever possible, and never in the playroom. The child needs to feel that his bed, room, and playroom are safe places. For example, take the child to the treatment room for painful suture removal or a lumbar puncture. If there is a playroom, post a sign on the door to remind health team members that it is off limits for all painful procedures.
- Express a positive attitude toward injuries, procedures, pain, and blood. Keep wounds clean and neat, and comment on any progress or good prognosis, e.g., say that an incision looks good. Explain the need for procedures. If the sight of blood cannot be avoided, assure the child that it is normal, perhaps remarking that it is a good red color. Let him know when a procedure is over or when bleeding has stopped. Explore any misconceptions about pain or blood, e.g., indications that he will die or be disfigured or that all of his blood could run out of a hole made by a needle stick. Discuss when the child will look just like he did before or be able to return home or go to school.
- Discuss with the child what he does and does not want done to relieve his pain, and why. Two useful items to ask about are the presence of a parent and the use of Band-aids. Regardless of age, most children want a parent, especially the mother, present when they hurt. If this is not possible, talk with the child about his family, friends, and pets. As for Band-aids, they seem to have a magic power for very young children, and even an adolescent may want a Band-aid to shield a wound from sight or to avoid seeing a drop of blood from a needle stick. For ongoing pain or following a painful procedure, the younger child may want a Band-aid not only on himself but also on his doll or some other object.

Patient Examples

Band-aids seem to help in a variety of painful circumstances. Young children who have pain under a plaster cast that has been applied to a broken limb may request that a Band-aid be placed on the cast. Following open heart surgery, one young child seemed distressed and would not cooperate with procedures until the nurse complied with his request to use Band-aids to cover the transparent dressing over his incision. Another child, 3½ years old, was terminally ill and being cared for at home, receiving morphine at various doses over 100 mg/hr. The mother reported to the nurse that her daughter was fully alert and comfortable and had requested that a Band-aid be placed on the infusion pump because "that's where the feel good comes from" (Wiley, 1988).

- Discuss with the child his reactions to pain. Explain that during procedures it may be necessary for him to help by being very still, but that he can usually cry or scream if he wishes. In spite of the fact that adults are often disturbed by behaviors such as screaming or crying, some children find them helpful or need permission to act that way without being considered a sissy. However, be alert to the possibility that the child may want very much *not* to cry or scream, and explain tactics such as deep breathing that may help him avoid crying.
- Praise the child's responses to pain and offer a symbol of courage. During or after the procedure, you may say, "You help so much by trying to be still," or, "You are really able to scream and let us know when its hurting." Offer to let the child keep any clean and safe articles involved in the procedure, e.g., a cotton ball or a syringe without the needle.
- Carefully observe the neonate's, especially the preterm infant's responses to eye contact, touch, or being talked to. A child this age may easily be overloaded with sensory stimuli even from simple manipulations such as feeding and certainly from a painful event. Frequent rest periods may be needed to allow for recovery from stress and use of self-regulatory behaviors (Als, 1982). Painful procedures probably should be performed as quickly as possible and the premature infant allowed to recover before inflicting additional pain or stimulation. This might decrease the intensity of the physiological response, e.g., smaller increase in heart rate.

An appreciation of the prominent features of the ways children tend to think about and react to pain at different ages aids in communication. The reader is referred to other resources for summaries and detailed accounts of the child's concepts of pain during the major stages of cognitive development and responses to pain at various ages.*

Play

Play is a special tool for communicating with children. In relation to pain, play may involve learning about painful procedures before and after they occur such as handling a syringe, participating in activities such as handing tape to the nurse, or being involved in some other way such as floating objects in the fluid used for soaking a wound. Materials for play may include those actually used in the procedure, replicas available in toy stores or from specialty groups (e.g., Pediatric Projects, resource sec-

---

*Als, 1982; Als et al, 1986; Hurley and Whelan, 1988; McGrath and Unruh, 1987; Piaget, 1930; Ross and Ross, 1988; Whaley and Wong, 1989; Wong and Whaley, 1986.

tion, p. 296), books, pictures of equipment, or the child's doll or stuffed animal.

Play is important business for the child. Whenever possible, use play both before and after a painful experience. Prior to a painful event, play may be used as a rehearsal. After a procedure or during ongoing pain, play serves to promote understanding of what is occurring or what has already happened. The possible benefits of play are (Wong and Whaley, 1986):

- Facilitates mastery over an unfamiliar situation.
- Provides opportunity to learn about parts of the body and diseases.
- Corrects misconceptions about the use and purpose of equipment and procedures.
- Provides distraction.
- Promotes relaxation by providing a means for release of tension and expression of feelings.

Patient Example

Over a period of about 1 month Eric, 4 years old, experienced numerous venipunctures for the purpose of administering fluids and medications and obtaining blood samples. Fortunately, it was possible for Eric to play with the equipment prior to the first venipuncture, which was for the purpose of starting a continuous IV infusion. Using a clean needle connected to clean IV tubing and an IV bottle with plain water, the nurse showed Eric how to insert the needle in a rag doll's arm and how the fluid came down the tubing into the doll, explaining that the doll was sick for a little while and could not drink water. The nurse also explained that it only hurt when the needle was inserted, not while the tube remained in place. She emphasized that the doll helped by staying very still while the needle was being inserted, but could move around afterward. The nurse suggested several ways to keep the needle from hurting so much and asked Eric which the doll should do. Eric decided the doll should take a deep breath and blow it out slowly like a kiss. Under the supervision of the nurse, Eric performed the procedure on the doll, blowing for the doll, and the tube (without the needle) was secured in place with a Band-aid. When the venipuncture was performed on Eric, he was able to cooperate by remaining still, and he blew kisses to his doll, which was nearby. Thereafter, prior to each venipuncture, Eric prepared his doll, blew during the procedure, and comforted the doll afterward, often explaining to the doll why the venipuncture needed to be done.

ASSESSMENT

Assessment of pain in children from birth through adolescence will include a discussion of the following:
- Assumptions and beliefs about the existence of pain in children and the possible indications of pain.
- A multidimensional approach to assessment of pain.
- Specific pain scales that may be useful with children who are verbally fluent.

Assumptions and Beliefs

Assessment of pain in children, especially the very young, requires active use of educated assumptions and guesses. Based on certain assumptions, guesses are made, action is taken, and the outcome is evaluated, recognizing that once again certain assumptions must be made.

The pain sensation is subjective and cannot be proved or disproved in any age group. Thus in the absence of absolute proof, our approach to pain assessment in the child is based on the following basic assumptions or beliefs:
- All children, including neonates, have the ability to feel pain.
- Anything that causes pain in adults also causes pain in children.
- Some things that do not cause pain in adults may cause pain in children.
- Assessment encompasses responses at the moment and over time. Assessments are made at regular intervals and compared, and a written record is kept.
- In determining the presence (not absence) of pain, priority is given to any information directly communicated by the child; i.e., self-report of pain is the most valuable method of identifying pain.
- Self-report of absence of pain is viewed with suspicion and explored further if pathology or other behaviors indicate that pain might be present. Children, like adults, may deny pain or refuse analgesia for many reasons.
- Children respond to pain not only in a variety of physical and physiological ways but also without exhibiting any observable responses. Lack of response does not necessarily mean lack of pain.

In the assessment of pain in neonates, preverbal children, children who are not fluent verbally, and those who are reluctant to admit pain, the following additional assumptions and approaches are especially important:
- In the absence of the ability and willingness for self-report of pain, detection of the possibility of pain requires attention to multiple facets with special attention to *changes* in responses.
- Opinions about the child's pain are sought from parents and others.
- An ongoing, open dialogue about the child's pain is encouraged in the hope that increasingly accurate assessments and insights will occur.
- There is no way to be sure that a child does or does not have pain—it is always a guess.
- There is no way to be sure that pain relief measures are or are not effective—this, too, is always a guess.

A Multidimensional Approach to Pain Assessment in Children

For those children who cannot communicate verbally about their pain, observations must be made of physiological signs and nonverbal behavior, including vocalizations such as crying or groaning, along with knowledge of pain associated with procedures and pathological processes. Few guidelines exist for which behaviors are most indicative of pain. The meaning of the direction of change in response—e.g., increased or decreased pulse—is not always clear. Further, since most research on pain, especially in the very young, has been related to brief procedural pain such as responses to injections or circumcision, very little is known about the child's response to prolonged or chronic pain that may last hours, days, or months.

Currently several easily used and apparently reliable and valid instruments or tools are available for assessment of pain in children 3 years and older. However, even in children with the ability to communicate verbally, assessment can be seriously hampered by simple problems such as failure to establish what the specific words mean to the child. Or, the child may deliberately conceal pain because he fears the consequences of pain; e.g., fear that an injection will be given to relieve pain or fear that pain will result in a longer hospital stay.

The need for reliable and valid tools for assessment of pain in the neonate and very young child is one of the most pressing problems in management of pain in this group. Lack of sufficient data to construct simple and accurate tools for this youngest and most defenseless group of children has probably seriously hampered development of pain relief strategies, and even prevented an awareness of the need for pain relief.

However, *the absence of reliable and valid pain assessment tools for the very young is perhaps not as important as the willingness to believe that the very young do indeed have pain,* even if we cannot measure it with the seeming accuracy with which we measure pain in older children and adults. Despite having tools available for several years to assess pain in adults, pain continues to be undertreated. Thus while an assessment tool for the very young is needed, the existence of one would not necessarily assure that pain would be relieved.

While assessment or measurement of pain is absolutely essential if the effectiveness of pain relief methods is to be identified, simple awareness that the very young are capable of feeling pain may be sufficient data on which to base a systematic attempt to relieve the pain. For example, some physiological parameters (e.g., heart rate) in neonates may be measured in response to procedural pain. Regardless of the direction of change, i.e., increased or decreased rate, the fact that a change occurs may be sufficient evidence that pain is probably perceived. Based on this observation in the individual neonate, the nurse can attempt pain relief, using measures such as narcotics or a pacifier, and monitor whether or not this facilitates a return to baseline observations.

However, relying exclusively on behavioral or physiological response has serious limitations. Fatigue alone, due to pain or other reasons, may diminish the intensity of the infant's response to pain. Adults may sleep in spite of severe pain—so may a child. Likewise, in adults autonomic arousal, e.g., increased heart rate, in response to pain may occur briefly but subside in a few moments—this may also happen in a child. Further, at a young age children become aware that nonverbal behaviors are a means of communication. Thus the child may be observed to behave in one way when he knows others are present, and in another manner when he thinks he is not being observed. This can easily be misunderstood as some form of attention seeking or manipulation. However, just as an adult stops talking about pain when others leave the room and are unable to hear him, so may a child stop crying about pain when he believes he is alone and there is no one there to hear him.

KEY POINT: **Although research clearly shows that newborns have a specific response to pain involving crying, heart rate changes, and facial expressions, as pain increases in duration these responses are less and less useful in indicating the presence or severity of pain.**

Thus with neonates and even with children who are verbally fluent, the task of assessing pain is not always straightforward. Relying only on any *single* measure or indication of pain, e.g., self-report, physiologic changes, facial expression, known physical cause, or crying may be dangerously limiting.

KEY POINT: **In some children assessment of pain requires a multidimensional approach.**

Components of a multidimensional assessment of pain in neonates and older children are:
- Initiate discussions about pain. Include the child, if possible, parents, and other caregivers. Do not assume that the presence of pain will be spontaneously reported. Emphasize to the parents and to the child, if the child is capable of self-report of pain, that the health team members do not always know when a child is hurting. Remind the child at regular intervals that he must tell you when he hurts. Preschool children can usually understand when they are told that their help is needed in finding out about their pain. Help the parents become sensitive to behaviors the child may use to express pain, and explain that severe pain may exist in the absence of any obvious behavioral indication, especially if pain is prolonged.
- Obtain a self-report, if possible, by talking or playing with the child. Use whatever words the child uses to denote pain. Consider using one or more of the pain scales described later, or encourage the child to make his own scale such as drawings of faces. This approach is obviously impossible or of no value if the child is preverbal, unconscious, or unable to speak, e.g., on a ventilator with a muscle relaxant, and some feel that

self-report is of no value in children younger than 4 years of age (McGrath, PJ, et al, 1985). The child, like the adult, is the only authority about his own pain, but he is not always able or willing to communicate about his pain. Because even the verbal child may deny pain, it is vital to use the following methods of assessment in addition to self-reports.

KEY POINT: When pancuronium bromide (Pavulon, a muscle paralyzing agent) is administered, extra attention must be given to assessing the need for anesthesia and analgesia since the patient's methods of communicating pain are severely limited.

• Identify the presence of pathological processes or occurrence of procedures that are known to cause pain in others, e.g., older children and adults who are willing to report pain. Keep in mind that sensitivity to pain may be greater in younger children so that some things that do not cause pain in adults may cause pain in premature neonates or infants.

• Notice vocalizations that may indicate pain, e.g., hiccoughs or sneezing in the neonate, and crying, grunting, moaning, screaming, and breath holding at any age.

• Observe facial expressions. Those associated with pain include a wrinkled forehead, tightly closed or widely opened eyes, tightly closed or widely open mouth, or any distorted facial expression. Although infants differ tremendously in their response to pain, a facial expression of pain seems to occur fairly consistently as an immediate response to pain. The typical facial expression of pain consists of brows lowered and drawn together, bulging forehead with vertical furrows between the brows, a broadened nasal root, eyes tightly closed, and an angular, squarish mouth (Johnston and Strada, 1986). An expression of anger (eyebrows drawn downward and inward) may occur in older infants and toddlers (Izard et al, 1983). Especially in the infant, note whether or not it is possible to elicit a smile.

• Observe body movements, e.g., splaying of hands in the neonate, clenched fists, rigid posturing, guarding of a body part, agitation, moving head from side to side, jerking or pulling back, kicking, waving arms, or curling and uncurling fingers, fidgeting, or clinging to the parent.

• Note changes in autonomical (physiological) responses, e.g., heart rate, especially an increase, although a decrease may occur in some neonates, especially an initial drop. Other changes in a child of any age may include respiratory rate, apnea, perspiring, pallor or gray-bluish coloring (especially circumoral in neonates), and a rise or fall in blood pressure. (The Valsalva maneuver occurs when neonates cry, and this increased intrathoracic pressure decreases blood flow to the heart which may cause bradycardia, preventing an increased heart rate in response to pain.)

• Ask about any changes in daily activities or behaviors, e.g., sleep disturbance, nausea or vomiting, decreased appetite, decreased activity, or increase in rest periods, irritability or low frustration tolerance, aggressive behavior such as hitting, restlessness, or an increase or decrease in social interactions.

• Consider a trial of an appropriate dose of analgesic and note the responses, as discussed above. This may be particularly helpful when the issue arises about whether the child's response is due to pain or anxiety. Sometimes the response is clearly in anticipation of pain, occurring before anything painful is done. At other times it is unclear whether the behavior is a result of pain or fear of pain. In a practical sense, distinguishing between the two need not be a limiting problem. Whether the child's reaction is due primarily to fear or pain, the child still needs help, and most approaches to pain also help decrease distress about pain. For example, distraction or narcotics may reduce the child's fear of pain *and/or* provide pain relief.

The fear and anxiety caused by pain is sometimes misunderstood as a behavior problem. Health team members may become upset by a child's hostile behavior, refusal to cooperate, regressive tendencies, or constant whimpering, but overlook the possibility that the behavior could be caused by pain (e.g., Nover, 1973). They may try to control this behavior with rewards or limit-setting rather than persisting with efforts to relieve pain. A trial dose of analgesic may help clarify the problem; e.g., the child may cooperate and stop whimpering when the pain is relieved.

The components of a multidimensional approach to assessment of pain in children are summarized in the box below.

Components of a Multidimensional Approach to Assessment of Pain in Children

Initiate discussions about pain. Include the child (if possible), parents, and other caregivers.

Obtain a self-report, if possible, by playing or talking with the child. Consider using one or more of the pain scales.

Identify presence of pathology or occurrence of procedures that are known to cause pain in others.

Observe:
• Vocalizations
• Facial expressions
• Body movements
• Autonomic responses
• Changes in daily activities and usual behaviors

Consider a trial dose of analgesic and note the child's responses.

Assessment Tools for Children with Verbal Communication Ability

Several instruments have been developed to obtain a self-report about pain intensity from children as young as 3 or 4 years old. This section includes only those tools that are easily used in the clinical setting and readily available, e.g., those tools for which permission to duplicate, where necessary, has been granted. These tools may be considered for use with children between the ages of 3 or 4 and 18 years.

Usually the specific tool selected for the individual child is simply the one that the child seems best able to use. Thus different tools may be used for different children. However, to avoid confusing the child and to maintain consistency in assessment, for a given child the same tool is ordinarily used over time. In some instances an entirely new tool may need to be constructed for the individual child. Research may support the validity of one assessment tool over another, and there is much wisdom in resisting the temptation to develop more tools. However, in attempting to relieve pain in the individual child, it makes sense to use whichever tool the child responds to readily and seems to understand.

General Guidelines

Before using any of the pain assessment scales, talk with the child about the following:

- Find out what words the child uses for pain, e.g., *ouch, hurt.*
- Ask the child to give two or three examples of pain (to identify the child's understanding and use of words pertaining to pain). If he has difficulty, ask him if he has ever fallen down, skinned his knee, hit his head, or had his finger pricked.
- Consider using a numerical scale only if the child can count to the highest number on the scale, e.g., 10 or 100. Verify this by asking the child to count to that number.
- Help the child practice with whatever pain assessment tool is selected by using the examples of pain given by him. Time may not permit this, but practice may increase the chances of a more accurate picture of the child's pain.

The specific directions given with each of the following scales are not limited to the precise ones used in research to establish the validity and reliability of the tools. Variations of the original directions are included here to foster flexibility in individualizing these tools in the clinical setting.

Numerical Scales

In general, numerical scales can be used by most children by age 9 to 10 years. The choice of numerical scale depends on the child's ability to count and his preference. Numerical scales may range from zero (meaning no pain) to 5, 10, or 100 (meaning the worst possible pain). How-

ever, children in school may view 100 positively, associating it with a perfect test score, and view zero negatively. This possibility should be discussed with children choosing a scale of 0 to 100, and consideration given to reversing the usual meaning of the scores, i.e., having 100 mean feeling perfectly OK with no pain.

Most children 7 years or older can probably use a visual analog consisting of a vertical line, rather than the usual horizontal line, going from 0 to 10 (see p. 22). Children do not seem to easily grasp that going from left to right on a horizontal line represents an increasing intensity of pain (Beyer and Aradine, 1987).

In addition to the general guidelines given above, including a discussion of painful experiences and asking the child to count to 10, the *specific guidelines* for using the vertical visual analog scale on p. 22 are:
1. Explain that 0 means no hurt (or whatever term the child uses for pain) and 10 means the worst possible hurt.
2. To verify the child's understanding of the scale, ask the child to point to or state a number that means the following:
   - No hurt.
   - The worst hurt.
   - A hurt he has already experienced, picking one of the examples he has given.
   - The hurt he feels now (specify which pain if more than one is possible).
3. For future rating, note whether the child needs to point to the scale or is able to verbalize the number.

Wong/Baker Faces Rating Scale

The six faces shown in the Wong/Baker scale have been used to assess pain in children ages 3 to 18 years. Research comparing this tool with others suggests that this faces scale is well liked by the children and one of the most accurate methods of assessing pain (Wong and Baker, 1988). The faces and specific directions for using them are presented in Figure 10-2. General guidelines stated above should also be used.

Eland Color Scale

The Eland Color Scale differs from many other pediatric pain assessment tools in that it yields information about the location of pain in addition to its intensity. It consists of figure drawings, back and front views, on which the child marks the location of pain. Intensity is indicated by the color the child uses to mark the location (Eland, 1981, 1985a, 1988a). The Eland Color Scale seems to be a sensitive instrument for identification of pain site. On numerous occasions the coloring of the figures has identified metastasis from cancer before objective evidence could be obtained (Eland, 1986). Specific guidelines for using the Eland Color Scale are summarized on p. 280 accompanying Figure 10-3, p. 281.

WONG/BAKER FACES RATING SCALE

1) Explain to the child that each face is for a person who feels happy because he has no pain (hurt, or whatever word the child uses) or feels sad because he has some or a lot of pain.

2) Point to the appropriate face and state, "This face is...":
0—"very happy because he doesn't hurt at all."
1—"hurts just a little bit."
2—"hurts a little more."
3—"hurts even more."
4—"hurts a whole lot."
5—"hurts as much as you can imagine, although you don't have to be crying to feel this bad."

3) Ask the child to choose the face that best describes how he feels. Be specific about which pain (e.g. "shot" or incision) and what time (e.g. now? earlier before lunch?).

■ (From Wong, D, and Whaley, L: Clinical Handbook of Pediatric Nursing, ed. 2, p. 373, St. Louis, 1986, The C. V. Mosby Company. Printed with permission of the publisher and authors who also give their permission for this to be duplicated and used in the care of children with pain.)

FIGURE 10-2 Wong/Baker Faces Rating Scale (can be duplicated for use in clinical practice).

Patient Example

An 8-year-old with small-cell sarcoma identified an area in her left upper chest using the color chosen for moderate pain. Appropriate scans and tests done at that time revealed no pathologic processes, but 2 months later lung metastasis was found in the exact area the child had been coloring (Eland, 1986).

Hester Poker Chip Scale

The original tool consisted of four white chips, each representing a piece of hurt, with four pieces being the most hurt (Hester, 1979). This was later modified to include four red chips for levels of pain and a white chip for no pain (Molsberry, 1979). This scale can probably be used by children as young as 4 years.

This tool has several variations. Either four or five chips may be used. All four or five chips may be the same color to represent varying intensities of pain, with no chips equaling no pain. Or four chips may be the same color to represent varying levels of pain and one a different color to represent no pain. To simplify matters, the following instructions assume that four chips of the same color are used.

In addition to the general guidelines given above, including a discussion with the child about his previous experiences with painful events, *specific guidelines* for using this assessment tool are:

1. Obtain four white poker chips, coins of the same size, or paper cutouts.
2. Caution: Take special care that the young ones do not swallow the chips.
3. Place the chips side by side on a surface in front of the child.
4. Using the child's terminology and any examples he volunteers, explain the following:
   • These are pieces or chips of hurt.
   • One chip means a little hurt.
   • Four chips mean the most or worst hurt.
   • No chips means no hurt.
5. Allow the child to handle the chips and play with them if he wishes. Choosing the number of chips that equals his pain must not be influenced by his desire to touch or have the chips.
6. Then ask the child if he hurts now. If not, tell him that means he would show you no chips. If he says he hurts, ask him to use the chips to show you how much he hurts.

Eland Color Scale: Directions for Use

After discussing with the child several things that have hurt the child in the past:

1. Present 8 crayons or markers to the child. Suggested colors are yellow, orange, red, green, blue, purple, brown, and black.

2. Ask the following questions, and after the child has answered, mark the appropriate square on the tool (e.g., severe pain, worst hurt), and put that color away from the others. For convenience, the word *hurt* is used here, but whatever term the child uses should be substituted. Ask the child these questions:

   • "Of these colors, which color is most like the worst hurt you have ever had, (using whatever example the child has given) or the worst hurt anybody could ever have?" Which phrase is chosen will depend on the child's experience and what the child is able to understand. Some children may be able to imagine much worse pain than they have ever had, while other children can only understand what they have experienced. Of course, some children may have experienced the worst pain they can imagine.

   • "Which color is almost as much hurt as the worst hurt (or, use example given above, if any), but not quite as bad?"

   • "Which color is like something that hurts just a little?"

   • "Which color is like no hurt at all?"

3. Show the four colors (marked boxes, crayons, or markers) to the child in the order he has chosen them, from the color chosen for the worst hurt to the color chosen for no hurt.

4. Ask the child to color the body outlines where he hurts, using the colors he has chosen to show how much it hurts.

5. When the child finishes, ask the child if this is a picture of how he hurts now or how he hurt earlier. Be specific about what earlier means by relating the time to an event, e.g., at lunch or in the playroom.

(Printed with permission of JM Eland, who also gives permission for this to be duplicated and used in the care of children with pain.)

■ May be duplicated for use in clinical practice. From McCaffery, M, and Beebe, A: PAIN: CLINICAL MANUAL FOR NURSING PRACTICE, St. Louis, 1989, The CV Mosby Company.

ELAND COLOR SCALE: FIGURES

Mark each box with color child selects:

No pain No hurt	Mild pain A little hurt	Moderate pain More hurt	Severe pain Worst hurt

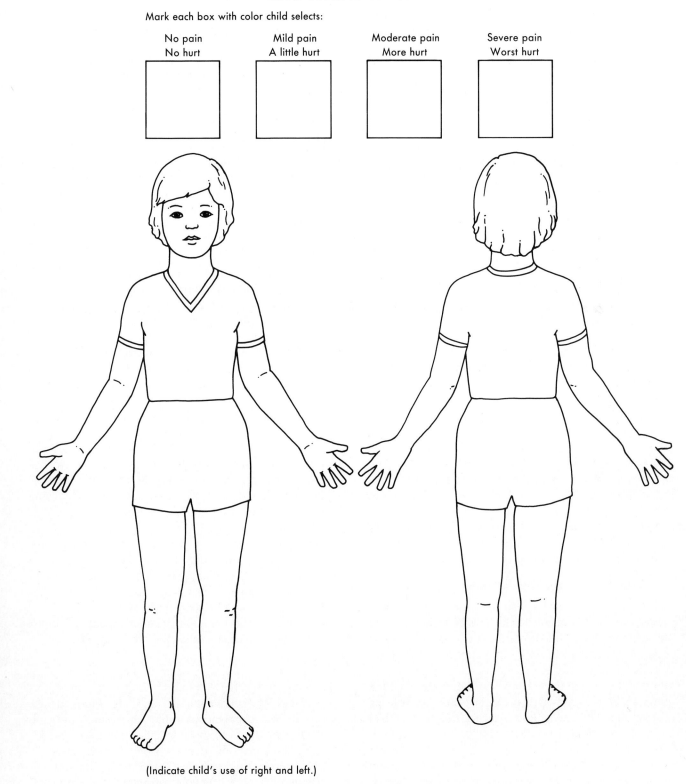

(Indicate child's use of right and left.)

FIGURE 10-3 Eland Color Scale: figures. (Printed with permission of the author, who also gives permission for this to be duplicated and used in the care of children with pain.)

APPROACHES TO PAIN RELIEF

Pharmacological and noninvasive methods of pain relief discussed in detail in previous chapters for use with adults are also appropriate for relieving pain in infants and children. Much of what has already been addressed also applies to children. The purposes of this section are to present:

- Special considerations related to needle sticks and procedural pain in children.
- Reminders of pertinent material already presented in Chapters 4 through 9.
- Modifications and additional considerations specific to the various age groups in children.

As was true with adults, several methods may need to be used for adequate pain relief and control of accompanying emotional states. For example, an 8-year-old child with a simple fracture of the arm may benefit from an oral narcotic, a nonnarcotic, distraction, relaxation, a cold pack, and various other pain relief methods, used at the same time or alternately.

Since assessment of the child with pain may be very complex, it is obviously difficult at times to individualize pain relief measures for children, especially neonates and the very young. For example, adjusting the dose of analgesic and interval between doses is not as easy to do with young children who cannot communicate verbally as it is with adults who can provide numerical ratings of their pain. In spite of this difficulty, every attempt must be made to tailor pain relief measures to the individual child.

We agree with others who have suggested that failure to try to provide pain relief for infants and children is both abusive and unethical. "Failure to relieve pain amounts to child abuse and must not be tolerated," says Rana (1987, p. 309). Stang et al (1988, p. 1511) point out that ". . . according to current ethical guidelines, surgical procedures cannot be performed on research animals without using anesthesia . . . are we not morally obligated to do the same for the young of our human species?"

Avoiding/Minimizing Needle Sticks

The most objectionable pain for children of all ages seems to be that of needle sticks. This is evident even in the newborn when he responds to his first heel lance (e.g., Owens and Todt, 1984). In a survey of 242 hospitalized children between the ages of 4 and 10 years, 49% said that the "needle" or "shot" was the worst of all the things, including surgical pain, that had hurt them during hospitalization. Some children giving this answer had multiple surgeries (Eland, 1981). Similarly, in another survey of children age 3 to 18 years, the most commonly reported painful events involved needles (Wong and Baker, 1988). Since needle sticks seem especially distressing and painful to children from birth through adolescence, this specific type of pain is addressed separately as a special issue in pain relief for children.

Needle sticks are frequently performed on children

for two main purposes: (1) to deliver medication, including analgesics, via IV, IM, and SC routes, and (2) for diagnostic or therapeutic procedures, such as injection of a local anesthetic or finger stick. Suggestions are made below for avoiding needle sticks or minimizing each of these types of needle sticks.

Alternatives to Needle Sticks for Delivery of Medications

Sticking children with needles is avoided whenever possible. It is especially important to avoid needle sticks for pain relief. It makes little, if any, sense to a young child to have his pain relieved by undergoing the painful and frightening experience of an injection. Further, the child's limited understanding of human physiology makes it unlikely that he will associate an injection in the hip or thigh with pain relief in another location at a later time. Additionally, the injection of the narcotic may momentarily be more distressing to the child than the ongoing pain. Many children deny pain to avoid such injections.

The following are alternatives to needle sticks performed to administer medications:

- *PO route, tablets or liquid.* For medication that tastes bad, ice chips or cold liquid may be used to numb the taste buds prior to taking the medication. Most nonnarcotic analgesics for relief of mild to moderate pain are given PO. Remember, even severe pain may be relieved using oral narcotics if the child can swallow and if nausea and vomiting can be controlled (see p. 88).
- *Troches* may be used for PO or sublingual administration of many medications, including narcotics. Troches are an excellent method of drug delivery if the child has difficulty swallowing pills or if crushing or liquifying results in a bad taste, although troches do not mask all bad tastes (Wong, 1987). Troches are artificially sweetened and may be scored for division into smaller doses. Essentially they are like a hard candy and may be chewed, sucked, or placed under the tongue. (For information on compounding drugs in troches, see p. 296, Resources for Children/Parents/Nurses.)
- Use *IV line* (not multiple venipunctures) for bolus doses or continuous infusions. All narcotics may be administered IV.
- *SC continuous infusion* or an SC needle left in place and covered with a dressing for intermittent injections (not multiple needle sticks). Medications must be approved for subcutaneous route and volume must be small enough not to cause irritation or tissue damage. Narcotics commonly delivered by SC route are morphine and hydromorphone (Dilaudid), not meperidine (Demerol) (see pp. 93-99 regarding SC continuous infusion). An SC needle left in place for intermittent injections does not eliminate the discomfort of the medication being injected, but it does eliminate the needle stick—children may object more to the needle stick pain

than to the pain of injecting medication. The pain of injecting the medication may be minimized by injecting slowly and partially relieved by some of the methods suggested below, e.g., ice or cold near the site.

- *Rectal* route may be preferable, in some cases, to IM or SC. Virtually any analgesic can be made into a suppository (see p. 92). Narcotics currently available commercially as rectal suppositories are hydromorphone, morphine, and oxymorphone (Numorphan). Nonnarcotics commercially available as rectal suppositories include aspirin, acetaminophen, and indomethacin (Indocin).
- *TAC* (Tetracaine, Adrenalin, Cocaine) may provide local anesthesia without the need to inject the tissues. Tetracaine is a local anesthetic with an onset of 5 to 10 minutes and a duration of anesthetic action of 30 to 60 minutes. Adrenalin provides vasoconstriction to reduce bleeding and lengthen duration of the anesthetic effects. Cocaine provides both local anesthesia and vasoconstrictive action. Application of TAC prior to suturing minor lacerations, e.g., in the emergency room, is especially useful for children ages 1 to 5 years. This liquid is prepared by the pharmacy as a controlled substance, usually in 5 ml portions: T = tetracaine, 0.5%, 25 mg/5 ml; A = adrenalin, 1:2000; C = cocaine, 11.8%, 590 mg/5 ml.

TAC may be administered by pouring it over the wound, slowly dripping it into the wound, or saturating a 2 × 2 gauze with it and applying this with firm pressure. If it is dripped into the wound, use a syringe without a needle, and demonstrate to the child that no needle or injection is involved. Wait 5 to 10 minutes and then test sensation in the wound by gently applying a 25-gauge needle to the wound surface, again assuring the child that no injection is planned. Avoid using TAC on the mucosa, penis, digit, or pinna of the ear because the vasoconstrictive action could cause tissue damage (Brown, 1984; Pryor, Kilpatrick, and Opp, 1980).

Some feel that the use of TAC could increase the risk of infection (Barker et al, 1982). However, thorough cleaning and flushing of the contaminated wound seems to reduce the occurrence of infection (Eland and Herr, 1988).

Minimizing Discomfort of Needle Sticks

When needle sticks must be performed, one or more of the following steps may decrease the pricking sensation:

- *Ice, cold, or Frigiderm* immediately before, during (if possible), and after needle stick, e.g., applied over site prior to needle stick, then to a site adjacent to or on the opposite side during the needle stick, returning to the site of the needle stick afterward. Frigiderm, a skin coolant, sprayed for 3 to 5 seconds on the injection site immediately before the injection significantly decreases the pain children report (Eland, 1981). However, ice cubes or a cold pack are often more readily available.

Be sure to explain to the child that he will feel something cold before the injection is given. If possible, allow the child to apply the cold pack or ice cube himself.

- *Offer distraction,* e.g., tell the child to "see if you can count to 20 before the injection is over," but also tell the child he may instead cry out, punch his pillow, or express his feelings in another way as long as he remains still enough for the injection to be given.
- Use the *ventrogluteal site* for IM injections whenever possible (see Figure 4-4 on p. 89). Injection into this muscle tends to hurt less than injection into the vastus lateralis muscle, rectus femoris muscle, or the posterior gluteal (dorsogluteal) muscle. The ventrogluteal site is sometimes not recommended for children younger than 3 years, but this is controversial (Eland, 1983, 1985).
- Always *be honest* with the child and forewarn him of the injection. Never sneak up on him. Tell him the injection will hurt, using descriptive terms such as a pinch or sting.
- *Allow the child to choose the site* for the injection, if possible, such as the right or left hip.
- *Offer a "badge of courage,"* such as a colorful bandage over the injection site, especially if it bleeds. Blood can be very upsetting to the child as well as to the parents.
- Help the child *relax the muscle.* For the dorsogluteal site, have the child lie on his abdomen with his legs and toes rotated inward. For the ventrogluteal site, place the child on his side with the upper leg flexed and in front of the lower leg (Whaley and Wong, 1989). Asking the child to wriggle his toes or take a deep breath may help him relax, too.
- To minimize the discomfort associated with actual injection of the medication itself, have the *medication near room temperature,* use *Z-track,* and *inject slowly.*

To promote the child's understanding of the benefits of an injection of analgesic, a clock or timer may be used to indicate the passage of time between the injection and the probable onset of pain relief. It is extremely difficult for a child to make a logical association between the fearful and painful injection and the desired pain relief.

Minimizing Traumatic Procedural Pain

Numerous diagnostic and therapeutic procedures that are performed on children can cause brief but significantly intense pain. Analgesics or anesthetics are not always used to relieve this pain. If they are used, they do not always produce adequate pain relief. Children age 7 to 17 years in one pediatric intensive care unit indicated that the worst stressors were painful invasive procedures (Tichy et al, 1988). This is of special interest because research shows that around the age of 7 years, there tends to be a dramatic decrease in behavioral response to painful procedures (Jay et al, 1983). Once again, we see that a lack of behavioral expression of pain does not necessarily mean a lack of pain.

Since the child's experience with the first procedure sets the tone for reactions to future ones, it is especially important that the best possible methods of pain relief are chosen initially. This includes not only pain relief during the procedure but also appropriate discussions and play before and after the procedure. In addition, if the child is very anxious and this cannot be alleviated with nonpharmacological approaches, a premedication such as midazolam (Versed) should be considered.

To cope with procedural pain, noninvasive pain relief methods, such as those illustrated so beautifully in the videotape "No Fears, No Tears" (see resource section, p. 296), may be extremely helpful in addition to analgesics and anesthetics (Kuttner, 1988). Some of these are discussed later in the chapter, e.g., blowing bubbles and telling the child's favorite story.

The following discussion is limited to a few suggestions for pharmacological approaches to minimizing the pain of procedures that last from a few minutes up to about 30 minutes, such as lumbar punctures, changing burn dressings, and bone marrow aspirations.

Avoid "DPT." For many years a concoction often referred to as "DPT" (Demerol [meperidine], Phenergan [promethazine], and Thorazine [chlorpromazine]) or "Lytic Cocktail," has been a popular method of pain relief for children, particularly as a premedication for painful procedures. It has been administered IM, IV, and PO. While DPT may sedate the child and make it easier to perform a painful procedure, sedation must not be confused with pain relief. For the following reasons, DPT is an irrational combination for relieving pain of any sort, particularly as a premedication for a brief painful procedure:

- Two phenothiazines are included, and both may increase hypotension and sedation, sustain respiratory depression, and actually increase pain perception (Howland and Goldfrank, 1986; Ros, 1987). (See also discussion on pp. 117-118.)
- The effect of "DPT" is often prolonged sedation or sleep, lasting for 7 hours or longer (Nahata, Clotz, and Knogg, 1985).
- While the duration of analgesia from IM or PO meperidine is relatively short, e.g., about 3 hours or less, it may last longer than needed for some brief procedures, and it is combined with phenothiazines that have a considerably longer duration (4 to 6 hours) than that required for a brief procedure.

Fentanyl. IV fentanyl is recommended for a variety of brief but very painful procedures such as repair of lacerations in the emergency room, reduction of fractures or dislocations, and bone marrow aspirations. Even for infants, IV fentanyl is considered by many to be a safe and ideal drug and to have numerous advantages over DPT (Billmire, Neale, and Gregory, 1985; Ros, 1987). It has a rapid onset (90 to 120 seconds), short duration of action (up to 40 minutes), and minimal side effects when it is administered in the following manner:

- Slow IV administration over 3 to 5 minutes, and
- Doses of 2 to 3 μg/kg.*

Virtually all problems with IV fentanyl, e.g., respiratory depression (including delayed respiratory depression), muscular rigidity, hypertension, and bradycardia, seem to arise from too rapid administration or large doses. When IV fentanyl is given as recommended above, side effects are rare. In one study of 2000 children from 1 to 12 years of age, IV fentanyl was used during repair of facial trauma and only three apneic episodes occurred. Nevertheless, the child must be monitored for respiratory depression, which may not peak for 15 minutes. As with all drugs capable of producing respiratory depression, oxygen, airway equipment, and naloxone should be readily available.

Regarding suggested doses of IV fentanyl for brief procedures, it is of interest that several researchers noted that higher doses seem to be required in infants and young children than in older children. For example, using 2 to 3 μg/kg, to calculate doses, Billmire, Neale, and Gregory (1985) found that children 18 to 36 months usually required the full dose and older children usually required less than the calculated dose. Using a broader dose range for calculation, Maunuksela, Rajantie, and Silmes (1986) found that infants under 2 years of age experienced no apparent analgesia from fentanyl 5 μg/kg.

Local anesthetics—"caines." Unfortunately, many painful procedures are performed without any local anesthesia. Yet infiltration of the skin with a local anesthetic is considered so safe that there is little if any reason ever to fail to use it in a newborn or older child whenever skin must be incised, e.g., for vascular access or circumcision (Stang et al, 1988; Yaster, 1987).

However, the stinging sensation of the local anesthetic is a major reason children dislike having procedures such as lumbar puncture or bone marrow aspiration performed under a local anesthetic. When a long-acting anesthetic such as lidocaine (Xylocaine) is used, stinging may last up to 60 seconds. However, the stinging associated with chloroprocaine (Nesacaine) lasts only about 2 to 3 seconds. Since numbness from chloroprocaine lasts about 15 minutes, a longer-acting local anesthetic such as bupivacaine (Marcaine) may need to be combined with it, resulting in stinging for 2 to 3 seconds and numbness for up to 10 hours (Eland, 1986). This long duration of numbness is especially helpful following a bone marrow aspiration since pain at the site of the procedure may last for several hours.

Anesthesiologists may be helpful resources when the nurse suggests that physicians use combinations such as the above. The help of anesthesiologists may also be

---

*μ or μg = microgram; 1000 μg = 1 mg.

enlisted to encourage surgeons to infiltrate surgical wounds with the long acting bupivacaine to reduce pain and narcotic need postoperatively. This may be especially helpful in the care of children and elderly persons, since the health team seems particularly reluctant to use narcotics in these age groups.

TAC, discussed above, is another method of using local anesthesia in a manner that minimizes the discomfort of painful procedures such as suturing or cleansing performed on open wounds.

Ketamine. Depending upon the dose administered, ketamine may produce anesthesia or analgesia. It has been used safely for procedural pain in children as young as 7 months and has been recommended for use during burn tanking and debridement, laryngoscopy, circumcision, and other less painful procedures (Forlini, Morin, and Treacy, 1987).

Ketamine anesthesia is dissociative. The eyes may remain open, and unpurposeful movement may occur. Although the patient is awake, constant supervision is necessary.

Prior to administration of ketamine, a drying agent such as atropine is given since ketamine produces a large amount of upper airway secretions. Also prior to administration, patients must be NPO for 6 hours (4 hours for infants), which may be a disadvantage in some situations, especially if calorie intake is a priority.

At recommended doses respiratory depression is absent or minimal, and the pharyngeal and laryngeal reflexes are retained. Low doses recommended for procedures lasting 5 to 30 minutes, such as burn dressing changes, are as follows (Martyn, 1987):
- IV (given over 60 seconds), 0.5 to 1.0 mg/kg. Higher doses up to 2 mg/kg may be given (Forlini et al, 1987).
- IM 1 to 3 mg/kg. Higher IM doses of 5 to 10 mg/kg may be given (Forlini et al, 1987).
- Rectally, 9 to 10 mg/kg.

With repeated doses, tolerance develops and larger doses are required.

Transcutaneous Electric Nerve Stimulation (TENS). For some types of localized pain accompanying procedures, TENS may be used in a manner similar to its use postoperatively (see pp. 161-164). The comfortable "conventional" TENS setting may be used with the electrodes on either side of the painful area. TENS has been successfully used with children to relieve pain associated with intravenous insertion and particularly painful subcutaneous injections, such as cytarabine (ARA-C) injections (Eland, 1988c).

Patient Example

An adolescent experienced considerable discomfort during the continuous infusion of amphotericin. He lay in bed rigidly and with occasional tears in his eyes. After TENS electrodes were placed above and below the IV site, he was lying in bed relaxed and smiling (Eland, 1988b).

Analgesics

Do children suffer pain because of underuse of analgesics? Inadequate pharmacological management of pain in children has been suggested for many years. Most studies that compare analgesic administration in adults and children with similar painful conditions show that less analgesic is given to children than to adults, but the studies do not actually assess whether or not pain is greater in the children than in the adults (e.g., Beyer, DeGood, Ashley, and Russell, 1983; Schechter, Allen, and Hanson, 1986). However, based on studies in which adults do report their pain in relation to analgesic administration, it is clear that in many situations adults suffer moderate to severe pain from underuse of narcotics (see p. 67). Thus even in the absence of children's reports of pain, the analgesic record strongly suggests that children are not only undertreated for pain but also are undertreated to a greater extent than adults.

In an early study (1977) Eland and Anderson reported that 25 children ages 4 to 8 years, hospitalized for surgical procedures, received only 24 doses of analgesics compared with 671 doses received by 18 adults who had similar surgical procedures. Thirteen of the 25 children were given no analgesic during their entire hospitalization. Among those receiving no analgesic were children who had traumatic amputation, excision of a malignant neck mass, and repair of atrial septal defect.

Later in a survey of burn units, respondents assessed pain the same in adults and children but choices of treatment of burn pain differed greatly for children. Some units tended to give relatively larger doses of morphine to children than to adults. However, while only 6 respondents stated they would not routinely premedicate the adult for tanking, 24 stated they would not routinely premedicate the child (Perry and Heidrich, 1982). Apparently there is a tendency to undertreat pain in children but there are also occasions when children may be treated for pain more aggressively than are adults. Analgesic administration is most certainly more variable in children than in adults.

Analgesic research in children. Compared with adults, there are fewer double-blind analgesic studies in children, and the pharmacokinetics of analgesics, e.g., half-life and absorption, are not as well understood in children. Some analgesics have not yet been approved for use in children, although that does not necessarily mean they cannot be used.

Certain warnings about using analgesics in children may unnecessarily discourage their use unless these statements are appropriately interpreted. Some drug information states that studies have shown the drug to be unsafe in children, but most state that studies establishing safety and effectiveness in children are *lacking*. For example, the PDR (Physician's Desk Reference, 1988) states, "Controlled clinical trials to establish the safety and effectiveness of MOTRIN in children have not been conducted" (p. 2139). This has not prevented the use of this drug in young children with rheumatoid arthritis or postoperative pain, nor should it, provided the physician is aware of the usual precautions suggested with this drug.

Physiological considerations influencing analgesic therapy in children. Maturational changes seem to have a striking effect on drug response but are still poorly understood (Stewart and Hampton, 1987). In relation to narcotic and nonnarcotic analgesics, the possibility of adverse side effects, a longer duration of action, and the need for lower doses in children compared with adults may be explained in part by some of the following physiological differences in children (Pagliaro and Pagliaro, 1986):

- Renal function. In the neonate, renal blood flow is lower and glomerular filtration rate is about half that of the normal adult. Thus drugs that are primarily excreted unchanged in the urine will have a much longer half-life. However, the renal system matures relatively rapidly and reaches a state of function comparable to that of the adult by the age of 6 to 12 months. Recent research shows that clearance of morphine reaches or surpasses the adult level by 1 month of age (Lynn and Slattery, 1987).
- Hepatic function. Since hepatic function is not fully developed at birth, some enzymes produced in the liver and responsible for drug metabolism are not available. Thus some drugs such as morphine will be metabolized more slowly in the neonate and have a longer duration of action (Lynn and Slattery, 1987).
- Protein binding. Many drugs bind to plasma proteins, leaving a portion of each drug circulating unbound or free. Only the free drug produces a pharmacological effect. Under the age of about 2 years, the mechanism for producing albumin, a major plasma protein, is not fully developed (Pagliaro and Pagliaro, 1986). Decreased circulating proteins potentially result in greater drug effect from higher concentrations of unbound drug, with a greater risk of toxic effects. Nonnarcotic analgesics that are protein bound and likely to be associated with greater pharmacological effect include ibuprofen, naproxen, indomethacin, meclofenamate, and piroxicam (Flower, Moncada, and Vane, 1985).
- "Immature" receptors. Some drugs seem to have a stronger or weaker effect on children than on adults. It has been suggested that this could be due to some drug receptors not being fully developed in children. For example, decreased numbers of receptors or decreased responsiveness of the receptors might result in a drug having a greater effect. However, currently there is no research to support this.

Many formulas have been introduced over the years for calculating pediatric doses, recognizing that there are many physiological differences in children and adults. However, it is vital to remember that those formulas for calculating analgesic doses have not been verified with research. They are merely guidelines.

Key Concepts in Analgesic Administration

The same key concepts that apply to adults receiving analgesics for pain also apply to the child: using a preventive approach, individualizing or titrating the dose and other aspects of the analgesic, and the patient controlling his own pain relief to the extent possible. These are discussed extensively in Chapter 4 (see pp. 48-54). The following is a brief overview of these concepts along with special considerations related to their application to children:

- Patient controlled analgesia (PCA). All analgesia is controlled by the patient to the extent possible since the patient is the only person who can feel the pain being treated. Whenever possible, the patient's report of his pain is used as the reason to begin use of analgesics and then to make adjustments in the analgesic dosage so that the safest and most complete pain relief possible is provided. Obviously neonates, young children, and some older children will not be able to report pain verbally. In the absence of direct patient control over analgesia, initiation and adjustment of analgesics must be based primarily on the following:
  - Nonverbal and physiological behaviors that indicate pain.
  - Known pathological process or cause of pain.
  - Safety.
  Using the above, parent control (as opposed to patient control) of analgesia may be possible. Further, trial doses of narcotic and/or nonnarcotic analgesics are indicated for children who cannot or will not report pain.
- Preventive approach. If pain is predictable, regularly scheduled doses should be instituted after determining the duration of action of the analgesic in the individual child. If an occurrence of pain can be predicted, an analgesic is given prior to the onset of pain, provided the patient's physical condition permits; e.g., if the child's condition is stable, a narcotic may be administered during surgery or in the recovery room before the child awakens. A plan to keep pain under control is particularly important in children since even the verbally fluent child may fail to report pain or deliberately conceal it. Remember that PRN orders may be implemented around the clock (ATC) if a flow sheet type of assessment indicates they are safe and needed.
- Titrate to effect. Based on the specific child's responses, the dose, interval between doses, choice of analgesic, and route of administration are individualized. When the child is unable to report pain, safety may be the major guide to titration of any of these aspects; e.g., if pain is suspected, the dose of narcotic may continue to

be increased until significant respiratory depression occurs.

Nonnarcotics (NSAIDs)

The specific details of nonnarcotic analgesic therapy are discussed in Chapter 4 (pp. 54-66), including indications, disadvantages, mechanisms underlying the effects of nonsteroidal antiinflammatory drugs (NSAIDs), adverse side effects, promising uses, and guidelines for their effective use, along with patient/family teaching tools that may be adapted for use with children and their parents. From this discussion, reminders of some important aspects that also apply to children are:

- Nonnarcotics relieve more pain than most people realize; acetaminophen 325 mg PO relieves about as much pain as codeine 15 mg PO.
- When pain is too severe to be relieved with nonnarcotics alone, continue to administer nonnarcotics along with narcotics since this provides safe, additive pain relief, and the combination narcotic plus nonnarcotic attacks pain in both the central and peripheral nervous systems. Further, the narcotic dose needed may be lower when a nonnarcotic is given at the same time.
- Types of pain that seem to be especially responsive to NSAIDs such as ibuprofen are:

Postoperative pain. Indomethacin (Indocin) rectally has been found effective in relief of postoperative pain in adults, and recent preliminary research suggests that IV infusion during the first 24 hours postoperatively is effective and safe in relieving pain and reducing the morphine requirement in children (Maunuksela, Olkkola, and Korpela, 1987).

Cancer pain.

Dysmenorrhea (painful menstrual cramps). Every adolescent girl needs to understand the value of nonprescription ibuprofen for this purpose.

When the child has both narcotic and nonnarcotic prescriptions for pain relief, there seems to be a tendency for nurses to select the nonnarcotic (e.g., Mather and Mackie, 1983). While nonnarcotics relieve more pain than most people realize, they do not usually provide sufficient relief for severe pain. However, as noted above, they may be given *along with narcotics* to relieve severe pain.

For children the recommended doses for both acetaminophen and aspirin are about 10 mg/kg every 4 hours, or up to 15 mg/kg of aspirin for children under two years of age (Benitz and Tatro, 1981). For practical purposes, approximate doses of aspirin and acetaminophen by age and weight are presented in Table 10-2. Use aspirin with caution in children with fever and dehydration because they are particularly prone to intoxication from relatively small doses of salicylate (Flower, Moncada, and Vane, 1985). For ingredients and formulations of nonnarcotics available for children without a prescription, see Table 10-4, p. 289.

To facilitate combining narcotics and nonnarcotics, notice that the same age and weight format is used in Tables 10-2 and 10-3. For example, if the child is four years old, Table 10-2 may be used to obtain the recommended dose of acetaminophen (240 mg) for this age, and Table 10-3 may be used to obtain the recommended dose of morphine IM for this age, between 1.6 and 4.4 mg. The two drugs may then be given at the same time for additive pain relief.

Reye's syndrome and salicylates. Since 1982 avoidance of salicylates in children and adolescents during respiratory illness or chicken pox has been suggested because of the possibility that use of salicylates might lead to the development of Reye's syndrome (encephalopathy and fatty degeneration of the viscera), a rare but often fatal syndrome. Since that time, salicylate use among children has declined, as has the incidence of Reye's syndrome.

Caution regarding salicylate use is still suggested by some who feel that the majority of Reye's syndrome cases may be attributed to salicylate use (Hurwitz et al, 1987). If caution is warranted regarding aspirin, then caution should also be taken with other salicylates, e.g., choline magnesium trisalicylate (Trilisate). However, others have reported a complete lack of association between the development of Reye's syndrome and ingestion of aspirin or other salicylates (Orlowski, Gillis, and Kilham, 1987).

Narcotics (Opioids)

A considerable amount of information related to narcotics has already been covered in Chapter 4 (pp. 66-113), including the mode of action, forms of undertreatment, reasons for undertreatment, equianalgesic doses, factors influencing selection of a narcotic, various routes of administration (e.g., oral, continuous subcutaneous infusion, spinal), and side effects, along with numerous patient/family teaching tools that may be adapted for use with children and their parents. Since narcotics are often administered parenterally, the reader is also reminded to review methods of avoiding or minimizing the pain of needle sticks (pp. 282-284). This section presents an overview of some important aspects of narcotic administration along with special considerations for children.

Undertreatment with Narcotics

Even when the existence and severity of pain in a child is acknowledged, health team members may still be tempted to undertreat with narcotics because of two issues, addiction and safety.

Addiction. The exaggerated and unfounded fear of causing *narcotic addiction* has been discussed previously (see pp. 67-71 and 268). This section focuses on how the nurse can assist parents, adolescents, and school-age children who show concern about taking narcotics and other drugs for pain relief. The following facts may help reassure them so that they can feel confident about using analgesics appropriately:

- Narcotic addiction is defined as a psychological dependence, a desire to use the drug for other than medically approved reasons. Pain relief is a legal and legitimate use of narcotic analgesics. Relief of pain is the primary reason the federal government has approved the use of narcotics. Tolerance to analgesia (requiring larger doses) and withdrawal symptoms are physiological problems that are separate from addiction.
- "Depending" on narcotics or pain relievers is not the same as "drug dependency," or psychological dependence. Parents may say they don't want their child to *depend* on drugs, failing to appreciate that there are situations where it is appropriate to depend on or to use narcotics to relieve pain, just as insulin is used to manage diabetes. Emphasize that narcotics are used to help the child feel normal or simply be himself. Without the narcotic he would feel pain and be affected by it, perhaps crying and unable to sleep or eat.
- The word *narcotic* is easily misunderstood because it is usually used by the government and the news media to refer to substances that can be abused. Not all of these are pharmacologically narcotic (opioid) analgesics, or pain relievers. For example, cocaine is a common drug of abuse and is frequently mentioned in daily news reports. Although it is legally classified as a narcotic, meaning that it is a federally controlled substance, it is actually completely unlike a narcotic analgesic. Cocaine is classified pharmacologically *not* as a narcotic but as a local anesthetic with a stimulant effect. Since cocaine is referred to as a narcotic and the abuse of it is often

TABLE 10-2 Approximate Doses* of Aspirin and Acetaminophen by Age and Weight

Age	Weight (lbs)	Weight (kg)	Dosage (mg) PO Acetaminophen	Dosage (mg) PO Aspirin	
0-3 months	6-11	2.5- 5.4	40	25 to 40 or 60 ⎫	
4-11 months	12-17	5.5- 7.9	80	60 to 80 ⎬ or 10-15 mg/kg, or as directed by the physician	
12-23 months	18-23	8.0-10.9	120	80 to 150 ⎭	
2-3 years	24-35	11.0-15.9	160	160	
4-5 years	36-47	16.0-21.9	240	240	
6-8 years	48-59	22.0-26.9	320	320	
9-10 years	60-71	27.0-31.9	400	400	
11-12 years	72-95	32.0-43.9	480	480	
12 years +			650 = adult dose	650 = adult dose	

*Not to exceed 5 doses a day.

TABLE 10-3 Approximate Calculations of Suggested *Initial* Doses of Morphine and Meperidine for Children with Moderate to Severe Pain

Age	Weight (lbs)	Weight (kg)	Dosage (mg) IM* q3-4h or IV continuous drip q2-4h Morphine	Meperidine†
0-3 months	6-11	2.5- 5.4	0.25 to 1.0	2.5 to 10
4-11 months	12-17	5.5- 7.9	0.55 to 1.6	5.5 to 14
12-23 months	18-23	8.0-10.9	0.8 to 2.2	8.0 to 19
2-3 years	24-35	11.0-15.9	1.1 to 3.2	11.0 to 29
4-5 years	36-47	16.0-21.9	1.6 to 4.4	16.0 to 39
6-8 years	48-59	22.0-26.9	2.2 to 5.4	22.0 to 48
9-10 years	60-71	27.0-31.9	2.7 to 6.4	27.0 to 57
11-12 years	72-95	32.0-43.9	3.2 to 8.8	32.0 to 75 or 80
12 years +			10+ = adult dose	75+ = adult dose

*IM is not the preferred route of administration for children.
†Meperidine is not a logical first choice of analgesic for most children.
The *purpose* of this table is to provide a quick reference for the usual initial dose of the most commonly administered narcotics, morphine and meperidine, by the most common routes, IM and IV, for children of various ages and weights. *Limitations* of this table are: (1) Dosage recommendations appear to be based more on observations of safety than effectiveness. A safe dose is not necessarily an effective one. (2) Age and weight are not well researched criteria for determining a safe and effective dose. (3) The lower range of the recommended dose is very conservative. Hence they may be safe but ineffective. The lower recommended doses must often be titrated up quickly to achieve satisfactory pain relief. (4) All initial doses must be immediately titrated up or down according to the individual child's response.
References: Goodman and Gilman (Jaffe and Martin, 1985), The pediatric drug handbook (Benitz and Tatro, 1981), and The Harriet Lane handbook (Rowe, 1987).

publicized, people may be unrealistically afraid of drugs that are pharmacologically classified as narcotics, e.g., morphine.

- The use of narcotics for pain relief almost never results in narcotic addiction. On the other hand, it is important to acknowledge to children and parents that drug abuse and addiction are problems in our society, and "street drugs" should be avoided. Medicine used for pain relief, however, is not a "street drug" and rarely results in feeling "high" or silly. (Referring to a narcotic as medicine instead of a drug may help make this point.)
- Narcotics are not nearly as appealing to most people as are other nonnarcotic drugs such as alcohol, marijuana, and cocaine. Adolescents who are familiar with "street" drugs often say they do not like the "feel" of narcotics given for pain relief.

Safety. There is an assumption that it is safer to withhold narcotics than to give them. Dealing with tiny doses of drugs and with the less physiologically stable systems in the very young may cause concerns about the immediate dangers of narcotics to override concerns about im-

TABLE 10-4 Common Nonprescription Analgesics for Children

Brands	Ingredients
Acephen Suppositories	120 mg, 650 mg acetaminophen
Arthropan Liquid	174 mg choline salicylate/ml (equivalent to 130 mg of aspirin)
Aspergum Chewing Gum	228 mg aspirin
Aspirin Suppositories	125 mg, 300 mg, 600 mg aspirin
Bayer Children's Aspirin	81 mg aspirin
Liquiprin Solution	48 mg acetaminophen/ml
St. Joseph Aspirin for Children Chewable Tablets	81 mg aspirin
St. Joseph Aspirin-Free Infant Drops	80 mg acetaminophen/0.8 ml (dropperful)
St. Joseph Aspirin-Free Liquid for Children	80 mg acetaminophen/2.5 ml (½ teaspoonful)
St. Joseph Aspirin-Free Tablets for Children	80 mg acetaminophen
Tempra Syrup	24 mg acetaminophen/ml
Tempra Drops	100 mg acetaminophen/ml
Tylenol, Children's Junior Strength Swallowable Tablets	160 mg acetaminophen
Tylenol, Children's Chewable Tablets	80 mg acetaminophen
Tylenol, Children's Elixir	32 mg acetaminophen/ml
Tylenol, Children's Drops	100 mg acetaminophen/ml

The brand names and ingredients of the above nonprescription (OTC, over-the-counter) analgesics were obtained from Van Tyle, WK: Internal analgesic products. In Handbook of nonprescription drugs, ed 8, pp 191-214, Washington, DC, 1986, American Pharmaceutical Association.

mediate pain relief and complications from unrelieved pain. However, under certain circumstances, pain may be hazardous. Pain may increase the incidence of intraventricular hemorrhage in premature infants, a major cause of death in this age group (Anand, Sippell, and Aynsley-Green, 1987; Beaver, 1987). Following tonsillectomy, pain may result in crying, which may precipitate bleeding (Krishnan, Tolhurst-Cleaver, and Kay, 1985).

Further, under careful observation, narcotic administration is probably much safer than is usually recognized (e.g., Beasley and Tibballs, 1987). For example, in children age 6 months to 15 years old receiving a total of 397 variable-rate IV narcotic infusions, respiratory rate dropped below the set minimum in only 2 patients. One responded to reduction in dose, the other required a small dose of naloxone (Dilworth and MacKellar, 1987). Research shows that infants older than 1 month of age are *not* more sensitive to the respiratory depressant effects of morphine than are adults (Lynn and Slattery, 1987). Use of a flow sheet (p. 27) to carefully document any changes accompanying narcotic administration may reveal that physiological responses, such as respiratory function, not only remain stable but actually show improvement.

Respiratory depression is one of the most feared side effects of narcotics, but naloxone (Narcan) provides reassurance. Although narcotic administration is always accompanied by a certain amount of risk, there is an antidote. Naloxone reverses almost all the undesirable side effects of narcotics, including respiratory depression. Following are reminders about the appropriate use of naloxone in children:

- The individual child's respiratory rate prior to a narcotic dose should be used for comparison purposes. Respiratory rates in children vary considerably.
- The average respiratory rates at rest for children are faster than those of adults, usually 30 to 35 per minute in newborns and infants, 25 to 30 per minute in toddlers, 20 to 25 per minute in preschool and school-age children, and 16 to 19 per minute in adolescents.
- The usual recommended dose of naloxone for neonates or young children is 0.01 mg/kg IV given over 2 to 3 minutes with subsequent doses of 0.1 mg/kg (Physician's Desk Reference, 1988). Large doses administered rapidly may precipitate not only severe pain but also nausea, vomiting, sweating, and increased blood pressure. In children who have become physically dependent, withdrawal syndrome may occur. Given IV, the onset of action is about 2 minutes, and slightly longer if it is administered IM or SC.

Choice of Narcotics

Findings regarding narcotic use in children plus reminders from material presented in this chapter and in Chapter 4 are:

- *Meperidine* is a *poor* first choice of narcotic analgesic for several reasons. The active metabolite normaperidine, a central nervous system stimulant, may accumulate and lead to seizures. Since meperidine is relatively short-acting, pain relief in young children may last much less than 3 hours, necessitating administration at inconveniently frequent intervals. The older child who can tell time may become a "clock-watcher" because pain returns long before he is allowed to have his next dose. For these and other reasons, "DPT" is a particularly irrational choice for relief of ongoing pain (see discussion on p. 284).

- *Nalbuphine* (Nubain) administered IV seems to have advantages over other narcotics. Like the other agonists-antagonists, it has a ceiling for respiratory depression, but unlike pentazocine (Talwin) and butorphanol (Stadol), it does not tend to produce psychomimetic effects (Bikhazi, 1978; Krishnan, Tolhurst-Cleaver, and Kay, 1985). Unlike buprenorphine (Buprenex), it can be completely reversed with naloxone if respiratory depression does occur. The recommended dose is essentially the same as that for morphine, i.e., 0.1 mg/kg or more (e.g., Wandless, 1987). Choice of dose is less critical with nalbuphine than morphine and other pure agonists because of nalbuphine's proved maximal respiratory depressant effect.

  Although the narcotic agonist-antagonists are pharmacologically narcotics, they are not always classified as narcotics by national and local governments. Consequently, health team members may be more willing to use these drugs because of less fear of narcotic addiction (an unfounded but nevertheless frequent fear).

- *Methadone or levorphanol*, especially orally, may be appropriate for some children since they are longer acting narcotics, and children tend to metabolize narcotics more rapidly than adults. Oral methadone for relief of cancer pain has been used successfully in children as young as 1 year of age (e.g., Martinson et al, 1982). A safe starting dose appears to be 0.1 mg/kg. However, the dose required for pain relief may be much larger in some children. Further, Miser and Miser (1985) report that unlike adults, children may show no evidence of drug accumulation.

- *Morphine and fentanyl* IV have been used safely in neonates. Narcotic analgesia in the neonate requires a vigilant approach. The half-life of narcotics in the neonate may be significantly longer than in the older child, and high-dose infusions or rapid administration via an IV bolus may cause seizures. Continuous IV infusion of morphine in newborns must be watched closely, even for several hours after the infusion is stopped, since the duration of action may be much longer than in older patients and the plasma concentration may continue to increase due to reabsorption of morphine (Koren et al, 1985). Nevertheless, these and other narcotics may be safely administered to neonates. Preliminary studies provide guidelines for initial and ongoing dosing of narcotics in premature neonates and infants (see anno-

tated references Beasley and Tibballs, 1987; Bell and Ellis, 1987; Hatch, 1987; Koren et al, 1985). Safe use of IV narcotics in neonates requires use of a flow sheet, gradual increases in doses, and avoidance of rapid bolus administration.

Dose

Most dosage recommendations for narcotic analgesics in children are not supported by double blind analgesic research in children. Recommendations are usually extrapolated from data on adults and appear to be based more on observations of what is safe rather than what is effective. Thus, as with adults, the initial recommended doses must be viewed merely as educated guesses. The initial dose must be immediately adjusted up or down according to the individual child's responses.

Standard pharmacology textbooks such as *Goodman and Gilman* (Jaffe and Martin, 1985), *The Pediatric Drug Handbook* (Benitz and Tatro, 1981), and *The Harriet Lane Handbook* (Rowe, 1987) give almost identical recommendations for initial doses of the two most commonly administered narcotic analgesics, morphine and meperidine:

- Morphine SC, IM, or IV—0.1 to 0.2 mg/kg/dose (maximum 15 mg), every 2 to 4 hours.
- Meperidine IM or IV—1 to 1.5 or 1.8 mg/kg/dose, every 3 to 4 hours.

NOTE: Although it is not stipulated, the IV dose should not be administered as a bolus; the recommended IV doses most likely refer to continuous infusion.

A quick guide to the usual recommended doses of morphine and meperidine IM or IV, using the above recommendations from standard pharmacology textbooks to calculate the dose according to weight, are presented in Table 10-3 (p. 288). Using this table the nurse may check a dose prescribed by the physician against the usual recommendations. For example, if morphine 2 mg IM is prescribed for a 4-year-old in severe pain and if this is not effective, the nurse may glance at the table and see at once that this dose is at the lower end of currently recommended doses. The nurse may report this information along with the child's response; e.g., "breathing well but still says he hurts very much," to obtain an order for an increase in dose.

Codeine is given PO, IM, or occasionally IV to young children (toddlers and preschoolers), rather often in some clinical settings. However, codeine is considered appropriate for mild to moderate pain, not severe pain, and tends to have dose-limiting side effects of nausea and constipation. Standard reference textbooks show less consistency regarding dosage recommendations for codeine. The two stated were:

- Codeine IV or PO—0.5 to 1.0 mg/kg/dose every 4 to 6 hours, to be used with acetaminophen orally (Rowe, 1987).
- Codeine IM or SC—0.5 mg/kg/dose every 4 to 6 hours;

PO dose is about ⅔ as potent as parenteral, i.e., the PO dose that provides analgesia equal to an IM dose must be about 1.3 higher (Benitz and Tatro, 1981). Other sources recommend the PO dose be 1.5 the IM dose (see equianalgesic chart, pp. 78-79).

Patient Example

A 3-year-old receives codeine 15 mg IM for moderate pain. It effectively relieves the pain, but the PO route is preferred. Using the more conservative 1.3 conversion factor (see above), the following calculations are a reasonable initial guess about the PO dose needed to obtain the same analgesia: 15 mg IM × 1.3 = 19.5 mg, or 20 mg codeine PO for approximately the same pain relief. Using data from Table 10-2, regarding oral non-narcotics, one may consider adding a dose of 160 mg acetaminophen, either for added pain relief or to allow a reduction of the codeine dose. When any of these doses are given for the first time, the child is observed and the dose is titrated up or down immediately.

Of course, any narcotics given to adults may also be given to children. A simple guide to doses for children 2 years and older is offered by Rogers (1985):
- 2 to 6 years—one-fifth to one-quarter the adult dose
- 7 to 12 years—half the adult dose
- 12 years or older—adult dose

Patient Example

Using the above suggestions along with the equianalgesic list and initial dose recommendations for adults (see pp. 78-79), an initial dose of methadone PO for an 8-year-old child with severe pain would be 10 mg, half the recommended PO adult dose of 20. If a conservative approach is desired, the dose can be lowered to 5 mg PO. The child is observed and the dose is titrated up or down, usually by 25% to 50%, within 2 to 4 hours. Since this drug may accumulate in the system, both dose and interval may need to be observed for a few days. It is possible that a lower dose and less frequent intervals will be possible.

To control severe pain such as sickle cell crisis, the IV route is preferred, using boluses to control the pain quickly and a continuous infusion to maintain a steady level of analgesia. Suggestions for initial doses of morphine or meperidine IV and a method of fairly rapid titration are offered by Cole and others (1986, see the annotated reference for details). However, meperidine is still regarded as a poor choice for severe pain if tolerance requires high doses, since the active metabolite normeperidine may accumulate and cause seizures (Howland and Goldfrank, 1986).

When tolerance to analgesia develops or when pain increases, doses of narcotic much higher than those recommended for an initial dose may be required. For example, for a 3½-year-old girl with extensive metastatic cancer, the dose of morphine IV escalated from 1.8 mg/hr to over 100 mg/hr in a 2-week period (Wiley, 1988). In a terminally ill 4-year-old the dose of IV morphine escalated from 48 mg/day to 4000 mg/day over a period of only 9 days (Eland, 1988b). In a 5-year-old boy with extensive gastrointestinal disease since birth, the safe and effective dose of IV morphine reached 225 mg/hr, and several months later toward the end of his life the dose reached 1000 mg/hr of IV morphine (Sentivany, 1988). Other examples of high doses given safely for relief of severe pain in children also appear in the literature (see annotated references Burne and Hurt, 1987; Rogers, 1985).

Route of Administration

The importance of avoiding the IM or SC route, and how to use other routes of administration, especially PO or continuous IV, have been discussed (pp. 282-283). Because babies and many young children have difficulty swallowing pills, it is common practice to dissolve them. To make this easier, remember that medication dissolves more quickly and more completely in *warm* water. If it has an unpleasant taste, suggest that the child suck on some ice for a few moments to numb the taste buds just before taking the medication.

Patient controlled analgesia (PCA) is an appropriate method of administering analgesics for some children. Successful use of PCA via the IV route has been reported in children as young as 11 years (Rogers, Webb, Stergios, and Newman, 1988; Schechter, Berrien, and Katz, 1988). Considering the adolescent's cognitive ability and need to maintain control, PCA by any route seems appropriate to the developmental needs and abilities of this age group. IV PCA may be possible in some children as young as 6 years, or the device may be operated by the parents. Eland (1988b) reports using IV PCA with a 4-year-old child.

Physical Dependence (Withdrawal)

Physical dependence may occur in adolescents and young adults after fairly brief narcotic administration, e.g., 6 to 21 days. After abrupt discontinuation of narcotic therapy, withdrawal syndrome may occur within 6 to 48 hours. This syndrome includes agitation, irritability, muscular jerks, abdominal pain, diarrhea, "gooseflesh," and itching (Miser et al, 1986). Withdrawal syndrome may also occur in the neonate when IV narcotics are abruptly discontinued. The following are essential to appropriate care:
- Be alert to withdrawal syndrome after 6 days or more of narcotic therapy.
- Reassure the patient and his family that physical dependency is not the same as addiction and does not lead to addiction. (The occurrence of physical dependence is unpredictable but is frequent compared to the infrequent occurrence of addiction.)
- If pain is resolved or if spinal analgesia is begun, gradual tapering of narcotics is indicated to prevent withdrawal symptoms.

Adjuvant Analgesics

Adjuvant analgesics have been discussed at length in Chapter 4 (pp. 113-123), including antidepressants, anticonvulsants, so-called potentiators, and considerations in treating sleep disturbances, anxiety, depression, muscle spasms, and aching or lancinating neuropathic pain. Guidelines for the use of adjuvant analgesics are not well established and continue to be researched. Following are brief reminders of important aspects of using adjuvant analgesics:

• Adjuvant analgesics usually are not a substitute for adequate doses of narcotic or nonnarcotic analgesics. Most of the time, aggressive titration of narcotic and nonnarcotic analgesics is indicated before adjuvant analgesics are tried.

• Appropriate indications for a trial of an adjuvant analgesic are those pain syndromes that do not respond to narcotics or nonnarcotics, such as phantom limb pain.

Dextroamphetamine, a central nervous system stimulant, is one of the adjuvant analgesics previously discussed. Although this drug may be used to treat hyperactivity in some children, it may cause stimulation in other children. Dextroamphetamine may be helpful in minimizing some of the side effects of narcotics, such as sedation, nausea and vomiting, and respiratory depression. There are some indications that it is analgesic or a potentiator of analgesia. For example, to counteract sedation from IV morphine in a 22-month-old child, dextroamphetamine 2.5 mg PO was used successfully (McManus and Panzarella, 1986).

Cutaneous Stimulation

Toddlers and older children may obtain pain relief from the types of cutaneous stimulation previously discussed in Chapter 5 (pp. 130-170), including superficial massage, pressure with or without massage, superficial heat or cold, ice massage, menthol applications, and TENS. However, special precautions apply to the neonate and infant.

Preterm and Full-Term Neonates

Stimulation of any sort, including stimuli felt as pleasant in infants and older children, should be administered cautiously to the neonate, especially the premature neonate. In a preterm infant, simple stroking of the skin may cause an intense physiological response. Hence, bathing by immersion in warm water rather than sponge bathing is recommended for preterm and full-term neonates (Als et al, 1986).

Cutaneous stimulation such as stroking above or below the site of pain is recommended for older children and adults for pain relief, but it does not appear to be helpful to neonates. For example, stroking the premature neonate's leg above the site of a heel lance may dramatically increase heart rate and other responses to pain. Research shows that the greatest percentage change in heart rate occurs during the first 10 seconds after application of stimuli such as touch and/or heel lance (Beaver, 1987). Hence, in the neonate, a convenient and quick method of assessing the effect of any stimulation, whether it is painful or intended to decrease pain, may be to observe immediate changes in heart rate.

Toddlers and Older Children

Special considerations in the use of certain cutaneous stimulation techniques for toddlers and older children are:

• *Cold and ice* applications are usually readily accepted by children, whereas adults are often reluctant to use them. Simply handing the injured child an ice cube can be distracting, and helping the child to rub it above or below the injury or contralaterally may also relieve pain. Children with headaches or undergoing orthodontic adjustments are often receptive to trying ice cube massage to the web of the hand (see p. 154).

A cold pack made from a disposable plastic glove may be especially useful with children since the fingers of the glove will cover small areas or get into narrow spaces between tiny body parts. The glove may be filled with ice chips and water, or placed in the freezer after filling with two-thirds water and one-third alcohol (alcohol keeps it from freezing into a hard mass). Further, if the cold pack must be sterile, sterile gloves may be used.

A recommended site for cutaneous stimulation, especially when the site of pain is not accessible, is between pain and the brain. A common method of increasing fluid intake in young children, e.g., postoperatively, is the Popsicle. Interestingly, this also serves the purpose of placing cold between pain and the brain.

Alternating applications of heat and cold is one of the most effective methods of pain relief with cutaneous stimulation. The child may be given both heat and cold packs, with instructions to alternate them at his own discretion. This may also distract him and give him a sense of control.

• *Menthol* products applied to the skin are usually well accepted by children. The odor may also add an element of distraction. Those products containing methyl salicylate should be avoided in children in whom aspirin and other salicylates are contraindicated.

• *TENS* reportedly is helpful to many children, although not to all, who have chronic nonmalignant pain (Beyer and Leven, 1987; Epstein and Harris, 1978). It may relieve some types of procedural pain, such as IV insertion, burn graft donor site pain, and prolonged pain from bone metastasis (Eland, 1988c).

Distraction

Children seem to be especially talented in the use of distraction, especially physical activity, to make pain more bearable. Therefore overuse of this technique must be avoided. Fatigue may occur easily, and pain persists in the presence of distraction, sometimes requiring analgesics in addition to distraction. For example, energetic distraction such as play is frequently followed by fatigue, irritability, and an increased awareness of pain, and analgesics are often indicated at that time.

Those distraction techniques discussed in Chapter 6 (pp. 172-186) that are especially appropriate for preschool and older children for brief painful procedures are sing and tap rhythm, active listening to recorded music or stories, anything funny, and pictures, particularly pop-up books. For children of all ages, maintaining normal sensory input is helpful in coping with ongoing pain. However, stimulation of all sorts must be used with caution in the very young.

Preterm infants. An infant at this age is easily overwhelmed by what is considered ordinary sensory stimuli. To decrease stress and promote self-regulation in the preterm infant, certain stimuli should be *avoided or minimized,* e.g., unnecessary touching, stroking, or taking out of the isolette. The preterm infant should be placed away from noises such as water faucets, telephones, radios, areas of heavy activity and traffic, and bright lights. Feeding may need to take place in a shielded isolette or quiet corner of the room with the infant swaddled and often should not be accompanied by talking to or looking at the infant. Care must be taken not to offer too many types of stimuli at the same time. Appropriate stimuli for the preterm infant include listening to soothing instrumental music and opportunities to grasp a finger roll or to suck (Als et al, 1986).

Preschool and older children. Preschool and older children often produce or initiate distraction to deal with pain. For painful procedures such as lumbar punctures, children 3 years of age and older may benefit from something as ordinary as squeezing someone's finger, clenching their fists, or engaging in an interesting conversation (McGrath and de Veber, 1986; Ross and Ross, 1984).

Out of 63 children between the ages of 6 to 19 years observed during bone marrow aspiration, 18 were bothered very little by the procedures. Fourteen were able to give significant clues about how they handled the procedure. Explanations included deliberate use of the following before and during the procedure: muscle contraction, e.g., clenching the fist or gripping the side of the table; screaming *prior* to pain, i.e., the needle injection; conversation, especially humorous and lively; religion, e.g., prayer; and fantasy, e.g., drinking a milkshake, and watching a television program (Hilgard and LeBaron, 1984).

For painful procedures, a pop-up book may be especially suitable for the toddler. It has the advantage of providing multiple new and novel stimuli that is helpful in recapturing the child's attention whenever he focuses on the painful procedure. The child may stop looking at the book at times and watch the painful procedure or make some remark about it, but attention is fairly easily returned with a new pop-up. Being able to name the pictures in the book may also give the child a sense of achievement. The effectiveness of this distraction usually increases with practice or with experience using it in repeated painful procedures. Children report that the pop-up surprises seem to help the procedure go more quickly (Kuttner, 1986).

For children from 3 years of age through adolescence, listening to music or a story through a headset is highly effective during a variety of brief painful procedures (Eland, 1988b; Kuttner, 1986). Naturally, allowing the child to select the story or music helps increase the effectiveness.

To use humor, keep in mind that a child's sense of humor differs from the adult's. For example, Looney Tunes are usually much funnier to school-age children than to adults.

Maintaining normal sensory input. For children confined to bed, especially in a hospital, avoiding boredom can be a challenge. Putting up mirrors so the child can see around the room and outside the room may help. Whenever possible, move the bed to the hallway, playroom, or outside. Provide physical exercise for the extremities with games such as throwing (with hands or feet) bean bags or wadded paper into the wastebasket. A daily project might be decorating the bed as a spaceship or with pictures drawn daily or cards received in the mail. For many adolescents, a telephone is a necessary lifeline to the rest of the world.

Relaxation

Relaxation primarily reduces distress rather than pain, and it is not usually an appropriate substitute for pain relief measures such as analgesics. However, it is a helpful coping mechanism for children and adults. Those relaxation strategies discussed in Chapter 7 (pp. 188-211) that are useful for children 3 or 4 years of age and older include the deep breath/tense, exhale/relax, yawn exercise; humor; slow rhythmic breathing; progressive relaxation; and remembering peaceful past experiences. It is especially helpful to tape record the recollection of the pleasant memories.

The presence of the parent, especially the child's mother, is helpful in reducing distress associated with pain in almost all age groups. As soon as the child is able to recognize the parent, probably in early infancy, encourage the parent to stay with the child during painful procedures or ongoing pain, allowing the parent to touch, stroke, and hold the child whenever possible. From infancy up to age 4 years, the parent's holding of the child during painful procedures, such as IMs or lumbar punctures, has been shown to result in less distress (Brown, 1984; Hallstrom, 1968).

As an example, to hold an infant or toddler during a lumbar puncture the parent, most often the mother, is usually standing for the convenience of the person performing the puncture. The mother holds the child upright against her chest. The child's head rests on her shoulder, and his legs are wrapped around her waist. A small pillow is placed between the child's abdomen and the parent to help arch the child's back. The parent talks or hums to the child during preparation and the procedure (Brown, 1984).

Preterm infants. Certain interventions appear to reduce stress and promote self-regulation in these infants during or between painful or other stressful events. Bedding and clothing may consist of a water mattress, sheepskin, and rolls of cloth to provide boundaries similar to those in the womb. When painful procedures are performed, an effort can be made to avoid interrupting deep sleep and to sequence activities to allow time in between. During the procedure the infant can be shielded from light and placed in as comfortable a position as is possible, such as supported in the prone or side-lying positions (not lying on the back). The infant can be swaddled, allowed to suck, and provided with something to grasp (see additional suggestions in Als et al, 1986).

In preterm and older infants, pacifiers have been shown to help reduce crying during circumcision (Gunnar, Fisch, and Malone, 1984). Pacifiers are also offered to infants and toddlers to help reduce stress of ongoing pain. Sometimes they contain sugar and whiskey.

Toddlers and older children. Blowing bubbles is an especially effective technique, providing both relaxation and distraction. Most children are familiar with this game. The child can count the bubbles as they float around the room, burst them, blow them around, or simply watch what happens to them. Or, blowing alone may be helpful. The child can be instructed to take a deep breath and slowly blow away anything that bothers him, such as hurt or scarey feelings. Ideally this is taught prior to a painful event (Kuttner, 1986).

Bubble blowing may evolve into a form of slow rhythmic breathing without the bubbles. During a painful procedure, particularly one where the child must be very still or a sterile field is required, the bubbles may not be possible, but the technique can then be done without the bubbles. The young child may not be able to be distracted or to relax during the actual painful procedure, but the bubbles or slow breathing may reduce anxiety prior to the procedure.

Imagery

Imagery techniques designed to relieve pain are discussed in Chapter 8 (pp. 212-230). Those that may be adapted for toddlers and older children include conversational imagery, breathing out pain, the ball of healing energy, and an individualized imagery technique.

Examples of possible conversational imagery with the older child are suggestions to imagine medication traveling through the body to the pain or imagine blowing out the hurt with each exhalation. For a headache, the child can be instructed to gently blow air, e.g., enough to cause thin paper to flutter, and imagine his headache getting smaller and smaller each time he blows out.

Retelling or playing a tape recording of the child's favorite story during a painful procedure can be particularly effective. Prior to a painful event, if possible, find out what story is the child's favorite, or ask if he has a favorite outing such as going to Disneyland. If the story or outing is unfamiliar to you, ask the child to tell you about it. During pain, the child can become involved in this, closing his eyes and pretending to be there in his imagination. The nurse can help the child become actively involved in this imagery by asking questions about what he sees, where he goes, and suggesting different possibilities, such as asking if the house in the story could be made of candy. The favorite story technique seems to be effective in reducing distress during painful procedures for children as young as 3 years of age, but does not significantly reduce pain (Kuttner, 1988). (This form of imagery seems to be distracting and relaxing, and it may also produce dissociation from the pain.)

Chronic Pain

Children suffer from almost all the various forms of chronic pain that occur in adults, e.g., recurrent acute pain as in migraine and chronic nonmalignant pain as in musculoskeletal problems. (See pp. 19-20 for classifications of chronic pain.) Of course, prolonged cancer pain occurs from infancy through adulthood, but some types of chronic pain are more common with children, e.g., recurrent abdominal pain. However, chronic pain in children, except for cancer pain, has received very little attention. Although there are numerous multidisciplinary pain clinics for adults, very few exist for children.

Cancer pain in children is treated according to the same principles involved in treating adults. A considerable amount of literature addresses relief of cancer pain in children, particularly procedural pain, e.g., bone marrow aspirations. Pharmacological approaches are similar to those recommended for adults, and are discussed earlier in this chapter.

Examples of chronic noncancer pain in children include colic, cystic fibrosis, hemophilia, burns, headaches, recurrent abdominal pain, reflex sympathetic dystrophy, juvenile arthritis (JA, juvenile rheumatoid arthritis, juvenile chronic polyarthritis), and sickle cell disease. Some of the approaches suggested in Chapter 9 (pp. 232-263) are helpful. For example, the number and severity of chronic migraine and nonmigrainous headaches may be reduced in adolescents by teaching them relaxation techniques (Larsson et al, 1987).

Recurrent abdominal pain is one of the most common types of chronic nonmalignant pain in children. Recently a simple approach proved effective in 52 children 5 to 15 years of age. Fewer attacks of recurrent abdominal pain occurred after only 6 weeks on a simple regimen of two corn fiber cookies per day (McGrath and Feldman, 1986).

Sickle cell crisis, on the other hand, must usually be relieved with IV narcotics (for specific guidelines see annotated reference Cole, Sprinkle, Smith, and Buchanan, 1986). IV PCA may be especially appropriate. Unfortunately, lack of knowledge of pharmacology and exaggerated fears of addiction have interfered with pain relief and research in this area (Schechter, Berrien, and Katz, 1988).

When pain is prolonged in the child, achievement of age-related developmental tasks may be hampered. For example, pain may adversely affect motor development in the infant, play in the toddler, and peer relationships in the adolescent. Special efforts are required to decrease the intensity of the pain and teach the child coping mechanisms such as relaxation and distraction. For example, a comprehensive program has been used for management of chronic nonmalignant pain in children from preschool age through adolescence. Increased adherence to rehabilitation programs has been successfully achieved with techniques such as guided imagery, relaxation, and modification of environmental factors that influence pain behaviors (Varni, Jay, Masek, and Thompson, 1986). An increase in nonpain behaviors and the ability to avoid crying during a procedure probably also increase the child's self-esteem.

Adolescents may tend to report more pain than school-age children (Beales, Kean, and Lennox-Holt, 1983). This may be especially true when pain is chronic and not the result of a visible injury. Past experience with chronic pain may contribute to increased expression of pain because chronic pain may affect the child's life in ways that increase the child's awareness of the meaning of pain, e.g., decreased activity of juvenile arthritis.

When a child of any age is very expressive in response to prolonged or recurrent pain, there is sometimes a temptation to ignore the child's behavioral responses in an effort to decrease the intensity or frequency of the behavior. Such an approach can easily lead to one of the historical problems in managing pain in adults—trying to minimize expression of pain without trying to relieve pain. This results from the health care system holding the health team responsible for controlling a patient's expression of pain without being held responsible for relieving the pain (see pp. 1-2).

In both children and adults with pain it is essential to remember the following about the relationship between behavioral expression and presence of pain:
- Lack of expression of pain does not necessarily mean lack of pain.
- Minimizing behavioral response to pain by ignoring the behavior does not relieve the pain. Adults may be more

comfortable if the child stops crying or clinging, but simply ignoring this behavior is not an appropriate way to change the behavior.
- If behavioral responses to pain are used by the child to gain attention or some other reward, the desired and appropriate rewards should be given to the child in situations other than pain.
- The best way to minimize behavioral response to pain is to relieve the pain or help the child learn ways of making the pain more tolerable.

The child's responses to pain must be met with appropriate attention and concern along with suggestions and efforts to relieve the pain or make it more bearable. When a child has pain, no matter how he expresses or responds to the pain, the child deserves our respect.

RESOURCES FOR CHILDREN, PARENTS, AND NURSES

American Academy of Pediatrics, Committee on the Fetus and the Newborn, 141 Northwest Point Blvd, Elk Grove Village, IL 60007. Write them to express your opinion to the medical community on the issue of withholding anesthesia from infants.

American Association of Critical-Care Nurses (AACN), Neonatal and Pediatric Special Interest Group. This group distributes a free brochure for parents of critically ill newborns or premature infants that suggests questions parents may wish to discuss with the health team regarding the issue of anesthesia for infants and lists the rights of the parents. Write: AACN, 1 Civic Plaza, Newport Beach, CA 92660; phone: 714-644-9310.

Biomedical Ethics Board, US Congress, 2311 Rayburn Bldg, Washington, DC, 20515. Write them to express your opinion to the government and the medical community on the issue of withholding anesthesia from infants.

The Candlelighters Childhood Cancer Foundation. This is an international network of groups of parents of children with cancer. Membership is also open to anyone interested in the control and cure of childhood cancer and in meeting the needs of families facing this experience. Various publications and activities are provided, including "Myths About Pain in Children" by Jo Eland, which may be ordered by asking for Progress Reports, vol 5, no 1, 1985 and enclosing $0.50. Write: 1901 Pennsylvania Ave, NW, Suite 1001, Washington, DC 20006; phone: 202-659-5136.

Children's Hospice International. They provide various materials for parents and health professionals regarding care of the dying child, especially in the home. Write: 501 Slaters Lane, #207, Alexandria, VA 22314; phone: 703-556-0421. Hotline to respond directly to children, their families, or their caregivers: 1-800-242-4453.

Crygone. This audio pacifier cassette combines womb sounds, e.g., amniotic fluid swoosh and mother's heart beat, with music and subliminal calming affirmations. Babies as young as premature infants seem to find these sounds relaxing and respond by ceasing to cry and going to sleep. It is suggested for any babies prone to prolonged crying periods, including colicky babies. An accompanying booklet for mothers con-

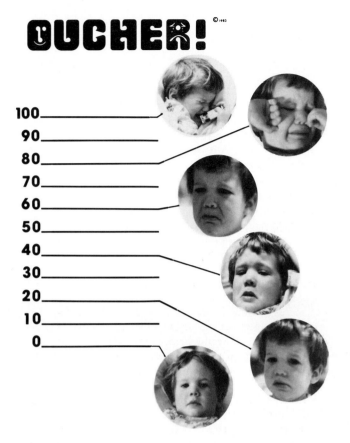

OUCHER! ©1983

100
90
80
70
60
50
40
30
20
10
0

FIGURE 10-4 The Oucher, copyright 1983 by the University of Virginia. Reprinted with permission.

tains tips on how to improve the baby's physical comfort. (Note: The manufacturers state that this is repeatedly effective, but no research is cited.) Approximately $16.95. Order from: Lee Enterprises, Suite 2406N, 5410 Palafox, Pensacola, FL 32505.

No Fears, No Tears: Children with Cancer Coping with Pain. Educational video prepared primarily for parents, but also appropriate for health team members. It features nine patients, ranging in age from 2½ to 15 years old, using noninvasive pain relief measures such as distraction and imagery as they undergo various painful procedures. A written guide accompanies the video. Available for purchase, approximately $45.00 (US) for both video and booklet. Write: Canadian Cancer Society, BC/Yukon Division, 955 W Broadway, Vancouver, BC, V5Z 3X8, Canada. Reprints of a publication reporting research on some of the techniques (Kuttner, 1988, below) is available by writing: Leora Kuttner, PhD, #204-1089 W Broadway, Vancouver, BC V6H 1E5, Canada.

The Oucher. Several studies (e.g., Beyer and Aradine, 1988) support the content and construct validity of this tool for self-reporting of pain intensity in white children ages 3 to 12 years. Although research on its use with nonwhite children has not been completed, the tool may be offered to these children. A small picture of this much larger posterlike scale is shown in

Fig. 10-4 (actual size is approximately 11 inches wide and 16 inches tall). The two scales, numerical and photographic faces, facilitate its use by children of varied ages and abilities. Those who can count to 100 may use the numerical scale, and those who cannot may use the six faces. Since this tool is copyrighted, the reader must order this. Parents may find it helpful in the home care of children with pain, or the tool might be posted in several places in a facility caring for children, e.g., treatment rooms where painful procedures are performed. For a copy of the Oucher scale, user's manual, and technical report, send $9.95 to Judith E Beyer, RN, PhD, Associate Professor, University of Colorado Health Sciences Center, School of Nursing, Campus Box C288, 4200 East Ninth Ave, Denver, CO 80262.

Pediatric Projects. A nonprofit group that develops and distributes medical toys and books that help children understand health care. Books for parents and health professionals are also available. For a free catalog, write: Pediatric Projects Incorporated, PO Box 1880, Santa Monica, CA 90406-1880; phone: 213-828-8963.

The Rainbow Dream. This audio cassette tape ($8.95), accompanied by a guide, tells a story that teaches relaxation and mental imagery to children. Write: Minneapolis Children's Medical Center, 910 E 26th St, Suite 410, Minneapolis, MN 55404; phone: 612-874-6798.

SleepTight. This consists of two separate units that produce an effect that feels and sounds like a car ride. One unit simulates the vibrating, rhythmic motion of a car. The other unit is battery powered and simulates the rushing sound of wind passing by a closed car window. Research on use of comparable vibration and/or sound for 60 infants with colic showed significant relief of colic severity in 97%, usually within 4 to 9 minutes (Loadman et al, 1987). It also reduces parental stress. To order, send $69.95 plus applicable sales tax and shipping charges, to: SleepTight, Inc, 3613 Mueller Rd, St Charles, MO, 63301; phone toll free: 1-800-325-3550; in Missouri call collect 314-946-5132.

Troches. A variety of drugs, including narcotics, may be compounded as troches. They are similar to hard candy and come in different flavors. They may be chewed, sucked, or placed under the tongue. This is an ideal formulation for children who have difficulty swallowing pills. For information about compounding drugs in troches (or suppositories) contact Technical Staff, Professional Compounding Centers of America, PO Box 368, Sugarland, TX 77487; phone: 1-800-331-2498.

SELECTED ANNOTATED REFERENCES THAT CITE RESEARCH OR GIVE CLINICAL SUPPORT

Als, H: Toward a synactive theory of development: promise for the assessment and support of infant individuality, *Infant Mental Health J* 3:229-243, Winter 1982. A theoretical model to understand and assess the individual preterm infant, 24-27 weeks postconception, is presented. The focus is on the dynamic, continuous interplay of various subsystems: autonomic, motor, state organizational, attentional-interactive, and self-regulatory. Specific interventions are suggested for accomplishing the goal of decreasing the stress accompanying manipulation of the infant and enhancing stabilization. Suggestions include introducing stimuli to the baby during a transition state and avoiding introduction of stimuli when the baby is soundly asleep or quietly alert, helping the infant into a flexed position, providing a soft, graspable roll for both hands, facing the baby away from a direct light source, avoiding the supine position, avoiding eye contact with certain infants during feeding, and being alert to cues that too much input is being provided. Such cues include the infant yawning, averting his gaze, sneezing, or hiccoughing. Tables of stress reactions and of self-regulatory behaviors are included.

Anand, KJS, and Hickey, PR: Pain and its effects in the human neonate and fetus, *N Engl J Med* 317:1321-1329, Nov 19, 1987. This review of the literature includes 201 references to pain in the human fetus and neonate. Based on the findings of numerous studies, the authors state some of the following conclusions in an attempt to help correct widespread misconceptions about the fetus or neonate not feeling pain. Cutaneous sensory receptors have spread to all cutaneous and mucous surfaces by the 20th week of gestation, and the density of nociceptive nerve endings in the skin of newborns is similar to or greater than that in adult skin. Also, by 20 weeks the fetal neocortex has a full complement of neurons, and several tests suggest functional maturity. Lack of myelination does not support the argument that neonates are not capable of pain perception. Even in the peripheral nerves of adults, nociceptive impulses are carried through unmyelinated fibers. Incomplete myelination merely implies a slower conduction velocity in the nerves, which is offset completely in the neonate by the shorter distances traveled by the impulses. They conclude, "Thus, human newborns do have the anatomical and functional components required for the perception of painful stimuli" (p 1323). Regarding memory of pain, they point out that even adults cannot remember pain, only the experiences associated with pain. Further, memory and learning depend on brain plasticity, which is known to be highest during the late prenatal and neonatal periods.

Studies of neonates undergoing painful procedures reveal changes in cardiovascular variables, transcutaneous partial pressure of oxygen, and palmar sweating. Local anesthesia for circumcision prevents changes in heart rate, blood pressure, and decreases in transcutaneous partial pressure of oxygen, but use of a pacifier during heel stick does not alter the preterm neonates cardiovascular or respiratory responses to pain. Detailed hormonal studies in preterm and full-term neonates undergoing surgery with minimal anesthesia document marked metabolic stress responses that can be inhibited by potent anesthetics such as halothane and fentanyl. In fact, preliminary evidence suggests that neonates having light anesthesia during major cardiac surgery have increased postoperative morbidity and mortality. Evidence for increased sensitivity to pain with decreased age includes several studies of the cry response to painful procedures in neonates and older infants (3 to 12 months). The authors conclude that the evidence shows that "marked nociceptive activity clearly constitutes a physiologic and perhaps even a psychological form of stress in premature or full-term neonates" (p 1320.)

Anand, KJS, Sippell, WG, and Aynsley-Green, A: Randomized trial of fentanyl anaesthesia in preterm babies undergoing surgery: effects on the stress response, *Lancet* 1:62-66, Jan 10, 1987. In a study of preterm infants undergoing ligation of patent ductus arteriosus (PDA) and anesthetized with nitrous oxide and d-tubocurarine, 8 with fentanyl (10 µg/kg IV) added

and 8 without fentanyl, major hormonal responses to surgery were significantly greater in the non-fentanyl than in the fentanyl group. Some responses remained greater in the non-fentanyl group on the third postoperative day. Compared with the fentanyl group, the non-fentanyl group were more likely to require an increase in ventilatory support after surgery and to have circulatory or metabolic complications. Two in the non-fentanyl group developed intraventricular hemorrhages during or soon after surgery. The authors conclude that the substantial stress response to surgery under anesthesia with nitrous oxide and curare can be prevented by the addition of fentanyl and this may improve postoperative outcome. They also conclude that the degree of analgesia in paralyzed and ventilated infants can be assessed reliably only by measurement of the biochemical and endocrine markers of stress. The authors cite studies showing that surgical stress responses last longer in preterm than in full-term babies and are greater in magnitude than those of adult patients. Further analysis of 40 published reports showed that 77% of newborn babies undergoing surgical ligation of PDA received either muscle relaxants alone or with nitrous oxide given intermittently.

Beasley, SW, and Tibballs, J: Efficacy and safety of continuous morphine infusion for postoperative analgesia in the paediatric surgical ward, *Aust NZ J Surg* 57:233-237, Apr 1987. Continuous infusion of morphine following major surgery in 121 nonventilated children resulted in few side effects with adequate pain relief as rated by the patient, if able, and the parents and nurses. The article includes the protocol for morphine infusion. A therapeutic range of 10-40 µg/kg/hr was used, usually starting at 20-25 µg/kg/hr. The age ranged from less than 1 year (13 infants, 4 weighing less than 5 kg) to 14 years. Only 26 of the 121 patients had complications attributed to morphine, the most frequent problem being vomiting (27 patients). Respiratory depression did not occur in any patient. The authors recommend continuous morphine infusion as a routine method of analgesia for children following major surgery.

Beaver, PK: Premature infants' response to touch and pain: can nurses make a difference? *Neonatal Network* 6:13-17, Dec 1987. Intraventricular hemorrhage (IVH) is a major cause of death among premature infants. Decreasing crying and hypoxic episodes may decrease the incidence of IVH. Thus, painful stimuli may be life threatening if they result in crying in these neonates. This study of 8 premature infants exposed to touch only, heel lance only, and heel lance plus stroking on the medial side of the same leg, revealed that the latter situation caused the greatest increase in heart rate and blood pressure and decrease in transcutaneous oxygenation. The greatest percentage of change from baseline for both heart rate and blood pressure occurred during the first 10 seconds after the stimuli. The author suggests that to reduce the magnitude of the premature's response to stimulation, stimulation might be done as quickly as possible and the infant allowed to recover before being exposed to the next set of stimuli.

Bell, SG, and Ellis, LJ: Use of fentanyl for sedation of mechanically ventilated neonates, *Neonatal Network* 6:27-31, Oct 1987. This article combines a good review of the literature with the authors' clinical experience. It is fairly common practice to use low to moderate doses (2-4 µg/kg) for sedation of the mechanically ventilated infant who is agitated and/

or in pain. Neonates' responses to noxious stimuli include agitation, cyanosis, bradycardia, hypoxia, and hypercarbia. Advantages of fentanyl for neonates is a faster onset and shorter duration than morphine. Given IV it has an almost immediate onset with peak respiratory depression occurring in 5-10 minutes. These authors have successfully used fentanyl for sedation and pain relief in both ventilated and nonventilated infants, e.g., for postoperative pain or one time doses for painful procedures such as insertion of a chest tube. For sedation they recommend fentanyl 2-4 μg/kg given IV over a minimum of 2 minutes (preferably over 15 minutes to avoid respiratory muscle rigidity), with frequency determined on an individual basis. Because fentanyl binds to tissues, the infant must be observed for rebound fentanyl plasma levels. As with all narcotics, there is a risk of seizure activity. Fentanyl should be avoided in patients who are hypotensive or have impaired hepatic function. During the initial administration of fentanyl to the ventilated infant, a respiratory therapist probably should be present to evaluate the need for changing ventilatory settings. When fentanyl is discontinued after prolonged use, the infants should be observed for signs of withdrawal syndrome.

Beyer, JE, and Aradine, CR: Patterns of pediatric pain intensity: a methodological investigation of a self-report scale, *Clin J Pain* 3:130-141, 1987. This study of 95 hospitalized children 3-12 years old supported the construct validity of a self-report scale called the Oucher, copyrighted in 1983 by The University of Virginia. (Construct validity is the degree to which an instrument measures the concept, e.g., pain under investigation.) For more information on the Oucher, see p. 296 and Figure 10-4.

Bikhazi, GB: Comparison of morphine and nalbuphine in postoperative pediatric patients, *Anesthesiol Rev* 5:34-36, July 1978. The method of pain assessment is not clear, but the author states that in 41 children 1 to 15 years of age who underwent circumcision, there was no significant difference between nalbuphine (a narcotic agonist-antagonist) and morphine on a milligram to milligram basis (0.1-0.12 mg/kg IM). Both were safe and effective methods of pain relief. He recommends nalbuphine because unlike morphine, it apparently has a ceiling on respiratory depression, and unlike pentazocine (another narcotic agonist-antagonist), it does not have psychomimetic effects.

Billmire, DA, Neale, HW, and Gregory, RO: Use of IV fentanyl in the outpatient treatment of pediatric facial trauma, *J Trauma* 25:1079-1080, Nov 1985. For repair of facial lacerations in 2000 children between the ages of 12 months and 12 years, a dose of 2 to 3 μg/kg body weight was administered slowly intravenously to provide sedation and analgesia. The rapid onset and short duration (30 to 40 minutes) of fentanyl make it advantageous for use in brief painful procedures where rapid recovery is desired. The IV dose was administered over 3 to 5 minutes since more rapid administration may result in paralysis of the respiratory muscles or apnea. Peak respiratory depression from fentanyl may not occur for 5 to 15 minutes. Only 3 apneic episodes occurred and all were successfully reversed with naloxone. Interestingly, the authors report that children 18 to 36 months usually required the full calculated dose while older children usually required less than the calculated dose. Facial pruritus was a minor problem. Few difficulties were encountered with nausea and vomiting, and

there were no episodes of delirium or muscular rigidity. Local anesthesia was used after fentanyl became effective. An additional benefit of using fentanyl was that the children were less fearful when they returned for suture removal.

Brown, SR: An anxiety reduction technique during lumbar punctures in infants and toddlers, *J Assn Pediatr Oncol Nurs* 1:24-25, Summer 1984. In 8 children between the ages of 1 and 4 years, a total of 25 lumbar punctures were performed with the mother holding the child upright in her arms with a pillow at the child's abdomen to help arch the back. The children exhibited minimal crying and movement, and the parents were pleased to be able to offer comfort.

Burne, R, and Hunt, A: Use of opiates in terminally ill children, *Palliative Med* 1:27-30, 1987. A review of the records of 21 children, ranging in age from infancy to 14 years, who received morphine or diamorphine (heroin) during terminal care, revealed that the highest four hourly doses were in the young age group, 1 to 4 years. The doses included the equivalent of 360 mg of morphine PO q4h in one child and 240 mg q4h in another. High doses also occurred in the age group 5 to 9 years, with one child receiving 150 mg q4h and another receiving 90 mg q4h. These doses were determined by titration according to the individual's response. Respiratory depression was not seen in any child. Routine administration of laxatives, but not antiemetics, is likely to be necessary in children receiving strong opiates.

Burokas, L: Factors affecting nurses' decisions to medicate pediatric patients after surgery, *Heart Lung* 14:373-379, July 1985. A self-administered questionnaire survey of 134 nurses employed in pediatric units revealed that only 12% reported complete pain relief as their goal; 61.2% reported relief as much pain as possible as their goal. About 50% of the PICU and ICN nurses indicated that the pain relief needs of their patients were not met. Nurses in this study were not influenced by their own previous pain experience, but having offspring who have experienced pain did influence nurses to chose to medicate pediatric patients more frequently after surgery. However, what influenced the nurses most was their goal in relieving pain. Those who believed in relieving as much pain as possible choose more often to give an analgesic rather than use nonpharmacological pain relief measures. Those nurses who did not expect complete pain relief more often chose nonpharmacological pain relief. A review of 40 charts of children who ranged in age from neonate to 10 years revealed that following surgery only two received all the doses of analgesic that could have been administered throughout their postoperative course. Five children ages 2 days to 5 years received no doses of narcotics; these included ruptured appendectomy in a 5-year-old and PDA ligation in 2 infants. Another five children ages 6 months to 10 years received only one dose of narcotic postoperatively.

Cole, TB, Sprinkle, RH, Smith, SJ, and Buchanan, GR: Intravenous narcotic therapy for children with severe sickle cell crisis pain, *Am J Dis Child* 140:1255-1259, 1986. The records of 38 children and adolescents (age range not specified) with 98 episodes of sickle cell vaso-occlusive crisis were reviewed, in which 76 episodes were treated with a continuous IV narcotic infusion. The authors used a protocol consisting of bolus IV injection of 0.15 mg/kg morphine or 1.0 mg/kg meperidine upon arrival at the hospital, followed by narcotic continuous infusion at a dose rate of 0.07 to 0.10 mg/kg/hr morphine or

0.5 to 0.7 mg/kg/hr meperidine, with bolus injections as needed, titrated upward by increments of about 25% q3h until satisfactory pain relief was achieved (usually based on ratings by patient or the parents). Patient comfort was usually achieved in a little over 3 hours after the protocol was initiated. Narcotic infusions usually continued for about 72 hours, and then some were stopped abruptly and others tapered with doses of oral acetaminophen with codeine. Seizures did not occur with meperidine, as had been reported by others, but the authors specify that they did not use phenothiazines as did the others because phenothiazines lower seizure threshold and do not enhance analgesia. Side effects of narcotic therapy were frequent, especially lethargy, but not serious. No addictive behavior was observed in any patients.

Dale, JC: A multidimensional study of infants' responses to painful stimuli, *Pediatr Nurs* 12:27-31, Jan-Feb 1986. Ten infants age 6 weeks to 6 months of age were videotaped during DPT injections. In response to the injections, all infants cried and initially opened their mouths wide. Nine infants kicked their legs. Eight infants had increased heart rates while two had decreases.

Dilworth, NM, and MacKellar, A: Pain relief for the pediatric surgical patient, *J Pediatr Surg* 22:264-266, Mar 1987. In 144 patients ranging in age from 6 months to 15 years who received 155 variable-rate IV narcotic infusions, respiratory rate dropped below the set minimum in only one patient. Reduction of drug dosage was sufficient and naloxone was not required. Restriction of movement troubled the 1 to 2 year old children and sometimes led to early termination of the IV. In an additional 242 infusions in children, only one patient suffered respiratory depression and required a small dose of naloxone. Contrary to the fears of medical and nursing staff, respiratory depression was very infrequent, promptly recognized, and easily corrected. The authors discuss other methods of postoperative pain relief and stress the importance of including this in pediatric surgical textbooks.

Dothage, JA, Arndt, C, and Miser, AW: Use of continuous intravenous morphine infusion for pain control in an infant with terminal malignancy, *J Assn Pediatr Oncol Nurs* 3:22-24, 1986. In a 10-month-old, 8-kg infant with prolonged cancer pain, the dose of IV morphine required to relieve pain seemed to be successfully titrated by using two independent observers (the mother and the nurse) who rated pain on a visual analog scale using behaviors that predictably varied with tumor size and analgesic administration. Behaviors that indicated pain and that improved with increased narcotic dose were holding the painful area, failure to move the painful limb, decrease in general activity, poor sleep, poor food intake, fretfulness, and crying. Physiological parameters, which have been shown to change in newborns in response to acute pain, were not reliable. At the time of his death the continuous IV infusion dose of morphine had remained at 0.25 mg/hr for 2 days. At this dose the mother could hold him without his crying out in pain, and he seemed to sleep comfortably, ate small amounts, and occasionally smiled at his parents.

Eland, JM: Children's pain: developmentally appropriate efforts to improve identification of source, intensity and relevant intervening variables. In Felton, G, and Albert, M, eds: Nursing research: a monograph for non-nurse researchers, pp 64-79, Iowa City, 1983, U of Iowa Press. This publication cites research data regarding the least painful injection site as being the ventrogluteal muscle. The vastus lateralis is more painful, and the rectus is the most painful of the three. (See also Eland, 1988a.)

Eland, JM: Minimizing pain associated with prekindergarten intramuscular injections, *Issues Comp Pediatr Nurs* 5:361-372, 1981. In a sample of 20 male and 20 female children between the ages of 4 years 9 months and 5 years 9 months the amount of pain expressed following DPT immunization was compared under four different conditions immediately prior to injection: Frigiderm sprayed on the injection site versus compressed air sprayed on the leg, and cognitive information versus no information about the spray and its purpose. The least pain occurred after Frigiderm spray, with or without cognitive information. Cognitive information made very little difference, possibly because the nurses giving the information did not believe the Frigiderm would help. Both Frigiderm and cognitive information seem indicated in procedures such as venipuncture and other injections. This article also includes data from a previous study, conducted in about 1974, of 242 hospitalized children between the ages of 4 and 10 who were asked, "Of all the things that have hurt you, which was the worst?" 49% answered "needle" or "shot." Six of the children giving this answer had undergone at least 25 surgical procedures.

Forlini, J, Morin, DM, and Treacy, S: Painless peds procedures, *Am J Nurs* 87:321-323, Mar 1987. The authors report on the use of the ultra–short-acting anesthetic ketamine for brief procedural pain in children as young as 7 months. Appropriate procedures include lumbar puncture, intrathecal chemotherapy, bone marrow aspiration, removal of an indwelling central catheter, laryngoscopy, burn debridement, circumcision, and dental work. Usually it is given IV, and loss of consciousness occurs in about 30 seconds and lasts approximately 10 minutes.

Franck, LS: A new method to quantitatively describe pain behavior in infants, *Nurs Res* 35:28-31, 1986. At 4 hours of age, the responses of 10 newborns to heelsticks were videotaped for analysis. The responses consisted of two components: immediate withdrawal of both legs followed by facial grimacing and crying. This is similar to the first and second pain experienced by adults. All infants demonstrated active avoidance of the stimulus, and seven used the unaffected leg to "swipe" at the site of pain. Eight of the neonates were able to quiet themselves within 3 minutes after the heelstick, which is probably an indication of gestational maturity. The author notes that many premature infants and neurologically damaged infants have difficulty recovering after stimulation.

Gaffney, A, and Dunne, EA: Children's understanding of the causality of pain, *Pain* 29:91-104, 1987. The responses of 680 Irish children, aged 5 to 14 years, showed that they frequently misinterpreted pain to be the result of transgressive or careless behavior. While this may be partly because parents use painful strategies to discipline children, it seems more likely that these misconceptions arise from the limited cognitive development of this age group. Transgression explanations offered by these children about the cause of pain included eating too much, running too much, carelessness, and disobedience.

Greene, RF, Miser, AW, Lester CM, Balis, FM, and Poplack, DG: Cerebrospinal fluid and plasma pharmacokinetics of morphine infusions in pediatric cancer patients and rhesus monkeys, *Pain* **30**:339-348, 1987. Morphine pharmacokinetics were studied during 21 infusions in 17 pediatric cancer patients with either mucositis or tumor-related pain. A wide dosage range (0.04 to 31 mg/kg/hr) was required for pain relief. No evidence for morphine accumulation was observed. The therapeutic usefulness of continuous long-term morphine infusions was supported. One infusion continued for 5 months (154 days).

Grunau, RVE, and Craig, KD: Pain expression in neonates: facial action and cry, *Pain* **28**:395-410, 1987. This study of 140 neonates, average age of 43.05 hours, revealed that responses to heel lance were complex and varied according to how the infant was handled. Facial activities of taut tongue and vertical stretch mouth were reliable measures. Individual differences in the responses of the infants were evident.

Haslam, DR: Age and the perception of pain, *Psychon Sci* **15**: 86-87, 1969. This is one of the few studies that addresses the issue of pain perception in relation to age in children. Using increasing pressure to the tibia to cause pain, the pain thresholds of 115 well school children aged 5 to 18 years were measured. The results indicated that pain threshold increases between the ages of 5 and 18, indicating that the perception of pain begins to decline at a very early age. In other words, between the ages of 5 and 18, the younger the child, the lower his pain threshold and the more pain he feels. (These findings are in direct opposition to the common belief that younger children feel less pain than older children and adults.)

Hatch, DJ: Analgesia in the neonate, *Br Med J* **294**:920, Apr 1987. This author notes that there is increasing acceptance that neonatal pain requires treatment. He states that narcotics are safe in babies being ventilated and suggests that severe pain in spontaneously breathing neonates may justify elective tracheal intubation and ventilation while opioids are given. He also suggests that infusion of narcotics may be safer than bolus doses.

Howland, MA, and Goldfrank, L: Meperidine usage in patients with sickle cell crisis, *Ann Emerg Med* **15**:1506-1507, Dec 1986. Meperidine cannot be considered a first-line analgesic for severe pain, especially if the development of tolerance requires high doses, because it is short acting and has an active metabolite, normeperidine, that may accumulate and cause CNS excitation, including seizures. Thus the use of meperidine with sickle cell patients is irrational. Another irrational use related to meperidine is "DPT" (Demerol, Phenergan, Thorazine) or the "Lytic Cocktail." Not only is meperidine a poor first choice as an analgesic, but these two phenothiazines may actually increase pain perception and increase the incidence of hypotension and sedation.

Izard, CE, Hembree, EA, Dougherty, LM, and Coss, CL: Changes in facial expressions of 2- to 19-month-old infants following acute pain, *Dev Psychol* **19**:418-426, 1983. In the first part of the study infants were videotaped while they received DPT immunization. The distress expression as an immediate response to pain (see Izard et al, 1980, below) was noted to decrease with age, and the anger expression (brows drawn downward and inward) as an immediate response to pain increased with age. In the second portion of the study the soothing time required following injection was studied. Infants differed significantly in the time required to soothe them and in the duration and pattern of their expressions.

Children who responded slowly to soothing showed a proportionately greater duration of anger expression than those who were soothed more rapidly. The distress and anger expression changed with age, as in the first study. Acute, unexpected pain seems to become an increasingly effective activator of anger with increasing age.

Izard, CE, Huebner, RR, Resser, D, McGinnes, G, and Dougherty, LM: The young infant's ability to produce discrete emotional expressions, *Dev Psychol* **16**:132-140, 1980. This article reports on a series of five studies. One finding concerned the facial expressions of infants during the first 6 months of life while they were receiving injections or having blood taken. The facial response to pain was characterized by lowering of the brow, broadening of the nasal root, an angular and squarish mouth, and tightly closed eyes. The facial response to anger was the same except that the eyes were open and staring. The reliability with which untrained observers identified the infants' various facial expressions confirms their social validity.

Jaffe, JH, and Martin, WR: Opioid analgesics and antagonists. In Gilman, AG, Goodman, LS, Wall, TW, and Murad, F, eds: Goodman and Gilman's The pharmacological basis of therapeutics, ed 7, pp 491-531, New York, 1985, Macmillan Publishing Co. On p 508, the dose of morphine for infants and children, IM or SC, is stated as 0.1 to 0.2 mg/kg (maximum 15 mg). By implication, this is meant to be an optimal initial dose. No references are cited.

Johnston, CC, and Strada, ME: Acute pain response in infants: a multidimensional description, *Pain* **24**:373-382, 1986. Responses of 14 infants, ages 2 and 4 months, undergoing routine immunization were observed. There was wide variability between infants, but facial expression was consistent among all the infants. The facial expression consisted of brows lowered and drawn together, bulging forehead with vertical furrows between the brows, a broadened nasal root, eyes tightly closed, and an angular, squarish mouth. The pattern of response was characterized by several phases: an initial drop in heart rate and a long, high-pitched cry followed by a period of apnea, rigid torso and limbs, and a facial expression of pain. This was followed by a sharp increase in heart rate, lower-pitched but dysphonated cries, less body rigidity, and a facial expression of pain, and finally a continued elevation in heart rate, lower-pitched and more rhythmic cries with a rising-falling pattern, and a return to normal body posture.

Katz, ER, Kellerman, J, and Siegel, SE: Behavioral distress in children with cancer undergoing medical procedures: developmental considerations, *J Consult Clin Psychol* **48**:356-365, 1980. An observational behavior rating scale was used to measure anxiety responses to bone marrow aspirations in 115 children with cancer, ages 8 months to 17 years and 9 months. A significant relationship was found between age and both quantity and type of anxious behavior, with younger children tending to respond with a greater variety of anxious behaviors over a longer period of time than older children. With advancing age the children responded with more withdrawal and muscle tension. These data clearly show that children do not "get used to" painful procedures.

Katz, ER, et al: Beta-endorphin immunoreactivity and acute behavioral distress in children with leukemia, *J Nerv Ment Dis* **170**:72077, 1982. Beta-endorphin levels were measured in 75 children with leukemia, ages 8 months to 18 years 4 months, undergoing routine lumbar puncture. Behavioral measures of distress included objective behavior, nurse ratings of anxiety, and self-reports of pain and fear. Results of the study support the hypothesis that pain and stress produce increased endorphin levels. In the children over 4 years of age, endorphin decreased with age, suggesting greater distress and pain in the younger children. Inconsistent results were obtained for children younger than 4 years of age, possibly because of antineoplastic chemotherapeutic variables. Interestingly, girls were found to have lower endorphin levels than boys, suggesting that boys may be biologically more adept at minimizing pain and stress because of their enhanced ability to produce endorphin. Alternatively, girls may have less need for endorphin because of better expressive abilities and less internal stress. All of these findings, of course, must be considered preliminary. Further research is needed.

Koren, G, Butt, W, Chinyanga, H, Soldin, S, Tan, Y-K, and Pape, K: Postoperative morphine infusion in newborn infants: assessment of disposition characteristics and safety, *J Pediatr* 107:963-967, 1985. Morphine plasma concentrations from bolus and continuous infusion IV for postoperative analgesia were studied in 12 neonates of gestational ages 35 to 41 weeks, weighing 2.2 to 4.21 kg, at postnatal ages ranging from 1 to 49 days. Plasma morphine concentrations tended to decrease in some patients receiving a constant infusion rate, suggesting improvement in morphine clearance rate. Elimination half-life of morphine (13.9 hrs, plus or minus 6.4 hrs) was significantly longer than in older children and adults (about 2 hrs). Morphine concentrations in neonates receiving 20 μg/kg/hr were 3 times higher than in older children receiving the same. Two infants who received 32 and 40 μg/kg/hr, respectively, developed generalized seizures. Apparently the newborn has greater sensitivity to morphine and a lower elimination rate. These authors suggest that infused dose of morphine in newborns should not exceed 15 μg/kg/hr. Because of the possibility of seizure, a loading bolus is not recommended. In several neonates, the authors report that serum concentrations of morphine increased despite cessation of the drug and they suggested this might be due to a mechanism that allows reabsorption of morphine.

Krishnan, A, Tolhurst-Cleaver, CL, and Kay, B: Controlled comparison of nalbuphine and morphine for post-tonsillectomy pain, *Anaesthesia* 12:1178-1181, 1985. Pain relief following tonsillectomy helps prevent crying and straining that might precipitate bleeding. Morphine 0.2 mg/kg IM, nalbuphine 0.3 mg/kg IM, and placebo were compared following tonsillectomy in 60 children between 4 and 12 years old. One of the drugs was administered 5 minutes before the conclusion of surgery. Pain, restlessness, and side effects were assessed 1 and 2 hours later. (It is not clear how pain was assessed.) No significant differences were found between the two narcotics. Drowsiness occurred but other side effects were uncommon. Nalbuphine may offer advantages compared with morphine in regard to safety. Choice of dose with nalbuphine is less critical than it is with morphine since nalbuphine has a proven maximal respiratory depressant effect.

Lynn, AM, Opheim, KE, and Tyler, DC: Morphine infusion after pediatric cardiac surgery, *Crit Care Med* 12:863-866, 1984. After cardiac surgery, 44 children, aged 14 months to 17 years, received a continuous IV infusion of morphine ranging from 10 to 50 μg/kg/hr, with the majority on 10 to 30 μg/kg/hr.

Lynn, AM, and Slattery, JT: Morphine pharmacokinetics in early infancy, *Anesthesiology* 66:136-139, 1987. Pharmacokinetic studies of morphine in ten infants showed longer elimination half-lives in those 1 to 4 days of age than in older infants 17 to 65 days of age, mean 6.8 hours and 3.9 hours, respectively. Clearance in the young ones was less than half that found in the older infants. The combination of lower clearance and longer elimination half-life in the newborns may explain the prolonged duration of action of morphine in very young infants. However, in infants older than 1 month of age, morphine clearance reaches or surpasses adult level, and they are not more sensitive to respiratory depressant effects of morphine than are adults.

Martinson, I, et al: Nursing care in childhood cancer: methadone, *Am J Nurs* 82:432-435, Mar 1982. Oral methadone doses for children ranging in age from 1 to 17 years included up to 10 mg q6h for a 1-year-old, 15 mg q6h for a 2-year-old, and up to 40 mg q8h for a 16- and 17-year-old. Children received methadone for 1 to 95 days.

McManus, M-J, and Panzarella, C: The use of dextroamphetamine to counteract sedation for patients on a morphine drip, *J Assn Pediatr Oncol Nurs* 3:28-29, 1986. These authors suggest that dextroamphetamine be considered in combination with morphine as a solution to the side effects, such as sedation, nausea, and respiratory depression. It also increases pain relief. It is available in tablets, elixir, or slow release capsules. They report on a 22-month-old whose pain was controlled with IV morphine but was heavily sedated. Adding dextroamphetamine 2.5 mg PO each morning enabled him to be awake and playing all day.

Miser, AW, Chayt, KJ, Sandlund, JT, Cohen, PS, Dothage, JA, and Miser, JS: Narcotic withdrawal syndrome in young adults after the therapeutic use of opiates, *Am J Dis Child* 140:603-604, June 1986. Five young adults, including one 14- and one 15-year-old, developed narcotic withdrawal 6 to 48 hours after abrupt discontinuation of narcotic therapy that had been administered for 6 to 21 days. The symptoms included agitation, irritability, muscular jerks, abdominal pain, diarrhea, burning sensations, "gooseflesh," and itching. Four of the patients, including the two adolescents, were successfully weaned without recurrence of withdrawal symptoms. The fifth patient was continued on methadone because of continuing pain. Important points include the fact that physical dependence on narcotics refers to an altered physiological state produced by prolonged or repeated exposure to a drug that results in withdrawal syndrome when the drug is abruptly discontinued. It is not addiction, defined as a behavioral pattern of drug use and overwhelming involvement with use of a drug. Further, cancer patients may frequently become physically dependent but rarely become addicted to narcotics. Families need to be assured that physical dependency is not synonymous with addiction. The etiology of physical dependence and the withdrawal symptoms that follow abrupt discontinuation of narcotics is not fully understood. However, continuous morphine infusion may more rapidly lead to physical dependence than an intermittent narcotic schedule. Several methods may be used to manage withdrawal symptoms. The authors chose to use oral methadone, a long-acting narcotic, given in a tapering schedule over approximately 5 days.*

Miser, AW, and Miser, JS: The use of oral methadone to control moderate and severe pain in children and young adults with malignancy, *Clin J Pain* 1:243-248, 1985. Based on this study of 19 patients, aged 4 to 23 years, receiving 22 courses of oral methadone, the safe starting dose appears to be 0.1 mg/kg q4h. Unlike reports of adult patients on methadone who often required a dose reduction due to accumulation, no patient in this study has evidence of drug accumulation. Days on methadone ranged from 2 to 267.

Nover, RA: Pain and the burned child, *J Am Acad Child Psychiatry* 12:499-505, July 1973. This is one of the early studies of children's reactions to pain. A case study of a 5-year-old boy with a 3% second and third degree burn on the leg and buttocks, but no sense of pain in the area due to a spinal cord anomaly, revealed this child reacted far less to the burn than other children who felt the sensation of pain. The child showed very little regressive tendency and no hostile behavior toward the staff. Consequently the author says that negative feelings of the staff toward the child were absent. (Apparently it was common for staff to react to burned children with judgments of "good and bad," failing to understand that the child's hostile behavior and lack of cooperation was due to pain.)

Owens, ME, and Todt, EH: Pain in infancy: neonatal reaction to heel lance, *Pain* 20:77-86, 1984. Responses in 20 2-day-old newborns to heel lance showed that crying and increased heart rate occurred consistently. Heart rate increased to an average of 179 beats per minute, a rise of 49 beats per minute, with this increase lasting an average of 3.5 minutes until a return to baseline.

Rogers, A: Narcotic drug therapy in children. In Management of cancer pain, pp 169-174, New York, 1985, Memorial Sloan-Kettering Cancer Center. The author reports that 4 children with cancer pain who had become tolerant to narcotics required doses as high as methadone 6 mg IV q2-3h (age 1½ years), morphine continuous IV infusion 24 mg/hr (age 4 years), Dilaudid continuous IV infusion 23 mg/hr (age 12 years), and methadone continuous IV infusion 55 mg/hr (age 12 years). General recommendations for initial narcotic doses compared with initial adult doses are one fifth to one quarter of that dose for ages 2 to 6 years, half that dose for ages 7 to 12 years, and the full adult dose thereafter. However, no research is cited to support these recommendations.

Rogers, BM, Webb, CJ, Stergios, D, and Newman, BM: Patient-controlled analgesia in pediatric surgery, *J Pediatr Surg* 23:259-262, Mar 1988. PCA (patient controlled analgesia) using IV boluses of morphine without continuous infusion, was evaluated in 15 children between 11 and 18 years old undergoing major abdominal or thoracic surgery. All were mentally alert, had no history of narcotic abuse, and were able to understand the instructions. Several different approaches to pain rating were used, and apparently satisfactory pain

*This reinforces the merit of an intermittent schedule of oral narcotics when this is possible. When IV narcotics are necessary, the health team should be alert to withdrawal syndrome and institute appropriate treatment. The higher likelihood of withdrawal syndrome with IV narcotics should not prohibit their use, since withdrawal can be successfully handled in several ways.

relief was obtained in all patients. Compared with 15 patients receiving the usual IM analgesia postoperatively, the 15 children on IV PCA self-administered about twice as much narcotic during the first 24 hours, but the dose was still well within the recommended therapeutic range. This finding is also typical of adult patients on IV PCA. No significant respiratory depression occurred. By the third day, the PCA patients were administering less analgesia than the comparison group receiving IM narcotics. (Authors' note: There was no evidence of narcotic abuse postoperatively in the group using IV PCA.) Only two patients did not like IV PCA, and both experienced burning at the site of infusion of morphine, which the researchers thought was due to rapid infusion of a relatively large bolus dose, i.e., greater than 2.5 mg. They conclude that the most satisfactory degree of analgesia is achieved with smaller doses of morphine at shorter lockout intervals. They suggest a loading dose of morphine 2 to 4 mg (0.05 to 0.10 mg/kg) and bolus doses of 1 to 2 mg (0.025 to 0.05 mg/kg) with a lockout interval of 10 to 15 minutes. (Authors' note: This study was done before most PCA pumps had the capacity for continuous infusion in addition to boluses. Based on the researchers' recommendations, a combination of continuous infusion with boluses as needed would probably be better than bolus alone.)

The advantages of PCA IV were that the child had control of analgesia and did not have to wait for nurses to bring doses. The children apparently had no difficulty understanding how to use PCA IV boluses. The researchers recommend PCA for patients 10 years of age or older and are now exploring the possibility of allowing responsible parents to use PCA IV to provide postoperative analgesia for younger children.

Ros, SP: Outpatient pediatric analgesia—a tale of two regimens, *Pediatr Emerg Care* 3:228-230, Dec 1987. The author compares the disadvantages of "DPT" (Demerol, Phenergan, Thorazine) with the advantages of IV fentanyl for brief painful procedures. A review of the literature reveals that there is no conclusive evidence that phenothiazines enhance the analgesic action of narcotics. In one study, DPT produced excessive central nervous system depression in the majority of patients, along with prolonged sedation or sleep, i.e., 7 hours or longer (Nahata, Clotz, and Knogg, 1985). Various other studies have shown that DPT results in sustained respiratory depression, hypotension, and lethargy.

By comparison, IV fentanyl (a narcotic analgesic reversible with naloxone) offers several advantages over DPT: rapid onset (90 to 120 seconds) and short duration of action (up to 40 minutes). Major complications of respiratory depression (including delayed respiratory depression), bradycardia, hypertension, and muscular rigidity have occurred only when fentanyl is used in large doses and/or rapidly injected. The author concludes that fentanyl in doses of 2 to 3 µg/kg is the preferred analgesic regimen for children undergoing painful procedures in the emergency department.

Ross, DM, and Ross, SA: Childhood pain: the school-aged child's viewpoint, *Pain* 20:179-191, 1984. Semistructured interviews of 994 children, age 5 to 12 years, revealed great diversity in children's preference for the timing of information about pain. The trend was for a preference toward having a longer rather than a shorter period between receiving information and the actual event. Parents in particular need to be aware of their child's preference. Only 213 children reported use of self-initiated strategies for coping with pain, with distraction and physical activity, such as fist clenching, being the more frequent.

Stang, HJ, Gunnar, MR, Snellman, L, Condon, LM, and Kestenbaum, R: Local anesthesia for neonatal circumcision: effects on distress and cortisol response, *JAMA* **259**:1507-1511, Mar 11, 1988. Although there is no absolute medical indication for routine circumcision of the newborn, it continues to be done in the United States and typically in the absence of anesthesia. Oddly, it is the only elective surgical procedure routinely performed without anesthesia. In a controlled, double-blind study of healthy male newborns, 60 subjects were randomly assigned to three groups for circumcision with lidocaine, saline, or no injection. The results revealed that dorsal penile nerve block was safe, easy, and effective in reducing behavioral distress and modifying the adrenocortical stress response. However, there was still discomfort and stress associated with circumcision. During the circumcision, babies in the lidocaine group cried 23% of the time, while babies in the saline and control groups cried 68% and 71% of the time, respectively, the latter two figures being striking increases in the percent of time crying compared with the injection period and the precircumcision nursery observation period. Overall, the lidocaine injection attenuated the adrenocortical response to circumcision, as compared with the response in the saline and no injection groups. Further, in the majority of instances, observers were able to correctly distinguish between infants who received saline and those who received lidocaine.

The process of injecting the lidocaine did not increase stress reactions and did not offset the beneficial effects of anesthesia. In fact, during the injection period (strapped on the restraint board 5 minutes before circumcision), the babies in the lidocaine and saline groups did not cry more than did the babies in the no-injection group. Thus the restraint itself caused as much crying as the injection. Several research studies are cited as evidence that the absence of crying following circumcision is the result of coping mechanisms, not a result of lack of postoperative pain. The authors state that if circumcisions are to be performed, they should be done as humanely as possible.

Stevens, MS: Which adolescents breeze through surgery? *Am J Nurs* **87**:1564-1565, Dec 1987. On the evening before elective surgery, interviews of 59 adolescents, aged 12 to 17 years, revealed that 40 were very frightened (a high-threat group), and 19 were mildly frightened or confident (a low-threat group). In the high-threat group, 60% reported frightening or painful previous hospitalizations and only 5% felt confident of their ability to manage pain, the remainder often saying that pain was out of their control and would have to be accepted.

Stewart, CF, and Hampton, EM: Effect of maturation on drug disposition in pediatric patients, *Clin Pharm* **6**:548-564, July 1987. Age-related changes in biotransformation (the chemical alterations that a substance undergoes in the body) are extremely complex. It is almost impossible to predict the effect of maturation on a biotransformation process based solely on the postnatal age of an infant. For most drugs, biotransformation is decreased in the neonate, increased from 1 to 5 years of age, and decreased after puberty, eventually reaching adult values. Maturational changes from infancy to adolescence have a more striking effect on drug response than do changes associated with aging. Still, biological maturation has a poorly understood effect on drug disposition. Children remain "therapeutic orphans," and many drugs marketed in the United States for adults have not been studied in children and thus carry the warning on the drug insert that safe drug usage has not been established for certain young age groups.

Williamson, PS, and Williamson, RN: Physiologic stress reduction by a local anesthetic during newborn circumcision, *Pediatrics* **71**:36-40, 1983. Circumcision in 2-day-old infants showed that penile nerve block attenuated heart rate increases and crying. Heart rate response to circumcision without anesthesia consisted of an average increase of 181 beats per minute, a rise of 54.1 beats per minute, with the average duration of increase lasting 3.5 minutes. There was more crying without anesthesia, and increased crying lasted up to several days.

Wong, DL, and Baker, CM: Pain in children: comparison of assessment scales, *Pediatr Nurs* **14**:9-17, Jan-Feb 1988. The validity, reliability, and preference of 6 pain assessment scales (simple descriptive, numeric of 0 to 10, faces, water glasses, chips, and colors) were investigated in 150 hospitalized children ages 3 to 18 years. With all scales, validity increased with advancing age. Reliability increased from the 3 to 7 year to the 8 to 12 year group, but decreased for most scales in the 13 to 18 year age group, suggesting the possibility that the younger children remembered pain more vividly than older children. The most preferred scale overall was the faces scale. Of the 116 events the children reported as painful, the most commonly reported were those involving needles, e.g., injections and venipuncture.

Wong, DL, and Whaley, LF: Clinical handbook of pediatric nursing, ed 2, St. Louis, 1986, The CV Mosby Co. This book is a practical guide to many aspects of caring for the child and his family. Specific information that is particularly helpful in caring for children with pain includes both general and age-specific guidelines for preparing children for procedures (pp 363 to 366), play activities for specific procedures (p 368), and suggestions for assessing and relieving pain in children (pp 372 to 378).

REFERENCES AND SELECTED READINGS

Als, H, Lawhon, G, Brown, E, Gibes, R, Duffy, FH, et al: Individualized behavioral and environmental care for the very low birth weight preterm infant at high risk for bronchopulmonary dysplasia: neonatal intensive care unit and developmental outcome, *Pediatrics* **78**:1123-1132, Dec 1986

Als, H, Lester, BM, Tronick, EZ, and Brazelton, TB: Toward a research instrument for the assessment of preterm infants' behavior (APIB). In Fitzgerald, H, Lester, BM, and Yogman, MW, eds: Theory and research in behavioral pediatrics **1**:35-63, New York, 1982, Plenum Press

Anand, KJS, and Aynsley-Green, A: Metabolic and endocrine effects of surgical ligation of patent ductus arteriosus in the human preterm neonate: are there implications for further improvement of postoperative outcome? *Mod Probl Paediatr* **23**:143-157, 1985

Anand, KJS, Brown, MJ, Causon, RC, Christofides, ND, Bloom, SR, and Aynsley-Green, A: Can the human neonate mount an endocrine and metabolic response to surgery? *J Pediatr Surg* 20:41-48, Feb 1985

Anand, KJS, et al: Studies on the hormonal regulation of fuel metabolism in the human newborn infant undergoing anesthesia and surgery, *Horm Res* 22:115-128, 1985

Anand, KJS, and McGrath, PJ: Neonatal pain and distress, Amsterdam, 1989, Elsevier Science Publishers, Inc (in press)

Anand, KJS, Sippell, WG, and Aynsley-Green, A: Randomized trial of fentanyl anaesthesia in preterm neonates undergoing surgery: effects on the stress response, *Lancet* 1:243-248, 1987

Aradine, CR, Beyer, JE, and Tompkins, JM: Children's pain perception before and after analgesia: a study of instrument construct validity and related issues, *J Pediatr Nurs* 3:11-23, Feb 1988

Axton, SE, and Fugate, T: A protocol for pediatric IV Meds, *Am J Nurs* 87:943-945, July 1987

Baker, CM, and Wong, DL: Q.U.E.S.T.: a process of pain assessment in children, *Orthopaed Nurs* 6:11-20, Jan-Feb 1987

Barker, W, Rodeheaver, GT, Edgerton, MT, and Edlich, RF: Damage to tissue defenses by a topical anesthetic agent, *Ann Emerg Med* 11:307-310, June 1982

Beales, JG, Kean, JH, and Lennox-Holt, PJ: The child's perception of the disease and the experience of pain in juvenile chronic arthritis, *J Rheumatol* 10:61-65, 1983

Benitz, WE, and Tatro, DS: The pediatric drug handbook, Chicago, 1981, Year Book Medical Publishers

Beyer, JE: The Oucher: a user's manual and technical report, Evanston, Ill, 1984, Judson Press

Beyer, JE, and Aradine, CR: Content validity of an instrument to measure young children's perceptions of the intensity of their pain, *J Pediatr Nurs* 1:386-394, Dec 1986

Beyer, JE, and Aradine, CR: Convergent and discriminant validity of a self-report measure of pain intensity for children, *Child Health Care* 16:274-282, Spring 1988

Beyer, JE, Ashley, LC, Russell, GA, and DeGood, DE: Pediatric pain after cardiac surgery: pharmacologic management, *Dimens Crit Care Nurs* 3:326-334, Nov-Dec 1984

Beyer, JE, and Byers, ML: Knowledge of pediatric pain: the state of the art, *Child Health Care* 13:150-159, Spring 1985

Beyer, JE, DeGood, DE, Ashley, LC, and Russell, GA: Patterns of postoperative analgesic use with adults and children following cardiac surgery, *Pain* 17:71-81, 1983

Beyer, JE, and Knapp, TR: Methodological issues in the measurement of children's pain, *Child Health Care* 14:233-241, Spring 1986

Beyer, JE, and Levin, CR: Issues and advances in pain control in children, *Nurs Clin North Am* 22:661-676, Sept 1987

Bradshaw, C, and Zeanah, PD: Pediatric nurses' assessments of pain in children, *J Pediatr Nurs* 1:314-322, Oct 1986

Broadman, LM, et al: Post-circumcision analgesia—a prospective evaluation of subcutaneous ring block of the penis, *Anesthesiology* 67:399-402, Sept 1987

Brown, L: Physiologic responses to cutaneous pain in neonates, *Neonatal Network* 6:18-22, Dec 1987

Brown, TG: Applying T.A.C. solution, *Nursing* 14:92, Jan 1984

Collins, L: Pain sensitivity and ratings of childhood experience, *Percept Mot Skills* 21:349-350, 1965

Craig, KD, McMahon, RJ, Morison, JD, and Zaskow, C: Developmental changes in infant pain expression during immunization injections, *Soc Sci Med* 19:1131-1137, 1984

Dale, J: A multidimensional study of infants' responses to painful stimuli, *Pediatr Nurs* 12:27-31, 1986

Duncan, A: The postoperative period, *Clin Anesthesiol* 3:619-632, July 1985

Eland, JM: The child who is hurting, *Semin Oncol Nurs* 1:116-122, May 1985a

Eland, JM: Pain in children. In Hockenberry, M, and Coody, D, eds: Pediatric hematology–oncology: perspectives in care, pp 394-406, St Louis, 1986, The CV Mosby Co

Eland, JM: Pediatrics. In Pain. Nursing now series, pp 108-118, Springhouse, Pa, 1985b, Springhouse Corp

Eland, JM: Persistence in pediatric pain research: one nurse researcher's efforts, *Recent Adv Nurs* 21:43-62, 1988a

Eland, JM: Personal communication, University of Iowa, Iowa City, Iowa, 1988b

Eland, JM: Pharmacologic management of acute and chronic pediatric pain, *Issues Comp Pediatr Nurs* 11:93-111, 1988c

Eland, JM and Anderson, JE: The experience of pain in children. In Jacox, A, ed: Pain: a sourcebook for nurses and other health professionals, pp 453-473, Boston, 1977, Little, Brown & Co

Eland, JM, and Herr, K: Does suturing have to hurt so much? *Child Nurse* 1988 (in press)

Epstein, MH, and Harris, J, Jr: Children with chronic pain: can they be helped? *Pediatr Nurs* 4:42-44, 1978

Favaloro, R: Adolescent development and implications for pain management, *Pediatr Nurs* 14:27-29, Jan-Feb 1988

Feychting, H: Premedication and psychological preparation, *Clin Anaesthesiol* 3:505-514, July 1985

Fisher, DM, Robinson, S, Brett, CM, Perin, G, and Gregory, GA: Comparison of enflurane, halothane, and isoflurane for diagnostic procedures in children with malignancies, *Anesthesiology* 3:647-650, Dec 1985

Flower, RJ, Moncada, S, and Vane, JR: Drug therapy of inflammation. In Gilman, AG, Goodman, LS, Rall, TW, and Mural, F, eds: Goodman and Gilman's The pharmacological basis of therapeutics, ed 7, pp 674-715, New York, 1985, Macmillan Publishing Co, Inc

Fowler-Kerry, S, and Lander, JR: Management of injection pain in children, *Pain* 30:169-175, 1987

Gaffney, A, and Dunne, EA: Developmental aspects of children's definitions of pain, *Pain* 26:105-117, 1986

Gunnar, M, Fisch, R, and Malone, S: The effects of pacifying stimulus on behavioral and adrenocortical responses to circumcision, *J Am Acad Child Adolesc Psychiatry* 23:34-38, 1984

Hallstrom, B: Contact comfort: its application to immunization injections, *Nurs Res* 17:130, 1968

Hatch, DJ, and Sumner, E: Neonatal anaesthesia, *Clin Anaesthesiol* 3:633-655, July 1985

Hawley, DD: Postoperative pain in children: misconceptions, descriptions and interventions, *Pediatr Nurs* 10:20-23, Jan-Feb 1984

Hester, NO: The preoperational child's reaction to immunizations, *Nurs Res* 28:250-254, 1979

Hester, NO, and Barcus, CS: Assessment and management of pain in children, *Pediatrics: Nurs Update* 1:2-7, 1986

Hickey, P, et al: Blunting of stress responses in the pulmonary circulation of infants by fentanyl, *Anesthesiol Analg* 64:1137-1142, 1985

Hilgard, JR, and LeBaron, S: Hypnotherapy of pain in children with cancer, Los Altos, Cal, 1984, William Kaufmann, Inc

Hockenberry, MJ, and Balogna-Vaughan, S: Preparation for intrusive procedures using noninvasive techniques in children with cancer: state of the art vs. new trends, *Cancer Nurs* 8:97-102, Apr 1985

Hurley, A, and Whelan, EG: Cognitive development and children's perception of pain, *Pediatr Nurs* 14:21-24, Jan-Feb 1988

Hurwitz, ES, Barrett, MJ, Bergman, D, Gunn, WJ, Pinsky, P, et al: Public Health Service study of Reye's syndrome and medications: report of the main study, *JAMA* 257:1905-1911, Apr 10, 1987

Jaffe, JH, and Martin, WR: Opioid analgesics and antagonists. In Gilman, AG, Goodman, LS, Rall, TW, and Mural, F, eds: Goodman and Gilman's The pharmacological basis of therapeutics, ed 7, pp 491-531, New York, 1985, Macmillan Publishing Co

Jay, SM, Ozolins, M, Elliott, C, and Caldwell, S: Assessment of children's distress during painful medical procedures, *J Health Psychol* 2:133-147, 1983

Jeans, ME: The measurement of pain in children. In Melzack, R, ed: Pain measurement and assessment, pp 183-189, New York, 1983, Raven Press

Kaiko, RF: Age and morphine analgesia in cancer patients with postoperative pain, *Clin Pharmacol Ther* 28:823-826, Dec 1980

Kavanagh, C: A new approach to dressing change in the severely burned child and its effect on burn-related psychopathology, *Heart Lung* 12:612-619, Nov 1983

Koehntop, D, et al: Pharmacokinetics of fentanyl in neonates, *Anesthesiol Analg* 65:227-232, 1986

Koren, G, et al: Pediatric fentanyl dosing based on pharmacokinetics during cardiac surgery, *Anesthesiol Analg* 63:577-582, 1984

Kuttner, L: Favorite stories: a hypnotic pain-reduction technique for children in acute pain, *Am J Clin Hypn* 30:289-295, Apr 1988

Kuttner, L: No fears, no tears: children with cancer coping with pain, Vancouver, BC, 1986, Canadian Cancer Society (Guide that accompanies video, see resource section, p 296)

Lacouture, PG, Gaundreault, P, and Lovejoy, FH: Chronic pain of childhood: a pharmacologic approach, *Pediatr Clin North Am* 31:1133-1151, 1984

Lamontagne, LL, Mason, KR, and Hepworth, JT: Effects of relaxation on anxiety in children: implications for coping with stress, *Nurs Res* 34:289-292, Sept-Oct 1985

Langer, JC, Shandling, B, and Rosenberg, M: Intraoperative bupivacaine during outpatient hernia repair in children: a randomized double blind trial, *J Pediatr Surg* 22:267-270, Mar 1987

Larsson, B, Daleflod, B, Hakansson, L, and Melin, L: Therapist-assisted versus self-help relaxation treatment of chronic headaches in adolescents: a school-based intervention, *J Child Psychol Psychiatry* 28:127-136, Jan 1987

Levy, DM: Observations of attitudes and behavior in the child-health center, *J Public Health* 41:182-190, 1951

Levy, DM: The infant's earliest memory of inoculation: a contribution to public health procedures, *J Genet Psychol* 96:3-46, 1960

Liebeskind, JC, and Melzack, R: The international pain foundation: meeting a need for education in pain management, *Pain* 30:1-2, 1987

Loadman, WE, Arnold, K, Volmer, R, Petrella, R, and Cooper, LZ: Reducing the symptoms of infant colic by introduction of a vibration/sound based intervention, *Pediatr Res* 21:182A, 1987

Lutz, WJ: Helping hospitalized children and their parents cope with painful procedures, *J Pediatr Nurs* 1:24-32, Feb 1986

Marshall, RE, Stratton, WC, Moore, JA, et al: Circumcision. I. Effects on newborn behavior, *Infant Behav Dev* 3:1-14, 1980

Martin, BB: Where are all the children, *Am J Hospice Care* 2:6-7, Mar-Apr 1985

Martin, RG: Drug disposition in the neonate, *Neonatal Network* 4:14-19, Feb 1986

Martyn, JAJ: Ketamine pharmacology and therapeutics, *J Burn Care Rehabil* 8:146-148, Mar-Apr 1987

Matheus, BA: Quick dissolve, *Nursing* 17:66, Sept 1987

Mather, L, and Mackie, J: The incidence of postoperative pain in children, *Pain* 15:271-282, 1983

Maunuksela, EL, Olkkola, KT, and Korpela, R: Intravenous indomethacin as postoperative analgesic in children: acute effects on blood pressure, heart rate, body temperature and bleeding, *Ann Clin Res* 19:359-363, 1987

Maunuksela, EL, Rajantie, J, and Silmes, MA: Flunitrazepam-fentanyl-induced sedation and analgesia for bone marrow aspiration and needle biopsy in children, *Acta Anaesthesiol Scand* 30:409-411, 1986

McCaffery, M: IV morphine for children, *Am J Nurs* 84:1153, Sept 1984

McGrath, PA, and de Veber, LL: The management of acute pain evoked by medical procedures in children with cancer, *J Pain Sympt Manag* 1:145-150, Summer 1986

McGrath, PA, de Veber, LL, and Hearn, MT: Multidimensional pain assessment in children. In Fields, HL, Dubner, R, and Cervero, F, eds: Advances in pain research and therapy, vol 9, pp 387-393, New York, 1985, Raven Press

McGrath, PJ, Johnson, G, Goodman, JT, Schillinger, J, Dunn, J, and Chapman, J: The CHEOPS: a behavioral scale to measure postoperative pain in children. In Fields, HL, Dubner, R, and Cervero, F, eds: Advances in pain research and therapy, vol 9, pp 395-402, New York, 1985, Raven Press

McGrath, PJ, Cunningham, SJ, Goodman, JT, and Unruh, A: The clinical measurement of pain in children: a review, *Clin J Pain* 1:221-227, 1985

McGrath, PJ, and Feldman, W: Clinical approach to recurrent abdominal pain in children, *Devel Behav Pediatr* 7:56-63, 1986

McGrath, PJ, and Unruh, AM: Pain in children and adolescents, New York, 1987, Elsevier Science Publishing Co, Inc

Mischel, HN, Fuhr, R, and McDonald, MA: Children's dental pain: the effects of cognitive coping training in a clinical setting, *Clin J Pain* 1:235-242, 1985

Miser, AW, McCalla, J, Dothage, JA, Wesley, M, and Miser, JS: Pain as a presenting symptom in children and young adults with newly diagnosed malignancy, *Pain* 29:85-90, 1987

Miser, AW, Dothage, JA, and Miser, JS: Continuous intravenous fentanyl for pain control in children and young adults with cancer, *Clin J Pain* 3:152-157, 1987

Molsberry, D: Young children's subjective quantifications of pain following surgery, Unpublished master's thesis, 1979, University of Iowa

Nahata, MC, Clotz, MA, and Knogg, EA: Adverse effects of meperidine, promethazine, and chlorpromazine for sedation in pediatric patients, *Clin Pediatr* 24:558-560, 1985

Orlowski, JP, Gillis, J, and Kilham, HA: A catch in the reye, *Pediatrics* **80**:638-642, Nov 1987

Owens, ME: Pain in infancy: conceptual and methodological issues, *Pain* **20**:213-230, Nov 1984

Pagliaro, LA, and Pagliaro, AM: Age-dependent drug selection and response. In Pagliaro, LA, and Pagliaro, AM, eds: Pharmacologic aspects of nursing, pp 130-139, St. Louis, 1986, The CV Mosby Co

Penticuff, JH: Neonatal nursing ethics: toward a consensus, *Neonatal Network* **5**:7-16, June 1987

Perin, G, and Frase, D: Development of a program using general anesthesia for invasive procedures in a pediatric outpatient setting, *J Assn Pediatr Oncol Nurs* **3**:8-10, 1985

Perry, S, and Heidrich, G: Management of pain during debridement: a survey of US burn units, *Pain* **13**:267-280, 1982

Physicians' desk reference, Oradell, NJ, 1988, Medical Economics Company, Inc

Piaget, J: The child's concept of physical causality, London, 1930, Routledge & Kegan-Paul

Poland, RL, Roberts, RJ, Gutierrez-Mazorra, JF, and Fonkalsrud, EW: Neonatal anesthesia, *Pediatrics* **80**:446, Sept 1987

Purcell-Jones, G, Dormon, F, and Sumner, E: Paediatric anesthetists' perceptions of neonatal and infant pain, *Pain* **33**:181-187, May 1988

Pryor, GJ, Kilpatrick, WR, and Opp, DR: Local anesthesia in minor lacerations: topical TAC vs lidocaine infiltration, *Ann Emerg Med* **9**:568-571, Nov 1980

Quinton, D, and Rutter, M: Early hospitalization and later disturbances of behaviour, *Devel Med Child Neurol* **18**:447-459, 1976

Rana, SR: Pain—a subject ignored, *Pediatrics* **79**:309, 1987

Rawlings, DJ, Miller, PA, and Engel, RR: The effect of circumcision on transcutaneous PO$_2$ in term infants, *Am J Dis Child* **134**:676-678, 1980

Ross, DM, and Ross, SA: Childhood pain, Baltimore, 1988, Urban & Schwarzenberg, Inc

Ross, DM, and Ross, SA: Pain instruction with third- and fourth-grade children: a pilot study, *J Pediatr Psychol* **10**:55-63, 1985

Rowe, PC, ed: The Harriet Lane handbook: a manual for pediatric house officers, ed 11, Chicago, 1987, Year Book Medical Publishers, Inc

Savedra, M: Coping with pain: strategies of severely burned children, *MCN* **5**:197-203, Fall 1976

Savedra, M, Gibbons, P, Tesler, M, Ward, J, and Wegner, C: How do children describe pain?: a tentative assessment, *Pain* **14**:95-104, 1982

Scanlon, J: Barbarism, *Perinatal Press* **9**:103-104, 1985

Schechter, NL, and Allen, D: Physicians' attitudes toward pain in children, *J Devel Behav Pediatr* **7**:350-354, 1986

Schechter, NL, Allen, DA, and Hanson, K: The status of pediatric pain control: a comparison of hospital analgesic usage in children and adults, *Pediatrics* **77**:11-15, 1986

Schechter, NL, Berrien, FB, and Katz, SM: The use of patient-controlled analgesia in adolescents with sickle cell pain crisis:

a preliminary report, *J Pain Sympt Manag* **3**:109-113, Spring 1988

Schultz, NV: How children perceive pain, *Nurs Outlook* **19**:670-673, Oct 1971

Sentivany, S: Personal communication, Children's Hospital at Stanford, Palo Alto, Calif, 1988

Smith, MS, and Womack, WM: Stress management techniques in childhood and adolescence: relaxation training, meditation, hypnosis, and biofeedback: appropriate clinical applications, *Clin Pediatr* **26**:581-585, Nov 1987

Stevens, B, Hunsberger, M, and Browne, G: Pain in children: theoretical, research, and practice dilemmas, *J Pediatr Nurs* **2**:154-166, June 1987

Steward, DJ: Paediatric diseases which may cause anaesthetic problems: prematurity. In Gomez, QJ, Egay, LM, and de al Cruz-Odi, MF, eds: Anaesthesia—safety for all, pp 189-193, New York, 1984, Excerpta Medica

Swafford, LI, and Allan, D: Pain relief in the pediatric patient, *Med Clin North Am* **52**:131-136, Jan 1968

Tichy, AM, Braam, CM, Meyer, TA, and Rattan, NS: Stressors in pediatric intensive care units, *Pediatr Nurs* **14**:40-42, Jan-Feb 1988

Tree-Trakarn, T, Pirayavaraporn, S, and Lertakyamanee, J: Topical analgesia for relief of post-circumcision pain, *Anesthesiology* **67**:395-399, Sept 1987

Ubell, E: Should infants have surgery without anesthesia? *Parade Magazine*, p 17, Apr 12, 1987

Varni, JW, Jay, SM, Masek, BJ, and Thompson, KL: Cognitive-behavioral assessment and management of pediatric pain. In Holzman, AD, and Turk, DC, eds: Pain management: a handbook of psychological treatment approaches, pp 168-192, New York, 1986, Pergamon Press

Varni, JW, Katz, ER, and Dash, J: Behavioral and neurochemical aspects of pediatric pain. In Russo, DC, and Varni, JW, eds: Behavioral pediatrics: research and practice, pp 177-224, New York, 1982, Plenum Press

Walsh, VR: Making medication tasteless, *Nursing* **17**:66, Sept 1987

Wandless, JG: A comparison of nalbuphine with morphine for post-orchidopexy pain, *Eur J Anaesthesiol* **4**:127-132, Mar 1987

Westfall, LK, and Pavlis, RW: Why the elderly are so vulnerable to drug reactions, *RN* **50**:39-42, 1987

Wetchler, BV: The role of anesthesia in outpatient surgery, *Today's OR Nurse* **4**:18-23, 62, Sept 1982

Whaley, L, and Wong, D: Essentials of pediatric nursing, ed 3, St. Louis, 1989, The CV Mosby Co

Wiley, F: Personal communication, University of California Medical Center, Los Angeles, Calif, May 1988

Woffard, LG: Pain in children with cancer: an assessment, *J Assn Pediatr Oncol Nurs* **2**:34-37, Spring 1985

Wong, D: Lozenges can be "Lifesavers," *Am J Nurs* **87**:1129-1130, Sept 1987

Yaster, M: Analgesia and anesthesia in neonates, *J Pediatr* **111**:394-395, Sept 1987

CHAPTER

11

Pain in the Elderly
Special Considerations

Tremendous advances have been made in the scientific understanding and clinical management of pain. However, the special needs and considerations of the elderly with pain is a neglected area. In 1984, for the first time in the United States, elderly people outnumbered adolescents (Harkins et al, in press). According to the Department of Health and Human Services, by 1990, 12.7% of the U.S. population, or 31.8 million people, will be over 65 years of age. By the year 2030, there will be approximately 65 million older Americans, two-and-one-half times their number in 1980 (American Association of Retired Persons and the Administration on Aging, 1987).

Despite the continuing growth of this segment of our population, research examining the effects of age on various pain control modalities is scarce. As a result, strategies for effective pain control in this population are at present based mostly on clinical experience and application of pain control methods shown to be useful with younger adults. There is a need for research in all areas of pain control for the elderly; too many questions remain unanswered.

PURPOSE AND LIMITATIONS OF THIS CHAPTER

The purpose of this manual is to present specific, clinical pain control strategies for the nurse in any health care

■ The authors would like to thank Susan C. Schafer, RNC, MS, Clinical Research Nurse, Pain Research Clinic, National Institutes of Health, Bethesda, Maryland, and Madelyn Miscally, RN, MSN, Geriatric Clinical Specialist, Bowman Gray School of Medicine, Winston-Salem, North Carolina for their review of this chapter, helpful comments and suggestions, and for supplying many of the patient examples.

setting. In this chapter, however, there are many gaps because the answers are simply not known yet. Our frustration as we prepared this chapter was the realization that although the elderly comprise *the fastest growing segment* of our population, the *least amount* of research on pain control exists in this age group. Thus we present this chapter with the hope that it will serve as a catalyst to stimulate thinking and generate exploration.

The primary purpose of this chapter is to address the areas of greatest need in the care of the elderly with pain:
- To raise questions about our lack of knowledge.
- To correct misconceptions.
- To prevent the perpetuation of misinformation that may ultimately interfere with effective assessment and treatment of pain in the elderly population.

A beginning step is to acknowledge that older patients may have different responses and needs than younger ones concerning assessment and interventions for pain control. It is beyond the scope of this chapter to present a thorough exploration of all the important aspects of gerontology.

Similar to the explosion of literature in pain control in children over the last several years, research in the elderly undoubtedly will continue to evolve. The authors look forward to developing this chapter further as more information on pain and the elderly becomes available.

For now, however, it is important for us to be particularly vigilant in applying scientific skills that include avoiding generalizations about elderly patients, being skeptical of assumptions that lack a research base, and continuously reminding ourselves that each person, regardless of age, reacts individually to any treatment modality.

MISCONCEPTIONS ABOUT PAIN IN THE ELDERLY

Many of the misconceptions previously discussed in Chapter 2 on assessment and Chapter 9 on chronic non-malignant pain apply to the older person with pain, and the reader is encouraged to review these. Following are misconceptions that are specific to the elderly. In addition, several misconceptions are restated from Chapter 9 because of their relevance to the older person with pain. Refer to Chapter 9 (pp. 236-240) and the annotated references (pp. 257-262) for more detailed discussion.

Misconception: Pain is a natural outcome of growing old.

Correction: Pain is in fact not an inevitable part of aging, and its presence necessitates assessment, diagnosis, and treatment similar to pain in any age group (Butler and Gastel, 1980; Harkins et al, 1984). This assumption can no longer be tolerated. Harkins et al (in press) suggest that this erroneous assumption may even be responsible for the lack of research on pain in the elderly.

The illogical nature of this misconception is best illustrated by the 101-year-old male participant in a study on aging as described by Butler and Gastel (1980). When he stated that his left leg hurt, the physician suggested that it was to be expected at age 101. The man then asked him to explain why his right leg, which was also 101 years old, did not hurt a bit.

Although pain is not an inevitable result of aging, the elderly are at greater risk for many disorders that may result in pain, e.g., arthritic disorders, cardiovascular diseases, osteoporosis, and cancer (Rowe and Besdine, 1982). The incidence of less common painful disorders such as postherpetic neuralgia and trigeminal neuralgia also are increased in elderly populations (Butler and Gastel, 1979). Further, injuries such as falls and hip fractures are more common in the elderly population and may result in chronic pain (Rubenstein and Robbins, 1984).

Is the lack of interest in pain in the elderly a reflection of our fear of aging? Butler and Gastel (1980) eloquently remind us that this neglect cannot continue. The elderly are "our future selves" (p. 297) and the quality of our own lives as we grow older may in fact depend on the extent of our efforts at understanding pain in the older generation.

Misconception: Pain perception, or sensitivity, decreases with age.

Correction: This assumption is unsafe. In addition to the fact that conflicting data exist, this generalization results in our missing important indications of pain. The consequences are needless suffering and undertreatment of both pain and the underlying causes.

Results of experimental studies on pain perception in the elderly fail to conclusively report age-related differences in pain perception (Clark and Mehl, 1971; Har-

kins et al, 1986; Harkins et al, in press; Harkins and Chapman, 1976).

Instances of atypical presentations of clinical pain include silent myocardial infarctions and the absence of abdominal pain in elders with peptic ulcer disease (Clinch et al, 1984; MacDonald, 1984). However, these reports of pain absence cannot be generalized to all disorders that may result in pain, or to all elders who may experience myocardial infarcts or ulcers. Further, if the elder has atypical absence of pain, this cannot be generalized to mean that pain will be absent in other conditions as well.

Failure to report pain must not be interpreted as absence of pain. The elderly may not report pain readily; however, this does not necessarily mean that they feel it any less. Further research is needed to understand all components of the pain experience in this segment of the population.

Misconception: The potential side effects of narcotics make them too dangerous to use to relieve pain in the elderly.

Correction: Narcotics may be used safely in the elderly if the person's response to medication is followed and evaluated closely and the pharmacokinetics in this population are recognized (Portenoy, 1987). Although the elderly may be more sensitive to narcotics, this does not justify withholding narcotics and failing to treat the pain. The potentially dangerous side effects of narcotics can be readily monitored with careful and frequent assessments of the individual's response to the narcotic, and usually avoided by adjustment of dose and interval between doses. If necessary, the most life-threatening side effect, respiratory depression, can be reversed by the antidote naloxone.

Misconception: If the elderly patient appears to be occupied, sleeps, or can be otherwise distracted from pain, then he does not have much pain.

Correction: The older patient need not act like he is in pain to be in pain. Lack of pain expression does not mean lack of pain (see pp. 12-14). The older person may have experienced pain for a long time and for many different reasons may minimize his expression of pain.

The elderly patient may not believe it is acceptable to show pain, so he may have a variety of ways to keep himself occupied or distracted from the pain. Assumptions about the presence or absence of pain cannot be solely based on a person's behavior.

Misconception: If the older person is depressed, especially if there is no known cause for the pain, then depression is causing the pain. Pain is a symptom of depression and would subside if the depression were effectively treated.

Correction: It is normal to be depressed because of chronic pain. Chronic pain may cause depression. Some types of depression are present prior to the onset of pain but are not likely the cause of pain. However, a preexisting depression does affect the person's ability to cope with the pain.

When the symptoms of chronic pain are compared with those of depression, the similarities between the two make it easy to see how they can become confused and how a patient can be mistakenly identified as being "only depressed" (see Table 9-1, Features of Chronic Pain and Depression, p. 238).

It is dangerous to assume that treatment of the depression is all that is needed to alleviate the pain. With this assumption, we run the risk of omitting a thorough pain assessment, not treating the pain, and ultimately allowing suffering to continue (refer to annotated references in Chapter 9: Ahles et al, 1987; Bouckoms et al, 1985; Hendler, 1984; Krishnan et al, 1985, Parts I and II; Pilowsky et al, 1985).

Misconception: Narcotics are totally inappropriate for all patients with chronic nonmalignant pain.

Correction: There is little evidence to support this view. However, this belief has been held for many years. This bias is compounded by the additional suggestion that side effects from narcotics are more pronounced in the elderly, and therefore they should be used only for severe acute episodes of pain.

Several studies have shown that prolonged narcotic therapy for selected patients with chronic nonmalignant pain can be a safe and humane alternative to no treatment. Portenoy and Foley (1986) reported on 38 patients, 25 to 82 years of age, in which 19 patients were maintained on narcotics for 4 or more years. Most researchers suggest that prolonged narcotic therapy for chronic nonmalignant pain be considered after other reasonable attempts to control pain have been unsuccessful and only in patients without a history of drug abuse (see annotated references in Chapter 9: Crook and Tunks, 1985; Halpern and Robinson, 1985-86; Portenoy and Foley, 1986).

ASSESSMENT OF PAIN

At the present time, pain assessment tools specifically tailored for the elderly are lacking, as is research examining the special considerations when questioning this population about pain. The many unanswered questions and lack of information on specific strategies make this section particularly difficult to present to the reader. For the present, we must recognize our lack of knowledge, but never stop asking questions that promote our exploration of this area.

Factors That Influence Assessment

Following are factors to consider concerning the assessment process in the elderly. Those elders who are active with minimal memory and cognitive problems may not require any adjustments in the assessment process already discussed in Chapter 2 (pp. 20-33). However, for others, these problems will present special needs and may influence the patient's report of pain. Although these factors are by no means an all-inclusive list, they are proposed to define our lack of knowledge and to stimulate thought in this area.

Communication Problems

Some elders may have hearing or vision problems that may complicate their ability to report their pain experience or apply pain-control strategies. In some cases, we may not be aware of these problems and may have to determine them through the use of open-ended questions and observations. For example, requests to "Describe what the pain feels like," or "Read me the prescription label on your bottle of pills" may alert the nurse to these problems.

For those patients in whom self-report about pain is not clear or possible, the nurse may need to rely on reports from family or caregiver. Observations of changes in level of functioning may be an indication of pain, e.g., a change in gait or guarding of a part of the body. Asking the family what they notice about the patient's level of activity during the day may be helpful. Are there any changes in the way the elder moves or any decrease or increase in activity?

Patient Example

A couple in their mid 70s living at home receive regular visits from the home health nurse. The husband is unable to articulate thoughts and feelings because of a stroke. Although the wife has periods of mild memory loss, she still functions well with household activities. The wife reports that her husband has headaches and asks if there is any medication she can give him. Because of the wife's mild cognitive impairment, the nurse tries to confirm the accuracy of her pain report. She asks the wife how she knows about her husband's pain. The wife describes her husband's grimaces and rubbing his head and face. The nurse observes this behavior during her visit, and together they plan strategies to control the husband's headaches (Kelly, 1988).

The older patient with confusion or dementia in addition to pain presents a particularly complex situation. Some patients with dementia may be able to tell you that they hurt; however, they may be unable to describe the pain. Detailed questions may result in their becoming frustrated.

Patient Example

Mrs. P., 84 years old with severe memory deficit, repeatedly tells the visiting nurse that she has pain and points to her upper abdominal area. She asks over and over "Why do I have pain?" The nurse tries to ask detailed questions about the pain; however, Mrs. P. is not able to answer them and instead becomes frustrated and anxious. Although the patient has a history of ulcer disease, the nurse decides that a further workup is needed. The

FLOW SHEET—PAIN

Age: 92 years

Patient Mrs. W.   Date 5/11

~~Pain rating scale used~~ Behaviors indicating pain: Continuous grunting, eyes tightly closed, legs pulled in toward abdomen, picks at bed covers.

Purpose: To evaluate the safety and effectiveness of the analgesic(s).

Analgesic(s) prescribed: Trilisate liquid 1 teaspoon (500 mg) bid; MS Contin 30mg PO q24h

Time	Possible ~~Pain rating~~ behaviors	Analgesic	R	P	BP	Level of arousal	Possible ~~Other~~ comfort behaviors	Plan & comments

FIGURE 11-1 Example of how the flow sheet from p. 27 may be adapted for the noncommunicating elder.

VIII. Effects of the pain. Ask "If you had a 50% reduction in pain daily, what would you be doing?"

Pain Flow Sheet

The pain flow sheet (p. 27) provides a quick and easy tool to evaluate the safety and effectiveness of analgesics and other pain control measures. The flow sheet may be adapted for use in the noncommunicating elder. Ask the family or someone who knows the patient well to help you list behaviors that might indicate pain and those that indicate comfort. Figure 11-1 shows an example of how the flow sheet may be modified for a noncommunicating elder.

Daily Diary

The daily diary (p. 30) may be kept by the patient or family and may be especially helpful in gathering data when the pain picture is confusing and the elder is at home. Although every hour does not need to be recorded, it is important to note when medication is taken, or when the level of activity alters a previous pain rating. The Patient/Family Teaching Point for use of Daily Diary (p. 31) may be duplicated for patients and family members.

PAIN CONTROL INTERVENTIONS

Chapters 4 through 8 discuss in detail pharmacological and nonpharmacological pain control measures. Therefore the purpose of this section is to build on this infor-

mation and present an overview of research, clinical strategies, and unanswered questions concerning effective pharmacological and noninvasive pain control methods for the elderly.

Pharmacological Interventions

This section addresses the following issues:
- Physiological changes as a result of aging and the resulting pharmacological implications as they apply to analgesics.
- Key concepts of analgesic therapy.
- Nonnarcotic analgesics.
- Narcotic analgesics.
- Adjuvant analgesics.

Physiological Changes Influencing Drug Therapy

". . . Aging is a unique and individual process that occurs at different rates in different individuals" (Pagliaro and Pagliaro, 1983, p. 1). Knowledge of how this process affects the distribution, metabolism, and elimination of drugs provides a framework for understanding altered pharmacological responses to analgesics in the elderly. With more research, our knowledge of the most effective ways to monitor and adjust analgesic therapy will be refined.

Distribution of Drugs

Factors that affect the distribution of drugs are altered by increasing age and include the following (Ouslander,

1981; Pagliaro and Pagliaro, 1986; Reidenberg, 1982; Schmucker, 1984; Westfall and Pavlis, 1987):

• Changes in body composition. An increase in the proportion of body fat may cause delayed onset and accumulation with repeated dosing of drugs that are fat soluble, e.g., diazepam (Valium) and methadone (Dolophine). Heart, kidney, and muscle mass decrease with age. As a result, a usual adult dose may need to be decreased to avoid toxic drug levels in the blood and tissue.

• Serum proteins. Many drugs bind to plasma proteins, leaving a portion of each drug circulating unbound or free for pharmacological activity. Although the normal aging process probably does not reduce serum proteins, malnutrition and chronic disease, observed more often in this population, may contribute (Lamy, 1983; Mitchell and Lipschitz, 1982). Decreased circulating proteins potentially result in greater drug effect from higher concentrations of unbound drug, with a greater risk of toxic effect. Nonnarcotic analgesics that are protein bound and likely to be associated with greater pharmacological effect include: ibuprofen (Motrin), naproxen (Naprosyn), indomethacin (Indocin), meclofenamate (Meclomen), and piroxicam (Feldene) (Flower, Moncada, and Vane, 1985).

Metabolism of Drugs

The liver is the major site of drug metabolism. However, the effect of aging on hepatic metabolism is complex, difficult to predict, and has not been well studied in humans (Greenblatt et al, 1982; Ouslander, 1981). It appears that the capacity of the liver to metabolize drugs may not be uniformly affected by aging and that most drugs are normally metabolized in the older population (Ouslander, 1981; Pagliaro and Pagliaro, 1986). Although it cannot be generalized to all other drugs, the rate of some forms of hepatic metabolism may be decreased in specific drugs, e.g., acetaminophen (Pagliaro and Pagliaro, 1986). The practical application of this finding may be to allow for the longer period of metabolism of the drug dose by anticipating the need for a longer interval between doses.

Excretion of Drugs

As a result of age, both structural and functional changes occur in the kidney. These include a decrease in renal mass, renal blood flow, glomerular filtration rate, and tubular secretion. Dehydration and heart failure occur rather frequently in ill elderly patients and may further reduce renal function (Lonergan, 1988; Ouslander, 1981; Pagliaro and Pagliaro, 1983). Consequently, drugs or the active metabolites of drugs that are eliminated by the kidney may remain in the body longer, resulting in prolonged therapeutic and/or toxic effects.

The clinical importance of poor kidney function is apparent with the narcotic meperidine (Demerol). An active metabolite of meperidine, normeperidine, may accumulate with repeated doses, causing central nervous system excitation (Kaiko, 1983). This appears to be more likely to occur in patients with compromised renal function (American Pain Society, 1987).

Research documenting renal metabolism of drugs in the elderly is just beginning; it is suggested that there will be increasing evidence of the importance of the kidney in the elimination of opiates and other drugs (Hanks and Aherne, 1985; Lonergan, 1988).

Clearance of Drugs

Kaiko and associates (1982) report that morphine clearance from the plasma decreases with age. As a result, morphine may remain in the body longer and at higher concentrations, suggesting that its effects could be greater and last longer in the elderly as opposed to younger patients. Therefore in clinical situations, this finding alerts us to the fact that individual patients' responses need to be assessed for adjustments that may include lower doses of narcotic given less frequently.

Drug Receptors

It has been suggested that a decreased number of drug receptors or decreased responsiveness of these receptors in the elderly may account for increased sensitivity to drug effects (Pagliaro and Pagliaro, 1986). However, there is little data to suggest that aging is accompanied by a decrease in number or effectiveness of drug receptors (Schmucker, 1984).

KEY POINT: In attempting to explain the effect of aging on the pharmacokinetics of drug therapy for pain, it is clear that this is an underdeveloped area of research.

The impact of the above potential physiological changes is not totally clear, and the difficulty in predicting individual responses remains. The following principles, e.g., titrating to effect by adjusting drug dose and interval according to individual response, remain vital strategies for effective pain control in all ages.

Key Concepts in Analgesic Therapy

The following three concepts have already been discussed at length in Chapter 4 (pp. 48-50). The reader is encouraged to refer to Chapter 4 for detailed guidelines and patient examples. The concepts are summarized briefly here as a reminder of their importance, and any variations specific to the elderly are noted:

1. Use a Preventive Approach

Use a preventive approach and stay on top of the pain. A preventive approach means that the analgesic is given or taken before pain occurs or before it increases, that is:

• ATC (around the clock at regularly scheduled intervals). This schedule is appropriate if the pain occurs consistently and predictably throughout a 24-hour period.

For some elderly patients a q4h or q6h schedule of pain medication may be easily forgotten or confused. It may be helpful in this situation to schedule the medication around specific activities throughout the day, as long as they occur consistently.

Patient Example

Mr. S. is taking Percocet 1 tablet for rib and back pain from metastatic prostate cancer. After a careful assessment, the home health nurse notes that he takes it irregularly and only when the pain becomes unbearable. The nurse encourages Mr. S. to try a new schedule for a trial of 3 to 4 days: take a Percocet before each meal and at bedtime. By linking the pain pill schedule with specific activities he does every day, Mr. S. is able to readily remember when to take the pain medicine. After a trial of 2 days, he is amazed at the difference in his comfort level, and he continues with this schedule.

- PRN (as needed, requires nursing assessment and evaluation), for pain that cannot be predicted. However, it should be used preventively, as soon as pain begins and before it gets out of control. An analgesic prescribed "PRN for pain" may be implemented on an ATC schedule for ongoing pain (see pp. 53-54).

2. Titrate to Effect

Adjust and individualize the analgesic for each patient. This involves tailoring analgesics by adjusting the following:
- Dose. Although it has been found that the elderly may be more sensitive to narcotics (Kaiko et al, 1982), this finding cannot be generalized to rule out the use of narcotics or to mean that all elderly patients need lower doses of analgesics. If greater sensitivity is noted in an elder, analgesics must be monitored and adjusted more vigilantly.

At first, it was suggested that age be the main criterion for choosing an initial analgesic dose (Bellville et al, 1971); however, current research suggests that age influences frequency of dosing more than dosage (Kaiko et al, 1982).

The only safe and effective way to administer an analgesic is to monitor the individual's response to the drug. For some elderly patients, it may be appropriate to administer a relatively low starting dose of medication (Portenoy, 1987). It is important that this dose is then immediately adjusted up or down depending on the patient's response. Interestingly, height, weight, and body surface are not accurate guides for narcotic dose requirements in the elderly (Bellville et al, 1971).

Patient Example

Mrs. L., 60 years old with end-stage breast cancer and metastasis to the spine, was admitted to the hospital for pain control. Upon admission, she was confused, so assessment was difficult. She was started on morphine continuous IV infusion at 2mg/hr. Within 2 days, the dose was titrated up to 900 mg/hr IV. She was comfortable on this dose, alert, and able to interact with her family before she died (Mahoney and Zukor, 1988).

The above patient situation is an excellent example of titrating up quickly if the patient is breathing well but the pain is uncontrolled. Adjusting the dose according to the individual's response may also involve titrating down if the patient's respiratory rate drops, or if pain control or side effects are excessive.

Use a flow sheet and look at patient responses, in the following order:
a. First, respiratory function.
b. Second, pain rating, descriptive phrase, or nonverbal behavior.
c. Third, based on the above, determine what should be done with the number of milligrams of analgesic the patient is receiving. *The last thing you look at are milligrams being given, look at effect first.*

- Interval between doses. Older patients may experience a longer duration of action of narcotics (Kaiko, 1980; Kaiko et al, 1982). Therefore increasing age should prompt close monitoring of the frequency of narcotic administration. For example, in the elderly, sustained-release morphine may last longer than 12 hours, in some instances up to 24 hours.

Again the key here is monitoring each patient individually; the flow sheet may be a particularly helpful tool for this.
- Route. Adjust the route of drug administration according to the individual patient's needs, remembering that even severe pain may be controlled with oral narcotics. These needs might include such considerations as convenience, side effects, cost, and onset of analgesia. The present discussion is limited to potential problems with the IM and continuous subcutaneous infusion route in the elderly. Refer to Chapter 4 (pp. 87-107) for detailed discussion of other routes of administration, remembering that the oral route is preferred. When this is not possible, the IV route may be appropriate.

Absorption of IM injections and continuous subcutaneous infusions are important factors when determining appropriate routes of administration for the elderly. Drug absorption is highly variable and likely to be diminished for a number of reasons. As a result, the drug may not be readily absorbed and there may be delayed onset of action (Lukacsko, 1987). Following are factors that interfere with absorption:
—Degenerated muscle from inactivity, poor nutrition, or dehydration.
—Absorption of IM narcotics may be poor, especially in the immediate postoperative period (Austin et al,

1980). In the elderly, especially in this postoperative period, peripheral circulation may be diminished. Circulatory problems may then result, and insufficient plasma concentration of drugs may be particularly significant.

—Variability in absorption poses a specific danger in the postoperative period when an IM dose is repeated. For instance, as a result of poor absorption, the first IM dose may not provide pain relief for the elderly person. The dose may be repeated. As circulation improves, the initial dose may be absorbed just as the second dose is taking effect. The result may be an elderly patient who is in pain just before the second dose, and afterward is more likely to be sedated or have respiratory depression.

• Choice of drug. The choice of analgesic may in large part be influenced by its potential adverse effects. The following considerations that influence drug selection in the elderly are discussed in the section on narcotic analgesics:

—Hazards of meperidine (Demerol).
—Problems with agonists/antagonists.
—Problems with narcotics with long duration.

Other factors may influence an elderly patient's willingness to accept the health team's choice of analgesic. Following is an example that illustrates the concern about cost of medication.

Patient Example

Mrs. A., 70 years old, is evaluated by the Pain Management Team for a more effective analgesic regimen. After discussing changing her medication to Percocet, Mrs. A. stated that she had just paid for a prescription of Darvocet-N. Even though she understood that the Percocet would probably give her better pain control, she wanted to finish the Darvocet-N before switching to a new medication (Wenzl, 1988).

3. Patient Controlled Analgesia (PCA)

In its broadest sense, the key concept of PCA may be defined as the patient's self-administration of all forms of pain control by methods that consider safety as well as the patient's ability and willingness to exercise control. The elder who feels the pain is the person who must have, to the extent possible, control of all measures to relieve it.

Some elderly patients may be unable or unwilling to exercise control. They may look to the physician or nurse for direction concerning all aspects of health care. In one study of 48 postoperative orthopedic patients, aged 16 to 79, a supply of Tylox was placed at the bedside of 26 patients. The older patients with Tylox at the bedside took significantly fewer pills than their counterparts who were given Tylox by the nurses (Jones, 1987).

Other elders may have mental status changes and be unable to determine or direct pain relief. In this case, the patient's indications of pain are carefully monitored and the form and/or the amount of pain control is adjusted according to the individual patient.

Nonnarcotic Analgesics (NSAIDs)

The following principles of nonnarcotic therapy have been discussed at length in Chapter 4: indications, disadvantages, mechanism underlying effects of NSAIDs, adverse side effects, promising uses, and guidelines for their effective use along with patient teaching tools that may be readily adapted for use with the elderly patient.

It is beyond the scope of this chapter to discuss the long-term use of antiinflammatory medications for the chronic treatment of highly inflammatory conditions such as rheumatoid arthritis. The interested reader is referred to other sources for this information (Baskin and Goldfarb, 1983; Gall, 1982; Lamy, 1986; Morgan and Furst, 1986; Polisson, 1987; Schlegel and Paulus, 1986).

Reminders of the important aspects of using nonnarcotics as analgesics include:

• Nonnarcotic analgesics are often undervalued as effective pain relieving medications. For example, two regular aspirin or acetaminophen (650 mg) relieve as much pain as codeine 30 mg PO, meperidine (Demerol) 50 mg PO, and propoxyphene hydrochloride (Darvon-N) 100 mg.

• Combining a nonnarcotic with a narcotic is a simple yet frequently overlooked strategy. It provides a safe and logical method of pain control.

• When NSAIDs are used for brief episodes of pain, the incidence or severity of side effects may not compare to those seen with long-term treatment. For example, when indomethacin (Indocin) is given rectally over 3 days for postoperative pain, side effects are likely to pose less of a problem than when indomethacin is given orally over several months.

In the elderly patient, there may be a concern about increasing side effects if a narcotic dose is increased. Adding an NSAID to the narcotic instead of increasing a narcotic dose may result in increased analgesia without increasing side effects (Weingart et al, 1985).

Dosage of Nonnarcotic Analgesics

One study of 17 healthy men and women from 65 to 78 years of age found that age had minimal effect on the absorption, distribution, metabolism, and excretion of ibuprofen (Motrin). Therefore Albert et al (1984) suggest that the dosage of ibuprofen does not need to be adjusted for age.

Side Effects of Nonnarcotic Analgesics

Cognitive dysfunction, i.e., memory loss, inability to concentrate, confusion, and personality change, was noted in eight patients over 65 years of age who took naproxen (Naprosyn) or ibuprofen (Motrin) over a period of 1 year. These symptoms cleared in all of the patients within 2 weeks after stopping the NSAID (Goodwin and Regan, 1982). Particularly noteworthy is the fact that none of the patients volunteered information about side effects. Instead, knowledge of adverse symptoms came from family members' remarks or as a result of direct questioning of the patient. One of the patients was relieved to learn that the distraction and memory loss she experienced were a result of the naproxen. She assumed she was "becoming senile" and that her family would have to put her in a nursing home.

Impaired renal function is another common side effect of NSAIDs in the elderly (Polisson, 1987; Schlegel and Paulus, 1986). Patients at increased risk for this side effect include those with (Schlegel and Paulus, 1986):

- Reduced cardiac output associated with congestive heart failure.
- Hepatic disease with cirrhosis and ascites.
- Diuretic-induced volume depletion.
- Atherosclerotic cardiovascular disease who are receiving concurrent diuretic therapy.

Upon initiation of NSAIDs, especially for chronic use, monitoring of renal function, electrolytes, and mental status is important. Following are important nursing care guidelines for using nonnarcotics as analgesics in the elderly:

- Discuss the possible side effects of NSAIDs with the patient and family.
- Initiate questions about symptoms of cognitive dysfunction or mood alterations.

Narcotic Analgesics (Opioids)

The following principles of narcotic therapy have been discussed in detail in Chapter 4 (pp. 66-113): mode of action, reasons for undertreatment, equianalgesic doses, selection of appropriate narcotics, selection of appropriate route of administration, and side effects, in addition to numerous patient examples and patient/family teaching tools.

Following are reminders of important aspects of narcotic analgesics that are particularly pertinent to the elderly:

1. Hazards of Meperidine

Although meperidine (Demerol) is a frequently prescribed IM narcotic, several characteristics of this drug make it an undesirable choice:

- Tissue irritation with the potential for severe muscle tissue fibrosis with frequent injections (Jaffe and Martin, 1985). This problem may be compounded in the elderly patient with decreased muscle mass.
- Possible neuropsychiatric effects, such as disorientation, bizarre feelings, and hallucinations. These occur frequently with parenteral meperidine (Miller and Jick, 1978).
- Toxicity, due to the accumulation of an active metabolite, normeperidine, which is a central nervous system stimulant (Kaiko et al, 1983; Szeto et al, 1977). Because

decreased renal function increases the likelihood of this side effect, elderly patients may be particularly vulnerable (Portenoy, 1987).

2. Problems with Agonists/Antagonists

Because all four drugs in this group, nalbuphine (Nubain), butorphanol (Stadol), pentazocine (Talwin), and buprenorphine (Buprenex), have a limit on the amount of respiratory depression they cause, it may be particularly tempting to prescribe this group of drugs for the elderly. However, pentazocine and butorphanol may both cause psychotomimetic effects such as confusion and hallucinations (American Pain Society, 1987). Although respiratory depression with buprenorphine is rare, it is the only one in which narcotic-induced respiratory depression is not readily reversed with naloxone (Narcan). Therefore of the four, nalbuphine may seem a logical first choice (pp. 85-86).

However, if the narcotic antagonist property of nalbuphine, butorphanol, and pentazocine is not understood, the following difficulties may occur in relation to "pure" narcotic agonists such as codeine, morphine, propoxyphene hydrochloride (Darvon), and meperidine:

- They may precipitate withdrawal in someone who has been taking a "pure" narcotic for a week or more.
- They may reverse analgesia of "pure" narcotics if an agonist/antagonist is given at the same time or alternately.

3. Problems with Narcotics with Long Half-Lives

The half-life of a narcotic refers to the time it takes for the drug to fall to half its initial plasma concentration. Methadone (Dolophine) and levorphanol (Levo-Dromoran) both have long half-lives, therefore the plasma levels of these drugs slowly rise over many days after initiating a dosing schedule. As a result, the risk of delayed toxicity is much greater than with drugs of shorter half-life such as morphine or hydromorphone (Dilaudid). In the elderly population where sensitivity to narcotics may be increased, the use of methadone or levorphanol must be approached with caution and particularly vigilant monitoring of the patient's response. If these drugs are used, refer to Chapter 4 (pp. 81-83) for suggestions on dosing.

4. Side Effects of Particular Concern: Confusion and Constipation

In some patients, polypharmacy (simultaneous administration of many medications, both prescription and over-the-counter), multiple medical problems, and age-related physiological changes with pharmacological impact may present a complex interrelationship contributing to many side effects, especially confusion and constipation. Frequently, narcotic analgesics are automatically blamed. While cognitive impairment in the elderly patient may be drug-induced (Larson et al, 1987), investigation into its cause should not be limited to narcotics.

Constipation may be of particular concern to some elderly patients. Many have probably established their own patterns for treating it. New suggestions for handling this side effect may not be followed. Therefore if possible, it is important to augment whatever strategies the patient currently uses. Refer to p. 114 for patient/family teaching point and p. 109 for suggested regimens.

It is important to tell patients that constipation is an expected side effect of narcotics and some adjuvant analgesic medications and that it can be prevented.

Patient Example

Mrs. T., 60 years old, began a course of amitriptyline (Elavil) for foot and abdominal pain from diabetic neuropathy. She stopped the drug on her own because of constipation. She was never told to expect it or how to prevent it. When she learned that this was an expected side effect and how to prevent it, she resumed the amitriptyline (Schafer, 1988).

Adjuvant Analgesics

The following principles of adjuvant analgesic therapy have been discussed at length in Chapter 4 (pp. 113-123): appropriate uses, disadvantages, so-called potentiators, adjuvant analgesics for sleep disturbances, anxiety, depression, shocklike pain, sedation, and muscle spasms.

Following are reminders of important aspects of using adjuvant analgesics:

- Adjuvant analgesics are not a substitute for adequate doses of narcotics or nonnarcotic analgesics. Aggressive titration of these analgesics to control pain comes first.
- The choice of an adjuvant analgesic is appropriate when there is: (1) a component to the pain that narcotics alone cannot address, e.g., depression, sleeplessness, or anxiety, and (2) a pain syndrome that may not respond to narcotics, e.g., phantom limb pain, post-herpetic neuralgia, or causalgia.
- While adjuvant analgesics are a logical consideration in the management of pain, their role and guidelines for use are still being established.

Precautions and Side Effects

Adjuvant analgesics must be used with caution in the elderly. Sedation, confusion, and constipation may be compounded by the sedative and anticholinergic effects of many of the adjuvant medications (Portenoy, 1987). Low starting doses, in some cases one half to two thirds that of doses normally used, are suggested for these medications (Cunha, 1986; Peabody et al, 1986; Portenoy, 1987). Any increase in dosage should be gradual.

If an elderly patient taking a narcotic and adjuvant analgesic reports unacceptable side effects, decrease or discontinue the adjuvant medication first. After evaluating the patient's response, it may then be necessary to change the narcotic (Portenoy, 1987).

Orthostatic hypotension (a severe drop in blood pressure when changing from a lying to a standing position) is one of the most common and serious cardiovascular complications of the tricyclic medications (Peabody et al, 1986). This complication may directly affect the elder's mobility by potentially resulting in injury from falls.

In the elderly patient, there is a tendency to use the benzodiazepines to sedate the agitated patient or better control his behavior (Meyer, 1982). This is particularly true for the anxious patient with uncontrolled pain. The long half-life of many of these drugs makes them a poor choice in the elderly patient. Although increased sensitivity of the elderly to this group of drugs needs further exploration, the following question alerts us to potential problems: "Do the benzodiazepines have an effect in producing accidental injury in the elderly?" (Meyer, 1982, p. 1021).

Noninvasive Interventions

Cutaneous stimulation (Chapter 5, pp. 130-170), distraction (Chapter 6, pp. 172-186), relaxation (Chapter 7, pp. 188-211), and imagery (Chapter 8, pp. 212-230) have previously been discussed, and the reader is referred to the corresponding chapters for detailed discussions, annotated references, and patient/family teaching points.

Rather than review the previously discussed concepts, this section presents special considerations in using selected techniques for the elderly patient.

Cutaneous Stimulation: Use of Cold and Menthol

Cold may be very effective for conditions that are traditionally treated with heat, e.g., low back pain and arthritis. However, the elderly person may be particularly reluctant to try the local application of cold. They may associate cold weather or dampness with increased pain; therefore it is helpful to clarify that the application of cold to a small body area does not necessarily produce the same results as cold damp weather. For an added sense of warmth and comfort while cold is being applied, suggest the use of a heating pad on other parts of the body.

A topically applied substance containing menthol is a type of external analgesic that may be particularly appealing to an elderly person. Menthol-containing preparations may have been a popular home remedy for this generation. In our present age of frequent medication use and a highly technical approach to health care, elderly patients may assume that menthol is an inappropriate and unscientific pain control measure, especially for use in the hospital setting. Initiating conversation about menthol products and encouraging the patient to use what has worked for him before may foster a sense of control and open-mindedness that can be applied to other pain control strategies.

Distraction: Listening to Music, Life Review, and the Use of Pets

Listening to music can provide powerful distraction from pain (Glynn, 1986; Herth, 1978). Selection of music according to the preference of the patient is crucial to its effectiveness. For some elderly, this may mean selecting music from a different era. For example, "Stardust" and "Moonlight and Roses" were very popular songs from the 20s and 30s. Elders may choose to listen to music that they grew up with or music that brings back pleasant memories.

Patients with a hearing aid may find it difficult to use a headset. If there is a problem using the two together, it may be helpful to use the speech and hearing department of a hospital as a resource. It is also important to note that problems with hearing aids are often the result of dead batteries, simple to correct, yet frequently overlooked.

Life review may be used as a means of distraction for the elder experiencing pain (Dietsche, 1979; Murray et al, 1980; Ryden, 1981). A tendency of the elderly to self-reflect and reminisce may be viewed as part of cognitive loss or onset of senility. However, Butler (1963) discovered the significance of these activities, recognized them to be a normal process, and named them life review.

Life review is defined as "a naturally occurring, universal mental process characterized by looking back over the life lived and recalling either pleasurable memories or unresolved conflicts which can be surveyed and integrated" (Murray et al, 1980, p. 284). While talking with an elderly patient, you may note recurrent themes that he frequently talks about. When using life review as a distraction technique for pain, ask the patient to tell you more about that particular event or period of time. To initiate reflecting or reminiscing behavior, ask the patient to look back over his life and tell you what stands out in his mind (Ryden, 1981).

Patient Example

Mrs. L., 79 years old with pancreatic cancer, was admitted to the hospital for severe abdominal pain, nausea, and vomiting. During one of her daily visits, the geriatric clinical nurse specialist found her lying in bed with her eyes tightly closed. Mrs. L. stated that she could not talk right now because the pain was so bad. After Mrs. L. received additional pain medication, the nurse asked if she could sit with the patient. Mrs. L. began to talk about her life. She talked about her childhood and an early marriage to an abusive husband. She talked of raising her own children in addition to some of her brothers and sisters. She stated that she was proud of her accomplishments even though there had been some bad times. The nurse reinforced the fact that she certainly made the best of many difficult situations. Mrs. L. then said that her pain was much better and that she was tired and needed to rest. She thanked the nurse for staying and said that it really helped to talk (Miscally, 1988).

Some community agencies on aging provide a "Pets on Wheels" program to benefit nursing home residents or elders who are home-bound. Volunteers bring pets such as dogs or cats to visit residents on a regular schedule. The unconditional love from a pet can be a soothing distraction, especially for those whose lives have always included animals.

Relaxation/Imagery

The term relaxation may be unacceptable to the elderly patient. It may be more appropriate to encourage the patient to tell you what brings them "peace of mind or comfort." For some patients this may mean reading poetry or the bible.

Other patients may respond to specific techniques by being encouraged to release any contractions in their muscles. One study of 20 adults aged 56 to 89 examined the effects of a jaw relaxation technique (dropping the lower jaw, relaxing the tongue, and using coordinated breathing) on the postoperative comfort level of patients with fractured hips. The use of this technique increased the level of the patients' postoperative comfort (Ceccio, 1984).

Griffin (1986) reports on the successful use of imagery in her gerontological practice. One of her techniques, the use of an "inner advisor," is explained to patients as a way to "help you get in touch with YOU again" (p. 806).

Patient Example

Mrs. J., a 67-year-old widow, developed abdominal pain 3 months after her husband died. She identified a ball of fire aiming rays at her stomach causing the pain. Weekly sessions with the nurse enabled her to stand up to this ball of fire and talk to it. Over a 2-month period, it shrank and finally disappeared. Although the pain was gone 1 year later, Mrs. J. continued to use a variation of this technique to increase her energy and help her sleep soundly (Griffin, 1986).

THE FUTURE

Much remains to be done about pain in the elderly. Beginning attempts are necessarily frustrating because we:

- Identify what we do not know.
- Tentatively apply to the elderly what we know about effective pain control measures used for younger patients.
- Attempt to formulate questions that are sensitive to the needs of the elderly.

In the years to come, it is our hope that the following quote will be no longer applicable: "... Pain is most poorly managed in those most defenseless against it—the young and the elderly" (Liebeskind and Melzack, 1987, p. 66).

SELECTED ANNOTATED REFERENCES THAT CITE RESEARCH OR GIVE CLINICAL SUPPORT

Albert, KS, Gillespie, WR, Wagner, JG, et al: Effects of age on the clinical pharmacokinetics of ibuprofen, *Am J Med* 77:47-50, July 13, 1984. The pharmacokinetics of one dose of 400, 800, and 1200 mg of ibuprofen (Motrin) were studied after administration to 17 healthy men and women aged 65 to 78 years. The findings were then compared with those in a similar study in young males aged 22 to 35 years. According to the results, advanced age has minimal influence on the absorption, distribution, metabolism, and excretion of ibuprofen. Therefore the authors suggest that the dosage does not need to be adjusted for elderly patients.

Bellville, JW, Forrest, WH, Miller, E, and Brown, BW: Influence of age on pain relief from analgesics, *JAMA* 217:1835-1841, Sept 27, 1971. This is a particularly meaningful study because it used well-controlled conditions to determine the correlation between age and analgesia. Seven hundred twelve patients received 10 mg of morphine IM or 20 mg of pentazocine IM or both for acute postoperative pain and were studied for correlations between the degree of pain relief and patient characteristics such as age, height, weight, body surface, operative site, and variations among hospitals. Age proved to be the most important variable in that the older age group reported more pain relief following IM administration of an analgesic. No difference was found between the incidence of side effects reported by patients 58 and older and those reported by patients younger than 58. No correlation was found between the sedation score and age. The authors suggest therefore that their findings concerning age cannot be explained purely on the basis of altered drug absorption and distribution, otherwise they would have expected to be able to correlate age with the sedative side effects. The authors state that it is more important to adjust dosage of a narcotic in relation to a patient's age than in relation to height, weight, or other patient characteristics.

Faherty, BS, and Grier, MR: Analgesic medication for elderly people post-surgery, *Nurs Res* 33:369-372, 1984. One hundred forty-two patients from 25 to 107 years old following abdominal surgery were studied to determine if elderly patients receive less analgesic medication than younger patients, and, if so, how the physician's prescriptions and the nurse's administration contribute to this finding. The data from this study indicate that older postsurgical patients have less analgesic medication prescribed and administered. The smaller amounts of analgesic medication given to elderly patients may have been influenced by the smaller amounts prescribed for this age group. However, nurses also administered a smaller percentage of the smaller amount prescribed for the elderly patients. Of the 83 patients who were 55 years or older, 50 (60.2%) received less than 50% of the dose prescribed.

Harkins, SW, Kwentus, J, and Price, DD: Pain and the elderly. In Benedetti, C, Chapman, CR, and Morrica, G, eds: Advances in pain research and therapy, pp 103-121, vol 7, New York, 1984, Raven Press. A review article examines age differences in pain perception under conditions staged in the laboratory and as a result of pathology. The authors conclude that any changes in pain sensitivity and perception related to age are difficult to document and may in fact be of little significance. Acute and chronic pain are reviewed with comments about the sensitivity of the elderly to narcotics and nonsteroidal antiinflammatory medications. Depression and chronic pain, pain and dementia, and social environment and pain are briefly discussed.

Harkins, SW, Price, DD, and Martelli, M: Effects of age on pain perception: thermonociception, *J Gerontol* 41:58-63, 1986. Forty-four young (20 to 36 years), middle-aged (45 to 60 years), and elderly (65 to 80 years) volunteers received noxious heat stimuli to several areas on the forearm. The participants used visual analog scales to rate the intensity and unpleasantness of the heat stimuli. The researchers found minimal differences with age between how strong the pain felt and the unpleasantness of the pain. There were more similarities in pain perception than differences among age groups.

Kaiko, RF: Age and morphine analgesia in cancer patients with postoperative pain, *Clin Pharmacol Ther* 28:823-826, 1980. The responses of 947 postoperative cancer patients receiving 8 and 16 mg doses of IM morphine were studied. Age was the significant factor associated with duration of analgesia, i.e., the older patient had a longer duration of analgesia than the younger patient. Seventy-one percent of patients age 70 to 89 years continued to experience pain relief 4 hours after morphine IM. However, only 28% of patients age 18 to 29 years felt pain relief after 4 hours. The results of this study suggest that age is a significant factor for anticipating the duration of morphine analgesia and therefore the frequency of administration.

Kaiko, RF, Wallenstein, SL, Rogers, A, et al: Narcotics in the elderly, *Med Clin North Am* 66:1079-1089, 1982. A report of three studies designed to further develop the observations of Bellville and colleagues (discussed above). Seven hundred fifteen patients who received 8 mg and 16 mg doses of morphine were studied to determine the following factors: the significance of age relative to dose and demographic and pain variables, age and peak vs. duration of morphine analgesia, and age and morphine plasma levels. Of the variables examined, age, race, sex, pretreatment intensity, character, and site of pain, the difference in age was associated with the greatest difference in analgesia. The patients who were particularly aged responded to morphine as though they had received three to four times the dose given to young adult patients. Age-related increase in analgesia is primarily a function of an increase in duration rather than an increase in peak analgesic effect. These studies in combination with previous ones suggest that morphine clearance decreases with age. The authors' data suggest that age be used as the criteria for choosing initial dosing frequency. They stress that pain be managed by adjustment of dose and dosing frequency according to individual patients' response.

Nolan, L, and O'Malley, K: Prescribing for the elderly. Part I. Sensitivity of the elderly to adverse drug reactions, *J Am Geriatr Soc* 36:142-149, 1988. The article reviews the inpatient and outpatient studies which report the relationship of adverse drug reactions to increasing patient age. While the incidence of adverse drug reactions may be greater in the elderly, there is no evidence to conclusively link these reactions to the biological effects of aging. It is suggested that polypharmacy is more consistently associated with adverse drug reactions, and that severe illness, multiple pathology, and its associated high level of prescribing is more important than age.

Portenoy, RK, and Kanner, RM: Patterns of analgesic prescription and consumption in a university-affiliated community hospital, *Arch Intern Med* 145:439-441, 1985. The records of 208 medical and 103 surgical patients were reviewed. The type of analgesic and psychotropic medications, dosage, and dosing intervals were noted. The older patients in this study were prescribed and took fewer narcotics. Two thirds of the patients were more than 60 years old, yet only half of the analgesics prescribed went to this group. More than 50% of the 18- to 40-year-old patients took an analgesic, in contrast to only 19% of those older than 80. Only 20% of the older group who took an analgesic used a narcotic, compared to 88% of the younger group. The authors suggest that the age-related differences in both prescribing patterns and consumption of analgesics may be a result of concern about increased risk of side effects in older patients. However, they state that there is inadequate information on this. The data also suggest additional findings concerning treatment of cancer pain, polypharmacy, and prescribing of psychotropics.

Roy, R, and Thomas, M: Elderly persons with and without pain: a comparative study, *Clin J Pain* 3:102-106, 1987. Two hundred five people, ages 60 to 89, who were ambulatory and capable of participating in a variety of activities were surveyed to assess prevalence of pain problems in the healthy elderly and how they compared with elderly without pain. Seventy percent of the people studied reported some kind of problem with pain, and yet disability due to pain was almost nonexistent. There were no signs of depression in this group, and all people in the group were part of an organization that promoted community involvement and organized social activities. Under these circumstances, pain and disability during the older years can be mutually exclusive.

REFERENCES AND SELECTED READINGS

Amadio, P, Cummings, DM, and Amadio, PB: Pain in the elderly: management techniques, *Pain Manag* 1:33-41, 1987

American Association of Retired Persons and the Administration on Aging: A profile of older Americans, 1987, The Association

American Pain Society: Principles of analgesic use in the treatment of acute pain and chronic cancer pain: a concise guide to medical practice, Washington, DC, 1987, The Society

Austin, KL, Stapleton, JV, and Mather, LE: Multiple intramuscular injections: a major source of variability in analgesic response to meperidine, *Pain* 8:47-62, 1980

Avorn, J: Drugs and the elderly, *Harvard Medical School Health Letter* 9:3-4, June 1984

Baskin, SI, and Goldfarb, AH: Age-associated changes of nonnarcotic analgesics. In Goldfarb, PB, and Robers, J, eds: CRC handbook on pharmacology of aging, pp 113-125, Florida, 1983, CRC Press

Butler, RN: The life review: an interpretation of reminiscence in the aged, *Psychiatry* 26:65-76, 1963

Butler, RN, and Gastel, B. Care of the aged: perspectives on pain and discomfort. In Ng, LK, and Bonica, J, eds: Pain, discomfort and humanitarian care, pp 297-311, New York, 1980, Elsevier North Holland

Ceccio, CM: Postoperative pain relief through relaxation in elderly patients with fractured hips, *Orthoped Nurs* 3:11-19, 1984

Clark, WC, and Mehl, L: Thermal pain, *J Abnorm Psychol* 78: 202-212, 1971

Clinch, D, Banerjee, AK, and Ostick, G: Absence of abdominal pain in elderly patients with peptic ulcer disease, *Age Ageing* 13:120-123, 1984

Cunha, UV: Antidepressants: their use in nonpsychiatric disorders of aging, *Geriatrics* 41:63-72, 1986

Dietsche, LM: Facilitating the life review through group reminiscence, *J Gerontol Nurs* 5:43-46, 1979

Eland, JM: Pain management and comfort, *J Gerontol Nurs* 14:10-15, 1988

Engelking, C: Comfort issues in geriatric oncology. In Frank-Stromberg, M, and Welch-McCaffery, D, eds: *Semin Oncol Nurs* 4:198-207, Aug 1988

Fakouri, C, and Jones, P: Relaxation rx: the slow stroke back rub, *J Gerontol Nurs* 13:32-35, 1987

Ferrell, BA, and Ferrell, BR: Assessment of chronic pain in the elderly, *Geriatr Med Today* (in press)

Flower, RJ, Moncada, S, and Vane, JR: Drug therapy of inflammation. In Gilman, AG, et al, eds: Goodman and Gilman's the pharmacological basis of therapeutics, pp 674-715, ed 7, New York, 1985, Macmillan Publishing

Foreman, MD: Acute confusional states in hospitalized elderly: a research dilemma, *Nurs Res* 35:34-38, 1986

Freund, G: Drug and alcohol-induced dementia. In Wood, WG, and Strong, R, eds: Geriatric clinical pharmacology, pp 95-105, New York, 1987, Raven Press

Gall, EP: Analgesic and anti-inflammatory agents. In Conrad, KA, and Bressler, R, eds: Drug therapy for the elderly, St Louis, 1982, The CV Mosby Co

Gioiella, EC, and Bevil, CW: Nursing care of the aging client, pp 291-310, Norwalk, Conn, 1985, Appleton-Century-Crofts

Glynn, NJ: The therapy of music, *J Gerontol Nurs* 12:6-10, 1986

Goodwin, JS, and Regan, M: Cognitive dysfunction associated with naprosyn and ibuprofen in the elderly, *Arthritis Rheumatism* 25:1013-1015, 1982

Greenblatt, DJ, Sellers, EM, and Shader, RI: Drug disposition in old age, *N Engl J Med* 306:1081-1088, May 6, 1982

Griffin, M: In the mind's eye, *Am J Nurs* 86:804-806, 1986

Hanks, GW, and Aherne, GW: Morphine metabolism: does the renal hypothesis hold water? *Lancet* 1:221-222, Jan 26, 1985

Harkins, SW, and Chapman, CR: Detection and decision factors in pain perception in young and elderly men, *Pain* 2:253-264, 1976

Harkins, SW, Kwentus, J, and Price, DD: Pain and suffering in the elderly. In Bonica, J, ed: Clinical management of pain, Philadelphia, Lea and Febiger (in press)

Herth, K: The therapeutic use of music, *Supervisor Nurs* 9:22-23, 1978

Jaffe, JJ, and Martin, WR: Opioid analgesics and antagonists. In Gilman, AG, Goodman, LS, Rall, TW, and Murad, F, eds: The pharmacological basis of therapeutics, pp 532-581, ed 7, New York, 1985, Macmillan Publishing

Johnson, J: Drug treatment for sleep disturbances: does it really work? *J Gerontol Nurs* 11:9-12, 1985

Jones, L: Patient-controlled oral analgesia, *Orthoped Nurs* 6: 38-41, 1987

Kaiko, RF, Foley, KM, Grabinski, PY, et al: Central nervous system excitatory effects of meperidine in cancer patients, *Ann Neurol* 13:180-185, 1983

Kelly, N: Personal communication, 1988. This patient example was given to us by Nancy Kelly, RN, MSN, Geriatric Intake and Assessment Nurse, East Boston Neighborhood Health Center, Boston, Mass. We are appreciative of her willingness to share this example.

Kwentus, JA, Harkins, SW, Lignon, N, and Silverman, JJ: Current concepts of geriatric pain and its treatment, *Geriatrics* 40: 48-57, 1985

Lamy, PP: The elderly, undernutrition, and pharmacokinetics, *J Am Geriatr Soc* 31:560-562, Sept 1983

Lamy, PP: Pain management, drugs and the elderly, *Am Health Care Assoc J* 10:32-36, July 1984

Lamy, PP: Adverse drug reactions and the elderly: an update. In Ham, RJ, ed: Geriatric medicine annual 1986, pp 128-154, Oradell, NJ, 1986, Medical Economics Books

Larson, EB, Kukull, WA, Buchner, D, and Reifler, BV: Adverse drug reactions associated with global cognitive impairment in elderly persons, *Ann Intern Med* 107:169-173, 1987

Liebeskind, JC, and Melzack, R: The international pain foundation: meeting a need for education in pain management, *Pain* 30:1-2, 1987

Linderborn, KM: The need to assess dementia, *J Gerontol Nurs* 14:35-39, 1988

Lonergan, ET: Aging and the kidney: adjusting treatment to physiological change, *Geriatrics* 43:27-33, 1988

Lukacsko, P: A guide to the parenteral management of moderate to severe pain, *Hosp Pharm* 22:361-412, Apr 1987

MacDonald, JB: Presentation of acute myocardial infarction in the elderly, *Age Ageing* 13:196-200, 1984

Mahoney, L, and Zukor, J: Personal communication, 1988. This patient example was given to us by Ms. Mahoney, RN, and Ms. Zukor, RN, staff nurses on the medical oncology unit, Stanford University Hospital, Stanford, Calif.

Mather, LE, Tucker, GT, Pflug, AE, et al: Meperidine kinetics in man, *Clin Pharmacol Ther* 17:21-30, 1975

McCaffery, M: Narcotic analgesia for the elderly, *Am J Nurs* 85:296-297, 1985

Meyer, BR: Benzodiazepines in the elderly, *Med Clin North Am* 66:1017-1035, 1982

Miller, RR, and Jick, H: Clinical effects of meperidine in hospitalized medical patients, *J Clin Pharmacol* 18:180-189, 1978

Miscally, M: Personal communication, 1988. This example was given to us by Madelyn Miscally, RN, MSN, Geriatric Clinical Nurse Specialist, Bowman Gray School of Medicine, Winston-Salem, NC. Ms. Miscally was also a reviewer and consultant for this chapter. We are very appreciative of her willingness to share her expertise on care of the elderly.

Mitchell, CO, and Lipschitz, DA: Detection of protein-calorie malnutrition in the elderly, *Am J Clin Nutr* 35:398-406, 1982

Morgan, J, and Furst, DE: Implications of drug therapy in the elderly, *Clin Rheumat Dis* 12:227-243, 1986

Murray, R, Huelskoetter, M, and O'Driscoll, D: The nursing process in later maturity, pp 284-293, Englewood Cliffs, NJ, 1980, Prentice-Hall

Ouslander, JG: Drug therapy in the elderly, *Ann Intern Med* 95:711-722, 1981

Pagliaro, LA, and Pagliaro, AM: Introduction. In Pagliaro, LA, and

Pagliaro, AM, eds: Pharmacological aspects of aging, pp 1-6, St Louis, 1983, The CV Mosby Co

Pagliaro, LA, and Pagliaro, AM: Age-dependent drug selection and response. In Pagliaro, LA, and Pagliaro, AM, eds: Pharmacological aspects of nursing, pp 130-139, St Louis, 1986, The CV Mosby Co

Peabody, CA, Whiteford, HA, and Hollister, LE: Antidepressants and the elderly, *J Am Geriatr Soc* 34:869-874, 1986

Petrucci, K: Personal communication, 1988. This patient example was given to us by Kerry Petrucci, RN, MSN, Nurse Gerontologist, Clinical Center Nursing, National Institutes of Health, Bethesda, Md. We appreciate her willingness to share this example.

Polisson, RP: Selecting a NSAID for elderly patients, *Hosp Ther* 12:17-32, 1987

Portenoy, RK: Postherpetic neuralgia: a workable treatment plan, *Geriatrics* 41:34-48, 1986

Portenoy, RK: Optimal pain control in elderly cancer patients, *Geriatrics* 42:33-44, 1987

Portenoy, RK, and Foley, KM: Chronic use of opioid analgesics in nonmalignant pain: report of 38 cases, *Pain* 25:171-176, May 1986

Reidenberg, MM: Drugs in the elderly, *Med Clin North Am* 66:1073-1078, 1982

Rowe, JW, and Bresdine, RW, eds: Health and disease in old age, Boston, 1982, Little, Brown & Co

Rubenstein, LZ, and Robbins, AS: Falls in the elderly: a clinical perspective, *Geriatrics* 39:67-78, 1984

Ryden, MB: Nursing intervention in support of reminiscence, *J Gerontol Nurs* 7:461-463, 1981

Schafer, SC: Personal communication, 1988. This patient example was given to us by Susan Schafer, RNC, MS, Clinical Research Nurse, Pain Research Clinic, National Institutes of Health, Bethesda, Md. Ms. Schafer was also a reviewer and consultant for this chapter. We are very appreciative of her willingness to share her expertise on pain in the elderly.

Schlegel, SI, and Paulus, HE: Non-steroidal and analgesic therapy in the elderly, *Clin Rheumat Dis* 12:245-273, 1986

Schmucker, DL: Drug disposition in the elderly: a review of the critical factors, *J Am Geriatr Soc* 32:144-149, 1984

Strumpf, NE, and Evans, LK: Physical restraint of the hospitalized elderly: perceptions of patients and nurses, *Nurs Res* 37: 132-137, 1988

Sturgis, ET, Dolce, JJ, and Dickerson, PC: Pain management in the elderly. In Carstensen, L, and Edelstein, BA, eds: Handbook of clinical gerontology, pp 190-203, New York, 1987, Pergamon Press

Szeto, H, Inturrisi, C, Houde, R, et al: Accumulation of normeperidine, an active metabolite of meperidine, in patients with renal failure or cancer, *Ann Intern Med* 86:738-741, 1977

Thomas, MR, and Roy, R: Age and pain: a comparative study of the "younger and older" elderly, *Pain Manag* 1:174-179, July-Aug 1988

Thorsteinsson, G: Chronic pain: use of TENS in the elderly, *Geriatrics* 42:75-82, 1987

Todd, B: Narcotic analgesia for chronic pain, *Geriatr Nurs* 7:53-55, Jan-Feb 1986

Travis, SS: Observer-rated functional assessments for institutionalized elders, *Nurs Res* 37:138-143, 1988

Triozzi, PL, Goldstein, D, and Lazlo, J: Supportive care of the patient with cancer. In Cohen, HJ, ed: *Clin Geriatr Med* 3:505-516, Aug 1987

Weingart, WA, Sorkness, CA, and Earhart, RH: Analgesia with oral narcotics and added ibuprofen in cancer patients, *Clin Pharm* 4:53-58, Jan-Feb 1985

Wenzl, C: Personal communication, 1988. This patient example was given to us by Carol Wenzl, RN, MSN, and is from her practice as Clinical Coordinator, Pain Management Team, Mercy Health Center, Oklahoma City, Okla. The authors appreciate her sharing this with us.

Westfall, LK, and Pavlis, RW: Why the elderly are so vulnerable to drug reactions, *RN* 50:39-42, 1987

Whall, A: Psychotropic medications and side effects in the elderly, *J Gerontol Nurs* 10:35, 1984

Williams, MA, Ward, SE, and Campbell, EB: Confusion: testing versus observation, *J Gerontol Nurs* 14:25-30, 1988

CHAPTER

12

Evaluation: The Total Picture

How well have we done with controlling a patient's pain? Is it the best we can do? These are vital questions to ask as we evaluate the effectiveness of our nursing actions.

Evaluation is a process that helps us measure a patient's progress or lack of progress toward a mutually set goal (Carpenito, 1983). As a component of the nursing process, evaluation provides information that may result in a readjustment or revision of the plan of care.

In each of the chapters on pain relief measures, specific suggestions are made for the initial and ongoing assessment or evaluation of the various pain relief methods. The flow sheet, p. 27, is one of the basic formats used to accomplish ongoing evaluation. It is a tool that promotes identification of necessary modifications, implementation of the modifications, followed by the continuous process of evaluation or assessment of the safety and effectiveness of the pain control measure.

This chapter addresses the total plan for pain control, specifically its effectiveness, comprehensiveness, and need for modification for the individual patient. Evaluation of the person with pain includes a review of the following points:
• Evaluation of the overall plan of care.
• Implementation of a checklist of pain control measures.
• Patient's assimilation of the pain experience.
• Failure to relieve pain.

EVALUATION OF THE OVERALL PLAN

The patient may be using analgesics, distraction, cold packs, relaxation, and a number of other specific methods of pain relief. But what is the total effect of all of these approaches? Each method may have been successful when it was evaluated separately; however, the following are key questions to ask when evaluating the overall plan:

• How successful are all the methods when one views the patient's life overall, 24 hours a day, day after day?
• To what extent is pain relieved throughout a 24-hour period?
• What effect have the pain relief measures had on the patient's quality of life or ability to function? Is the patient able to do the things he values or desires, e.g., get a good night's sleep or go to work? Have any of the pain relief measures interfered with this?
• Is the total plan for pain relief feasible, or is it consuming the person's day at the expense of other activities?

Patient Example

Mr. L., 65 years old with prostate cancer and widespread bone metastasis, is taking a narcotic and a nonsteroidal antiinflammatory drug on a regular schedule. At home he alternates a heating pad with cold packs in the morning. He uses a transcutaneous electrical nerve stimulator (TENS) for his back pain. In the afternoon and evening he uses biofeedback with a relaxation tape. In order to sleep, he uses relaxation with a guided image for pain relief. Despite these multiple modalities, Mr. L. rates his pain at 6 to 8 on a 0 to 10 scale (0 = no pain, 10 = worst pain) and finds that most of his time is spent in pain relief activities. His one main interest is to continue his oil paintings of the lake and woods behind his house. However, he is "too exhausted" and "hurts too much" to be able to stand at his easel.

Upon evaluation of Mr. L.'s day, it was apparent to the community health nurse that the narcotic needed to be increased and that some of the nonpharmacological methods needed to be omitted or tailored to allow the patient to pursue what was important to him. A 50% increase in Mr. L.'s narcotic allowed him to paint for several hours each day, and he was able to omit the use of heat and cold and one of the relaxation techniques. With better pain control, his mood and sleep improved also.

IMMEDIATE HELP WITH UNRELIEVED PAIN

How Can I Avoid Making This Situation Worse?

Time involved: Reading time, 2 minutes; implementation time, initial part within 3 to 5 minutes, follow-up contact may range from 30 seconds to 5 minutes each time.

Sample situation: The patient is still in pain, maybe even worse than when you first tried to help him. Perhaps you have done all you know how to do. Maybe you know that more can be done, but the methods are not available or you cannot get key people to cooperate. For whatever reason, at this moment, you have reached the limit of what you can do to reduce the pain.

Possible solution: Provide continued contact and concern.

Expected outcome: Hopefully the patient feels you believe that he hurts. You acknowledge that at this time you are unable to provide further pain relief measures; however, the patient is not abandoned to suffer alone with unrelieved pain.

You may not think so now, but there is a lot that can be done. However, it probably will not be easy. Ask yourself, "How can I avoid making this situation worse?"

Don'ts

Do not tell the patient it is not as bad as he thinks.
Do not tell the patient he would feel better if only he would act, think, or feel a certain way.

Do not sneak or rush away from the patient.
Do not show anger or disgust toward the patient.
Do not blame the patient for feeling pain.
Do not tell the patient he should count his blessings or otherwise be grateful.
Do not tell the patient that this is his problem that he now must handle on his own.
Do not tell the patient that others have lived through this or handled it better.
Do not tell the patient that he has a low pain tolerance.

Dos

Do tell the patient that you believe that he hurts.
Do explain why further pain control measures are not being provided, e.g., that this is all we know or are able to do right now.
Do show your concern by making a plan for continued contact, e.g., return regularly to the room or telephone regularly.
Do offer reasonable hope such as the patient's condition may improve with time or a new approach may become apparent.

Although it is appropriate to use multiple methods of pain control, we may overuse these methods to avoid pharmacological adjustments. At times the use of too many methods may completely control a person's life. In this case, evaluation of the overall plan of care resulted in a revision of pain control methods in order to address an important patient goal.

IMPLEMENTATION OF A CHECKLIST OF PAIN CONTROL MEASURES

If pain is not well controlled, have we tried everything that is indicated for this patient? To determine this, a checklist may be helpful (see pp. 326-327). Not all pain relief measures are indicated for every patient, but a checklist may help assure that everything appropriate for the individual patient has been considered. Use the checklist to ask these questions:

• Did we try this pain relief measure? If not, why not?
• If a pain relief measure was tried and was successful, is it still being used?
• If a pain relief measure was attempted and was not successful, is there any reason to try it again, perhaps with some modification? Further, some conditions change, so that something previously inappropriate or unsuccessful might be tried again.

ASSIMILATION OF THE PAIN EXPERIENCE

If pain is well controlled, or if pain has subsided and pain relief measures are no longer needed, does the patient need help with the intellectual and emotional incorporation of the painful experience?

Some patients may need to talk about their experience with pain. They may feel that they "performed poorly" or that they are failures because they were not able to "endure" a procedure without acting "like a baby." Others may have some unresolved issues about how they were treated when they hurt.

The process of assisting the patient to assimilate a pain experience involves encouraging him to express what he remembers about the pain sensation, his emotions, thoughts, reactions, how other people related to him, and how he felt about these. Listening to the patient describe his experience and providing support for his reactions may help him emotionally assimilate feelings that may linger long after the pain sensation has stopped.

Patient Example

A month after a sudden onset of severe back pain requiring hospital admission, Mrs. B. talked to the office nurse about her pain experience. She remembered how ex-

Text continued on p. 328.

Checklist of Possible Pain Relief Measures

Purpose: Use the following checklist to determine if all appropriate pain relief measures have been attempted for the individual patient, especially if pain is not well controlled overall or for certain periods of time. This list may be especially useful as a guide for discussing the patient in rounds or team conference. In addition to explanatory comments, codes for the comment column could include:

NA = not appropriate.

NS = not satisfactory, or tried but not successful.

√ = done or in progress.

? = may be appropriate, need to assess.

Comments: **Pain relief measures:**

Analgesics. Goal is reduction in pain intensity, elimination of pain if possible. Regardless of the type of pain, some type of analgesic is almost always appropriate. Remember all analgesics should be used according to the following principles:
• Patient control—to the extent patient is willing and able and within limits of safety.
• Preventive approach.
• Individualizing drug choice, route, dose, and interval.
• More than one type may be needed, e.g., narcotic + nonnarcotic.

_____ Nonnarcotic, e.g., PO tablets or liquids, rectal.

_____ Narcotic, e.g., PO tablets or liquids, buccal, sublingual, rectal, IM, SC, IV, spinal.

_____ Antidepressants, especially for dull aching neuropathic pain and for sleep disturbances.

_____ Anticonvulsants, especially for sharp, shooting neuropathic pain.

_____ Other adjuvant analgesics—beware of potentiators:

_____

_____

Cutaneous stimulation. Usually decreases the intensity of pain. Remember to consider the following:
• Sites other than pain, e.g., opposite side, between pain and brain, beyond pain, trigger points, acupuncture points.
• Combining sensations, e.g., menthol and cold, or alternating sensations, e.g., heat and cold.

_____ Superficial massage—body, hands, feet.

_____ Pressure/massage.

_____ Vibration.

_____ Heat, dry or moist.

_____ Cold, dry or moist.

_____ Alternating heat and cold.

_____ Ice, brief application or massage.

_____ Menthol application, e.g., Ben-Gay.

_____ TENS (Transcutaneous Electrical Nerve Stimulation).

_____ Other: _____

_____

Continued.

Checklist of Possible Pain Relief Measures—cont'd.

Distraction: Usually makes pain more tolerable; it does not make pain go away. Remember to consider the following:
- Use of all major sensory modalities, i.e., auditory, visual, and tactile-kinesthetic.
- Patient's energy level and ability to concentrate, e.g., avoid distraction that might be too difficult or tiring.
- Time limitation, i.e., distraction cannot be used continuously for hours of severe pain.

_____ Structured distraction strategies during brief episodes of pain such as painful procedures, e.g., visual concentration and rhythmic massage, sing and tap rhythm, and active listening to recorded music.

_____ Serious belly laughter prior to a brief episode of pain, particularly useful if distraction is difficult to perform during pain and if pain is predictable.

_____ Normal sensory input throughout the day—not only makes pain more tolerable but encourages return to normal activity.

_____ Other: _____

Relaxation. Reduces distress associated with pain; rarely relieves pain; not a substitute for appropriate methods of pain relief, e.g., analgesics. Remember to consider the following:
- Amount of time required to learn and perform the technique.
- Importance of relaxation in overall plan of pain control if pain is chronic.
- Patient's need to dissipate energy if very tense, e.g., need for progressive relaxation vs. a meditative technique.

_____ Simple techniques patient may quickly learn to use for brief periods throughout day, e.g., deep breath/tense, exhale/relax, yawn; heartbeat breathing; jaw relaxation; slow rhythmic breathing.

_____ Taped relaxation technique with nonlyrical music in background, e.g., peaceful past experiences, progressive relaxation.

_____ Simple massage, touch, warmth, or other technique that allows patient to be passive recipient (useful for patient who is confused, agitated, sedated, or fatigued).

_____ Other: _____

Imagery. May reduce pain and perhaps distress associated with pain. Remember to consider the following:
- May seem very strange to the patient.
- Rarely a substitute for other appropriate pain relief measures, e.g., analgesics.

_____ Subtle, conversational imagery—may be simple and quickly done, e.g., descriptive words about pain and how it is relieved.

_____ Symptom substitution—may be simple, quickly done, and not likely to seem strange to patient, e.g., holding ice and trying to focus on cold instead of pain.

_____ Tape of imagery technique developed by patient or of a standardized imagery technique, e.g., ball of healing energy. May be done by patient or others, e.g., friend, family, or nurse.

_____ Other: _____

Other Resources

_____ Consultation or referral, e.g., nurse specialist, pharmacist, anesthesiologist, or pain clinic.

_____ Support group, e.g., National Chronic Pain Outreach.

_____ Other: _____

cruciating the pain was every time she tried to move. She found herself totally dependent and very frightened. She told the nurse how ashamed she felt about screaming when the staff tried to get her on a bedpan. She remembered becoming "hysterical" because the pain was so bad and no one seemed to be helping her. She told the office nurse that she felt like somebody else, that she had never reacted in this way before.

The nurse encouraged her to describe what upset her the most about the situation. Mrs. B. discussed her feelings of helplessness, hopelessness, and anger about the way she was treated. The nurse reinforced the fact that one of Mrs. B.'s discs in her spine had compressed several nerves in that area, and there was very good reason for her to hurt and to show her pain. Mrs. B. could not believe she still had such strong feelings about this experience. On her next office visit 2 weeks later, Mrs. B. expressed thanks to the nurse for listening to her. She said how much it had helped her to talk about the experience, and that now she was not dwelling on the pain memories as much.

FAILURE TO RELIEVE PAIN

When this happens, perhaps our greatest failure is to abandon the patient. When a patient is still in pain, one of the most important actions a nurse may take is not to do something, but to simply be with the patient (McCaffery, 1981). Although pain may not be controlled, we still have something to offer the patient and his family (see Immediate Help on p. 325):

- Acknowledge to the patient that you know he hurts. Sometimes when efforts are unsuccessful in controlling pain or when further efforts are not made to relieve pain, the patient may think we no longer believe he has pain, that he must be imagining how bad his pain is, that he must be crazy, or that it is all in his head. *We need to assure the patient that we know he still hurts.*

- Acknowledge the reason for not providing further pain relief measures. It may be helpful to explain to the patient that we have done all we know to do, or all we are able to do right now.

- Provide continued contact and concern: This is particularly important for patients dealing with prolonged pain. Tell the patient when you will return and for how long. Even on a busy acute care clinical unit, the nurse probably can manage to commit to returning every hour for a few seconds.

If the patient is being followed at home, set a specific time each week when you will call to see how he is doing. Why? So the patient is not abandoned to suffer alone. In the authors' practices, patients have repeatedly stated that when efforts to control their pain were unsuccessful, what meant the most to them was the continued contact and concern, e.g., a weekly phone call, from the nurse.

- Offer reasonable hope. A statement that is usually honest is "Maybe things will change or I'll think of something else to do."

The science of pain is relatively new, and as a result, we simply do not know enough to relieve or control pain adequately in all patients. When this occurs, we are often tempted to avoid the patient. In spite of our frustration, a willingness to remain with the patient is often more valuable to the person than we realize.

REFERENCES AND SELECTED READINGS

Carpenito, LJ: Nursing diagnosis application to clinical practice, Philadelphia, 1983, JB Lippincott

McCaffery, M: When your patient is still in pain, don't just do something: sit there, *Nursing* 11:58-61, June 1981

Study Guide

OBJECTIVES OF THE STUDY GUIDE

Participation in the directions given for the study guide will enable you to:

1. Gain skill in using the selected assessment tools and pain relief measures.
2. Become familiar with some practical aspects of using selected assessment tools and pain relief measures with patients in the clinical setting.
3. Evaluate the effectiveness of selected noninvasive pain relief measures on yourself and your partner, noting any differences.
4. Identify the characteristics of the pain relief possible with specific noninvasive pain relief measures, e.g., decreased intensity of pain or increased tolerance for pain.

CHAPTER 1—PERSPECTIVES ON PAIN: HISTORY, CURRENT STATUS, AND DEVELOPING THE NURSE'S ROLE (pp. 1-5)

The purpose of this section is to encourage nurses who care for patients with pain to think about their own philosophy of pain control and to address the issue of patients' rights. It is important to understand that there are no right or easy answers. Exploration of the issues and acknowledgment of their importance is a beginning step.

It may be helpful to discuss your thoughts and reactions to the following with a colleague or fellow student.

1. Think back to a "problem" pain patient that you cared for; if you cannot recall one, reread the patient example on p. 3 concerning John. Identify the conclusions that you reached as a result of the patient's behavior. What are these conclusions based on? Do you believe that the patient is the final authority about assessment of his pain and all methods of pain control? Determine the appropriateness of your conclusions using this belief as a foundation.

Common answers: When a patient's behavior becomes a problem, exploration with the patient usually shows that his pain is not controlled and his medication is inadequate. Regarding the patient example on p. 3, watching the clock helps him stay on top of the pain and prevents it from becoming unbearable. Explore with the patient why he "prefers the needle to the pill." The answer usually is that the shot relieves the pain quicker and better than the

pill. In fact, this statement makes sense, that is, injections do have a faster onset of action than pills, and because a PO dose equivalent to 50 mg IM Demerol was not used in this situation, it is logical that the IM dose gives John better pain relief. However, even in the absence of pharmacological knowledge, the patient's statement about his pain and the effectiveness of the analgesic must be accepted.

2. Mrs. T. is scheduled for a cholecystectomy the next day. She anxiously tells you that she is afraid of the postoperative pain and that she is so scared of shots that she will "just suffer" rather than ask for them. Other patients on your unit receive IV narcotics with capabilities to self-bolus. Transcutaneous electrical nerve stimulation (TENS) applied in the operating room is another technique successfully used for many patients with similar surgeries. However, you know that Mrs. T.'s surgeon refuses to use either of these methods for his patients, and he insists that IM injections are the best method of pain relief. After talking with Mrs. T., you know these other methods of pain control could make a difference in her comfort and anxiety level. What are your choices in this situation? Do you do anything?

Common answers: An important role for the nurse is to assist patients to exercise their rights in situations where they are vulnerable. Has Mrs. T. talked to the surgeon about her fear of shots? Has she asked him for alternative methods of pain control? If she has not, you might suggest that you be present when she asks about these other methods. This encourages the patient to take responsibility for her concerns, and it also allows the nurse to be the patient's advocate and suggest other options if the surgeon does not answer her questions.

3. Tommy, a 20-month-old toddler with end-stage cancer, is receiving a continuous infusion of morphine at home. Although the dose is keeping him comfortable, he sleeps day and night. The parents are appreciative that their son's pain is finally controlled. However, as time passes, they tearfully talk with you about wanting to interact with their son during the short time they have before he dies. What are your responsibilities in this situation to Tommy? To his parents? What are your options?

Common answers: While you are mindful of the parents' concerns, the nurse must also try to state what is in the best interest of Tommy, who cannot speak for himself. The parents need to know what the consequences may be if the morphine dose is reduced, e.g., Tommy's pain may be out of control again. It is important to explore all possible options with the parents.

4. Mr. H., hospitalized for a recent stroke, is unable to talk or communicate in any way. His wife tells you repeatedly how worried she is about his arthritis pain which increased in severity over the last month at home. Cold packs to his knees in combination with Motrin 800 mg qid were the only way he could maintain minimal walking around the house. She is concerned now that he has not received these pain relief measures, that the pain is unbearable, and that he is suffering. The physician told her that Mr. H. probably is not aware of the pain now, and not to worry about it. She is convinced by his facial expression that he is suffering. What is the nurse's role in this situation?

Common answers: The wife probably knows her husband better than any of the members of the health care team. She is acting on behalf of her husband who cannot speak for himself. The nurse must support the wife in her role as advocate for her husband.

CHAPTER 2—ASSESSMENT (pp. 6-33)

To learn more about assessment of pain, try the following:

1. Complete the "Initial Pain Assessment Tool" (p. 21) by interviewing a patient. Compare this tool with one that you are already using in your practice setting. Combine the best parts of both for a tool that is easy and practical for your individual clinical setting.

If you are not currently using any tool, discuss with your colleagues how an assessment tool might be implemented in your practice setting.

2. Complete a "Flow Sheet" (p. 27) on a patient with a complicated pain medication regimen. Explore with colleagues how this might be implemented in your clinical setting.

3. Ask a patient or family member to keep a daily diary (p. 30). Does this tool help your assessment, planning, and evaluation for the patient?

CHAPTER 3—THE PROCESS OF NURSING PEOPLE WITH PAIN (pp. 34-41)

The following questions will help the nurse integrate pain theories and nursing diagnosis into clinical practice.

1. Using the endorphin theory, what would you say to a patient to explain how transcutaneous electrical nerve stimulation (TENS) works?

Common answers: Some types of TENS may increase your own natural narcotics, called endorphins. TENS may also increase input in the large nerves and help prevent pain impulses traveling on small nerves from reaching the brain.

2. A patient asks you, "How does listening to music help my pain?"

Common answers: Listening to music is a form of distraction. Distraction overloads a specific part of the brain with more input than it needs. This action sends impulses that keep the pain impulses from reaching the brain.

3. If pentazocine (Talwin) can reverse the analgesia of morphine, would pentazocine (Talwin), nalbuphine (Nubain), or butorphanol (Stadol) reverse the analgesia of our own natural narcotics?

Common answers: Probably not, because our own natural narcotics probably bind much tighter to the receptor sites than the systemic narcotics that we administer.

4. If a patient talks to you about morphine being a "bad drug," using the endorphin theory, what could you reply?

Common answers: Morphine may seem like less of a "bad drug" if we realize that it is comparable to our own natural narcotics that we were born with. So we really are only giving something that is very similar to what our bodies already have, but we just do not have enough of it, like a diabetic without enough insulin.

5. Both morphine and nalbuphine (Nubain) relieve pain, but how are they different?

Common answers: Both morphine and nalbuphine (Nubain) act at the central nervous system level by attaching to opiate receptor sites, but they attach to different sites. The site where nalbuphine (Nubain) attaches does not tend to cause euphoria, respiratory depression, or constipation like morphine does.

6. Practice formulating nursing diagnoses associated with pain on patients in your clinical setting.

Possible examples:

1. Chronic pain related to metastasis to the spine from breast cancer.
2. Sleep pattern disturbance related to increase in pain intensity at night.
3. Bathing/hygiene self-care deficit related to inability to bathe self secondary to increased pain with movement.
4. Fear related to belief that narcotic analgesic will become ineffective if dose escalation is too rapid.

CHAPTER 4—PHARMACOLOGICAL CONTROL OF PAIN: A MULTIDISCI-PLINARY APPROACH (pp. 42-129)

Practice questions using the equianalgesic chart (pp. 78-79): These questions assist the reader with the *calculation* of equianalgesic doses of medication. (For specific steps for changing route of medication, e.g., IM to PO, refer to pp. 106-107.)

1. The analgesia of meperidine (Demerol) 75 mg IM would require _____ mg meperidine PO.

2. The analgesic of morphine 10 mg would require _____ mg nalbuphine (Nubain) IM.

3. The analgesia of meperidine (Demerol) 75 mg IM would require _____ mg morphine IM.

4. The analgesia of meperidine (Demerol) 100 mg IM would require _____ mg morphine PO.

5. The analgesia of hydromorphone (Dilaudid) 4 mg IV per hour would require _____ mg Dilaudid PO q4h.

6. The analgesia of morphine 90 mg PO q3h would require _____ mg q12h of sustained-release morphine.

7. The analgesia of morphine 15 mg PO would require _____ mg levorphanol (Levo-Dromoran) PO.

Answers and considerations: All *initial* calculations are essentially "educated guesses" for the appropriate dose. Adjustments to the initial dose must follow quickly and are based on the patient's pain rating, respiratory function, level of alertness, and level of pain that is acceptable to the patient.

In each of these situations there may be more than one answer. For each individual patient there may be circumstances which lead you to try a slight variation of the exact calculations, e.g., the elderly cancer patient may be initially switched to a dose a little lower than the equianalgesic dose.

1. 300 mg meperidine PO.

However, this dose is not recommended because of the increased chance of accumulation of normeperidine. This knowledge is important, however, since it is a reminder that the analgesia of IM meperidine is about 4 times that of PO meperidine.

2. 10 to 20 mg nalbuphine IM.

Since there is some disagreement about the equianalgesic dose and since 20 mg causes very little more respiratory depression than 10 mg, many suggest starting with a higher dose. However, nalbuphine is a narcotic agonist-antagonist and is not recommended if the patient has been on pure narcotics long enough to develop physical dependence since nalbuphine would cause withdrawal-like symptoms. But if the patient is started on nalbuphine rather than a "pure" narcotic, he can be easily changed to a "pure" narcotic later, perhaps one with a slightly high dose initially until the antagonist effect is completely gone.

3. 10 mg morphine IM.

4. 40 to 80 mg morphine PO.

Explanation: 75 mg IM meperidine = 30 to 60 mg PO morphine. You would try the lower dose if the patient is elderly or very sensitive to narcotic changes.

Following is an example of the calculation process when the lower PO dose is chosen:

—75 mg IM meperidine = 30 mg PO morphine.
—100 mg IM meperidine = x mg PO morphine.
—75/30 = 100/x.
—75x = 3000.
—x (mg morphine PO) = 40.

Refer to pp. 106-107 for considerations when changing from IM to PO.

5. 80 mg hydromorphone PO q4h.

Explanation: The IM dose is used as the equivalent of the IV dose in this example.

Following is the calculation:

—1.5 mg IM(IV) hydromorphone = 7.5 mg hydromorphone PO.
—4 mg IV hydromorphone = x mg PO hydromorphone.
—1.5/7.5 = 4/x.
—1.5x = 30.
—x (mg hydromorphone PO) = 20 q1h; 80 q4h.

6. 360 mg sustained-release morphine q12h.

Following is the calculation:

—8 doses of 90 mg morphine q3h = 720 mg/24 hours
—720 divided by 2 = 360 q12h.

7. 1 mg levorphanol PO.

Explanation: 60 mg morphine PO = 4 mg levorphanol PO. You would probably decide to use the 60 mg and not the 30 mg equivalent if the patient is young and has a history of needing to start with higher equivalent doses and then be adjusted down once the pain is controlled.

Following is the calculation:

—60 mg morphine PO = 4 mg levorphanol PO.
—15 mg morphine = x mg levorphanol.
—60/4 = 15/x.
—60x = 60.
—x (mg levorphanol PO) = 1.

CHAPTER 5—CUTANEOUS STIMULATION (pp. 130-171)

The following format for practicing with cold (pp. 145-152) may be adapted to experiment with most of the other types of cutaneous stimulation discussed in Chapter 5:

• Pressure/massage (p. 141).
• Vibration (p. 143).
• Superficial heat (p. 145).
• Ice application/massage (p. 152).
• Menthol application (p. 155).
• TENS (p. 158).

Practice with Local Application of Cold

Equipment needed:

A cold pack and cloth to wrap it. A small plastic bag with ice inside and a washcloth will suffice.

Instructions:

I. Choose a partner (work in pairs). It is even more fun and informative if you have a group of 10 or more practicing in pairs. (However, if necessary, you can do this by yourself.)

II. Decide who will be the nurse (experimenter) and who will be the patient (subject). Whenever possible, take the time to practice both roles, i.e., give each partner a chance to be the nurse and the patient.

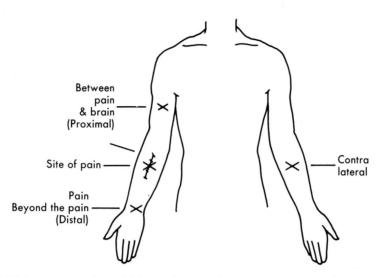

FIGURE SG-1 Examples of sites (*x*) for application of cutaneous stimulation for pain relief: site of pain, between pain and brain (proximal), beyond the pain (distal), and contralateral (opposite side).

III. The nurse finds a way to inflict moderate pain on the patient. A simple method of inflicting pain is to use the thumb and index finger to grasp and apply pressure to muscle or subcutaneous tissue, like pinching, but in a manner that produces a dull ache. Keep in mind the following:
   —For this experiment with cold, inflict pain on a leg or arm, at a point midway, e.g., the forearm rather than the finger tip, since you will experiment with placement of cold distal to the pain.
   —Inflict only moderate pain, not severe. No bleeding or bruising either.
   —The patient (subject) always has the right to tell you to stop.
IV. Perform the following sequence of instructions:
   A. Nurse inflicts moderate pain at a midpoint on the extremity. Hold this pressure/pain steady for the remainder of the experiment.*
   B. Before applying the cold, get a pain rating on a scale of 0 to 10 (0 = no pain, 10 = worst possible pain).
   C. Apply cold to the four sites listed below, one at a time, keeping the cold on the site until the patient feels cold as intensely as is comfortable. Get a pain

rating, and then apply cold to the next site. *Do not allow the cold to become painfully cold.* (Keep track of the results using question #1 below.) The experiment goes more quickly if cold is applied with a minimum of wrapping since it becomes colder faster. The four sites (see Figure SG-1 for examples) are:
   1. Contralateral—opposite side of body corresponding to pain site.
   2. Proximal—between pain and the brain.
   3. Distal—beyond the pain.
   4. Over the site of pain (the fingers applying the painful pressure will also probably have to be covered with the cold pack since you cannot get under the fingers).
   D. Do this again, switching roles so that the nurse now becomes the patient.
Questions/Answers:
1. What were the pain ratings?
   a. Before application of cold _____.
   b. Cold applied contralaterally (opposite side) _____.
   c. Cold applied proximal to the pain (between pain and brain) _____.
   d. Cold applied distal to pain (beyond pain) _____.
   e. Cold applied to site of pain _____.
2. Did cold relieve pain when it was placed at any site other than the site of pain? Which distant sites worked? Which worked the best?
   Common answers when this is practiced in a large group: A few people, up to about one half, will find that

*In clinical practice, a pain relief measure is applied prior to the onset of pain whenever possible. However, the experiment with cold can be done more quickly if pain is inflicted before the cold is applied. The effect of cold lasts several minutes or longer after it is removed, so it takes several minutes to feel the pain in the absence of cold if cold is applied prior to pain.

cold works at one or more sites distant from the pain. Cold will not necessarily work for an individual at all three sites distant from the pain. But, if the group is large enough, each site distant from pain will work for a few people. The distant site that works best varies between people.

3. Did cold relieve pain when it was placed at the site of pain? How effective was it at this site compared to the others?

     Common answers when this is practiced in a large group: Cold applied to the site of pain tends to work for more people than cold applied to any of the other sites, but cold does not work at the site of pain for everyone. Cold tends to relieve more pain when it is applied to the site of pain than when it is applied to other sites, but again, not always.

4. Was cold ineffective at all sites? Did it make pain worse?

     Common answers when this is practiced in a large group: Cold is ineffective for a very few people. Sometimes, although not commonly, cold makes pain worse.

5. Was cold more effective at any sites distant from the pain than it was over the site?

     Common answers when this is practiced in a large group: Almost always there are a few people who say that cold applied to one or more of the distant sites relieved pain better than cold applied to the site of pain. Frequently the patient will explain that when cold is applied to the site of pain, he feels both cold and pain. But when cold is applied away from the pain, one of two things may happen: (1) after a few moments it is like a switch suddenly goes off—the pain is gone and only the cold is felt, or (2) after a few moments attention gradually shifts to a focus on the cold instead of the pain, although the pain may still be felt to some extent.

6. What have you learned that will help you take care of a patient with pain?

     Common answers when this is practiced in a large group: Cold probably works best for most people when it is applied to the site of pain. Cold may relieve pain at sites other than the site of pain. Therefore when you cannot get to the site of pain, e.g., a sterile field, it is reasonable to try contralateral, proximal, and distal sites. All three can be tried at the same time in the clinical setting. Occasionally, when applying cold to the site of pain does not help or makes pain worse, it will be more effective to use distant sites. For a few people cold will not help regardless of where it is applied. These people have at least given cold a chance, and now should consider other methods of cutaneous stimulation. Some people simply prefer heat. When cold is effective, it relieves pain rapidly. For every patient, consider obtaining a physician's prescription for "application of cold or heat anywhere as needed to relieve pain."

CHAPTER 6—DISTRACTION (pp. 172-187)

The following format for practicing the distraction strategies of "Sing and Tap Rhythm" (p. 177) and "Active Listening to Recorded Music" (p. 177) may be adapted to experiment with most of the other types of distraction discussed in Chapter 6:
- Visual concentration and rhythmic massage (p. 176).
- Slow rhythmic breathing (p. 176).
- Taking laughter seriously (p. 178).
- Describing a series of pictures (p. 179).

Practice with "Sing and Tap Rhythm" or "Active Listening to Recorded Music"

Equipment needed:
- No equipment needed for "Sing and Tap Rhythm."
- For "Active Listening to Recorded Music," obtain a battery-operated tape recorder or cassette player with an earphone or headset and a tape of music, usually something fast and lively, but you may choose comedy routines or any type of music you like.

Instructions:

I. Choose a partner (work in pairs). It is even more fun and informative if you have a group of 10 or more practicing in pairs. (However, if necessary, you can do this by yourself.)

II. Decide who will be the nurse (experimenter) and who will be the patient (subject). Whenever possible, take the time to practice both roles, i.e., give each partner a chance to be the nurse and the patient.

III. The nurse finds a way to inflict moderate pain on the patient, unless the patient is already in pain. Methods of inflicting pain include:
   —Press the shank of a pencil or pen into the nailbed.
   —Use thumb and index finger to grasp and squeeze the trapezius (shoulder) muscle.
   —Use thumb and index finger to grasp and apply pressure to muscle or subcutaneous tissue, like pinching, but done in a manner that produces a dull ache.
   Keep in mind the following:
   —Inflict only moderate pain, not severe. No bleeding or bruising either.
   —The patient (subject) always has the right to tell you to stop.

IV. Decide which distraction strategy you are going to use, "Sing and Tap Rhythm" or "Active Listening to Recorded Music." Read about the distraction strategy you are going to use, p. 177.

V. Become acquainted with what you will be doing. Learn how to operate the tape player or recite to each other a few lines of the song each of you intends to sing in your role as patient.

VI. Perform the following sequence of instructions:
   A. Nurse helps the patient begin to use the distraction strategy without any pain being in-

flicted* (unless patient already has pain). Reminders to the patient:

—Start listening to the music or start singing the song by whispering or mouthing out the words.

—Focus your eyes on an object, e.g., a picture, or make eye contact with the nurse. If you prefer to close your eyes, have a mental picture or image that blocks out the pain.

—Tap out the rhythm.

B. While the patient continues to use the distraction, the nurse begins to gradually inflict increasing pain until the patient indicates a need to do more about the pain, i.e., either sings faster or turns up the volume. When this happens, hold the pressure/pain steady for the remainder of the experiment.

C. After a few moments, the nurse tells the patient to stop the distraction but the nurse continues the same amount of pressure/pain.

D. When the patient has stopped the distraction, tell the patient to focus on the pain and ask, "How does the pain feel now without the distraction compared to what it felt like with the distraction?" After he answers, release the pressure/pain.

E. Do this again, switching roles so that the nurse now becomes the patient.

Questions/Answers.

1. Did the distraction strategy help with the pain?

Common answers when this is practiced in a large group: About 80% to 90% of the group will say distraction helped.

2. If distraction did not help you with the pain, or if distraction was ineffective at first, why do you think it did not work for you? What could be done to make it work?

Common answers when this is practiced in a large group: Some do not like the song or music. It is not uncommon to find that a different song or tape works better. The patient's initial choice may be wrong for him. Sometimes the subject cannot get his mind off the pain. If singing does not provide enough distraction, switch to listening to a tape since that seems to have more appeal to most people and is a more demanding stimulus. Possibly pain was simply too severe for distraction to work, or so severe that a simpler distraction was needed, e.g., eye contact and counting backwards from 10 with the nurse. Or, it could be that the patient does not ordinarily use distraction, so ask what he usually uses to help himself with pain.

In some situations there are too many disturbances.

A room with noises and people talking can divert a person from the distraction strategy.

Some people kept watching the infliction of pain. In this experiment, as in the clinical setting, it is not unusual to find that the patient wants to monitor a painful event first before he is willing to direct his attention elsewhere. This, of course, should be respected. Sometimes the patient needs to watch to obtain information that assures him he is in good hands or is otherwise safe. Information also gives some patients a sense of control.

3. If distraction helped you with pain, how would you explain in simple terms how it helped?

Common answers when this is practiced in a large group: "It distracted me." "I was thinking of something besides the pain." "It took my mind off of pain." "When you concentrate on the distraction, you pay less attention to the pain and it doesn't bother you as much."

4. When distraction helped with the pain, did it make the pain go away?

Common answers when this is practiced in a large group: Virtually everyone says that distraction does not make the pain go away.

5. What have you learned that will help you take care of a patient with pain?

Common answers when this is practiced in a large group: A structured distraction strategy will help the majority of patients get through a brief episode of pain, making it more tolerable. The nurse might explain the potential benefits of distraction to the patient by saying, "When you concentrate on the distraction, you pay less attention to the pain and that makes the pain more bearable."

Distraction does not work for everyone, but sometimes a few minor modifications will enable the patient to benefit from it, e.g., avoid diverting the patient's attention from his distraction, or wait to use distraction until the patient has monitored the situation to his satisfaction.

Distraction does not make the pain go away. When patients are distracted from pain, they are not acting like they are in pain, yet they still have pain. Perhaps now it is easier to understand why a patient who is laughing at a TV program may still ask for a "pain pill."

Pain returns quickly once the distraction is stopped. This helps explain why all the lights go on and patients ask for "pain shots" after a big ball game on TV is over or visiting hours end.

CHAPTER 7—RELAXATION (pp. 188-211)

The following format for practicing the "Meditative Relaxation Script" (pp. 202-203) may be adapted to experiment with most of the other types of relaxation discussed in Chapter 7:

---

*A preventive approach is used here, i.e., the pain relief measure is started before the pain is felt. Ideally, this is what is also done in actual clinical practice.

- Deep breath/tense, exhale/relax, yawn (p. 199).
- Humor (p. 199).
- Heartbeat breathing (p. 200).
- Jaw relaxation (p. 200).
- Slow rhythmic breathing (p. 201).
- Peaceful past experiences (p. 201).
- Progressive relaxation script (pp. 204-205).
- Simple touch, massage, or warmth (p. 206).

Practice with "Meditative Relaxation Script"

Equipment needed:
The following is helpful, but not necessary: comfortable chair or bed with good support for legs (see figure on p. 197); tape recorder with microphone and blank tape.
Instructions:

 I. Note what time it is and record this in question #1 below.

 II. Choose a partner (work in pairs). It is even more fun and informative if you have a group of 10 or more practicing in pairs. (However, if necessary, you can do this by yourself.)

 III. Decide who will be the nurse (experimenter) and who will be the patient (subject). Whenever possible, take the time to practice both roles, i.e., give each partner a chance to be the nurse and the patient.

 IV. Familiarize yourselves with the following:

  —"Meditative Relaxation Script," read pp. 202-203 and ask the questions listed below.

  —Distress scale, Figure 7-1, see p. 195. If the patient is already in pain, also note the pain scale. (In this experiment, pain will not be artificially inflicted, since relaxation is best learned in the absence of pain and anxiety, and relaxation often does not reduce pain.)

  —How to record on the tape player.

  —Contents of Table 7-1, p. 196, regarding possible problems and their solutions, just in case you have any difficulty.

 V. As you read the script together, the nurse asks the patient the following questions and modifies the script accordingly. (The questions are preceded by the same number of asterisks as are used in the script so that you can easily locate the appropriate sections of the script.)

  *Do you know how you feel when you relax, e.g., heavy, light, or weightless?

  **Which method of breathing would you like to use? Do you need to find out by trying a few now?

  ***Do you want to change the sequence of body parts mentioned? Omit any body parts? Do you want this part shortened or lengthened?

  ****Can you remember a place you have been that was very peaceful, secure, or comforting? If so, give as detailed a description as you can, including any sights, colors, objects, sounds, touch and tempera-ture sensations, smells, or tastes that were especially important to you.

  *****If you want to use this tape primarily as a sleep aid, do you want to omit the ending?

  Are there any other changes you would like to make?

 VI. If you are going to tape this for the patient, try to include "easy listening," non-lyrical music in the background.

 VII. The nurse performs the following sequence of instructions:

  A. Ask the patient to rate his present distress, using the distress scale. Use the pain scale, too, if applicable. Also take the patient's pulse. Record these, using question #1, p. 336.

  B. Help the patient get ready to relax by covering the following points:

   —Empty your bladder, if needed.

   —Loosen clothing, and consider removing anything uncomfortable, e.g., take off your glasses, remove your contact lenses.

   —Put down anything that you are holding.

   —Get into a comfortable position.

   —Provide support under the neck and for elevating the legs, if possible, as in the figure on p. 197.

   —Do not cross your arms or legs since they may feel heavy and you may feel prickly sensations from reduced circulation.

   —Support your arms, perhaps on the arms of the chair or at your side if you are lying down. Do not let your arms dangle.

   —Try to create a quiet environment. This is often difficult, so if there are noises in the room, simply take about 30 seconds now to listen carefully to them so you can identify them, respond to them if necessary now, and then be better able to ignore them later. Consider a "Do not disturb" sign, taking the telephone off the hook, and possibly some background noise, e.g., quiet music or a fan, to override other noises.

   —If the room is cold or if you are cold-natured, cover yourself.

  C. Before you read the relaxation script, gently move a few of the patient's body parts with appropriate support, e.g, bend the arms at the elbow, but support the forearm, to help the patient identify for himself the presence or absence of tension. Ask the patient if he feels any tension and record his response in question #1, p. 336.

  D. Read and record the meditative script, with the background music, if possible, while the patient listens and participates. Read slowly in a quiet monotone with pauses at intervals, especially between paragraphs and when you see "..." within the script. Call the patient by name from time to time.

E. At the end of the relaxation script, but before ending the relaxation experience with the last paragraph, do the following, completing question #1 below:

—Tell the patient you will take his pulse rate.

—Then ask the patient to use the distress scale to rate his distress (and pain, if applicable).

—Tell the patient you will gently move a few body parts with appropriate support, e.g., bend the arms at the elbow and support the forearm, to help the patient identify for himself the presence or absence of tension. Ask the patient if he feels any tension and record his response in question #1.

F. Read the last paragraph of the script now to help the patient become fully alert again. If you decided not to put this last paragraph on the tape because the patient wanted to use the tape to go to sleep, turn off the tape before you read it.

G. Encourage the patient to begin to move about slowly; do not just jump up and start some vigorous activity.

H. Consider doing all of this again, switching roles so that the nurse now becomes the patient and receives her own personal tape.

Questions/Answers:

1. When did you begin this practice session with relaxation? _____

When did you finish? _____

Record the patient's responses in the following blanks.

	Prior to relaxation:	Immediately before ending relaxation:
Pulse rate:	_____	_____
Distress score:	_____	_____
Pain score, if applicable:	_____	_____
Tension reported from movement of body parts:	_____	_____

2. How long did this take?

Common answer: 30 to 60 minutes. It will probably take about this long with an actual patient.

3. Did the patient feel less distress? more relaxed? less pain?

—If not, why does the patient think there was no improvement? Does the nurse have any ideas?

—If yes, what does the patient think helped the most?

Common answers when this is practiced in a large group: The majority of people who participate in the relaxation exercise find that it produces relaxation,

even when no time has been taken to personalize the script in advance. However, it does not necessarily relieve pain except for a select few, e.g., those who have tension headache. At the conclusion of the relaxation experience when they open their eyes, many of them begin to smile and they appear well rested. Among the few people who find it ineffective, some of them already practice a relaxation technique to which they are conditioned, and it is actually inappropriate for them to try another technique. What participants like best about the script varies from one to another.

4. The nurse asks the patient how well the script was read and what suggestions the patient can make about how the nurse can improve her performance.

Common answer: The patient usually thinks the nurse performed very well. If the patient has any suggestions, they often concern script content and not the nurse's reading of it.

5. Both patient and nurse listen to at least a portion of the recorded tape. How well does the nurse think she has done?

Common answer: The nurse is surprised at how well she has done.

6. What have you learned that will help you take care of a patient with pain?

Common answer: Most people experience relaxation and reduced distress in response to a fairly standardized, permissive meditative relaxation script that has been only minimally individualized.

Even if you knew very little about relaxation before you began this practice session, you now know enough to record a somewhat personalized, and probably very effective, meditative tape for a patient.

This is a relatively time-consuming nursing activity, taking up to 1 hour. However, for a patient who has chronic pain, this investment of time may be worth the effort. The patient may very well find the tape helpful several times a day, daily, for months. But the benefits of relaxation must be respected by others. If relaxation helps the patient with pain, it cannot be concluded that the patient's pain is caused by anxiety.

CHAPTER 8—IMAGERY (pp. 212-231)

The following format for practicing the "Ball of Healing Energy" (p. 225) may be adapted to experiment with most of the other imagery techniques discussed in Chapter 8:

• Subtle conversational imagery (p. 218)
• Simple, brief symptom substitution (p. 219)
• Emptying the sandbag (p. 223)
• Breathing out pain (p. 224)
• Opening around pain (p. 226)
• Individualized imagery technique for pain relief (pp. 226-227)

Practice with "Ball of Healing Energy"

Equipment needed:
No equipment is needed unless you decide to tape-record the imagery technique.

Instructions:

I. Choose a partner (work in pairs). It is even more fun and informative if you have a group of 10 or more practicing in pairs. (However, if necessary, you can do this by yourself.)

II. Decide who will be the nurse (experimenter) and who will be the patient (subject). If there is time for only one person to be the patient and if someone actually has mild to moderate pain, allow that person to be the patient. Whenever possible, take the time to practice both roles, i.e., give each partner a chance to be the nurse and the patient.

III. If the person playing the role of patient does not have pain, decide whether or not you want to experiment with imagery in the presence of pain. If you are not at all familiar with imagery, you may decide to forego the pain and concentrate only on familiarizing yourself with imagery. If you want to inflict mild to moderate pain, consider the following methods:

—Press the shank of a pencil or pen into the nailbed.

—Use thumb and index finger to grasp and squeeze the trapezius (shoulder) muscle.

—Use thumb and index finger to grasp and apply pressure to muscle or subcutaneous tissue, like pinching, but in a manner that produces a dull ache.

Keep in mind the following:

—Inflict only mild to moderate pain, not severe. No bleeding or bruising either.

—The patient (subject) always has the right to tell you to stop.

IV. Familiarize yourselves with the following:

—"Ball of Healing Energy," read p. 225.

—Contents of Table 7-1, p. 196, and Table 8-2, p. 218, regarding possible problems and their solutions, just in case you have any difficulty.

V. As you read the script together, the nurse asks the patient about the following and modifies the script accordingly:

—If the patient does not have pain and none is inflicted, ask the patient to decide on an area of the body to use for the "area that hurts," mentioned in the script.

—Ask the patient to give you a description of the characteristics he has ascribed to the ball of healing energy, e.g., a white light or a religious symbol.

—Are there any other changes the patient would like to make?

VI. The nurse directs the following sequence of instructions:

A. Help the patient get into a comfortable, well-supported position.

B. Make the environment as quiet as possible.

C. If the patient already has pain, get a pain rating on a scale of 0 to 10 (0 = no pain, 10 = worst possible pain) and record the answer in question #1 below. If pain is to be inflicted, do so now, and obtain a pain rating.*

D. Read the script while the patient listens and participates. Read slowly in a quiet monotone with pauses at intervals, especially between paragraphs and when you see "..." within the script. Call the patient by name from time to time.

E. If pain was present at the beginning of the script, then when you finish the script, ask the patient to rate the pain as he remembers it during the script and also as it is now, recording your answers in question #1 below.

F. Consider doing all of this again, switching roles so that the nurse now becomes the patient.

Questions/Answers:

1. If the patient had pain, actual or inflicted, record the following pain ratings:
Before imagery began: _____.
During imagery: _____.
Immediately after imagery: _____.

2. Did the patient feel less pain? If not, why does the patient think there was no improvement? Does the nurse have any ideas?

Common answers when this is practiced in a large group: The majority of people who participate in this imagery find that it provides some form of pain relief. It may reduce the intensity of pain or it may make pain more tolerable because of distraction. Reasons given for why it did not relieve pain include feeling strange about doing imagery, not being able to take it seriously, having severe pain that interfered with concentration on the imagery, or experiencing difficulty with figuring out a pathway for moving the healing force. The latter problem may be resolved by discussing the possible ways to imagine maneuvering the ball around inside or outside of the body.

3. Did the patient experience any special feelings before, during, or after the imagery? What did you (both the nurse and patient) think about imagery before you tried it? What do you think about it now?

Common answers when this is practiced in a large group: People may say they felt ridiculous or weird because it was so different from anything they had ever done. In fact, it is not unusual to hear some laughter beforehand. A few people may voice surprise that it

---

*In clinical practice, a pain relief measure is used prior to the onset of pain whenever possible. However, the effect of imagery on pain may continue for several minutes or longer after it is stopped, so it may take some time to feel the full intensity of pain without the effects of imagery. Thus to make it easier for the patient in this experiment to evaluate the effectiveness of imagery, pain is inflicted prior to the imagery technique.

worked. Some will say it was not all that strange to them because they had tried something similar before, e.g., in a weight loss or stress reduction program. Those who used religious or spiritual symbols may say they had a religious or comforting experience.

4. The nurse asks the patient how well the script was read and what suggestions the patient can make about how the nurse can improve her performance.

Common answer: The patient thinks the nurse performed very well. If the patient has any suggestions, they usually concern script content and not the nurse's reading of it.

5. What have you learned that will help you take care of a patient with pain?

Common answers: Imagery may provide a form of pain relief for some people, but the results of imagery are unpredictable, even for the same person from time to time. Imagery for pain relief may be difficult to suggest to patients who have never had a comparable experience. Or, if imagery is new to you, you may not be able to talk about it with much confidence.

To introduce the idea of imagery, the nurse might say, "Have you ever had any experiences with using visualization or imagery, such as prayer or to help people relax or stop smoking?" If the answer is negative, then the nurse might say, "I know a lot of people think imagery is kind of crazy or unscientific. I thought so once myself (or, some people I've talked to thought I was nuts to bring up imagery). Anyway, as strange and unlikely as imagery for pain relief may sound, I'd be glad to talk with you about it, if you wish."

Imagery may be a relatively time-consuming nursing activity, requiring 15 to 60 minutes, depending on the technique selected. However, for a patient who has chronic pain or a patient who wants to feel in control of his pain, this investment of time may be well worth the effort. If imagery is tape-recorded, the patient may use the tape several times a day, daily, for months. But the benefits of imagery must be respected by others. If imagery helps the patient with pain, it cannot be concluded that the patient's pain is his imagination.

CHAPTER 9—CHRONIC NONMALIGNANT PAIN: SPECIAL CONSIDERATIONS (pp. 232-263)

To learn more about caring for patients who have chronic nonmalignant pain, you may use two of the forms in that chapter for an actual or hypothetical patient:

1. Copy the form "Planning for the Future: Review of Pain Relief Measures," p. 246, and complete it for an actual patient currently hospitalized for an exacerbation of chronic nonmalignant pain who is to be discharged from the hospital within 24 hours. (If no such patient is available, you might complete it for a patient you remember or a hypothetical patient.)

Common findings: Prescriptions for analgesics may have changed frequently, and many of the analgesics may not have been given as often as they could have been in spite of the patient being in pain. It may be difficult for you or the patient to remember the effects of some analgesics, and this information may not have been charted. The patient may report that what was done to relieve his pain was much less effective than you realized. It probably will be obvious that certain analgesics relieved more pain than others. A plan for future episodes of similar pain probably will include beginning with the most effective analgesics and giving them as often as possible and, if it was not done, trying the regular use of a strong nonnarcotic.

2. Copy the form "Important Information About a Pain Management Clinic," pp. 252-253, and try to complete it for an actual patient with chronic nonmalignant pain who wants to consider such a program, or simply complete the form for your own use to gather information in case your future patients are interested. Pain clinics or centers are accustomed to health professionals calling or visiting to obtain information. Other members of the health team may wish to accompany you if you attend a lecture or tour the facility.

If you do not know of a pain management program near you, contact the American Pain Society (see p. 5) or CARF (see p. 257) to locate one.

Common findings: This probably is not as easy as it seemed. You begin to understand the difficulties a patient faces when he tries to select a program that meets his needs. Many unexpected problems may arise. In some areas it is very difficult to locate an appropriate pain program nearby. If you do not live near a pain program, getting information long distance or by mail may take a very long time. The program may be expensive. The program may offer only limited services, and sometimes the exact services or exact goals of the program are not clear. It may become obvious that the program is new and that the staff is also new, perhaps with very little experience. There may be a long wait before a patient can be evaluated or admitted. In some instances, simply getting answers to these questions may prove to be a lesson in assertiveness. However, most well-established, comprehensive programs will be happy to answer your questions.

CHAPTER 10—PAIN IN CHILDREN: SPECIAL CONSIDERATIONS (pp. 264-307)

To learn more about caring for children with pain, you may engage in the following two exercises:

1. Copy the form "Parent Interview Regarding Child's Pain/Hurt," pp. 272-273. Talk with the parent of a well or sick child and discuss as many portions as possible, taking notes if appropriate.

Common findings: A systematic guide to discussing the child's pain with the parents reveals much more important information than the usual ongoing conversations with parents. It is, however, sometimes difficult for both nurse and parents to find the time to cover all the questions on the form. Therefore, it is wise to use it in an ongoing manner.

2. To become more familiar with narcotic doses recommended for children, use the equianalgesic chart for adult doses for moderate to severe pain, pp. 78-79, along with Rogers' (1985) suggestions for calculating narcotic doses for children from ages 2 to 12 years, p. 291, and do the following:

- For each age group (2-6 years, 7-12 years, and over 12 years), calculate IM and/or PO doses of hydromorphone, fentanyl, methadone, levorphanol, nalbuphine, and codeine.
- Calculate doses of IM morphine and meperidine and compare them with the ranges of doses for IM morphine and meperidine suggested in Table 10-3, p. 288. For example, a suggested adult dose for morphine is 10 mg IM. For a child 7 to 12 years old, Rogers recommends ½ the adult dose, which would be 5 mg. For this age range, Table 10-3 suggests approximately 2.2 to 8.8 mg morphine IM. This illustrates that recommendations differ and careful observation of the child's reponse to a dose is mandatory, immediately changing the dose if it is unsafe or does not relieve pain.

CHAPTER 11—PAIN IN THE ELDERLY: SPECIAL CONSIDERATIONS (pp. 308-323)

To learn more about assessment and relief of pain in the elderly, try the following:

1. Complete the "Initial Pain Assessment Tool" (p. 21) for an alert elderly patient and one who is confused or unable to communicate. Integrate the concepts of a multi-dimensional approach (p. 312). Compare this tool with one that you are already using for older patients. Combine the best parts of both for a tool that is easy and practical for your individual clinical setting.

2. Complete a "Flow Sheet" (p. 27) on an elderly patient who cannot communicate (see example, p. 313). What modifications can you and family members make in the Flow Sheet to record behaviors that indicate pain and those that indicate comfort?

CHAPTER 12—EVALUATION: THE TOTAL PICTURE (pp. 324-328)

Copy the checklist of possible pain relief measures (pp. 326-327) and fill it out on a patient.

Common findings: You may discover that a lot has already been done for the patient. However, you may also realize that some pain control methods that would be appropriate for the patient to try have never been considered.

Index

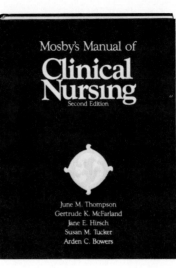

MOSBY'S MANUAL OF CLINICAL NURSING, 2nd Edition (5157-3)

By June M. Thompson, R.N., M.S.; Gertrude K. McFarland, R.N., D.N.Sc., F.A.A.N.; Jane E. Hirsch, R.N., M.S.; Susan M. Tucker, R.N., B.S.N.; and Arden C. Bowers, R.N., M.S.

The first edition of MOSBY'S MANUAL OF CLINICAL NURSING was voted nursing's "#1 most indispensable reference" in an *American Journal of Nursing* poll, and the second edition is even better than the first. No student should be without this comprehensive reference for planning nursing care.

- Part I, "Clinical Nursing Practice," is organized by body systems and covers virtually every condition, disease, or disorder you are likely to encounter. Complete nursing care is presented for all medical conditions and medical interventions.
- NEW! Part II, "Diagnostic Procedures," contains nursing care associated with every significant diagnostic test. The tests are presented by category and are also alphabetically indexed for easy access.
- Part III, "Nursing Diagnoses," has all NANDA-accepted nursing diagnoses including the 16 new diagnoses accepted at the Eighth NANDA Conference held in March 1988.
- Nursing care is concisely organized according to the nursing process.
- An assessment for each disease provides a checklist to ensure comprehensive nursing assessment.
- Comprehensive nursing interventions with rationales are linked to every possible nursing diagnosis for every disease to allow for individualized care.
- Patient teaching in the nursing care of each disease encourages you to build teaching interventions right into care plans.
- An evaluation section for each disease provides specific data to help determine when your nursing goals have been met, or when they need to be revised.

This useful text provides nurses and students with everything they need to plan and implement high quality nursing care. To order, call toll-free 800-221-7700, ext. 15A. We look forward to hearing from you!